FOURTH EDITION

PARAMEDIC CARE

VOLUME 2 | PARAMEDICINE FUNDAMENTALS

PRINCIPLES & PRACTICE

BRYAN E. BLEDSOE, DO, FACEP, FAAEM, EMT-P

Professor of Emergency Medicine
Director, Prehospital and Disaster Medicine Fellowship
University of Nevada School of Medicine
Attending Emergency Physician
University Medical Center of Southern Nevada
Medical Director, MedicWest Ambulance
Las Vegas, Nevada

ROBERT S. PORTER, MA, EMT-P

Senior Advanced Life Support Educator
Madison County Emergency Medical Services
Canastota, New York

RICHARD A. CHERRY, MS, EMT-P

Director of Training
Northern Onondaga Volunteer Ambulance
Liverpool, New York

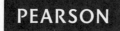

Boston Columbus Indianapolis New York San Francisco Upper Saddle River
Amsterdam Cape Town Dubai London Madrid Milan Munich Paris Montreal Toronto
Delhi Mexico City São Paulo Sydney Hong Kong Seoul Singapore Taipei Tokyo

Library of Congress Cataloging-in-Publication Data
Bledsoe, Bryan E. (Date)
  Paramedic care : principles & practice / Bryan E. Bledsoe,
    Robert S. Porter, Richard A. Cherry. — 4th ed. p. ; cm.
  Includes bibliographical references and index.
  ISBN-13: 978-0-13-211217-8 (v. 2 : alk. paper)
  ISBN-10: 0-13-211217-5 (v. 2 : alk. paper)
  I. Porter, Robert S. (Date) II. Cherry, Richard A. III. Title.
  [DNLM: 1. Emergencies. 2. Emergency Medical Services.
    3. Emergency Medical Technicians. 4. Emergency Treatment. WB 105]
  616.02'5—dc23
                                        2011034904

Publisher: Julie Levin Alexander
Publisher's Assistant: Regina Bruno
Editor-in-Chief: Marlene McHugh Pratt
Senior Managing Editor for Development: Lois Berlowitz
Editorial Project Manager: Sandra Breuer
Assistant Editor: Jonathan Cheung
Director of Marketing: David Gesell
Marketing Manager: Brian Hoehl
Marketing Specialist: Michael Sirinides
Managing Editor for Production: Patrick Walsh
Production Liaison: Faye Gemmellaro
Production Editor: Heather Willison, S4Carlisle Publishing Services
Manufacturing Manager: Ilene Sanford

Creative Director: Blair Brown
Cover and Interior Design: Kathryn Foot
Interior Photographers: Nathan Eldridge, Michael Gallitelli, Michal Heron, Ray Kemp/Triple Zilch Productions, Richard Logan, Scott Metcalfe
Cover Image: © corepics/Shutterstock
Managing Photography Editor: Michal Heron
Editorial Media Manager: Amy Peltier
Media Project Manager: Lorena Cerisano
Composition: S4Carlisle Publishing Services
Printer/Binder: Courier/Kendallville
Cover Printer: Lehigh-Phoenix Color/Hagerstown

Notice

The author and the publisher of this book have taken care to make certain that the information given is correct and compatible with the standards generally accepted at the time of publication. Nevertheless, as new information becomes available, changes in treatment and in the use of equipment and procedures become necessary. The reader is advised to carefully consult the instruction and information material included in each piece of equipment or device before administration. Students are warned that the use of any techniques must be authorized by their medical advisor, where appropriate, in accordance with local laws and regulations. The publisher disclaims any liability, loss, injury, or damage incurred as a consequence, directly or indirectly, of the use and application of any of the contents of this book.

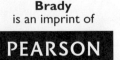
Brady
is an imprint of

www.bradybooks.com

10 9 8 7 6 5 4 3 2 1
ISBN 10:   0-13-211217-5
ISBN 13: 978-0-13-211217-8

DETAILED CONTENTS

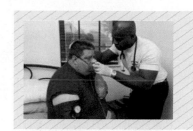

CHAPTER 2 • Human Life Span Development 121

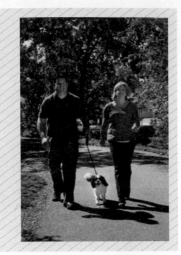

CHAPTER 3 • Emergency Pharmacology 136

CHAPTER 4 ● Intravenous Access and Medication Administration 226

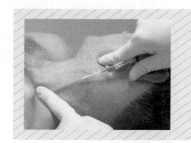

CHAPTER 5 ● Airway Management and Ventilation 294

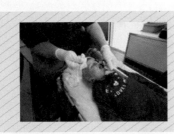

Today's paramedics require a solid background in basic sciences, including physiology, pathophysiology, and pharmacology. In Volume 2, we have followed the *National EMS Education Standards* and the accompanying *Paramedic Instructional Guidelines* to provide the appropriate introductory material in *Volume 2, Paramedicine Fundamentals*.

This volume provides paramedic students with the basic scientific information and skills that they will need throughout their practice and that they will apply to both medical patients and trauma patients. The first three chapters concern the scientific underpinnings of pathophysiology, life span development, and pharmacology. The final two chapters of this volume deal with the skills of intravenous access and medication administration and the skills of airway management and ventilation.

OVERVIEW OF THE CHAPTERS

CHAPTER 1   Pathophysiology provides a detailed description of basic pathophysiology. The first part of the chapter introduces the concept of disease, including predisposing factors to disease and classifications of disease. The next parts of the chapter discuss disease at the chemical level, the cellular level, the tissue level, and the organ level. Finally, the chapter details the body's defenses against disease and injury.

CHAPTER 2   Human Life Span Development provides an overview of physiologic and psychosocial developmental and age-related changes from infancy to late adulthood.

CHAPTER 3   Emergency Pharmacology is a comprehensive chapter covering the various medications used in medical practice, especially paramedic practice. It presents an overview of pharmacology, followed by a discussion of drug classifications.

CHAPTER 4   Intravenous Access and Medication Administration is presented in three parts, the first part detailing principles and routes of medication administration; the second part concerning intravenous access, blood sampling, and intraosseous infusion; and the final part giving an overview of medical mathematics and dose calculation.

CHAPTER 5   Airway Management and Ventilation presents the crucial prehospital skill of airway management. The first part of the chapter deals with respiratory anatomy, physiology, and assessment. The chapter then goes on to address both basic manual and advanced airway management techniques. In addition, this chapter details patient positioning, oxygenation, ventilation techniques, suction, rapid sequence intubation, surgical airways, the difficult airway, and other airway and ventilation issues and techniques.

ACKNOWLEDGMENTS

CHAPTER CONTRIBUTORS

We wish to acknowledge the talent, dedication, and commitment of the following people who contributed to Volume 2.

Darren Braude, MD, MPH, EMT-P
Professor of Emergency Medicine
University of New Mexico School of Medicine
Albuquerque, NM: Chapter 5

William E. Gandy, JD, LP, NREMT-P
Adjunct Faculty
University of Nevada School of Medicine
Tucson, AZ: Chapter 5

INSTRUCTOR REVIEWERS

The reviewers of *Paramedic Care: Principles & Practice, Fourth Edition, Volume 2* have provided many excellent suggestions and ideas for improving the text. The quality of the reviews has been outstanding, and the reviews have been a major aid in the preparation and revision of the manuscript. The assistance provided by these EMS experts is deeply appreciated.

John L. Beckman, AA, BS
FF/EMT-P I/C
Addison Fire Protection District
Technology Center of DuPage
Addison, IL

Bryon Bellinger, NREMT-P, BA, RN
Lead Instructor Paramedic Specialist Program
Indian Hills Community College
Ottumwa, IA

Brian Bird, AS, EMS
Firefighter/Paramedic
Santa Fe Fire Department
Santa Fe, NM

L. Kelly Kirk, III, AAS, BS, EMT-P
Director of Distance Education, Paramedic
Randolph Co. Community College/ Davidson County EMS
Asheboro, NC/Lexington, NC

Gregory M. Reardon, BS, NREMT-P
Paramedic, Adjunct Faculty Cecil College/Maryland Fire and Rescue Institute
Baltimore Washington International Airport Fire and Rescue Department
Baltimore, MD

Billy Respass, NCEMT-P
EMS Programs Instructor
Beaufort County Community College
Washington, NC

Mike Smertka, EMT-P
Assistant EMS Instructor
Graduate Student of Medicine/Medical University of Silesia
Katowice, Poland

Kelly Weller, MA, RN, LP, EMS-C
EMS Program Director
Lone Star College-Montgomery
Conroe, TX

We also wish to express appreciation to the following EMS professionals who reviewed the third edition of Paramedic Care: Principles & Practice. Their suggestions and perspectives helped to make this program a successful teaching tool.

Mike Dymes, NREMT-P
EMS Program Director
Durham Technical Community College
Durham, NC

Ginger K. Floyd, BA, NREMT-P
Assistant Professor
Austin Community College EMS Professions
Austin, TX

Darren P. Lacroix, AAS, EMT-P
Del Mar College
Emergency Medical Service Professions
Corpus Christi, TX

Greg Mullen, MS, NREMT-P
National EMS Academy
Lafayette, LA

Deborah L. Petty, BS, EMT-P I/C
Training Officer
St. Charles County Ambulance District
St. Peters, MO

B. Jeanine Riner, MHSA, BS, RRT, NREMT-P
GA Office of EMS and Trauma
Atlanta, GA

Aaron Weitzman, BS, NREMT-P
Lieutenant (ret.)
Faculty, Emergency Medical Services
Baltimore City Community College
Baltimore, MD

Brian J. Wilson, BA, NREMT-P
Education Director
Texas Tech School of Medicine
El Paso, TX

PHOTO ACKNOWLEDGMENTS

All photographs not credited adjacent to the photograph or in the photo credit section below were photographed on assignment for Brady/Prentice Hall/Pearson Education.

Organizations

We wish to thank the following organizations for their valuable assistance in creating the photo program for this edition:

Bound Tree University
Dublin, OH. www.boundtreeuniversity.com

Canandaigua Emergency Squad
Canandaigua, NY

Flower Mound Fire Department
Flower Mound, TX

Children's Hospital St. Louis/BJC Health Care
St. Louis, MO

Christian Hospital/BJC Health Care
St. Charles, MO

Tyco Health Care/Nellcor Puritan Bennet
Pleasanton, CA

Wolfe Tory Medical
Salt Lake City, UT

Winter Park Fire-Rescue
Winter Park, FL
Chief James E. White
Deputy Chief Patrick McCabe

City of Winter Park, FL
Kenneth W. Bradley, Mayor

Technical Advisors

Thanks to the following people for providing technical support during the photo shoots in Winter Park, FL, for this edition:

Andrew Isaacs, EMS Captain
Tod Meadors, EMS Captain
Dr. Tod Husty, Medical Director

Richard Rodriguez, EMS Captain
Jeff Spinelli, Engineer-Paramedic

Models

Thanks to the following people from the Flower Mound Fire Department, Flower Mound, Texas, and from Winter Park Fire-Rescue, Winter Park, Florida, who provided locations and/or portrayed patients and EMS providers in our photographs.

FAO/Paramedic Wade Woody
FF/Paramedic Tim Mackling
FF/Paramedic Matthew Daniel
FF/Paramedic Jon Rea
FF/Paramedic Waylon Palmer
FF/EMT Jesse Palmer
Captain/EMT Billy McWhorter
Linda Kirk, Director, Winter Park Towers,
    Winter Park, FL

Andrew Isaacs
Richard Rodriguez
Tod Meadors
Jeff Spinelli
Mark Vaughn
Victoria Devereaux
Teresa George

BRYAN E. BLEDSOE, DO, FACEP, FAAEM, EMT-P

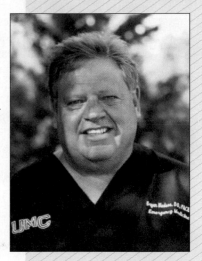

Dr. Bryan Bledsoe is an emergency physician, researcher, and EMS author. Presently he is Professor of Emergency Medicine and Director of the EMS Fellowship program at the University of Nevada School of Medicine and an Attending Emergency Physician at the University Medical Center of Southern Nevada in Las Vegas. He is board-certified in emergency medicine. Prior to attending medical school, Dr. Bledsoe worked as an EMT, a paramedic, and a paramedic instructor. He completed EMT training in 1974 and paramedic training in 1976 and worked for six years as a field paramedic in Fort Worth, Texas. In 1979, he joined the faculty of the University of North Texas Health Sciences Center and served as coordinator of EMT and paramedic education programs at the university.

Dr. Bledsoe is active in emergency medicine and EMS research. He is a popular speaker at state, national, and international seminars and writes regularly for numerous EMS journals. He is active in educational endeavors with the United States Special Operations Command (USSOCOM) and the University of Nevada at Las Vegas. Dr. Bledsoe is the author of numerous EMS textbooks and has in excess of 1 million books in print. Dr. Bledsoe was named a "Hero of Emergency Medicine" in 2008 by the American College of Emergency Physicians as a part of their 40th anniversary celebration and was named a "Hero of Health and Fitness" by *Men's Health* magazine as part of their 20th anniversary edition in November of 2008. He is frequently interviewed in the national media. Dr. Bledsoe is married and divides his time between his residences in Midlothian, TX, and Las Vegas, NV.

ROBERT S. PORTER, MA, EMT-P

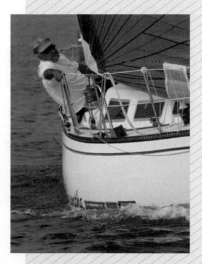

Robert Porter has been teaching in emergency medical services for 38 years and currently serves as the Senior Advanced Life Support Educator for Madison County (New York) Emergency Medical Services. Mr. Porter is a Wisconsin native and received his bachelor's degree in education from the University of Wisconsin. He completed his paramedic training at Northeast Wisconsin Technical Institute in 1978 and earned a master's degree in health education at Central Michigan University in 1990.

Mr. Porter has been an EMT and an EMS educator and administrator since 1973 and obtained his certification and national registration as an EMT-Paramedic in 1978. He has taught both basic and advanced EMS courses in the states of Wisconsin, Michigan, Louisiana, Pennsylvania, and New York. Mr. Porter conducted one of the nation's first rural paramedic programs and developed a university-based, two-year paramedic program. Mr. Porter served for more than ten years as a paramedic program accreditation-site evaluator for the American Medical Association and is a past chair of the National Association of EMTs—Society of EMT Instructor/Coordinators. Mr. Porter also served for 15 years as a flight paramedic with the Onondaga County Sheriff's Department air medical service, AirOne. He has authored Brady's *Paramedic Care: Principles & Practice, Essentials of Paramedic Care, Intermediate Emergency Care: Principles & Practice, Tactical Emergency Care,* and *Weapons of Mass Destruction: Emergency Care,* as well as the workbooks accompanying this text. When not writing or teaching, Mr. Porter enjoys offshore sailboat racing and home restoration.

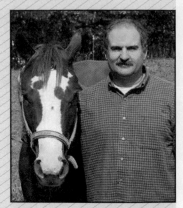

RICHARD A. CHERRY, MS, EMT-P

Richard Cherry is the Director of Training for Northern Onondaga Volunteer Ambulance (NOVA) in Liverpool, New York, a suburb of Syracuse. He recently retired from the Department of Emergency Medicine at Upstate Medical University where he held the positions of Director of Paramedic Training, Assistant Emergency Medicine Residency Director, Clinical Assistant Professor of Emergency Medicine, and Technical Director for Medical Simulation. His experience includes years of classroom teaching and emergency fieldwork. A native of Buffalo, Mr. Cherry earned his bachelor's degree at nearby St. Bonaventure University in 1972. He taught high school for the next ten years while he earned his master's degree in education from Oswego State University in 1977. He holds a permanent teaching license in New York State.

Mr. Cherry entered the emergency medical services field in 1974 with the DeWitt Volunteer Fire Department, where he served his community as a firefighter and EMS provider for more than 15 years. He took his first EMT course in 1977 and became an ALS provider two years later. He earned his paramedic certificate in 1985 as a member of the area's first paramedic class.

Mr. Cherry has authored several books for Brady. Most notable are *Paramedic Care: Principles & Practice, Essentials of Paramedic Care, Intermediate Emergency Care: Principles & Practice,* and *EMT Teaching: A Common Sense Approach.* He has made presentations at many state, national, and international EMS conferences on a variety of teaching topics. He and his wife, Sue, run a summer horse-riding camp for children with special needs on their property in West Monroe, New York. He also plays guitar in a Christian band.

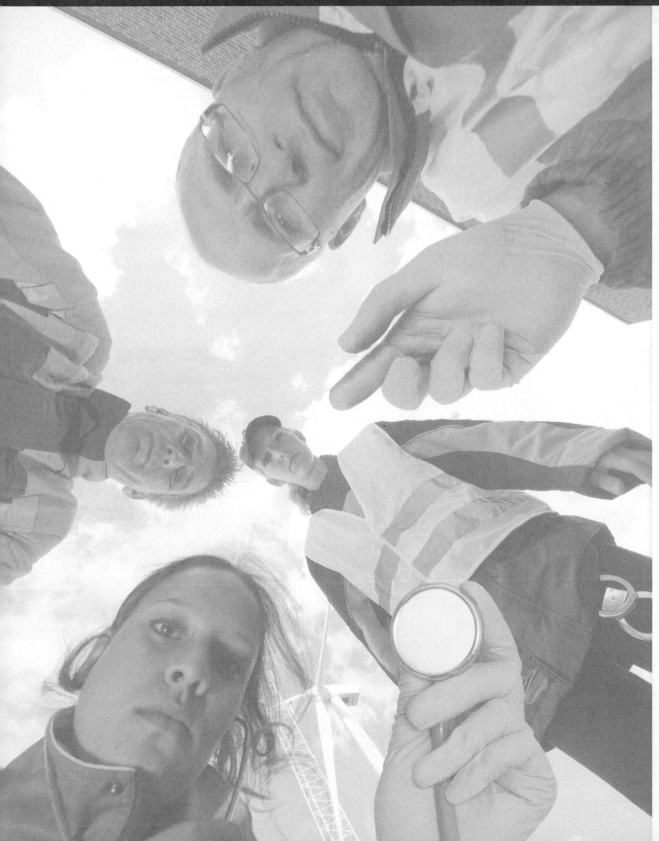

Welcome to

PARAMEDIC CARE PRINCIPLES & PRACTICE

FOURTH EDITION

A Guide to Key Features

Emphasizing Principles

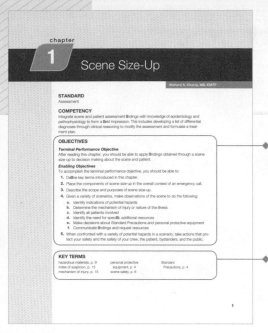

CHAPTER OBJECTIVES

Terminal Performance Objectives and a separate set of Enabling Objectives are provided for each chapter.

KEY TERMS

Page numbers identify where each key term first appears, boldfaced, in the chapter.

TABLES

A wealth of tables offers the opportunity to highlight, summarize, and compare information.

TABLE 4-2	Common Infectious Diseases	
Disease	**Mode of Transmission**	**Incubation Period**
AIDS (acquired immune deficiency syndrome)	AIDS- or HIV-infected blood via intravenous drug use, semen and vaginal fluids, blood transfusions, or (rarely) needlesticks. Mothers also may pass HIV to their unborn children.	Several months or years
Hepatitis B, C	Blood, stool, or other body fluids, or contaminated objects.	Weeks or months
Tuberculosis	Respiratory secretions, airborne or on contaminated objects.	2 to 6 weeks
Meningitis, bacterial	Oral and nasal secretions.	2 to 10 days
Pneumonia, bacterial and viral	Oral and nasal droplets and secretions.	Several days
Influenza	Airborne droplets, or direct contact with body fluids.	1 to 3 days
Staphylococcal skin infections	Contact with open wounds or sores or contaminated objects.	Several days
Chicken pox (varicella)	Airborne droplets, or contact with open sores.	11 to 21 days
German measles (rubella)	Airborne droplets. Mothers may pass it to unborn children.	10 to 12 days
Whooping cough (pertussis)	Respiratory secretions or airborne droplets.	6 to 20 days
SARS (severe acute respiratory syndrome)	Airborne droplets and personal contact.	4 to 6 days

PHOTOS AND ILLUSTRATIONS

Carefully selected photos and a unique art program reinforce content coverage and add to text explanations.

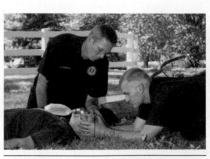

● **Figure 3-3** During the primary assessment of your patient, you will look for and immediately treat any life-threatening conditions.

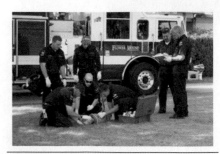

● **Figure 3-7** As leader of the EMS team, the paramedic must interact with patients, bystanders, and other rescue personnel in a professional and efficient manner.

CONTENT REVIEW

▶ Steps of Primary Assessment

- Form a general impression
- Stabilize cervical spine as needed
- Assess baseline mental status
- Assess and manage airway
- Assess and manage breathing
- Assess and manage circulation
- Determine priorities

CONTENT REVIEW

Screened content review boxes set off from the text are interspersed throughout the chapter. They summarize key points and serve as a helpful study guide—in an easy format for quick review.

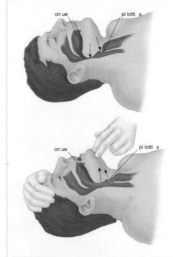

● **Figure 2-4** The head-tilt/chin-lift maneuver in an adult.

SUMMARY

This end-of-chapter feature provides a
concise review of chapter information.

 SUMMARY

The scene size-up is the initial step in the patient care process. Sizing up the scene and situation begins at your initial dispatch and does not end until you are clear of the call. As the call unfolds, you should be making constant observations and adjustments to your plan of action. Remember that your safety and the safety of your partner are paramount—it is hard to effectively treat both yourself and others.

Scene size-up should be practiced so much that it becomes second nature to you. It is like noticing veins on people in public after you begin starting IVs. (You have all done it—looked across the room at the back of someone's hand and noticed what nice veins they had.) Sizing up a scene is no different. After a while you begin to notice mechanisms of injury and other important details almost subconsciously. But be careful and do not get complacent! Always make it a point to pause for just a few seconds and consciously look around the scene before proceeding into any situation.

Scene size-up is not a step-by-step process, but a series of decisions you make when confronted with a variety of circumstances that are often beyond your control. It is a way to make order out of chaos, keep yourself and your crew safe, and ensure that all necessary resources are focused on patient care and outcomes. With time and experience, you will learn to perform a scene size-up quickly and focus on important issues. Your careful size-up lays the foundation for an organized and timely approach toward patient care and scene management.

REVIEW QUESTIONS

These questions ask students to review and
recall key information they have just learned.

REVIEW QUESTIONS

1. Which of the following is *not* a component of the scene size-up?
   a. Standard Precautions
   b. mechanism of injury
   c. primary assessment
   d. location of all patients

2. The HEPA mask is designed to protect you from _____.
   a. tuberculosis
   b. AIDS
   c. hepatitis
   d. meningitis

3. The top priority in any emergency situation is _____.
   a. patient assessment
   b. bystander cooperation
   c. customer service
   d. your personal safety

4. As you approach a scene, something just does not seem right. It is not anything you can put your finger on, just a sense that something is wrong or is about to happen. What should you do about it?
   a. Wait until law enforcement arrives before entering.
   b. Ignore your feelings and enter the scene.
   c. Enter the scene with something with which to protect yourself.
   d. Call out for the patient to come outside.

5. You are responding to a shooting at a well-known bar. How should you approach the scene?
   a. Stage outside the bar until the police arrive.
   b. Wait for another ambulance or rescue crew before entering.
   c. Just enter the scene.
   d. Stage your ambulance a few blocks away until law enforcement arrives.

6. You arrive on the scene and see that a power line lies close to your pediatric patient. You are fairly sure the line is live and decide to move it with a dry piece of equipment. Which of the following should you use?
   a. a wooden-handled ax
   b. a fallen tree branch
   c. a nylon rope
   d. none of the above

7. When you and your partner arrive at a multiple-patient incident, you should _____.
   a. begin assessing and treating the first patient you encounter
   b. establish command and begin triage
   c. provide intensive emergency care to the most critical patient
   d. start at opposite ends and begin assessing patients

REFERENCES

This listing is a compilation of source material
providing the basis of updated data and research
used in the preparation of each chapter.

REFERENCES

1. U.S. Department of Transportation/National Highway Traffic Safety Administration. *National EMS Scope of Practice Model*. Washington, DC, 2006.
2. National Registry of Emergency Medical Technicians. *2004 National EMS Practice Analysis*. Columbus, OH: National Registry of EMTs, 2005.
3. American College of Surgeons. *Verified Trauma Centers*. [Available at: http://www.facs.org/trauma/verified.html]
4. Feldman, M. J., J. L. Lukins, P. R. Verbeek, et al. "Use of Treat-and-Release Directives for Paramedics at a Mass Gathering." *Prehosp Emerg Care* 9 (2005): 213–217.
5. American College of Emergency Physicians. "Interfacility Transportation of the Critical Care Patient and Its Medical Direction." *Ann Emerg Med* 47 (2006): 305.
6. Harkins, S. "Documentation: Why Is It So Important?" *Emerg Med Serv* 31 (2002): 93–94.
7. Lerner, E. B., A. R. Fernandez, and M. N. Shah. "Do Emergency Medical Services Professionals Think They Should Participate in Disease Prevention?" *Prehosp Emerg Care* 13 (2009): 64–70.
8. Poliafico, F. "The Role of EMS in Public Access Defibrillation." *Emerg Med Serv* 32 (2003): 73.
9. Streger M. R. "Professionalism." *Emerg Med Serv* 32 (2003): 35.
10. Klugman, C. M. "Why EMS Needs Its Own Ethics. What's Good for Other Areas of Healthcare May Not Be Good for You." *Emerg Med Serv* 36 (2007): 114–122.
11. Touchstone, M. "Professional Development. Part 1: Becoming an EMS Leader." *Emerg Med Serv* 38 (2009): 59–60.
12. Bledsoe, B. E. "EMS Needs a Few More Cowboys." *JEMS* 28 (2003): 112–113.

FURTHER READING

This list features recommendations for books and
journal articles that go beyond chapter coverage.

FURTHER READING

Bailey, E. D. and T. Sweeney. "Considerations in Establishing Emergency Medical Services Response Time Goals." *Prehosp Emerg Care* 7 (2003): 397–399.

Bledsoe, B. E. "Searching for the Evidence behind EMS." *Emerg Med Serv* 31 (2003): 63–67.

Heightman, A. J. "EMS Workforce. A Comprehensive Listing of Certified EMS Providers by State and How the Workforce Has Changed Since 1993." *JEMS* 5 (2000): 108–112.

Jaslow, D. J., J. Ufberg, and R. Marsh. "Primary Injury Prevention in an Urban EMS System." *J Emerg Med* 25 (2003): 167–170.

National Academy of Sciences, National Research Council. *Accidental Death and Disability: The Neglected Disease of Modern Society*. Washington, DC:

U.S. Department of Health, Education, and Welfare, 1966.

Page, J. O. *The Magic of 3 AM*. San Diego, CA: JEMS Publishing, 2002.

Page, J. O. *The Paramedics*. Morristown, NJ: Backdraft Publications, 1979. [No longer available for purchase except as a used book. Entire book can be viewed online at www.JEMS.com/Paramedics.]

Page, J. O. *Simple Advice*. San Diego, CA: JEMS Publishing, 2002.

Persse, D. E., C. B. Key, R. N. Bradley, et al. "Cardiac Arrest Survival as a Function of Ambulance Deployment Strategy in a Large Urban Emergency Medical Services System." *Resusc* 59 (2003): 97–104.

CASE STUDY

This feature at the start of each chapter draws students into the reading and creates a link between text content and real-life situations.

CASE STUDY

On a quiet afternoon, paramedic Dean Barker hears the tones for a person slumped over the steering wheel of his car. He and his partner, Kyle Peeper, a new EMT, respond immediately. En route, Dean emphasizes to his rookie partner the need to put safety first and not to rush in without a quick evaluation of the scene. His partner nods agreeably but is obviously both excited and nervous about his first real emergency call.

When they arrive, Dean notices a very unusual and troubling scene. Dean grabs his partner and stops him from jumping out of the vehicle. He asks him to stop and look around. "Tell me what you see," he says. His partner nervously answers, "Right, OK, I see one car parked alongside a cemetery and it looks like someone might be inside. There seems to be a white cloud inside the car and I smell a strong odor of sulfur or rotten eggs. I also see a sign on the driver's side window with what looks like a hazard emblem on it."

"So, is there anything we should do before jumping out and entering this scene? What is our first priority? asks Dean. "Patient care." answers his partner. "No, safety first. We'll park our vehicle upwind from the car and I'll make a quick report to dispatch and call for more help. We already know this is more than we can handle by ourselves."

Dean assumes the role of incident commander; he calls for the fire department's hazmat team, cordons off the area, and alerts all responding personnel that the potential for fire and explosion exists. There also may be a need to evacuate the area. Waiting for the fire department to arrive seems like hours to his energetic partner. Dean asks him what they can do until they arrive. Kyle responds that they can shut down the road and secure the scene from bystanders.

When the hazmat team arrives, they read the signs that someone left on three of the four windows. They appear to be suicide notes and a warning to rescuers of the toxic atmosphere inside the car. The hazmat team begins the arduous process of identifying the toxic substance, containing the exposure, and decontaminating the victim and all rescuers. Dean and his partner are released and head back to the station.

Kyle asks Dean what the substance was inside that car and asks why they didn't try to extricate and resuscitate the driver. Dean calmly explains that the white cloud and rotten-egg odor strongly suggested a deadly asphyxiant, hydrogen sulfide, and if they had opened the door to extricate him, they would have been just as dead as their victim. This day a rookie learned a crucial lesson—on an EMS call, nothing is more important than his safety. Nothing.

YOU MAKE THE CALL

A scenario at the end of each chapter promotes critical thinking by requiring students to apply principles to actual practice.

YOU MAKE THE CALL

On a rainy and windy evening, you hear the tones for a car crash on the interstate highway just five minutes from the station. You are the only ambulance dispatched along with fire department rescue and fire apparatus. On arrival you see three cars smashed up, one on its side, smoke rising from the crash, and what looks like fluid leaking from one vehicle. By the time you arrive, traffic is backed up for three blocks. You realize that the decisions you make in the first few minutes will have a major effect on safety, patient care, and overall operations.

Describe how you would size up this scene. Make sure you cover the following areas:

- Vehicle placement
- Initial radio report
- Assuming incident command
- Safety
- Hazard control
- Standard Precautions
- Location and triaging of patients
- Resource determination
- Mechanisms of injury

See Suggested Responses at the back of this book.

PROCEDURE SCANS

Visual skill summaries provide step-by-step support in skill instruction.

Procedure 5–22 ● Reassessment

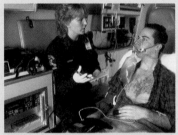

5-22a ● Reevaluate the ABCs.

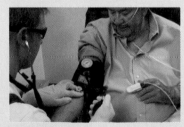

5-22b ● Take all vital signs again.

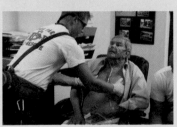

5-22c ● Perform your focused assessment again.

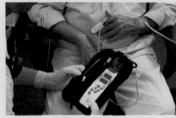

5-22d ● Evaluate your interventions' effects.

Special Features

PATHO PEARLS

Offer a snapshot of pathological considerations students will encounter in the field.

PATHO PEARLS

Patient assessment actually starts as soon as you approach the scene. Clues about the patient's underlying pathophysiology might be evident from such things as positioning of the vehicle, downed power lines, or the appearance and actions of bystanders. However, your safety, and that of your fellow rescuers, is always paramount. Never approach a scene that appears unsafe. With time, you will develop a "sixth sense" about emergency scenes and bystanders.

As you begin the patient encounter, process all that you see into your patient assessment and care. For example, consider this scenario: A car with two 16-year-old girls fails to negotiate a turn on a country road and overturns into a flowing creek adjacent to the road. Although the ambient temperature is in the 60s, you know that the temperature of the water in this area often is in the 40s. Thus, you should immediately suspect the possibility of hypothermia.

As the girls are removed from entrapment, no obvious injuries are noted. Vital signs are normal other than slight tachycardia. However, peripheral pulses are weak and the skin is pale and cool. Is it shock? Is it hypothermia? Is it both? Your index of suspicion is high for both hypothermia and blunt force trauma. You follow local protocols with regard to immobilization, fluid therapy, and monitoring. Once in the ambulance and wrapped in blankets, both girls start to show signs that blood flow to the skin is improving. By the time you reach the hospital, their skin has a normal color and their pulse rates are normal.

Following a comprehensive assessment in the emergency department, the girls are discharged to their parents with no apparent injuries. Thus, your instincts were right. The potential for shock was a greater risk to the girls than the potential for hypothermia, and you had to treat based on this risk. But hypothermia turned out to be the principal problem. Integrating information from the scene size-up, patient history, and patient examination gave you a clear picture of the patients' underlying pathophysiologic process.

CULTURAL CONSIDERATIONS

Provide an awareness of beliefs that might affect patient care.

CULTURAL CONSIDERATIONS

Eye contact is a major form of nonverbal communication. Short eye contact is often seen as friendly, whereas prolonged eye contact may be interpreted as threatening. Thus, timing is an important factor in how a person interprets eye contact.

One's culture also influences how eye contact is interpreted. Eye contact can mean respect in one culture and disrespect in another. Often, Asians will avoid eye contact even when they have nothing to hide. Eye contact between people of different sexes is problematic in Muslim cultures, in which a prolonged look in the face of a member of the opposite sex might be misinterpreted. Because of this, people in Middle Eastern countries might look a person of the same sex in the eye and not look into the eyes of a person of the opposite sex.

If you work in a culturally diverse community, you should learn the customs of eye contact and other forms of nonverbal communication of those you might encounter during the course of your work.

LEGAL NOTES

Present instances in which legal or ethical considerations should be evaluated.

LEGAL CONSIDERATIONS

Gatekeeper to the Health Care System. *The EMS system is often the initial point of contact for a person entering the health care system. Thus, to a certain extent, a paramedic frequently functions as a sort of gatekeeper to the health care system as a whole.*

Part of a paramedic's responsibility is to ensure that a patient is taken to a facility that can appropriately care for the patient's condition. Today, hospitals have become more specialized. That is, some hospitals have chosen to provide certain services and not provide others. For example, one hospital may elect to specialize in cardiac care, another in stroke care, another in burn care, and so on. This is especially true in communities with multiple hospitals. Because of this, it is essential that paramedics understand the capabilities of the hospitals in the system where they work. Also, with overcrowding in modern emergency departments, diversion of ambulances by hospitals whose emergency departments are full has become commonplace.

For all these reasons, local EMS system protocols must be available to guide prehospital personnel in ensuring that each patient is delivered to a facility that can adequately care for the patient's condition.

ASSESSMENT PEARLS

Offer tips, guidance, and information to aid in patient assessment.

ASSESSMENT PEARLS

Chest pain is a common reason that people summon EMS. However, the causes of chest pain are numerous. In emergency medicine or EMS, we often look to exclude the most serious causes before determining whether chest pain is of a benign origin. Internal organs do not have as many pain fibers as do such structures as the skin and other areas. Pain arising from an internal organ tends to be dull and vague. This is because nerves from various spinal levels innervate the organ in question. The heart, for example, is innervated by several thoracic spinal nerve segments. Thus, cardiac pain tends to be dull and is sometimes described as pressure. It also tends to cause referred pain (i.e., pain in an area somewhat distant to the organ), such as pain in the left arm and jaw. Dull pain that is hard to localize (or to reproduce with palpation) may be due to cardiac disease. One sign often seen with patients suffering cardiac disease is Levine's sign. With Levine's sign, the patient will subconsciously cle[...] pain. Levine's sign is a[...] (e.g., angina or acute c[...]

ASSESSMENT PEARLS

Assessing skin abnormalities in dark-skinned people can be a challenge. Try the following techniques:

Jaundice Look for a yellow color in the sclera and hard palate.

Erythema Look for an ashen color in the sclera, conjunctiva, mouth, tongue, lips, nail beds, palms, and soles.

Pallor Feel for warmth in the affected area.

Petechiae Look for tiny purplish dots on the abdomen.

Cyanosis Look for a dull, dark coloring in the mouth, tongue, lips, nail beds, palms, and soles.

Rashes Feel for abnormal skin texture.

Edema Look for decreased color and feel for tightness.

Student Workbook

A student workbook with review and practice activities accompanies each volume of the Paramedic Care series. The workbooks include multiple-choice questions, other exercises, case studies, and special projects, along with an answer key with text page references.

REVIEW OF CHAPTER OBJECTIVES

Tied to chapter objectives, content summaries review important information and concepts.

CASE STUDY REVIEW

An in-depth analysis at the start of each chapter highlights essential information and applied principles.

CONTENT SELF-EVALUATION

Multiple-choice, matching, and short-answer questions test reading comprehension.

SPECIAL PROJECTS

Experiences have been designed to help students remember information and principles.

PATIENT SCENARIO FLASHCARDS

Flashcards present scenarios with signs and symptoms and information to make field diagnoses.

DRUG FLASHCARDS

A special set of flashcards represents drugs commonly used in paramedic care.

MyParamedicLab

www.myparamediclab.com

WHAT IS MYPARAMEDICLAB?

MyParamedicLab is a comprehensive online program that gives you the opportunity to test yourself on basic information, concepts, and skills to see how well you know the material. From the test results, the program builds a self-paced, personalized study plan unique to your needs. Remediation in the form of e-text pages, illustrations, animations, exercises, and video clips is provided for those areas in which you may need additional instruction or reinforcement. You can then work through the program until material is learned and mastered. **MyParamedicLab** is available as a standalone program or with an embedded e-text.

    MyParamedicLab maps objectives created from the National EMS Education Standards for the Paramedic level to each learning module. With **MyParamedicLab**, you can track your own progress through the entire course. The personalized study plan material supports you as you work to achieve success in the classroom and on certification exams.

HOW DO STUDENTS BENEFIT?

MyParamedicLab helps you:

- Keep up with the new, complex information presented in the text and lectures.
- Save time by focusing study and review on just the content you need.
- Increase understanding of difficult concepts with study material for different learning styles.
- Remediate in areas in which you need additional review.

KEY FEATURES OF MYPARAMEDICLAB

Pre-Tests and Post-Tests Using questions aligned to Paramedic Standards, quizzes measure your understanding of topics and expected learning outcomes.

Personalized Study Material Based on the topic pre-test results, you will receive a personalized study plan highlighting areas where you may need improvement. Study tools include:

- Skills and animation videos
- Links to specific pages in the e-text
- Images for review
- Interactive exercises
- Audio glossary
- Access to full chapters of the e-text

HOW DO INSTRUCTORS BENEFIT?

- Save time by providing students with a comprehensive, media-rich study program
- Track student understanding of course content in the program Gradebook
- Monitor student activity with viewable student assignments

What Resources Are Available to Instructors?

Visit **www.bradybooks.com** to log onto Brady's Resource Central website for the Paramedic Care series. Your Brady sales representative will assist with access codes. At Resource Central instructors will find a wealth of curriculum management material to support class presentations, student assessment, and administrative functions.

Where Do I Get More Information?

Contact your local Brady representative for more information.

Pathophysiology

Bryan Bledsoe, DO, FACEP, FAAEM, EMT-P

STANDARD
Pathophysiology

COMPETENCY
Integrates comprehensive knowledge of pathophysiology of major human systems.

OBJECTIVES

Terminal Performance Objective
After reading this chapter you should be able to describe the pathophysiology of common patient disorders encountered by paramedics in the prehospital setting.

Enabling Objectives
To accomplish the terminal performance objective, you should be able to:

1. Define key terms introduced in this chapter.
2. Describe the relationship between homeostasis and health.
3. Explain how the predisposing factors of age, gender, genetics, lifestyle, and environment impact the development of disease.
4. Explain the basis of infectious, immunologic, inflammatory, ischemic, metabolic, nutritional, genetic, congenital, neoplastic, traumatic, physical, iatrogenic, and idiopathic classifications of diseases.
5. Describe the basic chemical structures that make up the body.
6. Differentiate between covalent, ionic, and hydrogen bonds.
7. Recognize the six major chemical elements and four major chemical compounds that make up the human body.
8. Describe the nature and roles of carbohydrates, proteins, nucleic acids, lipids, and water in the body.
9. Explain acid-base production, imbalances, and homeostasis in the body.
10. Explain the basic structure and function of a typical human cell and each of its components, including the following:
    a. plasma membrane
    b. cytoplasm
    c. nucleus
    d. ribosomes
    e. endoplasmic reticulum
    f. Golgi apparatus
    g. lysosomes
    h. vacuoles

    i. peroxisomes

    j. mitochondria

    k. cytoskeleton

11. Explain the movement of water and solutes into and out of cells under various intracellular and extracellular conditions, including osmosis, diffusion, facilitated diffusion, active transport, endocytosis, and exocytosis.

12. Describe the fluid and electrolyte composition of the cellular environment.

13. Explain fluid and electrolyte homeostasis and the effects of fluid and electrolyte imbalances.

14. Explain the movement of water between fluid compartments in the body.

15. Describe the composition and function of blood, including both plasma and formed elements.

16. Predict the physiologic effects of infusing various types of intravenous fluids.

17. Explain the processes of cellular respiration and energy production to include:

    a. glycolysis

    b. the citric acid cycle

    c. electron transport

    d. fermentation

18. Describe cellular responses to stress.

19. Describe the embryonic origins of body tissues.

20. Discuss the basic structure and function of epithelial, connective, muscle, and nervous tissues.

21. Describe the process of neoplasia, including factors associated with cancer.

22. Describe the risk factors and basic nature of the following types of disorders:

    a. immunologic diseases, including rheumatic fever, allergies, and asthma

    b. common cancers

    c. type I and type II diabetes mellitus

    d. hematologic disorders, including disorders of coagulation and hemochromatosis

    e. cardiovascular disease

    f. renal disorders

    g. rheumatic disorders

    h. gastrointestinal disorders

    i. neuromuscular disorders

    j. psychiatric disorders

23. Describe the physiology of perfusion.

24. Explain the etiologies and pathophysiology of hypoperfusion.

25. Describe the body's compensatory mechanisms in the face of hypoperfusion.

26. Predict the signs, symptoms, and consequences of untreated or inadequately treated shock.

27. Explain each of the following mechanisms of shock:

    a. cardiogenic

    b. hypovolemic

    c. neurogenic

    d. anaphylactic

    e. septic

28. Describe the evaluation and treatment goals for patients with cardiogenic, hypovolemic, neurogenic, anaphylactic, and septic shock.

29. Describe the pathophysiology of multiple organ dysfunction syndrome (MODS).

30. Describe the basic characteristics of bacteria, viruses, fungi, parasites, and prions that act as human pathogens.

31. Describe the body's three lines of defense against pathogens.

32. Explain the function of the immune system.

33. Describe the process of inflammation.

34. Explain the pathophysiology of hypersensitivity reactions and deficiencies in immunity and inflammation.

35. Describe the impact of age and stress on disease.

36. Describe the stress response.

KEY TERMS

ABO blood groups, p. 92
acid-base reaction, p. 25
acidosis, p. 28
acids, p. 25
acquired immunity, p. 88
active transport, p. 35
acute, p. 9
adenosine triphosphate (ATP), p. 21
adipocytes, p. 63
adipose tissue, p. 63
aerobic metabolism, p. 76
afterload, p. 73
AIDS, p. 111
albumin, p. 45
alkalosis, p. 28
allergy, p. 107
amino acids, p. 18
amylopectin, p. 17
amylose, p. 17
anabolism, p. 23
anaerobic metabolism, p. 76
anaphylaxis, p. 82
anencephaly, p. 8
anion, p. 14
antibiotics, p. 86
antibodies, p. 88
antigens, p. 88
antigen-antibody complexes, p. 93
antigen-presenting cells (APCs), p. 97
antigen processing, p. 96
apoptosis, p. 56
atom, p. 12
atomic number, p. 12
atrophy, p. 56
autoimmune disease, p. 9
autoimmunity, p. 107
B lymphocytes, p. 89
bacteria, p. 86

basement membrane, p. 61
bases, p. 25
basophils, p. 104
benign, p. 10
buffer, p. 27
carcinogenesis, p. 68
carcinoma-in-situ, p. 58
cardiac contractile force, p. 73
cardiac output, p. 74
cardiogenic shock, p. 80
carrier proteins, p. 35
cartilage, p. 63
cascade, p. 101
catabolism, p. 23
catecholamines, p. 73
cation, p. 14
cell, p. 30
cell-mediated immunity, p. 89
cell membrane, p. 31
cellular adaptation, p. 54
cellular respiration, p. 51
cellulose, p. 17
centrioles, p. 50
chemoreceptors, p. 28
chemotactic factors, p. 100
chemotaxis, p. 100
chromatin, p. 47
chromosomes, p. 47
chronic, p. 9
cilia, p. 51
cisternae, p. 48
citric acid cycle, p. 52
clinical presentation, p. 9
clonal diversity, p. 93
clonal selection, p. 93
coagulation system, p. 102
coenzymes, p. 20
cofactors, p. 20
collagen, p. 62
colloid, p. 45
compensated shock, p. 79
complement system, p. 101

complications, p. 9
compound, p. 15
concentration gradient, p. 33
congenital metabolic diseases, p. 19
connective tissues, p. 60
contraction, p. 106
cortisol, p. 114
covalent bond, p. 13
cristae, p. 50
crystalloids, p. 45
cytokines, p. 96
cytoplasm, p. 31
cytoskeleton, p. 50
cytotoxic, p. 57
debridement, p. 105
decompensated shock, p. 79
degranulation, p. 99
dehydration, p. 39
delayed hypersensitivity reactions, p. 107
denaturation, p. 18
deoxyribonucleic acid (DNA), p. 20
diagnosis, p. 9
diapedesis, p. 103
disaccharides, p. 17
disease, p. 6
dissociate, p. 40
dissociation reaction, p. 24
dynamic steady state, p. 112
dysplasia, p. 57
dysplastic, p. 66
ectoderm, p. 60
edema, p. 43
electrolyte, p. 40
electrons, p. 12
electron shells, p. 13
electron transport chain, p. 52
element, p. 12
endocrine secretions, p. 61

CASE STUDY

Medic 14 is dispatched to 1514 Houston on the outskirts of downtown. Paramedics quickly recognize the address as the Union Gospel Mission. It is a shelter for the homeless and the location of many EMS calls. Upon arrival, the crew is met by Reverend Williams, the aged gentleman who has operated the shelter for as long as anybody can remember. He recognizes Armando, the senior paramedic, and tells him, "It's Bill Jamison again. He looks bad this time." Paramedics roll the stretcher to the elevator only to learn that it is again broken. They grab the essential bags and climb four flights of stairs to reach Bill's room.

Bill is a chronic inebriate well known to virtually all EMS providers in the city. He is a former wrecker driver who used to interact with paramedics on accident scenes. However, his disease, alcoholism, eventually took his job, his family, his home, and now his health. EMS providers and the local county hospital have watched Bill's steady and predictable decline to his current condition. Bill is found prone on the floor in a dirty sleeping bag. He is unresponsive with snoring respirations. Paramedics know that Bill has type II diabetes and is often noncompliant with his medications. He is often found to be hypoglycemic—as a result of either his alcoholism or his medication.

They gently roll Bill to a supine position, and he moans slightly. His airway, though, is patent and his vitals are stable. They notice multiple bruises and a nosebleed. Bill has virtually all the stigmata of alcoholism and is now jaundiced. Armando says, "I'll bet he is hypoglycemic again." Armando's partner and rookie paramedic, Sam, begins to look for a vein. Reverend Williams holds a flashlight to help illuminate the dark and odorous room. No vein is identifiable. Armando switches places with Sam and takes a look. He too sees no veins. They then begin to discuss whether to give glucagon intramuscularly or place an intraosseous (IO) line. Armando decides on the IO. The line is placed without incident, and Bill awakens with half of an amp of $D_{50}W$. Bill is transported to University Hospital without incident.

On the way back from the hospital, Sam asks Armando why he chose the IO instead of the intramuscular glucagon. Armando explains, "Glucagon is a hormone that stimulates the release of glucose from carbohydrate storage sites, such as glycogen in the liver. Because of Bill's liver disease and poor diet, he has little, if any, glycogen stores and glucagon is unlikely to work. Besides, I've tried it in the past and it never has worked." Sam pondered the statement for a minute and asked, "What was the bleeding from?" Armando answers, "Not sure really. I could not see a source. But, it is probably a bleeding disorder." "What do you mean?" inquires Sam. Armando responds, "Many of the clotting factors, especially prothrombin, are made and stored in the liver. As the liver fails, as is the case with old Bill, his body loses its ability to properly clot, and he is prone to bleeding. Actually, the bleeding points to severe or even end-stage liver disease." Sam thinks for a minute and states, "Wow. You can learn something from every call—even at the Union Gospel Mission." Armando smiles and gently nods.

INTRODUCTION

The human body normally maintains its internal environment in a steady state of balance that is termed **homeostasis**. A significant disruption in homeostasis often leads to disease. **Disease** is an abnormal structural or functional change within the body. The study of disease is called **pathophysiology** and can be defined as the functional changes that occur within living cells and tissues that are associated with, or result from, disease or injury. **Pathology** is the medical science that deals with all aspects of disease. There is an emphasis on the essential nature, causes, and development of abnormal conditions as well as with the structural and functional changes that result from disease processes. A physician who specializes in pathology is called a **pathologist**.

Before embarking on the study of pathophysiology, it is essential that you first master the related normal anatomy and physiology. Only through understanding how the body is normally structured and works can one understand abnormal processes. In order to be an effective health care professional, the paramedic must understand the basic principles of pathophysiology so that he can properly assess and treat the disease and injury processes that affect humankind.

This chapter is divided into six parts:

Part 1: Disease

Part 2: Disease at the Chemical Level

Part 3: Disease at the Cellular Level

Part 4: Disease at the Tissue Level

Part 5: Disease at the Organ Level

Part 6: The Body's Defenses against Disease and Injury

HIERARCHICAL STRUCTURE OF THE BODY

We start with the concept that all living things that share this big blue-and-green planet known as Earth interact with each other at some point and on some level. Scientists have organized Earth's biological life into levels. In this chapter we will examine the disease processes that arise from the human body's cells, tissues, organs, organ systems and, ultimately, the organism (body) itself.

Cells, the smallest unit of life, are made up of chemical *molecules* (which are made up of individual *atoms*). A group of similar cells that performs a common function is known as a *tissue*. A group of tissues working together to perform a similar function is called an *organ*. A group of organs working together to perform a common or similar function is referred to as an *organ system*. Finally, a group of organ systems functioning together is called an *organism*. A human being is an organism. Humans have 11 different organ systems.

The organism, or individual, is the unit of life that is capable of surviving and reproducing in the environment. Humans, like many other "higher" animals, are social creatures. That is, we tend to associate with others of our kind. Humans are unique in that we also use other organisms for work and companionship.

Life can also be organized and stratified beyond the individual. For example, all the organisms of the same species residing in a distinct geographic area (e.g., continent, city) are called a *population*. A *community* is the sum total of all living organisms occupying a defined geographic area. A community and its physical environment are referred to as an *ecosystem*. An ecosystem can vary in size, based on the construct being studied, but is self-contained. Any number of ecosystems may exist within a *biome*. A biome is a geographic area with similar climatic conditions, such as a desert biome, a forest biome, a grasslands biome, or a marine biome. Finally, all ecosystems, biomes, and by definition all living organisms, form a *biosphere*. A biosphere is the portion of the Earth where life is found. Our biosphere extends from the depths of the deepest oceans (where life can be found) to approximately seven miles above sea level.

CONTENT REVIEW

▶ Hierarchy of the Body

- Cells
- Tissues
- Organs
- Organ systems
- Organism

PART 1: Disease

All cells and tissues are vulnerable to the effects of disease or injury, which can adversely affect the biology of the cells or tissues in question. There are **predisposing factors** that may lead to disease. These factors tend to increase the body's vulnerability to a specific disease. For example, it has been demonstrated that prolonged exposure to cigarette smoke changes the cellular structure of the respiratory tract. Sometimes these changes can result in abnormal cell function and cancer. Thus, cigarette smoking is a predisposing factor to the development of lung cancer.

PREDISPOSING FACTORS TO DISEASE

Factors that lead to the development of disease include age, gender, genetics, lifestyle, and environment.

- *Age.* Humans at both ends of the age spectrum are especially vulnerable to disease. Infants, for example, are vulnerable because their immune system is immature and they have not developed the necessary defenses. We augment these defenses by providing timely immunizations to enhance the infant's immune system. As we age, there is a decline in immune function that places us at increased risk for disease in our later years. This is due to a general decline in homeostatic function.

- *Gender.* Gender also plays a role in disease development. For example, men tend to develop heart disease at a younger age than women. Women are predisposed to certain diseases, such as osteoporosis, as they age. Often, these differences in disease development are due to the effects of the sex hormones.

- *Genetics.* A major factor in the development of disease is genetics. Only in recent years has the human genetic code been mapped through the Human Genome Project. Researchers are finding, with increasing frequency, that many diseases are due to expression of specific genes.

  Certain diseases are more common in certain families. For example, one family may have a history of atherosclerotic heart disease that routinely kills male members in the fifth or sixth decade of life. Other families may routinely develop diabetes mellitus.

  Because our ethnicity and race are also genetically encoded, certain diseases are common in certain races. For example, people of African and Mediterranean descent tend to develop sickle cell disease. People of Native-American and Mexican descent tend to develop diabetes mellitus. Ashkenazi Jews (Jews of central European descent) are vulnerable to many diseases, such as cystic fibrosis and Tay-Sachs disease, among others. This is thought to be due to significant intermarriage within the group, resulting in a small gene pool. A small gene pool from intermarriage can result in expression of disease-causing genes that would likely not be expressed if the gene pool were more varied. In fact, genetic testing has shown that 40 percent of the current Ashkenazi population is descended from just four women.[1]

- *Lifestyle.* Another major factor in the development of disease is lifestyle. This is particularly evident in today's society. A century ago, people ate primarily unprocessed foods. Today, foods are processed, removing many of the healthful ingredients that protected our forefathers from some of the diseases that are common today. Heart disease was much less common in the nineteenth century when compared to the latter half of the twentieth and the first part of the twenty-first century.

  In addition, the modern population obtains considerably less exercise than earlier generations because of the availability of cars and other forms of mechanized transportation and the fact that many farm and industry jobs that demanded intense physical labor have been replaced by more sedentary occupations. When you combine a lack of exercise with a diet that is devoid of quality calories (but rather is high in fats and carbohydrates), you end up with obesity. Obesity is one of the biggest health problems in the United States and is quickly becoming as great a problem in other developed countries such as the United Kingdom, Australia, and Canada.

- *Environment.* Finally, our environment can predispose us to disease. Native-Americans have long believed that an individual's health and the health of the community are directly related to the environment. We now know that numerous environmental factors are associated with the development of disease. For example, exposure to asbestos has been directly linked to the development of an uncommon lung cancer called mesothelioma.[2] Pollutants have been linked to the development of significant birth defects (such as **anencephaly**) in babies born to Mexican mothers in the lower Rio Grande river valley in south Texas, presumably caused by chemicals dumped into the river upstream.[3] And, in the Ukraine, the incidence of cancers, specifically thyroid cancer, has increased dramatically following the nuclear disaster in 1986 at Chernobyl.[4] Cumulative exposure to toxic substances also plays a role in disease development.

Any of these factors, or a combination of them, can lead to the development of disease. The effects of these factors can sometimes be cumulative. For example, an older person who smokes and also has a family history of lung cancer may be at a risk of developing the disease that is significantly increased over a person who has just one of those risk factors—age, or smoking, or family history—but not two or three of them.

Risk Analysis

It is important to point out that some predisposing factors can be modified while others cannot. While we cannot control our genetics, gender, or age, we can certainly control our lifestyle and, to a lesser degree, our environment. Minimizing some of these predisposing factors can also slow the effects of age. In the near future, genetic engineering may allow us to manipulate genes to prevent their expression and subsequent disease development.

We also know that there is a kind of cross-pollination of pathophysiologic factors, where risk factors figure in more than one kind of disease, and diseases become risk factors for other diseases. For example, various studies have identified as risk factors for cardiovascular disease such things as smoking, elevated blood pressure, cholesterol levels ("good" cholesterol versus "bad" cholesterol), diet, family history, age, gender, weight, level of exercise, obesity, diabetes, kidney disease, and lung disease (Figure 1-1 ●).

Using data from large-population studies, one can actually predict, with some degree of accuracy, whether a given person will develop any particular disease and how rapidly that person will develop it. This data can, therefore, be used to modify the risk factors that can be modified, thus holding off disease development. For example, a 34-year-old male paramedic is 30 pounds overweight, gets little exercise, routinely eats fast

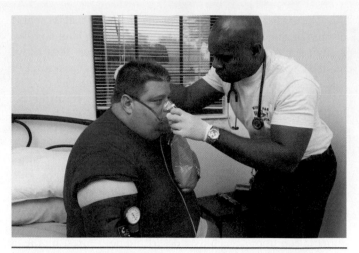

● **Figure 1-1** Obesity is one of many risk factors for cardiovascular disease.

foods, smokes half a pack of cigarettes a day, has a moderate family history of heart disease, and has mild hypertension. While he cannot modify his gender or genetics, he can increase exercise and decrease fast food intake. This will allow him to lose weight and improve the ratio of bad to good cholesterol. Concurrently, the weight loss can lead to reduction in his blood pressure. Abandonment of cigarette use further significantly decreases his risks for early development of heart disease. Together, these can modify or attenuate the development of cardiovascular disease, even though he is genetically predisposed to it. As he ages, he should stay abreast of practices that continue to minimize his risk for developing heart disease. For example, when he turns 50, he may be advised to begin taking an aspirin a day.

Risk analysis can now be used to look at a person's whole life. There are programs that can actually predict your life expectancy. These take into consideration health factors such as have been presented here. But, they also take into consideration environmental and lifestyle practices. High-risk behaviors such as scuba diving, skydiving, piloting single-engine aircraft, and rock climbing can statistically decrease projected life expectancy. Other more common behavioral practices that are risk factors include driving long distances, not wearing seat belts, carrying a handgun, practicing unsafe sex, illicit drug or significant alcohol use, and so on. Minimizing any of these risks can increase life expectancy and, in some instances, also enhance the quality of life.

DISEASE

Disease is an abnormal structural or functional change within the body. There is normally a defined sequence of events that leads to development of a disease. This is referred to as the **pathogenesis** of the disease. (The term derives from *pathogen*, defined as a microorganism capable of producing infection or disease). As already noted, there are a number of factors that can be identified that predispose a person to certain diseases. In some instances, predisposing factors cannot be identified. In this case, we say the disease is **idiopathic**.

The study of disease causes is termed **etiology**. Etiology comprises the occurrences, reasons, and variables of a disease. Etiology is often defined as consisting of *causality*, *contribution*, and *correlation*. Again using the example of smoking and lung cancer, we know that various factors are involved in the development of the disease. In some patients, the cause may be repeated exposure to cigarette smoke while in others it may be due to genetic expression. In the person who develops lung cancer from genetic expression, genetics is the cause but cigarette smoking and age may be contributing factors. It has been suggested, but not proven, that secondhand smoke may contribute to the development of lung cancer. In the example we have been using, secondhand smoke exposure in a lung cancer patient who had never smoked might be simply correlated to the condition. That is, it is a suspected factor but cannot be proven to either cause or contribute to the condition.

The manifestation of a disease is known as the **clinical presentation**. The clinical presentation includes both signs and symptoms of the disease. A **symptom** is what the patient tells you about the disease—a subjective complaint. Symptoms are often detailed when you obtain the patient's history. An objective finding that you can identify through physical examination is referred to as a **sign**. Some diseases have a specific constellation of commonly found signs and symptoms. These are referred to as a **syndrome**. However, some signs and symptoms are common among a variety of diseases and are referred to as being nonspecific symptoms, or generalized symptoms.

The process of identifying and assigning a name to a disease in an individual patient or a group of patients with similar signs and symptoms is termed **diagnosis**. A diagnosis is a generalization and an assumption that a disease will follow a prescribed course. However, just as people are different, all diseases are different, and each follows its own course. Some diseases have a sudden onset and are referred to as **acute** while others have a much slower onset and are referred to as **chronic** or **insidious**. The symptoms of a chronic disease are often milder and more difficult to initially identify.

When a disease such as diabetes mellitus is first identified, the primary problem is impaired glucose **metabolism**. However, as the disease progresses, other body systems can be affected. With diabetes, the eyes and kidneys can be adversely affected, causing both blindness and renal failure. Such abnormalities that result from the original problem are referred to as **complications**. When these resulting complications are common, or even expected, they are referred to as **sequelae** of the disease.

Many diseases are fairly well understood, and so we can predict their outcome. This expected outcome is referred to as the **prognosis**. For example, we know that hepatitis A has an incubation period of approximately 28 days and the disease lasts from two weeks to three months with relatively mild symptoms. Whenever the disease varies from the expected prognosis, it is important to reevaluate the patient to ensure that the diagnosis was correct and that complications are not occurring.

Classifications of Disease

There are various ways to classify diseases. The most common is by disease cause. On this basis, the following system of disease classification will be used in this text:

- *Infectious.* Infectious diseases are those that result from invasion of the body and colonization by a pathogenic organism. Most of these are microorganisms such as prions, viruses, bacteria, and fungi. Others are larger multicelled pathogenic organisms such as tapeworms and liver flukes.

CONTENT REVIEW

▶ Predisposing Factors to Disease

- Age
- Gender
- Genetics
- Lifestyle
- Environment

- *Immunologic.* Overreactions of the immune system, commonly called allergies or hypersensitivity, can cause diseases such as anaphylaxis. Sometimes the immune system fails to recognize certain tissues as belonging to the host and mounts an immune response as if the tissues were foreign. This phenomenon, referred to as **autoimmune disease**, is responsible for such conditions as rheumatic heart disease and rheumatoid arthritis. Inadequate immune system function makes the human more susceptible to pathogenic organisms and can result in overwhelming infection, such as that seen with acquired immune deficiency syndrome (AIDS).

- *Inflammatory.* Inflammatory diseases are those that result from the body's response to another disease process (primary disease). For example, pelvic inflammatory disease (PID) in a female is secondary to a bacterial infection in the reproductive tract—often gonorrhea or Chlamydia. The infection causes inflammation of the organs and supporting structures in the pelvis.

- *Ischemic.* Many diseases are due to diminished blood supply. Thus, the affected tissues may be deprived of oxygen and essential energy substrates, which can lead to cell death. Common examples of ischemic diseases include acute coronary syndrome (ACS), ischemic stroke, and ischemic bowel disease.

- *Metabolic.* Metabolic diseases result when there is a disturbance in the biochemical and metabolic processes within the body. Examples include diabetes mellitus, which results from decreased insulin secretion from the endocrine pancreas, and thyrotoxicosis that results from abnormally elevated levels of thyroid hormones that can markedly increase the basal metabolic rate, causing significant signs and symptoms.

- *Nutritional.* Nutritional diseases primarily result from a deficiency in one or all of the major nutritional sources (carbohydrates, proteins, fats). Vitamin deficiencies can also lead to nutritional diseases, because vitamins are required for normal metabolic processes. Examples of nutritional diseases are malnutrition and diseases that result from vitamin deficiency, such as scurvy and rickets.

- *Genetic.* Genetic diseases are those that are coded-for in a person's genetic material and thus are passed from parent to child. Examples of genetic diseases are hemophilia, Huntington's disease, and color blindness.

- *Congenital.* Certain diseases can result from problems that occur during fetal development. Most fetal development occurs during the first trimester of life. It is during this

▶ Disease Classified by Cause

- Infectious
- Immunologic
- Inflammatory
- Ischemic
- Metabolic
- Nutritional
- Genetic
- Congenital
- Neoplastic
- Trauma
- Physical agents
- Iatrogenic
- Idiopathic

period that the fetus is most susceptible to external factors that can adversely affect development (**teratogens**). However, many cases of congenital disease never have an identifiable cause. Examples of congenital diseases are cleft lip and palate, congenital heart disease, and Down syndrome (Figure 1-2 ●).

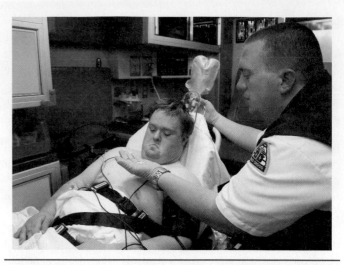

● **Figure 1-2** Down syndrome is a congenital disease. *(© Daniel Limmer)*

- *Neoplastic.* On occasion, certain cells will begin abnormal or uncontrolled cell growth. This process is referred to as **neoplasia**. The result is a tumor, or **neoplasm** (Figure 1-3 ●). A neoplasm can be **benign** (not cancerous, not able to spread to other tissues) or **malignant** (cancerous, able to spread), depending on the changes present in the cell line. Often the body's immune system is successful in removing cells that begin abnormal growth. However, when the cell growth is rapid, or if the cell is particularly resistant to removal by the body's defenses, the disease progresses and can eventually kill the patient. Fibroid tumors in the uterus, more accurately called uterine leiomyomas, are an example of a benign neoplastic process. Breast cancer (which usually arises from the breast ducts) is an example of a malignant neoplastic process.

- *Trauma.* External physical forces can mechanically change or disrupt the structure of the body and, as a result, affect body function. These external forces are referred to as **trauma**. An example might be blunt trauma to a kidney that fractures the kidney into multiple portions. This can cause the kidney to totally fail or to significantly decrease its ability to function.

- *Physical agents.* Myriad physical agents can adversely affect body structure and function. These include chemicals, poisons, ionizing radiation, extremes in temperature, changes in atmospheric pressure, and electrical shock. Examples of diseases caused by physical agents include transitional-cell bladder cancer, caused by exposure to chemicals such as ink, and ultraviolet keratitis (welder's flash) that results from looking at a welding arc that is producing ultraviolet radiation.

- *Iatrogenic.* Medical treatments for a disease can sometimes result in the development of other diseases or problems. A disease that occurs in this way is referred to as an **iatrogenic disease**. For example, a subclavian central intravenous line is placed into a patient to administer intravenous nutrition following a severe burn. During the line insertion, the dome of the lung is inadvertently punctured, resulting in a pneumothorax. This would then be termed an iatrogenic pneumothorax.

  Some procedures or treatments are so complicated or harsh that iatrogenic effects may be expected. The chances of developing iatrogenic complications are weighed against

PATHO PEARLS

The practice of medicine has become so complex that many patients actually die from the very treatments that are supposed to help them. It has been estimated that almost 200,000 patients a year suffer in-hospital deaths that are possibly preventable. Little is known about preventable out-of-hospital deaths. Further, a recent medical study found that medical errors caused up to 98,000 deaths annually and should be considered a national epidemic. Many of us forget that the primary dictum of medicine is primum non nocere (first, do no harm). We owe it to our patients, present and future, to ensure that our practices do not violate this dictum and bring them harm when they are seeking our help.

Neoplasia

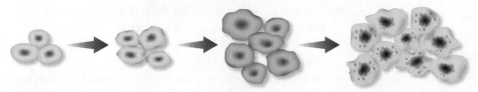

Abnormal or uncontrolled cell growth results in a tumor, or neoplasm.

● **Figure 1-3** How cancers grow. Factors such as genetic predisposition, smoking, pollution, and exposure to radiation or the sun's ultraviolet rays can trigger abnormal cell growth.

the perceived benefit of the treatment. An example is vaginal candidiasis following antibiotic therapy. The vagina normally has microorganisms present on its surface. These include both bacteria and fungi. The bacteria usually keep the fungi concentration low. However, if the patient is placed on potent antibiotics, the antibiotics can kill the normal vaginal bacteria (flora), which allows the fungus to proliferate, resulting in candidiasis. The disease is iatrogenic in that it resulted directly from medical treatment.

- *Idiopathic.* In many instances, as noted earlier, the specific cause of a disease is unknown. In this case, the disease is classified as idiopathic. Sometimes, a cause may be identified later. However, in many cases a specific cause is never found.

PART 2: Disease at the Chemical Level

To fully understand and appreciate anatomy, physiology, and pathophysiology, as a paramedic you must understand some basic chemistry and biochemistry as discussed in this chapter. Virtually every medical condition involves or affects biochemical mechanisms.

When did human life begin? This question has been a subject of discussion for thousands of years. In the sixth century B.C.E., pre-Socratic Greek philosophers spent a great deal of time discussing the possible origins of life. Although the true answer may never be known, the prevailing theory is that the universe was created almost 15 million years ago in a phenomenon referred to as the "Big Bang." The Big Bang theory (Figure 1-4 ●) was first put forth in 1927 by Belgian priest Georges Lemaître. He proposed that the universe began with the explosion of a primeval atom. Years later, the noted astronomer Edwin Hubble found experimental evidence to help validate Lemaître's theory. He found that distant galaxies in every direction were moving away from us at speeds proportional to their distance.

The theory of a Big Bang explained why distant galaxies were traveling away from Earth at great speeds. The theory also predicted the existence of cosmic background radiation (the energy left over from the explosion itself). The Big Bang theory received its strongest confirmation when, in fact, cosmic radiation was discovered in 1964 by Arno Penzias and Robert Wilson, who later won the Nobel Prize for this discovery. In 2006, a distant NASA space probe detected the light released just after the Big Bang. This cosmic afterglow, known as microwave background, is further support for the Big Bang theory. It is the oldest radiation ever detected, still traveling almost 14 billion years after it was emitted.

A related component to the origin of the universe is the origin of life as we know it. The prevailing scientific theory is that simple chemicals present in the primordial atmosphere and ocean combined to form larger, more complex chemicals. This theory is referred to as *chemical evolution.* Powered by the energy of the sun and other sources, the chemistry of the atmosphere and oceans changed over time. This ultimately led to the formation of complex chemicals that were able to *self-replicate* (produce identical copies of themselves). The ability of

The Big Bang Theory

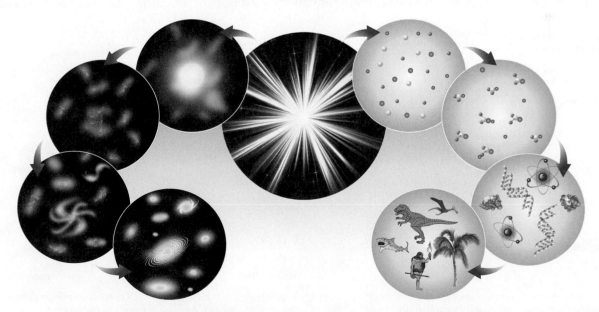

The Big Bang theory proposes that the universe began with the explosion of a primeval atom—resulting in both the formation of galaxies in a still-expanding universe and the origin of life from simple chemicals.

● **Figure 1-4** Development of the universe originating from a rapid expansion (explosion) of hot, dense primeval material is known as the "Big Bang theory."

a chemical to self-replicate marked the transition from chemical evolution to *biological evolution*. Once biological evolution began, *natural selection* began. (Natural selection is the tendency of traits that help a species to adapt and survive to become common in a population by being passed down to succeeding generations.) As these chemicals replicated and multiplied, they became more complex. The self-replicating chemical soon became surrounded by a membrane and cellular life began.

THE CHEMICAL BASIS OF LIFE

As stated previously, to understand pathophysiology, you must first understand normal anatomy and physiology. To understand normal anatomy and physiology, you must understand the chemical basis for life. In this section of the chapter we will summarize the basics of chemistry as they apply to pathophysiology. Then, we will detail the biochemical processes that are affected by injury and illness.

The fundamental chemical unit is the **atom**. Within the atom are particles, referred to as subatomic particles, which include electrons, protons, and neutrons. **Protons** and **neutrons** exist within the nucleus of the atom. **Electrons** are considerably smaller particles and orbit the nucleus (Figure 1-5 ●). Protons (p^+) have a positive electrical charge, neutrons (n) are electrically neutral, and electrons (e^-) have a negative electrical charge. Opposite charges attract and like charges repel. When the number of protons and the number of electrons are the same, the atomic charge is electrically neutral.

An **element** is a substance that cannot be separated into simpler substances. The number of protons in the nucleus of an atom (the **atomic number**) defines the element. Elements are

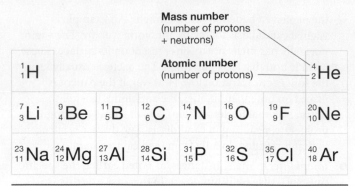

● **Figure 1-6** A portion of the periodic table of elements. Each element has an atomic number (the number of protons), a mass number (the total number of neutrons and protons), and a one- or two-letter symbol. *(Freeman, Scott, Biological Science, 4th Edition, © 2011. Reprinted and electronically reproduced by permission of Pearson Education, Inc., Upper Saddle River, NJ)*

usually classified by their atomic number in a scheme known as the *periodic table of elements* (Figure 1-6 ●).

Elements cannot be reduced to simpler substances by normal chemical means. That is, naturally occurring processes cannot break them down into more elemental structures. While each element contains a characteristic number of protons, the number of neutrons can vary. Elements that have the same number of protons but vary in the number of neutrons are referred to as **isotopes**, or variants of the same element. Some elements, such as uranium, can have multiple isotopes. While the number of protons in an atom's nucleus is referred to as the atomic number, the total number of neutrons and protons in an atom is referred to as the **mass number**.

Some combinations of neutrons and protons make the nucleus that contains them inherently unstable. These atoms are

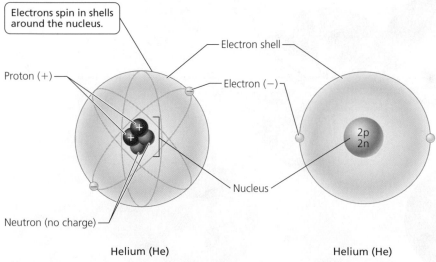

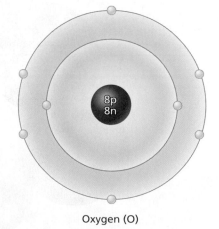

Helium (He)	Helium (He)	Oxygen (O)
(a) A three-dimensional representation of an atom of helium, showing protons and neutrons in the nucleus and electrons occupying a region around the nucleus.	**(b)** A two-dimensional representation of an atom of helium.	**(c)** A two-dimensional representation of an atom of oxygen.

● **Figure 1-5** Atoms can be represented in various ways. *(Goodenough, Judith and Betty A. McGuire, Biology of Humans: Concepts, Applications, and Issues, 3rd Edition, © 2010. Reprinted and electronically reproduced by permission of Pearson Education, Inc. Upper Saddle River, NJ)*

(a) Number of half-lives elapsed	Fraction remaining	Percentage remaining
0	1/1	100
1	1/2	50
2	1/4	25
3	1/8	12.5
4	1/16	6.25
5	1/32	3.125
6	1/64	1.563
7	1/128	0.781

(b)   Half-Lives of Isotopes of Americium
- Am241— 432.2 years
- Am242— 16.02 hours
- Am243— 7,380 years

● **Figure 1-7**   The half-life of a radioactive isotope is the time it takes for half the atoms of that substance to disintegrate into another form. The half-life of any radioactive isotope is unique to that isotope, so that a substance can be identified by discovering its half-life. (a) As half-lives elapse, smaller and smaller fractions of the original substance remain. (b) Half-lives can range from fractions of a second to billions of years. For example the element Americium has many isotopes with vastly different half-lives, three of which—americium 241, 242, and 243—are listed here.

called **radioactive isotopes** because their nuclei break down and emit radiation, or alpha, beta, and gamma rays, until the atom regains stability. This process is referred to as **radioactive decay**. The initial isotope is referred to as the parent and the resulting isotope is the daughter. The rate of radioactive decay is constant and specific for a given isotope. The rate of decay is usually measured in a unit called a half-life. A **half-life** is the time it takes for the parent isotope to decrease by one-half (Figure 1-7 ●).

Electrons rotate around the nucleus of the atom in a specific region referred to as an **orbital**. Each orbital has a specific shape and can hold two or more electrons. Orbitals occupy levels that are

defined based on their distance from the nucleus. These levels are referred to as **electron shells** and are numbered starting with the closest shell to the nucleus. Electrons first fill the electron shells closest to the nucleus and then progressively fill the more distant shells. The filling order of the more distant shells is complicated. The first shell can hold two electrons, and the second shell can hold eight electrons. The number of electrons a shell can hold increases with each level (2, 8, 18, 32, 50) (Figure 1-8 ●). The outermost shell of an atom is referred to as the **valence shell**. The electrons found in that shell are referred to as **valence electrons**. An atom is most stable when the valence shell is full. The only elements that have a full valence shell are the six that are called the **noble gases**: helium, neon, argon, krypton, xenon, and radon. Because their valence shell is full, the noble gases are extremely stable.

Chemical Bonding

Most atoms become stable by bonding to other atoms. For example, the simplest atom is hydrogen. Hydrogen contains only one electron. However, the first orbital shell can hold two electrons. Thus, to attain stability, hydrogen must find a second electron to fill the first shell. When two hydrogen atoms approach each other, they begin to share their two electrons, and then both atoms fill their valence shell and become stable.

Covalent Bonds

The equal sharing of electrons results in what is called a **covalent bond** that tends to hold the atoms together. A substance made up of atoms held together by one or more covalent bonds is referred to as a **molecule** (Figure 1-9 ●). Covalent bonds are the strongest of the three types of chemical bonds.

● **Figure 1-8**   Hydrogen, carbon, and oxygen atoms. Each concentric circle around the nucleus represents an electron shell. *(Goodenough, Judith and Betty A. McGuire, Biology of Humans: Concepts, Applications, and Issues, 3rd Edition, © 2010. Reprinted and electronically reproduced by permission of Pearson Education, Inc. Upper Saddle River, NJ)*

Hydrogen atom
(atomic number = 1)

Carbon atom
(atomic number = 6)

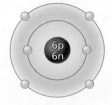

Oxygen atom
(atomic number = 8)

The shell closest to the nucleus can hold up to 2 electrons.

The next shell out can hold up to 8 electrons (the shell shown here has 6). Atoms with more than 10 electrons have additional shells.

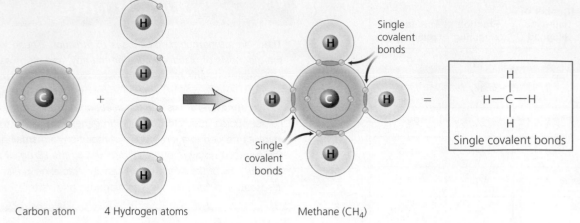

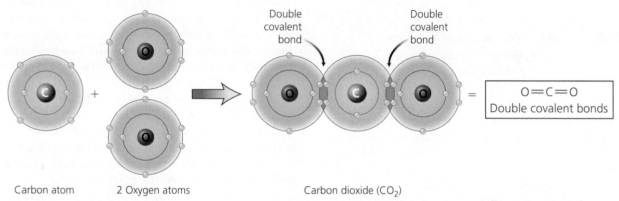

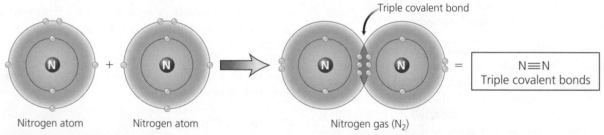

(a) The molecule methane (CH_4) is formed by the sharing of electrons between one carbon atom and four hydrogen atoms. Because in each case one pair of electrons is shared, the bonds formed are single covalent bonds.

(b) The oxygen atoms in a molecule of carbon dioxide (CO_2) form double covalent bonds with the carbon atom. In double bonds, two pairs of electrons are shared.

(c) The nitrogen atoms in nitrogen gas (N_2) form a triple covalent bond in which three pairs of electrons are shared.

● **Figure 1-9** Covalent bonds are formed when electrons are shared between atoms. Shown here are examples of single, double, and triple covalent bonds. The structural formula of each is shown at the far right. *(Goodenough, Judith and Betty A. McGuire, Biology of Humans: Concepts, Applications, and Issues, 3rd Edition, © 2010. Reprinted and electronically reproduced by permission of Pearson Education, Inc. Upper Saddle River, NJ)*

Ionic Bonds

In addition to covalent bonds, atoms can be held together when atoms with an electrical charge are attracted to each other. An atom or molecule that has acquired an electrical charge by either gaining or losing one or more is referred to as an **ion**. Neutral atoms have an equal number of protons and electrons. When an atom or molecule loses one or more electrons, the number of protons exceeds the number of electrons, thus giving the atom or molecule a net positive charge. (Remember that a proton has a positive charge while an electron has a negative charge.)

Conversely, when an atom or molecule gains one or more electrons, there are then more electrons than protons and the atom or molecule has a net negative charge. An atom or molecule with missing electrons and thus a net positive charge is called a **cation**. An atom or molecule with extra electrons and a net negative charge is called an **anion**. Because opposite charges attract, bonds form between atoms of opposite (positive/negative) charges. This kind of bond is referred to as an **ionic bond** (Figure 1-10 ●).

As with covalent bonds, ions will try to fill their outermost shell in order to reach stability. Thus, certain atoms tend to

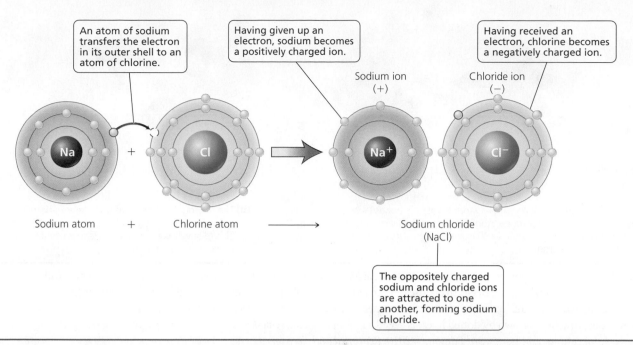

An atom of sodium transfers the electron in its outer shell to an atom of chlorine.

Having given up an electron, sodium becomes a positively charged ion.

Having received an electron, chlorine becomes a negatively charged ion.

Sodium ion (+)

Chloride ion (−)

Sodium atom   +   Chlorine atom   ⟶   Sodium chloride (NaCl)

The oppositely charged sodium and chloride ions are attracted to one another, forming sodium chloride.

● **Figure 1-10** An ionic bond involves the transfer of electrons between atoms. Such a transfer creates oppositely charged ions that are attracted to each other. *(Goodenough, Judith and Betty A. McGuire,* Biology of Humans: Concepts, Applications, and Issues, *3rd Edition, © 2010. Reprinted and electronically reproduced by permission of Pearson Education, Inc. Upper Saddle River, NJ)*

interact with other atoms to fill their outermost shell. Elements that are classified as **metallic elements** tend to lose electrons. Likewise, elements that are described as **nonmetallic elements** tend to gain electrons. Thus, most ionic bonds are between a metal and a nonmetal. The prototypical example of this is the ionic bonding of the atoms sodium (a metal) and chlorine (a nonmetal). Sodium is extremely reactive and occurs only in compounds in nature. Chlorine is also quite reactive and usually exists as a salt in nature. Sodium has one electron in its outer shell while chlorine has seven electrons in its outer shell. Thus, sodium (Na) must lose an electron to reach stability, and chlorine (Cl) must gain an electron to reach stability. When the two atoms come into close proximity, the sodium atom loses an electron to the chlorine atom, thus becoming a positively charged cation (abbreviated as Na^+). The chlorine atom, gaining an electron, becomes a negatively charged anion (abbreviated as Cl^-). The opposite ions are then attracted to each other, thus forming an ionic bond and becoming sodium chloride (NaCl), a salt (the main ingredient in common table salt).

Hydrogen Bonds

A hydrogen bond is the last type of chemical bonding. As already noted, the equal sharing of electrons forms a covalent bond. However, in selected cases, the sharing of electrons between two atoms is unequal. Thus, different parts of the same molecule can have an unequal charge. An unequal covalent bond is called a **polar bond**, and the molecule is referred to as a **polar molecule**. This relationship can be explained by looking at the water molecule. In water (H_2O), two hydrogen (H) atoms share their electrons with a single oxygen (O) molecule. But the electrons spend more time orbiting the oxygen atom compared to the hydrogen atoms. Thus, the oxygen atom has a slightly negative charge and each hydrogen ion has a slight

positive charge, thus making the entire water molecule polar. In nature, the hydrogen ions of a water molecule, because they have a slight positive charge, are attracted to the oxygen atom of other water molecules (because they have a slight negative charge). This attraction between a slightly positively charged hydrogen atom and a slightly negatively charged oxygen atom is referred to as a **hydrogen bond**. Hydrogen bonds are much weaker than either covalent bonds or ionic bonds. Collectively they are important in that they give water its special physical properties (Figure 1-11 ●).

Inorganic and Organic Chemicals

In general chemistry, chemicals are usually classified as organic or inorganic. **Inorganic chemicals** are chemicals that do not contain the element carbon. **Organic chemicals** are all the chemicals that do contain the element carbon. More than 90 percent of all known chemicals are organic, and most chemicals found in plants and animals are organic. Six elements (carbon, hydrogen, nitrogen, oxygen, phosphorus, and sulfur) make up approximately 98 percent of the body weight of most living organisms. Of these, the four major elements of living systems are carbon (C), hydrogen (H), oxygen (O), and nitrogen (N).

A **compound** is the chemical union of two or more elements. The four major compounds of living systems are carbohydrates, proteins, nucleic acids, and lipids. Molecules of these compounds are composed mostly of atoms from the four major elements, plus some additional elements, such as phosphorus (P), sulfur (S), iron (Fe), magnesium (Mg), sodium (Na), chlorine (Cl), potassium (K), iodine (I), and calcium (Ca) (Figure 1-12 ●).

Because of the diversity of the world of biochemistry, we will limit this discussion primarily to animals. Plants have very unique biochemical processes but these are not pertinent, for the most part, to the study of human pathophysiology.

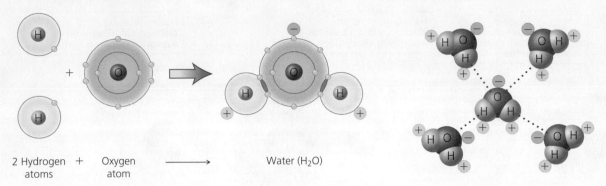

(a) Water is formed when an oxygen atom covalently bonds (shares electrons) with two hydrogen atoms. Due to unequal sharing of electrons, oxygen carries a slight negative charge and the hydrogen atoms carry a slight positive charge.

(b) The hydrogen atoms from one water molecule are attracted to the oxygen atoms of other water molecules. This relatively weak attraction (shown by dotted lines) is called a hydrogen bond.

● **Figure 1-11**   The hydrogen bonds of water. (a) Shown at left, water is formed when an oxygen atom covalently bonds with two hydrogen atoms. Because of unequal sharing of electrons, the oxygen atom has a slight negative charge and the hydrogen atoms have a slight positive charge. (b) Shown at right, the hydrogen atoms of one water molecule are attracted to the oxygen atoms of other water molecules. This relatively weak attraction (shown by dotted lines) is called a hydrogen bond. *(Goodenough, Judith and Betty A. McGuire, Biology of Humans: Concepts, Applications, and Issues, 3rd Edition, © 2010. Reprinted and electronically reproduced by permission of Pearson Education, Inc. Upper Saddle River, NJ)*

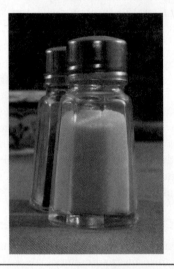

● **Figure 1-12**   Common table salt (sodium chloride, NaCl) is a compound of sodium and chlorine. Sodium is a silver-colored solid metal; chlorine is a yellow gas. Table salt is, obviously, neither a silvery metal nor a yellow gas but a grainy white compound that is quite different from its elements.

Classes of Biological Chemicals

There are four major classes of biological chemicals. These are the four major compounds already mentioned: carbohydrates, proteins, nucleic acids, and lipids (fats). Water, as well, plays an extremely important role in biological chemistry.

Carbohydrates

Carbohydrates are compounds that contain the elements carbon (C), hydrogen (H), and oxygen (O). Typically, the hydrogen and oxygen atoms occur in a 2:1 ratio. Carbohydrates provide the majority of calories in most diets. They are typically divided into the sugars and the polysaccharides.

Sugars   The **sugars** can be classified as either simple sugars (monosaccharides) or complex sugars (disaccharides).

Monosaccharides   The **monosaccharides** are simple sugars. Examples of monosaccharides are glucose, fructose, and galactose.

● **Glucose** is a six-carbon sugar and the principal energy source for the human body (Figure 1-13 ●).

● **Fructose** is a five-carbon sugar that is found in many plants and vegetables as well as honey.

● **Galactose**, also a six-carbon sugar, is primarily found in dairy products.

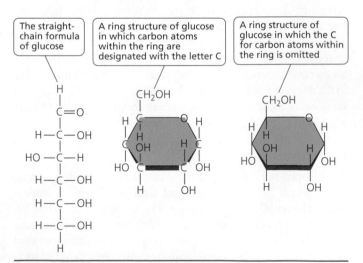

● **Figure 1-13**   Glucose is a monosaccharide, a six-carbon sugar that is the principal energy source for the human body. *(Goodenough, Judith and Betty A. McGuire, Biology of Humans: Concepts, Applications, and Issues, 3rd Edition, © 2010. Reprinted and electronically reproduced by permission of Pearson Education, Inc. Upper Saddle River, NJ)*

Sugars are the most important sources of energy for most cells. They are soluble in water.

Disaccharides The **disaccharides** are complex sugars. They are combinations of the simple sugars joined together by a glycosidic bond to form a double-sugar molecule. Examples of disaccharides are sucrose, lactose, and maltose.

- **Sucrose** is common table sugar. It is a combination of glucose and fructose (Figure 1-14 ●).

- **Lactose** is the principal sugar in milk. It is a combination of glucose and galactose.

- **Maltose** is a breakdown product of starch. It is a combination of two glucose molecules.

Sucrose and maltose are frequently encountered in the diet. As noted, maltose results from the degradation of starch.

Polysaccharides **Polysaccharides** are the second type of carbohydrates. Major polysaccharides are the starches, cellulose, and glycogen. Plants store glucose in the form of starches or cellulose. Animals store glucose in the form of glycogen. Starches and cellulose are major parts of the human diet.

Starches **Starches** are polymers of glucose. A **polymer** is a large organic molecule formed by combining many smaller molecules (**monomers**) in a regular pattern. In the case of starch, the smaller molecule is glucose. Thus, starches are long chains of glucose molecules connected by glycosidic bonds. Unlike the monosaccharides, starches are insoluble in water. This allows them to serve as storage reservoirs for glucose.

There are two types of starches:

- **Amylose** is a linear, unbranched chain of several hundred glucose molecules. (Portions of larger molecules, such as the glucose molecules that make up amylose, are called residues.)

- **Amylopectin** differs from amylose in that it is highly branched, not linear like amylose. The glucose residues in a molecule of amylopectin number several thousand.

Cellulose Like starch, **cellulose** is a polysaccharide polymer with glucose as its monomer. However, cellulose differs significantly from starch in its chemical properties. Cellulose is the most abundant organic molecule in the world and the major structural material of plants. For example, wood is largely cellulose, while cotton and paper are almost pure cellulose. Humans do not have the enzyme necessary to digest cellulose; thus, it passes through our gastrointestinal systems undigested. However, the fiber that cellulose provides is important in creating bulk and moving fecal matter through the large intestine.

Glycogen In terms of human pathophysiology, glycogen is certainly the most important polysaccharide. **Glycogen** (Figure 1-15 ●) is a glucose polymer much like amylopectin except that the branches tend to be shorter and less frequent. Glycogen is primarily stored in the liver and skeletal muscle. When needed, it is broken down to glucose in a process called

Glycogen

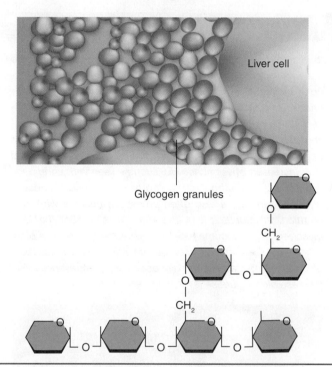

● **Figure 1-15** Glycogen is the storage polysaccharide in animals. It is stored primarily in the liver and in skeletal muscle.

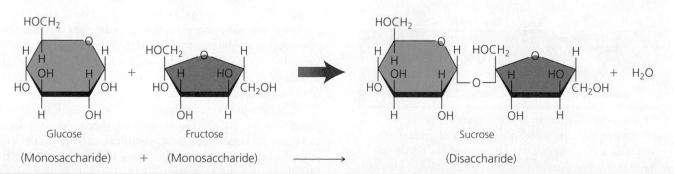

Glucose (Monosaccharide) + Fructose (Monosaccharide) → Sucrose (Disaccharide)

● **Figure 1-14** Sucrose is a disaccharide made when two monosaccharides, glucose and fructose, combine. (*Goodenough, Judith and Betty A. McGuire,* Biology of Humans: Concepts, Applications, and Issues, *3rd Edition, © 2010. Reprinted and electronically reproduced by permission of Pearson Education, Inc. Upper Saddle River, NJ*)

glycogenolysis. Glycogenolysis is controlled by the hormones glucagon and epinephrine. In persons with liver disease, such as chronic alcoholics, glycogen stores may be scant, and thus administration of glucagon is often ineffective in elevating the blood glucose level in hypoglycemia.

Proteins

Proteins, which are nitrogen-based complex compounds, are the basic building blocks of cells. Proteins are essential for the growth and repair of living tissues. They are the most abundant class of biological chemicals in the body (Table 1–1). Proteins consist of smaller building blocks called **amino acids.**

The amino acids are held together in proteins by **peptide bonds.** These bonds occur when two amino acid molecules join and a molecule of water is released. The shape and other properties of each protein are dictated by the precise sequence of amino acids it contains. Proteins consist of one or more

TABLE 1–1 | Protein Functions

Protein Type	Function
Antibodies and complement protein	Defense (destruction of disease-causing agents)
Contractile and motor proteins	Movement
Enzymes	Catalyze chemical reactions
Peptide hormones	Signal and control the activities of cells
Receptor proteins	Receive chemical signals from outside of the cell and initiate cellular response
Structural proteins	Support cells and tissues. Major factor in various body structures
Transport proteins	Move substrates across cell membranes and throughout the body

CLINICAL NOTE

It is common practice in EMS to administer glucagon to patients with hypoglycemia. Glucagon elevates the blood glucose indirectly by stimulating glycogenolysis. While usually effective, many patients, such as chronic alcoholics, have limited stores of glycogen because of their liver disease and associated malnutrition; thus, glucagon may be ineffective in this population. Decreased glycogen stores are also associated with increased physical activity, such as seen with endurance events (e.g., marathon races, football matches). Decreased glycogen stores are also often present in patients with malnutrition. In neonates it is important to remember that liver glycogen stores become rapidly depleted within hours of birth. When you suspect that your patient might have inadequate glycogen stores, administer glucose (orally or intravenously) to increase blood glucose levels (Figure 1-16 ●).

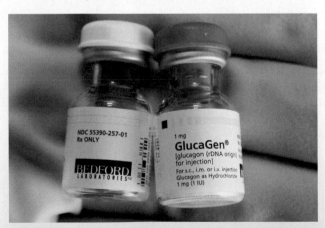

● **Figure 1-16** Glucagon administration may be ineffective in patients with limited stores of glycogen, such as alcoholics, because of liver disease and malnutrition. If you suspect your patient may have limited glycogen stores, administer glucose to increase blood glucose levels. (*Dr. Bryan E. Bledsoe*)

unbranched chains of amino acids. Thus, like the polysaccharides already discussed, proteins are polymers. There are 20 types of amino acids (monomers) that are synthesized in protein polymers.

The typical protein will contain 200–300 amino acid molecules. A protein chain containing less than 10 amino acids is often called a **peptide** while a chain of greater than 10 amino acids is called a **polypeptide.** Some proteins are extremely large, consisting of greater than 20,000 amino acid monomers (Figure 1-17 ●).

Proteins have four levels of structure: primary, secondary, tertiary, and quaternary. The precise sequence of amino acids in a protein is referred to as the primary structure. This sequence of amino acids in a protein is determined by the person's genes. The secondary structure of a protein results from bending and folding of the amino acid chain. The shape results from hydrogen bonding between parts of the chain. The overall three-dimensional shape of a protein is called the tertiary structure. Covalent, ionic, and hydrogen bonds all play a role in a protein's tertiary structure. Finally, some proteins will have more than one polypeptide chain. Each chain forms a subunit of the protein. The forces that hold the subunits together are the charges present on the side-chains. This level of protein structure is referred to as the quaternary structure (Table 1–2).

Changes in the environment of a protein can result in the protein losing its three-dimensional shape. Various factors can cause this, including heat, chemicals, and pH. These usually affect the secondary and tertiary structure, although they can also affect the primary structure. The loss of a protein's three-dimensional shape is called **denaturation**. The classic example of this is the act of cooking an egg. The egg white is primarily protein. When heat is applied, the proteins in the

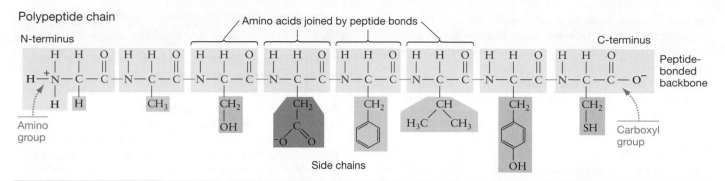

Polypeptide chain

N-terminus

Amino acids joined by peptide bonds

C-terminus

Peptide-bonded backbone

Amino group

Side chains

Carboxyl group

● **Figure 1-17** Amino acid monomers combine to form polymers consisting of long chains called polypeptides. *(Freeman, Scott, Biological Science, 4th Edition, © 2011. Reprinted and electronically reproduced by permission of Pearson Education, Inc., Upper Saddle River, NJ)*

egg white denature and lose their shape. This causes the egg white to change from a translucent substance to the white cooked egg.

Enzymes Most enzymes are proteins. **Enzymes** are substances that speed up chemical reactions. They accomplish this without being consumed in the process. Most chemical reactions that occur in the body occur too slowly to meet the needs of the body. Thus, we have multiple enzyme systems that speed these necessary chemical reactions—sometimes by as much as 10,000 to 1,000,000 times the rate such reactions would occur without the aid of the enzyme.

The substance an enzyme works on is called a **substrate**. The substrate binds to the enzyme, forming the **enzyme-substrate complex**. The substrate is then converted to the end product,

TABLE 1–2 | Protein Structure

Level	Description	Stabilized by	Example: Hemoglobin
Primary	The sequence of amino acids in a polypeptide	Peptide bonds	Gly — Ser — Asp — Cys
Secondary	Formation of alpha helices and beta-pleated sheets in a polypeptide	Hydrogen bonding between groups along the peptide-bonded backbone; thus, depends on primary structure.	One α-helix
Tertiary	Overall three-dimensional shape of a polypeptide (includes contribution from secondary structures)	Bonds and other interactions between side chains or between side chains and the peptide-bonded backbone; thus, depends on primary structure.	One of hemoglobin's subunits
Quaternary	Shape produced by combinations of polypeptides (thus, combinations of tertiary structures)	Bonds and other interactions between side chains, and between peptide backbones of different polypeptides; thus, depends on primary structure.	Hemoglobin, which consists of four polypeptide subunits

the enzyme then binds to another substrate, and the process begins again (Figure 1-18 ●). Some enzyme systems require **cofactors** to function. Cofactors are nonprotein substances that aid in the conversion of substrate to end product. Some cofactors are found in inorganic substances while others, such as vitamins, are organic. Organic cofactors are usually referred to as **coenzymes**.

Nucleic Acids

The class of molecules known as nucleic acids has two members: deoxyribonucleic acid (DNA) and ribonucleic acid (RNA). Adenosine triphosphate (ATP) is an important monomer of RNA.

DNA and RNA   **Deoxyribonucleic acid (DNA)** is the nucleic acid that contains the genetic instructions for life. It is composed of two long polymers called nucleotides that are joined by paired substances called nucleobases. There are four nucleobases in DNA, and the sequence of these encodes information known as the

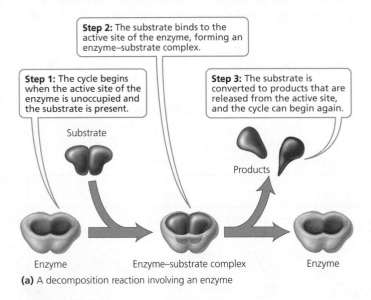

Step 1: The cycle begins when the active site of the enzyme is unoccupied and the substrate is present.

Step 2: The substrate binds to the active site of the enzyme, forming an enzyme–substrate complex.

Step 3: The substrate is converted to products that are released from the active site, and the cycle can begin again.

Substrate

Products

Enzyme   Enzyme–substrate complex   Enzyme

(a) A decomposition reaction involving an enzyme

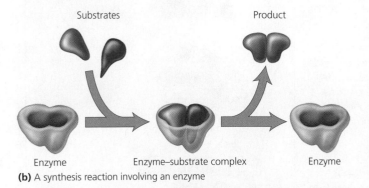

Substrates   Product

Enzyme   Enzyme–substrate complex   Enzyme

(b) A synthesis reaction involving an enzyme

● **Figure 1-18**   The working cycle of an enzyme. *(Goodenough, Judith and Betty A. McGuire, Biology of Humans: Concepts, Applications, and Issues, 3rd Edition, © 2010. Reprinted and electronically reproduced by permission of Pearson Education, Inc. Upper Saddle River, NJ)*

PATHO PEARLS

Free Radicals, a Side-Effect of Aging. *The effects of age are manifested throughout the body. Numerous metabolic processes, including metabolism as a whole, slow with age. This is due to multiple factors, including a loss in muscle tissue, but is also due to hormonal and neurologic changes.*

One of the side-effects of aging is the development of **free radicals.** *Free radicals are highly reactive molecules or atoms that have an unpaired electron in an outer orbital that is not contributing to molecular bonding (and is thus free). Atoms or small molecules that are free radicals tend to be the most unstable. The Free-Radical Theory of Aging (FRTA), advanced by Denham Harman more than 50 years ago, posits the following: Cells continuously produce free radicals, and constant radical damage eventually kills the cell. When radicals kill or damage enough cells in an organism, the organism ages. Aging occurs when energy-producing cells die, either when the mitochondria begin to die out because of free radical damage or when less functional mitochondria remain within these cells. (Free radicals will also be discussed in Chapter 5.)*

The body contains compounds called antioxidants that are molecules that eliminate radicals. Thus, elevated levels of antioxidants prevent much of the damage done by radicals. There are numerous antioxidant molecules found in the body, including superoxide dismutase, catalase, glutathione, and others. It has been postulated that administration of antioxidant substances can help delay the effects of aging. Vitamins A, C, and E, as well as several cofactors and minerals, have antioxidant properties. While the theory seems appropriate, clinical studies have failed to show any significant benefit on aging from the dietary addition of antioxidants (Figure 1-19 ●).

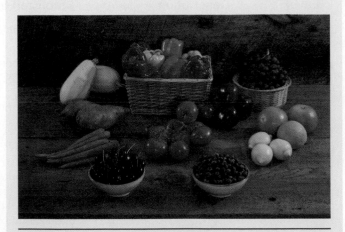

● **Figure 1-19**   Colorful fruits and vegetables (other than green) are rich in antioxidants although, contrary to popular belief, research has not shown that increasing their consumption has any cancer-preventing benefit. *(© Michal Heron)*

genetic code (Figure 1-20 ●). DNA contains segments referred to as genes that code for the specific amino acid sequence that makes up a specific protein. DNA is further organized into chromosomes. The number of chromosomes present in the cell nucleus varies with the type of organism (e.g., humans have 46, dogs have 78).

The other member of the class of nucleic acids is **ribonucleic acid (RNA)**, a chemical that is similar to DNA (Figure 1-21 ●). RNA plays a major role in protein synthesis, serving as a template for protein synthesis.

The fundamental building blocks of the nucleic acids, DNA and RNA, are **nucleotides**. Nucleotides are five-carbon sugar molecules that are bound to a nitrogen base and a phosphate group (Figure 1-22 ●). They form a long chain-like molecule. There are only five nitrogen bases: adenine, cytosine, guanine, thymine (found only in DNA), and uracil (found only in RNA). It is the sequence of these bases in both DNA and RNA that subsequently determines the sequence of amino acids in a protein.

DNA is a double-stranded helical chain while RNA is single-stranded. In DNA, the five-carbon sugar is deoxyribose; in RNA, the five-carbon sugar is ribose. RNA does not use the nitrogen base thymine, and DNA does not use the nitrogen base uracil. DNA has the capacity for self-replication (Table 1–3).

ATP **Adenosine triphosphate (ATP)** is a nucleotide that is one of the monomers of RNA. ATP is the principal source of

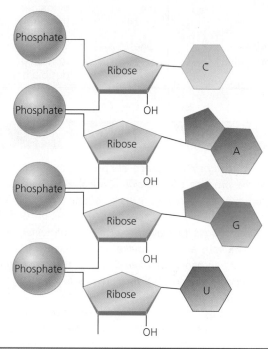

● **Figure 1-21** RNA is a single-stranded nucleic acid formed by the linking together of nucleotides composed of the five-carbon sugar ribose, a phosphate group, and one of four nitrogen-containing nucleobases: cystosine (C), adenine (A), guanine (G), and uracil (U). *(Goodenough, Judith and Betty A. McGuire, Biology of Humans: Concepts, Applications, and Issues, 3rd Edition, © 2010. Reprinted and electronically reproduced by permission of Pearson Education, Inc. Upper Saddle River, NJ)*

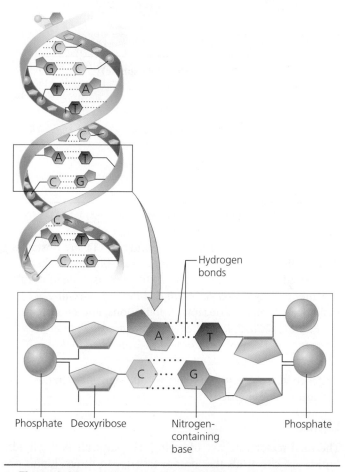

● **Figure 1-20** DNA is a nucleic acid in which two chains of nucleotides twist around one another to form a double helix (spiral). The two chains are held together by hydrogen bonds between the nitrogen-containing bases. Each nucleotide of DNA contains the five-carbon sugar deoxyribose, a phosphate group, and one of four nitrogen-containing nucleobases: adenine (A), thymine (T), cystosine (C), and guanine (G). *(Goodenough, Judith and Betty A. McGuire, Biology of Humans: Concepts, Applications, and Issues, 3rd Edition, © 2010. Reprinted and electronically reproduced by permission of Pearson Education, Inc. Upper Saddle River, NJ)*

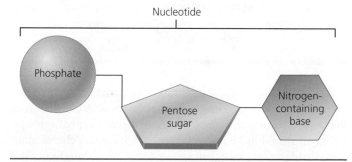

● **Figure 1-22** Nucleotides consist of a five-carbon (pentose) sugar bonded to a phosphate molecule and one of five nitrogen-containing bases: adenine, cystosine, guanine, thymine, and uracil. Nucleotides are the building blocks of the nucleic acids DNA and RNA. *(Goodenough, Judith and Betty A. McGuire, Biology of Humans: Concepts, Applications, and Issues, 3rd Edition, © 2010. Reprinted and electronically reproduced by permission of Pearson Education, Inc. Upper Saddle River, NJ)*

TABLE 1–3	RNA and DNA Structural Differences		
Characteristic	RNA	DNA
Sugar	Ribose	Deoxyribose
Bases	Adenine, guanine, cytosine, uracil	Adenine, guanine, cytosine, thymine
Number of Strands	One	Two, twisted to form a double helix

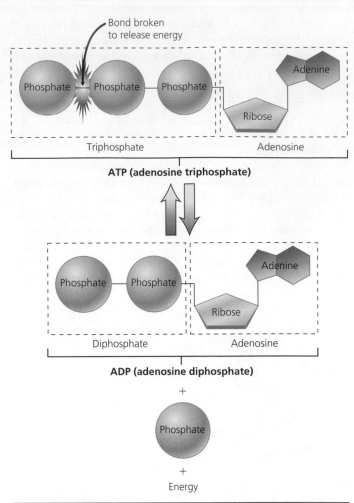

● **Figure 1-23** The nucleotide adenosine triphosphate (ATP) consists of the sugar ribose, the base adenine, and three phosphate groups. The phosphate bonds of ATP are unstable. When cells need energy, the last phosphate bond is broken, yielding adenosine diphosphate (ADP), a phosphate molecule, and energy. *(Goodenough, Judith and Betty A. McGuire,* Biology of Humans: Concepts, Applications, and Issues, *3rd Edition, © 2010. Reprinted and electronically reproduced by permission of Pearson Education, Inc. Upper Saddle River, NJ)*

energy for most of the energy-utilizing activities of the cells. Often called the "energy currency" of the cells, ATP consists of the base adenine, the sugar ribose, and three phosphate groups. Energy is stored in ATP when an energy-requiring chemical reaction adds an inorganic phosphate molecule, through covalent bonding, to adenosine diphosphate (ADP), forming ATP.

The phosphate bonds in ATP are highly unstable. Thus, when cells require energy, the phosphate bond is broken, liberating the stored energy, and the ATP then returns to ADP and an inorganic phosphate (Figure 1-23 ●). The liberated energy can then be used for chemical reactions occurring within the cell.

In humans, ATP also acts outside the cell. It is released from damaged cells and elicits pain. It is also released from the

stretched wall of the urinary bladder and signals when the bladder needs to be emptied.

Lipids

The final major category of biological chemicals is the lipids. **Lipids** are chemicals that do not dissolve in water. Lipids are nonpolar, while water is polar. Thus, water is not attracted to lipids, and lipids are not attracted to water.

In the human, lipids function in the long-term storage of biochemical energy, insulation, structure, and control. The lipids that pertain to human pathophysiology are triglycerides, phospholipids, and steroids (Figure 1-24 ●).

Triglycerides **Triglycerides** are rich sources of energy for the body. In fact, they provide approximately twice as much energy per gram as do proteins or carbohydrates. Triglycerides consist of one molecule of glycerol and three fatty acid molecules

Lipids

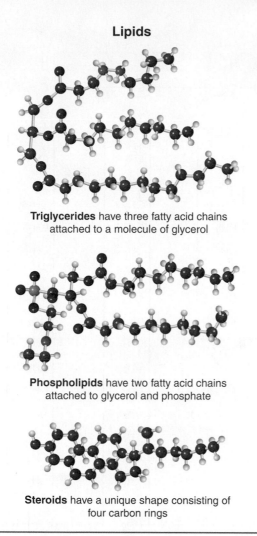

Triglycerides have three fatty acid chains
attached to a molecule of glycerol

Phospholipids have two fatty acid chains
attached to glycerol and phosphate

Steroids have a unique shape consisting of
four carbon rings

● **Figure 1-24**   The lipids that pertain to human pathophysiology are triglycerides, phospholipids, and steroids.

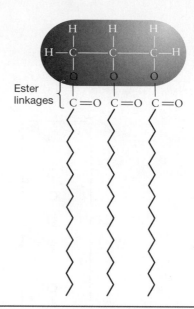

Ester linkages

● **Figure 1-25**   A triglyceride consists of a molecule of glycerol linked to three fatty acids. *(Freeman, Scott,* Biological Science, *4th Edition, © 2011. Reprinted and electronically reproduced by permission of Pearson Education, Inc., Upper Saddle River, NJ)*

(Figure 1-25 ●). Fatty acids are long carbon chains of carbon and hydrogen with an acid (carboxyl) group at one end.

Triglycerides can be classified as saturated or unsaturated. A **saturated fatty acid** has a single bond between each carbon atom, leaving room on the atom for two hydrogen atoms. Thus, the chemical is said to be saturated. When a double bond exists between carbon atoms, there is space for only one hydrogen atom, and thus the molecule is said to be an **unsaturated fatty acid**. Double bonds produce a bend in the fatty acid molecule and give it a different physical property (Figure 1-26 ●). Molecules with many of these bends cannot be packed as closely together as straight molecules, so these fats are less dense. As a result, triglycerides composed of unsaturated fatty acids melt at lower temperatures than those with saturated fatty acids. For example, margarine contains more saturated fat than corn oil. At room temperature it is solid while corn oil remains liquid.

Phospholipids   Another important lipid class is the **phospholipids**. These are extremely important in biological systems as they form the membrane that surrounds the cells. Structurally, phospholipids are similar to triglycerides in that they

contain a glycerol base. Instead of three fatty acid chains, they contain two fatty acid chains and a phosphate group that has a negative charge. Other smaller variable molecules are linked to the phosphate group. Thus, phospholipids have two distinct regions with different physical characteristics. The region with the two fatty acid chains, essentially the tail, is nonpolar and rejects water (hydrophobic). The phosphate region, essentially the head, is polar and thus attracts water (hydrophilic). This feature is what makes phospholipids an important part of biological membranes (Figure 1-27 ●). Two layers of phospholipids form the membrane. The hydrophobic tails are oriented to the inside of the membrane, and the hydrophilic heads are on the outside (Figure 1-28 ●). The tails form a protective region and hold the membrane together.

Steroids   The last major class of biological lipids is the **steroids**. Steroids have a unique shape. That is, they have a four-carbon ring as the backbone of their structure (Figure 1-29 ●). The basic unit is cholesterol, which is a component of plasma membranes and the base for synthesis of most of the steroid-class of hormones (i.e., estrogen, testosterone, cortisol, and aldosterone). The synthesis of steroid compounds by the body is termed form of anabolism. (**Anabolism** is the constructive phase of metabolism in which cells convert nonliving substances into living cytoplasm. Its opposite is **catabolism**, the destructive phase of metabolism in which cells break down complex substances into simpler substances with release of energy.) Steroids became a part of the human diet when the species went from a vegetarian to a carnivorous diet.

Water

Water has been called the "universal solvent." It is abundant in the body and plays a significant role in numerous biological processes. In fact, the physical properties of water are

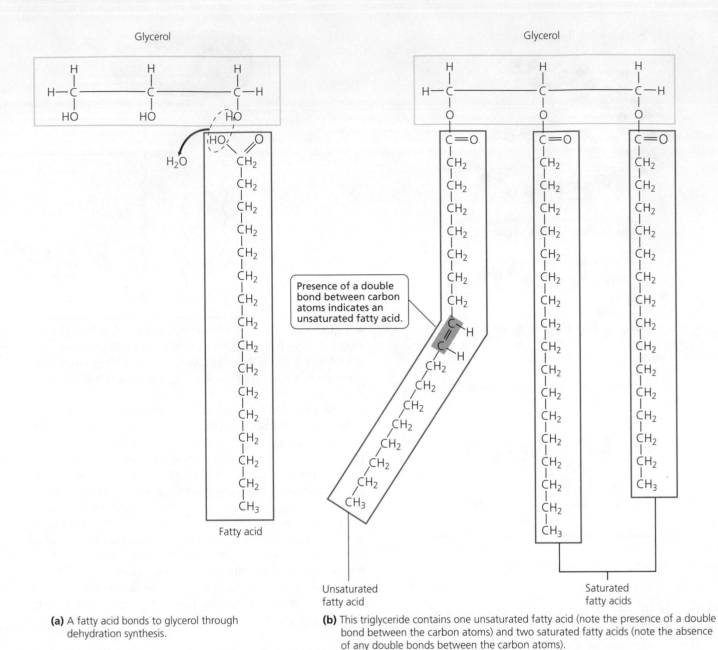

(a) A fatty acid bonds to glycerol through dehydration synthesis.

(b) This triglyceride contains one unsaturated fatty acid (note the presence of a double bond between the carbon atoms) and two saturated fatty acids (note the absence of any double bonds between the carbon atoms).

● **Figure 1-26** The triglyceride shown here contains one unsaturated fatty acid (note the double bond between the carbon atoms) and two saturated fatty acids (note the absence of any double bonds between the carbon atoms). *(Goodenough, Judith and Betty A. McGuire,* Biology of Humans: Concepts, Applications, and Issues, *3rd Edition, © 2010. Reprinted and electronically reproduced by permission of Pearson Education, Inc. Upper Saddle River, NJ)*

essential for life as we know it. As discussed earlier, water is a polar molecule and has the tendency to create hydrogen bonds, which causes water molecules to adhere to each other (Figure 1-30 ●). This gives water its liquid property. However, hydrogen bonds are the weakest of the chemical bond types. Consequently, the hydrogen bonds of water are frequently broken and re-formed.

Its polarity makes water an excellent solvent that can dissolve both polar and charged substances. Water also plays a major role in the transport of substances throughout the body and plays a significant role in maintaining a constant body temperature. Water has a high heat capacity, and therefore it can absorb a large amount of heat energy before the temperature

elevates. This property plays a major role in keeping the body cool. In addition to a high heat capacity, water has a high heat of vaporization, meaning that it takes a great deal of heat energy to make water vaporize. When water vaporizes, it carries away a significant amount of heat, thus cooling the body.

Acids and Bases

In solution, water has a tendency to break up into ions. That is, the water molecule is not a completely stable molecule. A water molecule, which is made up of hydrogen and oxygen atoms, can break apart into ions. This is a **dissociation reaction**. (A dissociation reaction is any reaction in which a compound or

A phospholipid

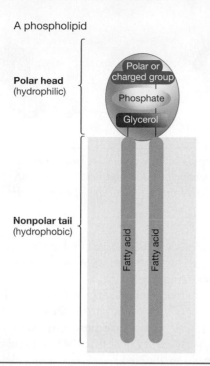

Polar head
(hydrophilic)

Polar or charged group

Phosphate

Glycerol

Nonpolar tail
(hydrophobic)

Fatty acid

Fatty acid

● **Figure 1-27**   The phospholipid has a nonpolar (hydrophobic) "tail" consisting of two fatty acids and a polar (hydrophilic) "head" consisting of a phosphate region. *(Freeman, Scott, Biological Science, 4th Edition, © 2011. Reprinted and electronically reproduced by permission of Pearson Education, Inc., Upper Saddle River, NJ)*

a molecule breaks apart into separate components.) This is reflected in the following equation:

$$H_2O \leftrightarrow H^+ + OH^-$$

This equation indicates that water dissociates into a hydrogen ion (H^+) and a hydroxide ion (OH^-). A hydrogen ion is a molecule that has lost its lone electron and is simply a proton. Substances that give up protons during chemical reactions are called **acids**. Likewise, substances that acquire protons during a chemical reaction are called **bases**. Any chemical reaction that results in the transfer of protons is referred to as an **acid-base reaction**.

Protons do not exist by themselves. In water, they actually associate with another water molecule to form a hydronium ion (H_3O^+). One of the water molecules gives up a proton and acts as an acid. The other water molecule accepts the proton and acts as a base. This process is reflected in the following equation:

$$H_2O + H_2O \leftrightarrow H_3O^+ + OH^-$$

By acting as a proton donor or proton acceptor, water has the unique ability to act as either an acid or a base. Most chemicals that are acids act only as acids, and most chemicals that are bases act only as bases. Acid-base reactions occur because of the number of protons present in the water solution at any given time.

The actual concentration of protons in water has been scientifically measured. In a sample of pure water at 25 °C (77 °F),

● **Figure 1-28**   Two layers of phospholipids form a biological membrane, with hydrophobic tails oriented to the inside of the membrane and hydrophilic heads oriented to the outside. *(Goodenough, Judith and Betty A. McGuire, Biology of Humans: Concepts, Applications, and Issues, 3rd Edition, © 2010. Reprinted and electronically reproduced by permission of Pearson Education, Inc. Upper Saddle River, NJ)*

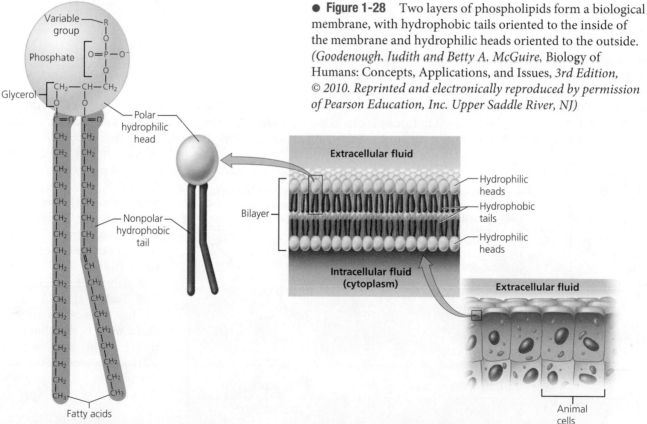

(a) A phospholipid consists of a variable group designated by the letter R, a phosphate, a glycerol, and two fatty acids. Because the variable group is often polar and the fatty acids nonpolar, phospholipids have a polar hydrophilic (water-loving) head and a nonpolar hydrophobic (water-fearing) tail.

(b) Within the phospholipid bilayer of the plasma membrane, the hydrophobic tails point inward and help hold the membrane together. The outward-pointing hydrophilic heads mix with the watery environments inside and outside the cell.

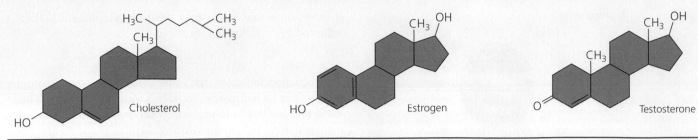

● **Figure 1-29** All steroids have a structure consisting of four carbon rings. Steroids such as cholesterol, estrogen, and testosterone differ in the groups that are attached to the four carbon rings. *(Goodenough, Judith and Betty A. McGuire, Biology of Humans: Concepts, Applications, and Issues, 3rd Edition, © 2010. Reprinted and electronically reproduced by permission of Pearson Education, Inc. Upper Saddle River, NJ)*

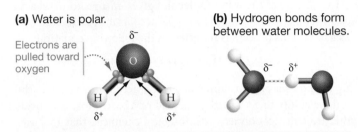

(a) Water is polar.

Electrons are pulled toward oxygen

(b) Hydrogen bonds form between water molecules.

● **Figure 1-30** Water is polar and participates in hydrogen bonds. *(Freeman, Scott, Biological Science, 4th Edition, © 2011. Reprinted and electronically reproduced by permission of Pearson Education, Inc., Upper Saddle River, NJ)*

the number of protons (in the form of H^+) is 1.0×10^{-7} M. (*M* represents **molarity**, or moles of solute per liter of solution. A **mole** is a measure of mass or weight used in chemistry. Mole is sometimes defined as "molecular weight.") Because the actual number of protons is so small, it is best to use a logarithmic representation. (A **logarithm** is a base number that is raised to a certain power. A common example is $2^3 = 8$. In other words, 2 to the third power—$2 \times 2 \times 2$—equals 8. In that example, 2^3 is a logarithm. With a positive exponent, like the ^{3} in 2^3, a logarithm

simplifies working with very large numbers. With a negative exponent, like the $^{-7}$ in 1.0×1.0^{-7}, a logarithm simplifies working with very small numbers.)

The accepted convention to express the degree of acidity or basicity (alkalinity) of a substance is to use the logarithmic **pH scale**. (A logarithmic scale is based on exponents or powers that raise the value of the base number rather than the base number itself.) The term pH comes from the French term *puissance d'hydrogéne* which literally means "power of hydrogen." In the pH scale, the greater the number of hydrogen ions, the higher the acidity.

The pH of a solution is the negative of the base-10 logarithm (log) of the hydrogen ion concentration $[H^+]$ and can be expressed in the following formula:

$$pH = -\log [H^+]$$

It can also be written as:

$$pH = \log \frac{1}{[H^+]}$$

The pH scale ranges from 0 to 14. A drop in the pH scale of 1 unit indicates a 10-fold increase in the hydrogen ion concentration, while a 2-unit drop indicates a 100-fold increase in the number of hydrogen ions, and so on. Pure water has a pH of 7.0 (1.0×10^{-7} M). Thus, a solution with a pH of 7.0 has an equal number of hydrogen ions and hydroxide ions. Substances with a pH of <7.0 are acidic, while substances with a pH >7.0 are basic. The normal pH of arterial blood is slightly basic, ranging from 7.35 to 7.45 (Table 1–4).

Just as there is a pH scale, there is also a **pOH scale**, although that scale is infrequently used in medicine. The pOH scale represents the number of hydroxide ions present in a solution. The pOH is the opposite of pH.

$$pH + pOH = 14$$

While the pOH of water is equal to the pH (7.0), when the pH goes up, the pOH comes down and vice versa.

TABLE 1–4 | The pH Scale and Hydrogen Ion Concentrations

pH		Example	Hydrogen Ion Concentration	
Acidic	0	Hydrochloric acid	10^{-0}	(1.0)
	1	Stomach secretions	10^{-1}	(0.1)
	2	Lemon juice	10^{-2}	(0.01)
	3	Cola drinks	10^{-3}	(0.001)
	4	White wine	10^{-4}	(0.0001)
	5	Tomato juice	10^{-5}	(0.00001)
	6	Coffee, urine, saliva	10^{-6}	(0.000001)
Neutral	7	Distilled water	10^{-7}	(0.0000001)
Basic	8	Blood, semen	10^{-8}	(0.00000001)
	9	Bile	10^{-9}	(0.000000001)

Buffer Systems

Free hydrogen ions are being constantly produced by the body, primarily from *glycolysis*, and result in the formation of carbon dioxide. These free hydrogen ions determine the body's pH. It is important to understand that all of the body's metabolic processes operate properly only when the pH is normal. In addition, all chemical reactions that depend on enzymes are susceptible to changes in pH. In fact, significant changes in pH can destroy these needed enzymes. Thus, biological systems function properly only within a very limited pH range.

Buffers are needed to counter the body's normal production of acids and to prevent significant variations in the body's pH. A **buffer** is a substance dissolved in water that counteracts changes in pH. When the hydrogen ion concentration increases, buffers remove excess hydrogen ions from the solution. Conversely, when the hydrogen ion concentration falls, buffers add hydrogen ions to the solution. The body has three major buffer systems:

- *Carbonic acid-bicarbonate buffer system.* The carbonic acid-bicarbonate buffer system is the most important buffer system in the extracellular fluid (ECF), including the blood. It is also the most rapidly acting of the three buffer systems.

- *Protein buffer system.* The protein buffer system works by way of selective amino acid monomers accepting or releasing hydrogen ions. This system plays a major role in pH regulation in both the ECF and intracellular fluid (ICF) compartments. It interacts significantly with the other buffer systems.

- *Phosphate buffer system.* The phosphate buffer system plays a role in buffering the pH of the ICF and the urine.

Carbonic Acid-Bicarbonate Buffer System   The pH of the blood is primarily regulated by the carbonic acid-bicarbonate buffer system. The primary role of this system is to buffer changes in pH caused by organic acids and fixed acids in the ECF. When carbon dioxide (CO_2) is added to water (H_2O), it forms carbonic acid (H_2CO_3). Carbonic acid, in turn, quickly dissociates into hydrogen ions (H^+) and bicarbonate ion (HCO_3^-). Carbonic acid is a volatile acid in that it will readily leave a solution and enter the atmosphere. In the lungs, carbonic acid breaks down into carbon dioxide and water. The carbon dioxide diffuses into the alveoli and is expelled with ventilation. In the peripheral tissues, carbon dioxide, a waste product of metabolism, combines with water to form carbonic acid. Carbonic acid then dissociates to release hydrogen ions and bicarbonate ions. This can be represented by the following equation:

$$CO_2 + H_2O \leftrightarrow H_2CO_3 \leftrightarrow H^+ + HCO_3^-$$

Water plays a significant role in the carbonic acid-bicarbonate system and is better represented by the following equation:

$$H_3O^+ + HCO_3^- \leftrightarrow H_2CO_3 + H_2O \leftrightarrow 2\,H_2O + CO_2$$

This reaction occurs spontaneously in body fluids. However, it occurs much faster in the presence of the enzyme *carbonic anhydrase.*

Carbonic anhydrase is found in red blood cells, the liver, kidneys, stomach, and other structures. Carbonic anhydrase promotes the rapid formation of water and carbon dioxide, thus making the reaction significantly faster.

$$CO_2 + H_2O \xleftarrow{\text{Carbonic Anhydrase}} H_2CO_3 \leftrightarrow H^+ + HCO_3^-$$

The carbonic acid-bicarbonate buffer system has several important limitations. First, it does not effectively protect the extracellular fluid from changes in pH that are due to changes in carbon dioxide levels. Since carbon dioxide is the weak acid in the carbonic acid-bicarbonate system, the system cannot protect against changes in the concentrations of one of its constituents (carbon dioxide). If this were to occur, elevated levels of carbon dioxide would mix with water, forming carbonic acid thus generating hydrogen ions (driving the equation to the right). This would be harmful, in that hydrogen ions would reduce the pH of the plasma.

Second, despite what has just been described, the carbonic acid-bicarbonate system can function only when the respiratory system and respiratory control centers are functioning normally. When the carbonic acid-bicarbonate buffer system buffers an organic or fixed acid, carbon dioxide is produced. This then elevates the partial pressure of carbon dioxide in the blood (**PaCO$_2$**). The respiratory centers in the brain must detect this increase and increase respirations accordingly to remove the excess carbon dioxide by exhaling it from the body. If this increase in respirations cannot occur, for whatever reason, the carbonic acid-bicarbonate system becomes considerably less effective. Stated another way, the buffer system cannot remove the hydrogen ions efficiently unless the respiratory system is functioning properly.

Third, the ability to buffer acids is limited by the amount of available bicarbonate ions. Every time a hydrogen ion is removed from the blood, it takes a bicarbonate ion with it. However, the body normally has an extremely large supply of bicarbonate ions, known as the *bicarbonate reserve.*

The normal pH of the blood can be calculated with the *Henderson-Hasselbalch equation* that states:

$$pH = 6.1^1 + \log\frac{\text{Base}}{\text{Acid}}$$

$$pH = 6.1 + \log\frac{HCO_3^-}{H_2CO_3} \quad \text{or} \quad pH = 6.1\,\log\frac{HCO_3^-}{\alpha^2 PaCO_2}$$

$$pH = 6.1 + \log\frac{20}{1}$$

$$pH = 6.1 + 1.3$$

$$pH = 7.4$$

This equation is based on that fact that the normal ratio of base to acid is 20:1.

---

[1]6.1 is the pK$_a$ of this system (the negative log of the ionization constant).
[2]Where α is the solubility coefficient of 0.226 mM/kPa.

CONTENT REVIEW

▶ Major Acid-Base Buffer Systems

- Carbonic acid-bicarbonate buffer system
- Protein buffer system
- Phosphate buffer system

CONTENT REVIEW
▶ Acid-Base Disorders
  • Respiratory acidosis
  • Respiratory alkalosis
  • Metabolic acidosis
  • Metabolic alkalosis

Protein Buffer System Protein buffers depend on the ability of select amino acids in the protein chain to react to changes in pH by accepting or releasing hydrogen ions. Proteins in the plasma play an important role in buffering pH changes in the blood. Similarly, protein fragments and amino acids play a role in buffering the pH of the interstitial fluid.

An important part of the protein buffer system is the *hemoglobin buffer system*. Red blood cells contain large quantities of hemoglobin and the enzyme carbonic anhydrase. Thus, they can have a significant effect on the pH of ECF. Carbon dioxide readily and rapidly diffuses into red blood cells that take in carbon dioxide from the plasma. There, they are rapidly converted into carbonic acid. When the carbonic acid dissociates, bicarbonate ions are excreted into the plasma (in exchange for chloride) in a phenomenon called the *chloride shift*. The remaining hydrogen ions are then buffered by the hemoglobin molecules present in the red blood cells. Overall, the hemoglobin buffer system plays a major role in preventing significant changes in ECF pH when the $PaCO_2$ is either rising or falling.

Phosphate Buffer System The last major buffer system is the phosphate buffer system, which is somewhat similar to the carbonic acid-bicarbonate buffer system. The phosphate buffer system uses the anion dihydrogen phosphate ($H_2PO_4^-$), which is actually a weak acid. Dihydrogen phosphate combines with hydrogen ion to form monohydrogen phosphate (HPO_4^{2-}). Monohydrogen phosphate is an anion and can be represented by the following equation:

$$H_2PO_4^- \leftrightarrow H^+ + HPO_4^{2-}$$

The phosphate buffer system can be represented by the following equation:

$$pH = 6.8^3 + \log \frac{Base}{Acid}$$

$$pH = 6.8 + \log \frac{HPO_4^{2-}}{H_2PO_4}$$

The phosphate buffer system is limited in the ECF but plays a major role in stabilizing the pH of urine.

Acid-Base Balance

As just presented, the acid-base balance must be tightly controlled. While the buffer systems described are effective in binding acids and rendering them harmless, these acids must then be removed from the body. Thus, excess hydrogen ions must be bound to water molecules and removed through the exhalation of carbon dioxide from the lungs or be removed from the body via secretion by the kidneys. The maintenance

---

[3]6.8 is the pK_a of this system (the negative log of the ionization constant).

of body pH is a constant balance between gains and losses of hydrogen ion that is achieved through the use of the buffer system, the respiratory system, and the kidneys. These systems secrete or absorb hydrogen ions, control the excretion of acids and bases, or create additional buffers when needed.

Whenever a change in pH occurs, the buffer systems react fastest. However, soon the respiratory system will be activated to help correct the problem through its direct effect on the carbonic acid-bicarbonate buffer system. This occurs primarily through a change in respiratory rate. **Chemoreceptors** in the carotid and aortic bodies sense changes in the PCO_2 in the circulating blood. Similar chemoreceptors are present in the medulla oblongata of the brain. When these receptors are stimulated, the respiratory rate increases, which leads to increased CO_2 loss through the lungs, which then increases the pH. Increasing or decreasing the respiratory rate will affect the PCO_2 that, in turn, affects the pH.

When the PCO_2 rises, the pH will fall, and the carbonic acid-bicarbonate equation will be driven to the right:

$$\uparrow H^+ + HCO_3^- \rightarrow H_2CO_3 \rightarrow \uparrow CO_2 + H_2O$$

Once enough carbon dioxide is lost to the environment, the respiratory rate returns to normal.

Conversely, when the PCO_2 of the blood falls, the chemoreceptors are inhibited, and the respiratory rate falls, thus causing a return of the PCO_2 to normal levels.

The renal system also plays a major role in acid-base balance. However, it tends to work more slowly than the other body systems. The renal effect is referred to as *renal compensation* and is due to the selective secretion or reabsorption of hydrogen ions or bicarbonate ions in response to changes in the plasma pH. In this way the kidneys effectively assist the lungs in maintenance of acid-base balance. When the pH falls, the kidneys respond by increasing the levels of bicarbonate to supply the carbonic acid-bicarbonate buffer system with adequate amounts of buffer. When the pH rises, bicarbonate ions are excreted from the body, thus removing the excess base. When the bicarbonate is lost from carbonic acid, hydrogen ions are liberated, thus further lowering the pH.

The pH can also be affected by movement of electrolytes from the inside of cells to the ECF. That is, sodium (Na^+) and potassium (K^+) ions can be exchanged for hydrogen ions (H^+) in the ECF, thereby moving the acid. Thus, potassium levels and hydrogen ion levels are a major aspect of pH (Table 1–5).

Acid-Base Disorders

Any significant deviation of pH outside the normal operating parameters (7.35–7.45) can be classified as an acid-base disorder (Table 1–6). The two major body systems involved in acid-base balance are the respiratory system and the renal system.

There are two classes of acid-base disorders: respiratory acid-base disorders and metabolic acid-base disorders. Of these, there are two types. **Acidosis** is an excess of acids in the body while **alkalosis** is an excess of base in the body. **Respiratory acid-base disorders** result from an inequality in carbon dioxide generation in the peripheral tissues and carbon dioxide elimination in the respiratory system. The hallmark of respiratory acid-base

TABLE 1–5 | Maintenance of Acid-Base Balance

System	Mechanism	Rate of Action
Buffer Pairs • Carbonic acid-bicarbonate • Proteins/Hemoglobin • Phosphate	Releases or absorbs hydrogen ions	Immediate
Respiratory System	Retain or remove CO_2 (H_2CO_3)	Minutes to hours
Electrolyte Shifts	Exchange Na^+ and/or K^+ for H^+ in ECF	Minutes to hours
Renal System	Secretion or absorption of H^+ and/or HCO_3^-, phosphate, and ammonia buffering.	Hours to days

pH within accepted values. With respiratory acidosis, there is an increase in PCO_2 and a decrease in pH. An elevation in the plasma CO_2 level is referred to as **hypercapnia**. The usual cause is **hypoventilation**. Hypoventilation can occur when the minute volume falls. The **minute volume** is the amount of air moved into and out of the respiratory tract in one minute. It is reflected in the following formula:

$$V_{min} = V_t \times \text{Respiratory Rate}$$

where V_{min} equals minute volume and V_t equals tidal volume (the amount of air moved through the respiratory system with each breath). Thus, a decrease in respiratory rate, tidal volume, or a combination of the two can cause respiratory acidosis.

disorders is a change in the PCO_2. Respiratory acid-base disorders can be classified as:

- Respiratory acidosis
- Respiratory alkalosis

The second class of acid-base disorders is the **metabolic acid-base disorders**. These result from the production of either organic or fixed acids or by conditions that affect the levels of bicarbonate in the ECF. Metabolic acid-base disorders can be classified as:

- Metabolic acidosis
- Metabolic alkalosis

Respiratory Acidosis

Respiratory acidosis occurs when the respiratory system cannot effectively eliminate all the carbon dioxide generated through metabolic activities in the peripheral tissues. Normally, the respiratory system reacts rapidly and corrects changes in carbon dioxide levels before the ECF pH is affected. However, in respiratory acidosis the respiratory system cannot maintain the

Respiratory Alkalosis

Respiratory alkalosis occurs when the respiratory system eliminates too much carbon dioxide through hyperventilation resulting in **hypocapnia**. **Hyperventilation** can result from emotional situations, metabolic disorders, medical conditions, environmental factors, or a combination of these. For example, anxiety, fear, or hysteria stimulates the respiratory centers in the brain resulting in what is referred to as **hyperventilation syndrome**. This results in excessive CO_2 elimination and thus a respiratory alkalosis. Fever and hyperthyroidism can cause respiratory alkalosis. These conditions increase the body's metabolic rate resulting in increased CO_2 elimination. Medical conditions such as congestive heart failure (CHF) and liver failure can cause increased CO_2 elimination. CHF can cause a respiratory alkalosis because of hypoxia-induced hyperventilation. Liver failure results in the accumulation of ammonia in the blood. Increased levels of ammonia can stimulate the respiratory center causing hyperventilation with resultant metabolic alkalosis. Ascension to a high altitude can cause hyperventilation. At higher elevations, oxygen levels are markedly decreased and the victim must increase respirations to ensure adequate oxygen levels until they become acclimated to the altitude or descend to lower levels.

Metabolic Acidosis

Metabolic acidosis is a deficiency of bicarbonate (HCO_3^-) in the body. It usually results from an increase in metabolic acids—primarily through anaerobic metabolism. When oxygen stores are low, energy production switches from aerobic metabolism to anaerobic metabolism. Anaerobic metabolism results in the production of pyruvic acid that is rapidly converted to lactic acid.

The kidney plays a major role in maintaining stable pH levels. The kidney can retain acids and excrete HCO_3^- as needed to maintain pH. Typically, bicarbonate levels in the body are stable. Thus, when there is an increase in metabolic acids, HCO_3^- buffers the excessive acid, keeping the pH neutral.

TABLE 1–6 | pH as a Function of Metabolism and Respiration

$$pH = \frac{\text{Base}}{\text{Acid}} \text{ thus pH} = \frac{\text{Bicarbonate (}HCO_3^-\text{)}}{\text{Carbonic Acid (}H_2CO_3\text{) or Carbon Dioxide (}CO_2\text{)}}$$

$$pH = \frac{\text{Metabolic Function}}{\text{Respiratory Function}}$$

$$pH = \frac{\text{Renal Compensation}}{\text{Respiratory Compensation}}$$

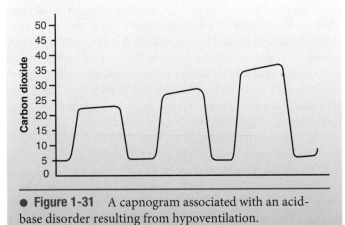

● **Figure 1-31** A capnogram associated with an acid-base disorder resulting from hypoventilation.

This results in a relative decrease in HCO_3^- because body stores remain stable—they are just bound to metabolic acids. Likewise, when the kidney retains acids, the total amount of acids increases while bicarbonate levels remain the same. This mechanism also results in a relative decrease in HCO_3^- levels. True HCO_3^- deficits result when the kidney excretes bicarbonate. Metabolic acidosis is a common problem and can be caused by disease processes such as diabetes, kidney disease, and similar conditions.

Metabolic Alkalosis

Metabolic alkalosis is relatively uncommon and is due to an increase in HCO_3^- levels or a decrease in circulating acids. Metabolic alkalosis results from an abnormal loss of hydrogen

ions (H^+), an increase in HCO_3^- levels, or a decrease in extracellular fluid levels. Vomiting (or nasogastric suctioning) is the most common cause of metabolic alkalosis. Stomach secretions are highly acidic—primarily hydrochloric acid (HCl). Vomiting or suctioning removes the HCl leaving a deficit in both H^+ and chloride ions (Cl^-). When this occurs, the bicarbonate anion shifts from the intracellular fluid (ICF) to the extracellular fluid (ECF) to replace the lost Cl^- ions, causing an increase in ECF HCO_3^- levels and thus a metabolic alkalosis. Several other conditions can cause metabolic alkalosis, all of which involve either the loss of H^+ or variations in circulating HCO_3^- levels.

This discussion of acid-base disorders is simply an overview of these conditions from a biochemical standpoint. They will be discussed in considerable detail in the respiratory and renal chapters of this text.

PART 3: Disease at the Cellular Level

THE CELL

The **cell** is the basic unit of all living organisms. The cell is capable of independent functioning and can typically be divided into two types: eukaryotic cells and prokaryotic cells. Distinction between the two is based on whether or not the cell has internal compartments, a nucleus and organelles, that are enclosed by membranes. The **nucleus** is the central portion of a cell that contains organelles and other components. **Organelles** are structures within the nucleus that carry out necessary biological processes. **Prokaryotic cells** do not contain a nucleus and do not contain organelles. Most prokaryotic cells are surrounded by a rigid cell wall. Many of the single-cell organisms, such as bacteria, are prokaryotes. **Eukaryotic cells** contain a nucleus and organelles. The cells of most multicellular organisms, including humans, are eukaryotes (Figure 1-32 ●).

THE PLASMA MEMBRANE AND CYTOPLASM

Cells are so small they can be visualized only with a microscope. Their small size is necessary, because they need a small surface-area-to-volume ratio that will allow movement of substances into and out of the cell.

Cells are surrounded by a **plasma membrane**. This membrane consists of several chemicals, of which the phospholipids are among the more important.

As discussed earlier, phospholipid molecules have two distinct regions with different physical characteristics. The region with the two fatty acid chains, essentially the tail of the molecule, is nonpolar and rejects water (is hydrophobic). The phosphate region, essentially the head of the molecule, is polar and attracts water (is hydrophilic). Two layers of phospholipids form the **cell membrane** referred to as a **lipid bilayer**. Some of the hydrophilic heads face outward toward the environment outside the cells. Other hydrophilic heads face inward toward the inner contents of the cell. In the middle of the membrane, the hydrophobic tails of outward and inward facing phospholipids face each other and hold the layers of the membrane together.

The hydrophilic heads of the phospholipid molecules on the outer layer of the plasma membrane are in contact with *extracellular fluid*. The hydrophilic heads of the phospholipid molecules on the inner layer of the plasma membrane are in contact with the **cytoplasm** (Figure 1-33 ●). Cytoplasm, also called *cytosol*, fills the inside of cells and consists of water, salts, organic molecules, and many enzymes that catalyze numerous biochemical reactions. The water component of the cytoplasm is referred to as *intracellular fluid*.

Throughout the lipid bilayer are proteins that serve numerous purposes. Some of these proteins span the entire membrane (*integral proteins*) while others may be embedded on the membrane surface (*peripheral membrane proteins*). The membrane proteins and their functions (Figure 1-34 ●) include:

● *Linkers.* Some membrane proteins attach the membrane to the cytoskeleton of the cell, thus allowing the cell to

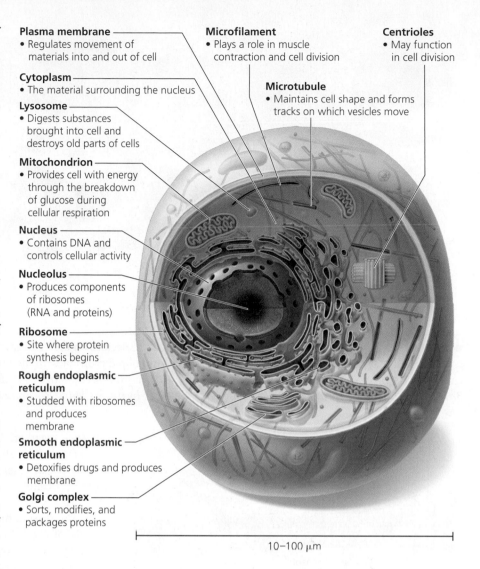

Plasma membrane
• Regulates movement of materials into and out of cell

Cytoplasm
• The material surrounding the nucleus

Lysosome
• Digests substances brought into cell and destroys old parts of cells

Mitochondrion
• Provides cell with energy through the breakdown of glucose during cellular respiration

Nucleus
• Contains DNA and controls cellular activity

Nucleolus
• Produces components of ribosomes (RNA and proteins)

Ribosome
• Site where protein synthesis begins

Rough endoplasmic reticulum
• Studded with ribosomes and produces membrane

Smooth endoplasmic reticulum
• Detoxifies drugs and produces membrane

Golgi complex
• Sorts, modifies, and packages proteins

Microfilament
• Plays a role in muscle contraction and cell division

Microtubule
• Maintains cell shape and forms tracks on which vesicles move

Centrioles
• May function in cell division

10–100 μm

maintain its shape and to secure the membrane in a certain place when needed.

● *Enzymes.* Some proteins function as enzymes and carry out the different steps of the metabolic reactions that take place near the cell membrane.

● *Receptors.* Some membrane proteins act as receptor sites for messenger molecules that signal the cell to start or stop a specific metabolic activity.

● *Transporters.* These proteins make the membrane **semipermeable**, also called *selectively permeable,* thus controlling the movement of substances into and out of the cell.

These varied membrane proteins give the cell membrane a mosaic quality. Yet even with the presence of proteins in the plasma membrane, the membrane still maintains a fluid quality. So the structure of the membrane is referred to as a *fluid mosaic*.

Plasma Membrane Functions

The plasma membrane has several functions in addition to the obvious function of separating the extracellular from the intracellular environment (Table 1–7). First, the plasma membrane plays a major role in the ability of cells to adhere to each other,

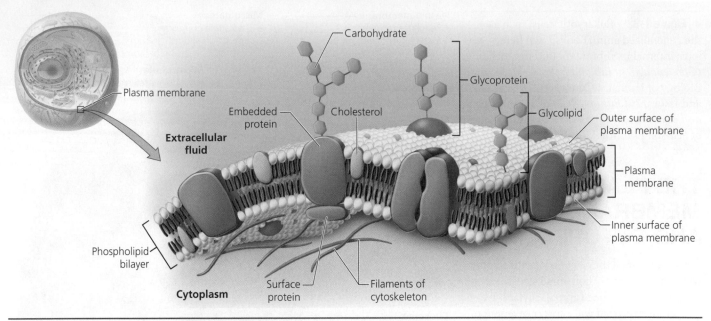

Carbohydrate

Glycoprotein

Plasma membrane

Embedded protein

Cholesterol

Glycolipid

Outer surface of plasma membrane

Extracellular fluid

Plasma membrane

Inner surface of plasma membrane

Phospholipid bilayer

Cytoplasm

Surface protein

Filaments of cytoskeleton

● **Figure 1-33**   The hydrophilic heads of the phospholipid molecules on the outer layer of the plasma membrane are in contact with extracellular fluid. The hydrophilic heads of the phospholipid molecules on the inner layer of the plasma membrane are in contact with the cytoplasm. *(Goodenough, Judith and Betty A. McGuire, Biology of Humans: Concepts, Applications, and Issues, 3rd Edition, © 2010. Reprinted and electronically reproduced by permission of Pearson Education, Inc. Upper Saddle River, NJ)*

Membrane Proteins

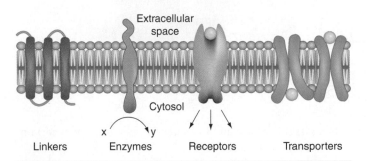

Extracellular space

Cytosol

x   y

Linkers   Enzymes   Receptors   Transporters

● **Figure 1-34**   Membrane proteins include linkers, enzymes, receptors, and transporters.

or stick together. This is primarily achieved through proteins (linkers) called *cell adhesion molecules (CAMs)* that extend out of the plasma membrane. CAMs hold cells together and play a role in cellular movement, tissue development, and healing (Figure 1-35 ●).

The plasma membrane helps with *cell-cell recognition*, the ability of a cell to distinguish one type of cell from another. Peripheral membrane proteins, often glycoproteins, differ from cell to cell and from species to species. Cell-cell recognition allows the body to recognize foreign cells, including cells that may cause infection or even cancer.

The plasma membrane maintains the structural integrity of the cell. It provides anchor sites for the interior cytoskeleton, which is both a muscle and a skeleton and is responsible for cell

TABLE 1–7 | Mechanism of Transport across the Plasma Membrane

Mechanism	Description
Simple diffusion	Random movement from region of high to region of low concentration
Facilitated diffusion	Movement from region of high to region of low concentration with the aid of a carrier or channel protein
Osmosis	Movement of water from a region of high water concentration (low solute concentration) to a region of low water concentration (high solute concentration)
Active transport	Movement from region of high to region of low concentration with the aid of a carrier or channel protein and energy, usually from ATP
Endocytosis	Materials are engulfed by the plasma membrane and drawn into the cell in a vesicle
Exocytosis	Membrane-bound vesicle from inside the cell fuses with the plasma membrane and spills contents outside the cell

movement and the organization of the organelles within the cell. (The cytoskeleton will be described in more detail later.)

The plasma membrane also plays a major role in communications between cells. Certain substances, such as hormones, will bind to the receptor proteins in the plasma membrane. The plasma membrane protein then relays the message of the bound substance to the interior of the cell, where it is transmitted to nearby molecules. Through a series of biochemical reactions, the message ultimately initiates the desired response by the cell.

Finally, the cell membrane regulates the movement of substances into and out of the cell. A large number of substances are routinely moved across the plasma membrane, but these are highly regulated by the cell. Because of this the plasma membrane is said to be *semipermeable*.

Simple Diffusion

Substances will move across a membrane from an area of higher concentration on one side to an area of lower concentration on the other side until the concentration of the substance is equal in both areas (a state of equilibrium) (Figure 1-36 ●). Even after the concentrations reach equilibrium, because of random movement, the substance continues to move back and forth across the membrane. However, the net rate of movement in each direction now remains the same. This process of passive movement across a membrane is called **simple diffusion**.

The plasma membrane essentially creates an intracellular environment separate from the extracellular environment. Thus, the concentration of substances inside the plasma membrane is often different from those outside the membrane. Smaller molecules, such as water, carbon dioxide, oxygen, ethanol, and urea, readily move across the plasma membrane. They pass either directly through the lipid bilayer or through pores created by certain integral proteins. The rate of transport for a particular molecule is proportional to the lipid solubility or hydrophobicity of the molecule in question. (Hydrophobicity is the tendency of a molecule to be repelled by water. An example is molecules of fat or oil that do not mix with water.)

● **Figure 1-35** Cell adhesion molecules (CAMs) extend out of the plasma membrane to bind cells to each other.

Oxygen, carbon dioxide, and ethanol are highly lipid soluble and therefore diffuse across the bilayer membrane almost as if it were not there. On the other hand, molecules that are large or contain a charge (are ionized) do not pass readily through the membrane and, in many cases, are repelled. The rate of diffusion is generally proportional to the **concentration gradient** across the membrane. (The concentration gradient is the difference in the number of molecules or ions of the substance on one side of the membrane from the number of molecules on the other.) The greater the concentration gradient the more rapid is the rate of diffusion. **Osmotic gradient** is a similar term but applies specifically to the movement of water across a semipermeable membrane. Another example of concentration gradient is the movement of oxygen. For example, oxygen concentrations are always higher outside a cell when compared to inside a cell. Therefore, oxygen diffuses down its concentration gradient (from higher to lower concentration) into the cell. Carbon dioxide, on the other hand, typically is at a higher concentration inside the cell and tends to diffuse out of the cell.

CONTENT REVIEW

► Types of Movement through a Cell Membrane

• Simple diffusion
• Osmosis
• Facilitated diffusion
• Active transport
• Endocytosis
• Exocytosis

Cell Adhesion Molecules

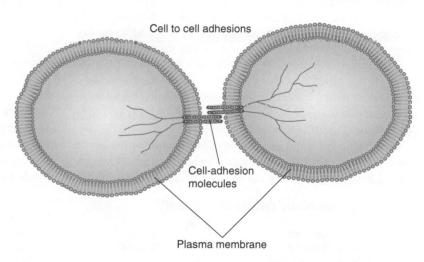

Cell to cell adhesions

Cell-adhesion molecules

Plasma membrane

Simple Diffusion

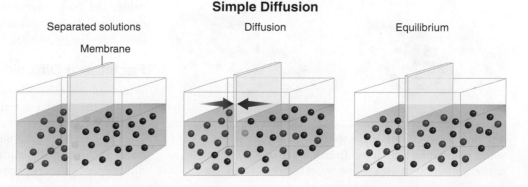

Separated solutions

Membrane

Diffusion

Equilibrium

● **Figure 1-36** Simple diffusion is the random movement of molecules from a region of higher concentration to a region of lower concentration. Solutes diffuse across the membrane until equilibrium is reached on both sides.

Osmosis

Osmosis is a specific type of diffusion. It is the movement of water molecules from an area of high water concentration to an area of low water concentration (Figure 1-37 ●). Semipermeable membranes, such as the cell membrane, allow the unrestricted movement of water across the membrane, at the same time restricting the movement of **solute** molecules and ions. It has been estimated that an amount of water roughly equivalent to 250 times the volume of the cell diffuses across the red blood cell membrane every second. Despite this large movement of water molecules, the cell does not lose or gain water, because equal amounts go in and out.

The concentration of water on different sides of a semipermeable membrane is a result more of the solutes present than of the amount of water present. That is, different concentrations of solute molecules on different sides of the membrane result in different concentrations of molecules of **free water** (water that is free of solute) on either side of the membrane. On the side of the membrane with higher free water concentration (which contains a lower solute concentration), more water molecules will strike the pores in the membrane in a given interval of time. The more membrane strikes there are the more molecules pass through the pores. This then results in a net diffusion of water from the compartment with high concentration of free water to that with a low concentration of free water. But, looking at it a different way, water molecules will diffuse from an area of lower *solute* concentration to an area of greater *solute* concentration.

Water is the universal *solvent* and necessary for many biochemical processes.

When the concentrations of solutions on both sides of a semipermeable membrane are equal, they are said to be **isotonic**. When a solution on one side of the membrane is more concentrated (has a greater quantity of solute) than the solution on the other side, the solution is said to be **hypertonic**. Conversely, when a solution on one side of a membrane is less concentrated than the solution on the other side, it is said to be **hypotonic** (Figure 1-38 ●).

Osmosis generates a pressure called **osmotic pressure**. If the pressure in the compartment into which water is flowing is raised to the equivalent of the osmotic pressure, movement of

Osmosis (Water Movement)

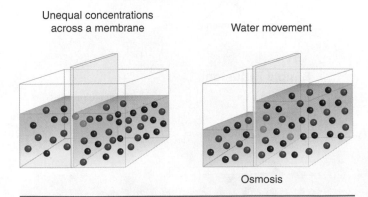

● **Figure 1-37**   Osmosis is a specific type of diffusion in which water molecules move from an area of high water concentration to an area of low water concentration.

Tonicity

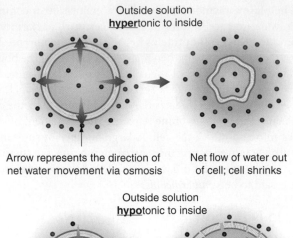

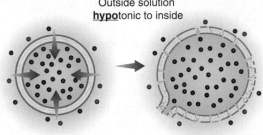

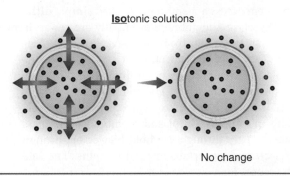

● **Figure 1-38**   Osmosis can shrink or burst a membrane-bound vesicle as water moves out of the vesicle to dilute a hypertonic outside solution or into the vesicle to concentrate an outside solution, always seeking to achieve isotonicity inside and outside the vesicle.

water will stop. (Osmotic pressure and its opposite, hydrostatic pressure, will be described in more detail later.) The concentration of solute particles in a solution is called the **osmolarity**. A similar measurement, the **osmolality**, is used to measure the concentration of particles in body fluids such as plasma and urine. The body's osmolality increases with dehydration and decreases with overhydration. Normal human osmolality ranges from 280–300 mOsm/kg.

Facilitated Diffusion

Water-soluble molecules and ionized molecules cannot move through the plasma membrane by simple diffusion. Because of this, their transport must be assisted, or "facilitated," by integral proteins in the plasma membrane through a process called **facilitated diffusion**. Facilitated diffusion, like simple diffusion, does not require an expenditure of metabolic energy.

The force driving facilitated diffusion, as with simple diffusion, is the concentration gradient. There are many important substances that are moved across the plasma membrane by facilitated diffusion, including glucose, sodium ions, and chloride ions. Glucose is water-soluble and sodium and potassium are ionized and are thus classified *as lipid-bilayer-excluded substances* (Figure 1-39 ●). That is, they cannot pass through the lipid bilayer by simple diffusion but rather, as just described, their passage across the plasma membrane must be assisted, or facilitated.

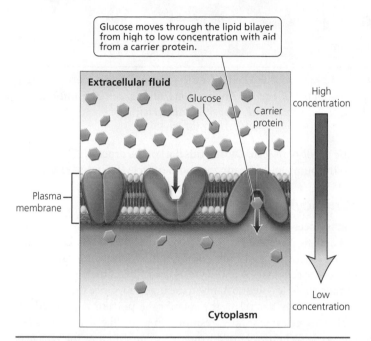

> Glucose moves through the lipid bilayer from high to low concentration with aid from a carrier protein.

Extracellular fluid

Glucose

Carrier protein

High concentration

Plasma membrane

Low concentration

Cytoplasm

● **Figure 1-39** Glucose is unable to diffuse across a plasma membrane by itself but can be moved across by a carrier protein embedded in the membrane, a process known as facilitated diffusion. (*Goodenough, Judith and Betty A. McGuire,* Biology of Humans: Concepts, Applications, and Issues, *3rd Edition,* © 2010. *Reprinted and electronically reproduced by permission of Pearson Education, Inc. Upper Saddle River, NJ*)

There are two major groups of integral membrane proteins involved in the process of facilitated diffusion:

● *Carrier proteins.* **Carrier proteins**, also called transporters, bind a specific type of solute and are induced to undergo a series of conformational changes that effectively carries the solute to the other side of the membrane. The carrier protein then releases the solute and, through another conformational change, is restored in the membrane to its original state. Typically, a given carrier will transport only a small group of related molecules.

● *Ion channels.* **Ion channels** are essentially hydrophilic pores through the membrane that open and allow certain types of solutes, usually inorganic ions, to pass through. (Note that the term **hydrophilic**, meaning attracted to water, is the opposite of the term **hydrophobic**, meaning repellent to water.) Typically, these ion channels are quite specific for a particular type of solute. Transport through ion channels is considerably faster than transport by carrier proteins. In addition, many ion channels are gated, which in effect controls the channel's permeability. When the gate is open, the ion channel transports the desired substance. When the gate is closed, no transport occurs. Ion channel gates can be controlled either by voltage across the membrane (voltage-gated channels) or by having a binding site for a *ligand* (a molecule that will bind to a site) which, when bound, causes the channels to open (ligand-gated channels). Ion channels are particularly important in excitable cells, like neurons and muscle cells, because they allow current flow to occur across the membrane (Figure 1-40 ●).

Active Transport

Sometimes it is necessary for a cell to move a solute across the plasma membrane against the concentration gradient. As with facilitated diffusion, this process, called **active transport**, uses a carrier protein but also uses energy in the form of ATP (Figure 1-41 ●). Thus, with active transport substances are moved from areas of lower solute concentration to higher solute concentration. This is especially important in regard to sodium and potassium ions. The concentration of sodium ions outside the cell membrane is much higher than inside the membrane.

Ion Channels

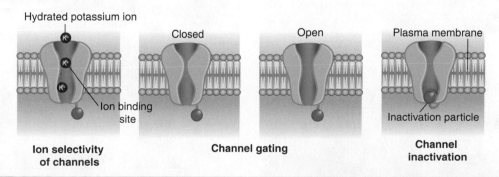

Hydrated potassium ion

Closed

Open

Plasma membrane

Ion binding site

Inactivation particle

Ion selectivity of channels

Channel gating

Channel inactivation

● **Figure 1-40** The function of a voltage-gated ion channel. (a) Several ways a channel can select for different ions are shown: (1) Negative charges at the opening of the channel repel anions and attract cations. (2) The pore diameter restricts the size of ions that can pass. (3) Ion-selective binding strips off water molecules so that ions can pass through. (b) Channel gating occurs when a portion of the channel changes conformation when the membrane potential changes, effectively swinging the gate open or shut. (c) Inactivation of the sodium channel occurs when an inactivating particle blocks the pore.

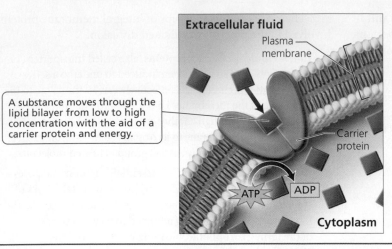 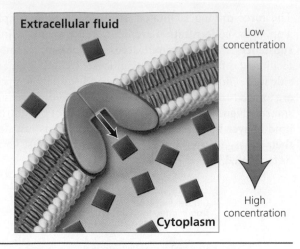

● Figure 1-41 Active transport moves a solute across the plasma membrane with the help of a carrier protein and energy in the form of ATP. *(Goodenough, Judith and Betty A. McGuire,* Biology of Humans: Concepts, Applications, and Issues, *3rd Edition,* © 2010. Reprinted and electronically reproduced by permission of Pearson Education, Inc. Upper Saddle River, NJ)

Conversely, the concentration of potassium ions is much higher inside the cell membrane than outside. The transport of sodium ions out of the cell and potassium ions into the cell, against the concentration gradient, is achieved by the **sodium-potassium pump**. The sodium-potassium pump is an enzyme (Na^+-K^+-ATPase) in the plasma membrane and is powered with ATP. Each of these enzymes binds three sodium ions on the inside of the cell membrane and transports them to the outside of the cell membrane. ATP is used in this step. Following that, two potassium ions are bound on the outside of the cell and transported to the inside of the cell. During this part of the process, ATP rebinds to the pump and is ready for another cycle (Figure 1-42 ●).

Endocytosis

Substances can also enter the cell through a process called **endocytosis**. With endocytosis, large molecules, single-cell organisms (bacteria), and fluid containing dissolved substances can enter the cell. During endocytosis, a section of the plasma membrane encircles the substance to be ingested. Once the substance is completely encircled, the membrane portion is pinched off from the cell membrane, resulting in a sac-like structure called a vesicle. When separated from the cell membrane, the vesicle is released into the cell.

Endocytosis is often divided into two categories: phagocytosis and pinocytosis. **Phagocytosis** is the process whereby the cell engulfs large particles or bacteria (Figure 1-43 ●). **Pinocytosis**

Sodium-Potassium Pump

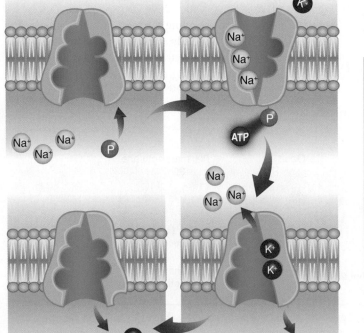

● Figure 1-42 The sodium-potassium pump.

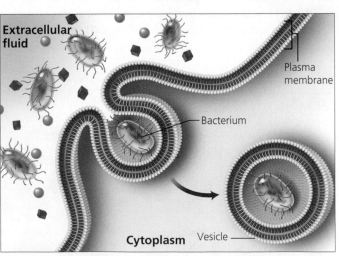

● Figure 1-43 Phagocytosis. The cell engulfs large particles or bacteria. *(Goodenough, Judith and Betty A. McGuire,* Biology of Humans: Concepts, Applications, and Issues, *3rd Edition,* © 2010. Reprinted and electronically reproduced by permission of Pearson Education, Inc. Upper Saddle River, NJ)

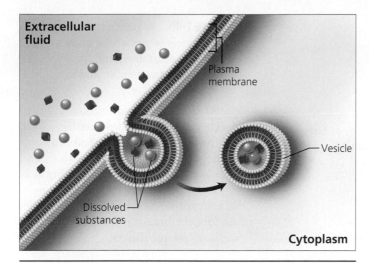

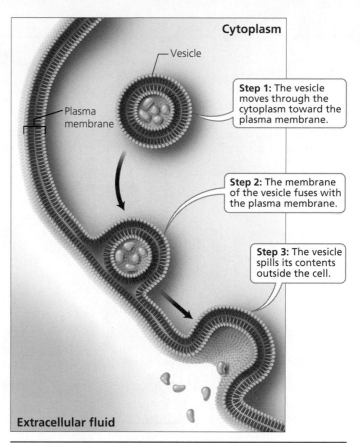

● **Figure 1-44** Pinocytosis. The cell engulfs droplets of extracellular fluid. *(Goodenough, Judith and Betty A. McGuire, Biology of Humans: Concepts, Applications, and Issues, 3rd Edition, © 2010. Reprinted and electronically reproduced by permission of Pearson Education, Inc. Upper Saddle River, NJ)*

is the process by which the cell engulfs droplets of fluid carrying dissolved substances (Figure 1-44 ●). Both mechanisms are necessary for cell survival.

Exocytosis

It is sometimes necessary for large molecules to leave the cells. For example, hormones are often large molecules that cannot readily pass through the cell membrane. As with endocytosis, large molecules can leave the cell by becoming encircled in a membrane vesicle. This process, called **exocytosis**, occurs in a fashion opposite to that of endocytosis. The membrane-bound vesicle containing the substance to be released from the cell approaches the cell membrane. There it fuses with the cell membrane, and its contents are released outside the cell (Figure 1-45 ●).

THE CELLULAR ENVIRONMENT: FLUIDS AND ELECTROLYTES

Many pathological conditions, both medical and traumatic, adversely affect the fluid and electrolyte balance of the body. Certain disease processes, such as diabetic ketoacidosis and heat emergencies, are associated with certain electrolyte abnormalities. Severe derangements in fluid and electrolyte status can result in death. For this reason, as a paramedic, you need to have a good understanding of the fluids and electrolytes present in the human body.

Water

Water is the most abundant substance in the human body. In fact, water accounts for approximately 60 percent of total body weight (the average for all ages). The total amount of water in the body at any given time is referred to as the **total body water (TBW)**.

● **Figure 1-45** Exocytosis. A membrane-bound vesicle is taken into the cell membrane and its contents are released to the exterior. *(Goodenough, Judith and Betty A. McGuire, Biology of Humans: Concepts, Applications, and Issues, 3rd Edition, © 2010. Reprinted and electronically reproduced by permission of Pearson Education, Inc. Upper Saddle River, NJ)*

In an adult weighing 70 kilograms (154 pounds), total body water would be approximately 42 liters (11 gallons) (Figure 1-46 ●).

Water is distributed among various compartments of the body (Table 1–8). These compartments are separated by cell membranes. The largest compartment is the *intracellular compartment*. This compartment contains the **intracellular fluid (ICF)**, which is all the fluid found inside body cells. Approximately 70 percent of all body water is found within this compartment. The *extracellular compartment* contains the remaining 30 percent of all body water. It contains the **extracellular fluid (ECF)**, all the fluid found outside the body cells.

There are two divisions within the extracellular compartment. The first contains the **intravascular fluid**—the fluid found outside cells and within the circulatory system. It is essentially the same as the blood plasma and accounts for about 5 percent of body water. The remaining compartment contains the **interstitial fluid**—all the fluid found outside the cell membranes, yet not within the circulatory system, making up about 25 percent of body water. For example, minute amounts of fluid are found in the synovial fluid that lubricates the joints; the aqueous humor of the eye; secretions including saliva, gastric juices, and bile; and so on.

Total body water and its distribution vary with age and physiologic condition. At birth, an infant's TBW is about 75 to 80 percent of its body weight, compared to the 65 percent TBW

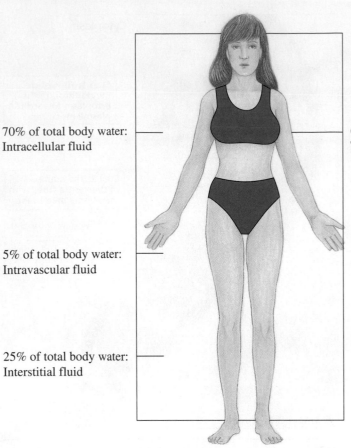

70% of total body water:
Intracellular fluid

5% of total body water:
Intravascular fluid

25% of total body water:
Interstitial fluid

60% of body weight:
Total body water

● **Figure 1-46**   Water comprises approximately 60 percent of body weight. The water is distributed into three spaces: intracellular, intravascular, and interstitial.

As the human body ages, the loss of muscle mass, increased percentage of fat, and the body's decreasing ability to regulate fluid levels lowers the TBW to around 45 to 55 percent. Due to a decreasing ability to regulate electrolytes and fluid levels, the elderly, like the very young, are at high risk for dehydration and disorders related to electrolyte imbalances.

Hydration

Water is the universal **solvent**. That is, most substances dissolve in water. When they do, chemical changes take place. For this reason, the water content of the body is crucial to virtually all of the body's biochemical processes. Normally, the total volume of water in the body, as well as the distribution of fluid in the three body compartments, remains relatively constant. This occurs despite wide fluctuations in the amount of water that enters and is excreted from the body on a daily basis. The water coming into the body is referred to as intake. The water excreted from the body is referred to as output. To maintain relative homeostasis, the intake must equal the output, as shown in the following text.

of the average adult. Infants have a higher TBW for two reasons. First, infants have less fat than adults. (Fat does not absorb water, so the less fat in the body, the more water.) Second, water is essential for the high rates of metabolism that are necessary to promote growth in the infant. The TBW slowly decreases to approximately 70 to 75 percent by age 1. Diarrhea is especially worrisome in the infant, because it can mean the loss of a significant percentage of TBW. In addition, body systems that compensate for fluid loss are still immature, so infants can rapidly become dangerously dehydrated and subject to electrolyte imbalances. By late childhood the TBW decreases to 65 to 70 percent.

By early adulthood, the TBW of males and females begins to differ. In adult males, TBW constitutes approximately 65 to 70 percent of the body weight, while in adult females the average TBW is 60 to 65 percent. The gender difference is the result of hormonal differences that result in the male's greater muscle mass and the female's greater percentage of body fat.

Intake

digestive system:

liquids	1,000 mL
food (solids)	1,200 mL
metabolic sources:	300 mL
TOTAL:	2,500 mL

Output

lungs (water vapor):	400 mL
kidneys (urine):	1,500 mL
skin (perspiration):	400 mL
intestines (feces):	200 mL
TOTAL:	2,500 mL

Several mechanisms work to maintain a relative balance between input and output. For example, when the fluid volume drops, the pituitary gland secretes antidiuretic hormone (ADH), which causes the kidney tubules to reabsorb more water into the blood and to excrete less urine. This process helps to restore the fluid volume to normal values.

Thirst also regulates fluid intake. The sensation of thirst normally occurs when body fluids decrease, stimulating

TABLE 1–8 | Body Fluid Compartments

Compartment	Percentage of Total Body Water	Volume in 70-kg Adult (42 liters total body water)
Intracellular fluid	70.0 percent	29.40 L
Extracellular fluid	30.0 percent	12.60 L
Interstitial fluid	25.0 percent	10.50 L
Intravascular fluid	5.0 percent	2.10 L

the person to take in more fluids orally. Conversely, when too many fluids enter the body, the kidneys are activated and more urine is excreted, thus eliminating excess fluid.

The body also maintains fluid balance by shifting water from one body space to another.

Dehydration **Dehydration**, an abnormal decrease in the total body water, can result from several factors:

- *Gastrointestinal losses* result from prolonged vomiting, diarrhea, or malabsorption disorders.

- *Increased insensible loss* is loss of water through normal mechanisms that is difficult to detect or measure (e.g., perspiration, water vapor from the lungs, saliva). These can be increased in fever states, during hyperventilation, or with high environmental temperatures.

- *Increased sweating* (also called perspiration or diaphoresis) can result in significant fluid loss. While sweating is a form of insensible water loss, it is a significant concern with many medical conditions or high environmental temperatures.

- *Internal losses* are commonly called "third-space" losses because fluid is lost from intravascular or intracellular spaces into the interstitial space. With dehydration, fluid is typically lost from the intravascular compartment into the interstitial compartment, which effectively takes it out of the circulating volume. This can occur with peritonitis, pancreatitis, or bowel obstruction. It can also occur in poor nutritional states in which there is not enough protein in the vascular system to retain water.

- *Plasma losses* occur from burns, surgical drains and fistulas, and open wounds.

Dehydration rarely involves only the loss of water. More commonly, there is also a loss of electrolytes. At the hospital, fluid replacement will be based on both fluid and electrolyte deficits once the patient's electrolyte abnormalities are determined through laboratory testing.

Clinically, the dehydrated patient will exhibit dry mucous membranes and poor skin **turgor**. There often is excessive thirst. As it becomes more severe, dehydration will be accompanied by an increased pulse rate, decreased blood pressure, and orthostatic hypotension (increased pulse and decreased blood pressure on rising from a supine position). In infants, the anterior fontanelle may be sunken and the diaper may be dry or reveal the presence of highly concentrated (dark yellow, strong-smelling) urine. The absence of tears in a crying infant, a capillary refill time greater than 2 seconds, dry mucosa, and a decrease in urinary output are signs that indicate severe dehydration. The treatment for dehydration is replacement of fluid.

Overhydration **Overhydration** can occur as well. The major sign of overhydration is edema. Patients with heart disease may manifest overhydration much earlier than patients without heart disease. In severe cases of overhydration, overt heart failure may be present. Treatment is directed at removing the excessive fluid.

CONTENT REVIEW

▶ Distribution of Fluid among Body Compartments

- Intracellular fluid (ICF)
- Extracellular fluid (ECF)
  - Intravascular fluid
  - Interstitial fluid

Electrolytes

How to Read Chemical Notation

To describe chemical substances and reactions, scientists use chemical notation, a kind of "shorthand." Every chemical element has a one- or two-letter abbreviation. Just four elements—hydrogen, oxygen, carbon, and nitrogen—make up over 99 percent of the body's atoms. These are called the "major elements." Nine "trace elements" account for the remaining less-than-1 percent.

Major Element	Symbol	Percent	Trace Element	Symbol
Hydrogen	H	62.0%	Calcium	Ca
Oxygen	O	26.0%	Chlorine	Cl
Carbon	C	10.0%	Iodine	I
Nitrogen	N	1.5%	Iron	Fe
			Magnesium	Mg
			Phosphorus	Ph
			Potassium	K
			Sodium	Na
			Sulfur	S

An atom is the smallest particle of an element. A molecule is a combination of atoms. The notation for a molecule combines the notations of the included elements. A subscript number after an element indicates the number of atoms of that element. If there is just one atom, there is no number. For example:

NaCl (Sodium chloride, or table salt. A sodium chloride molecule has 1 sodium atom and 1 chlorine atom.)

H_2O (Water. A water molecule has 2 hydrogen atoms and 1 oxygen atom.)

H_2CO_3 (Carbonic acid. A carbonic acid molecule has 2 hydrogen, 1 carbon, and 3 oxygen atoms.)

Ions

Each atom is made up of even smaller particles: electrons (that have a negative electrical charge), protons (that have a positive electrical charge), and neutrons (that are uncharged). Protons and neutrons are in the inner core, or nucleus, of the atom while electrons occupy outer orbits around the nucleus. Sometimes an atom of an element can lose one or more of its outer electrons or can capture one or more extra electrons from another element.

An ion is an atom that has lost one or more negatively charged electrons and now has a positive charge, or an atom that has gained one or more electrons and now has a negative charge. A superscript plus ($^+$) indicates a positively charged cation. A superscript minus ($^-$) indicates a negatively charged anion. For example:

Na^+ (A sodium ion has lost an electron and has a positive charge.)

Ca^{++} (A calcium ion has lost two electrons and has a double positive charge.)

Cl^- (A chloride ion has gained an electron and has a negative charge.)

Electrolytes are substances that form ions when they break down, or dissociate, in water. Remember that the body and its blood are mostly water. The ions formed by dissociation of electrolytes in the body's fluids are a major factor in body metabolism.

Chemical Reactions

Notations for chemical reactions use a plus sign ($+$) to indicate substances that are combined and an arrow ($\rightarrow$) to show the direction of the reaction. The reactants are usually on the left, with the product of the reaction on the right.

$$2H + O \rightarrow H_2O$$

(2 hydrogen atoms + 1 oxygen atom = 1 water molecule)

In some circumstances, a reaction may be reversible. That is, separate elements may synthesize (combine), or the synthesized substance may dissociate (break down) into separate components. A two-directional arrow ($\leftrightarrow$) shows that a reaction is reversible and can be read in either direction.

$$CO_2 + H_2O \leftrightarrow H_2CO_3$$

Read as: (carbon dioxide + water = carbonic acid) or (carbonic acid = water + carbon dioxide).

Notice that no atoms are gained or lost in a chemical reaction. In the previous example, the two oxygen atoms in CO_2 and the single oxygen atom in H_2O combine to equal the three oxygen atoms in H_2CO_3. The hydrogen and carbon atoms are also equal on both sides of the reaction.

Up and down arrows ($\uparrow\downarrow$) are used to indicate an increase or decrease in the substance that follows the arrows. For example:

$\uparrow H^+$ (an increase in hydrogen ions)

$\downarrow CO_2$ (a decrease in carbon dioxide)

Types of Electrolytes: Cations and Anions

The chemical substances present throughout the body can be classified as either electrolytes or nonelectrolytes. **Electrolytes** are substances that **dissociate** into electrically charged particles when placed into water. The charged particles are referred to as ions. Ions with a positive charge are called cations; ions with a negative charge are called anions.

An example of this would be the dissociation of the drug sodium bicarbonate when it is placed into water. Sodium bicarbonate is a neutral salt. When placed into water, it dissociates into two charged particles, as shown here.

$$NaHCO_3 \rightarrow Na^+ + HCO_3^-$$

sodium bicarbonate $\rightarrow$ sodium cation
        + bicarbonate anion neutral salt $\rightarrow$ cation + anion

Sodium bicarbonate is an example of an electrolyte that is taken into the body as a medication. However, there are many naturally occurring electrolytes present in the body.

The most frequently occurring cations include:

- *Sodium (Na^+).* Sodium is the most prevalent cation in the extracellular fluid. It plays a major role in regulating the distribution of water because water is attracted to and moves with sodium. In fact, it is often said that "water follows sodium." Sodium is also important in the transmission of nervous impulses. An abnormal increase in the relative amount of sodium in the body is called *hypernatremia*, while an abnormal decrease is referred to as *hyponatremia*.

- *Potassium (K^+).* Potassium is the most prevalent cation in the intracellular fluid. It is also important in the transmission of electrical impulses. An abnormally high potassium level is called *hyperkalemia,* while an abnormally low potassium level is referred to as *hypokalemia.*

- *Calcium (Ca^{++}).* Calcium has many physiologic functions. It plays a major role in muscle contraction as well as nervous impulse transmission. An abnormally increased calcium level is called *hypercalcemia,* while an abnormally decreased calcium level is called *hypocalcemia.*

- *Magnesium (Mg^{++}).* Magnesium is necessary for several biochemical processes that occur in the body and is closely associated with phosphate in many processes. An abnormally increased magnesium level is called *hypermagnesemia;* an abnormally decreased magnesium level is called *hypomagnesemia.*

The most frequently occurring anions include:

- *Chloride (Cl^-).* Chloride is an important anion. Its negative charge balances the positive charge associated with the cations. It also plays a major role in fluid balance and renal function. Chloride has a close association with sodium.

- *Bicarbonate.* Bicarbonate is the principal buffer of the body. This means that it neutralizes the highly acidic hydrogen ion (H^+) and other organic acids. (Buffering will be discussed in more detail later in this chapter.)

- *Phosphate.* Phosphate is important in body energy stores. It is closely associated with magnesium in renal function. It also acts as a buffer, primarily in the intracellular space, in much the same manner as bicarbonate.

Many other compounds carry negative charges. Among these are some of the proteins, certain organic acids, and other compounds. Electrolytes are usually measured in **milliequivalents** per liter (mEq/L). A milliequivalent is one thousandth (10^{-3}) of the relative weight of an element that has the same combining capacity as a given weight of another element (e.g., element, molecule, ion).

Nonelectrolytes are molecules that do not dissociate into electrically charged particles. These include glucose, urea, proteins, and similar substances.

Transport of Water and Electrolytes

In this section, we will review the concepts of diffusion, osmosis, active transport, and facilitated diffusion across a membrane—discussed earlier under "Plasma Membrane Functions"—as they concern the movement of water and electrolytes.

As noted earlier, the body's fluid compartments are separated by cell membranes. These membranes are called semipermeable or selectively permeable, meaning that they allow the easy passage of certain materials while restricting the passage of others. Compounds with small molecules, such as water (H_2O), pass readily through the membrane; larger compounds, such as proteins, are restricted. The movement of fluids through a membrane is enabled by the presence of pores (openings) in the membrane. Electrolytes do not pass through the membrane as readily as water. This is due not so much to the size of electrolyte molecules as to their electrical charge.

When solutions on opposite sides of a semipermeable membrane are equal in concentration, the relationship is said to be *isotonic.* When the concentration of a given solute (dissolved substance) is greater on one side of the membrane than on the other, it is said to be *hypertonic.* When the concentration is less on one side of the cell membrane, as compared to the other, it is referred to as *hypotonic.* This difference in concentration is known as the *osmotic gradient.*

The natural tendency of the body is to keep the balance of electrolytes and water equal on both sides of the cell membrane. This is an example of *homeostasis,* the body's normal tendency to maintain its internal environment in a steady state of balance. If one side of a cell membrane has an increased quantity of a given electrolyte (is hypertonic), there will be a shift of the electrolyte from that side and a shift of water from the other side to restore a balance in concentration—the balanced state.

The tendency of molecules to move from an area of higher concentration to an area of lower concentration is referred to as *diffusion* (or *simple diffusion),* a passive process that does not require energy (Figure 1-47 ●). The diffusion of a solute (usually an electrolyte) across a cell membrane from the area of higher

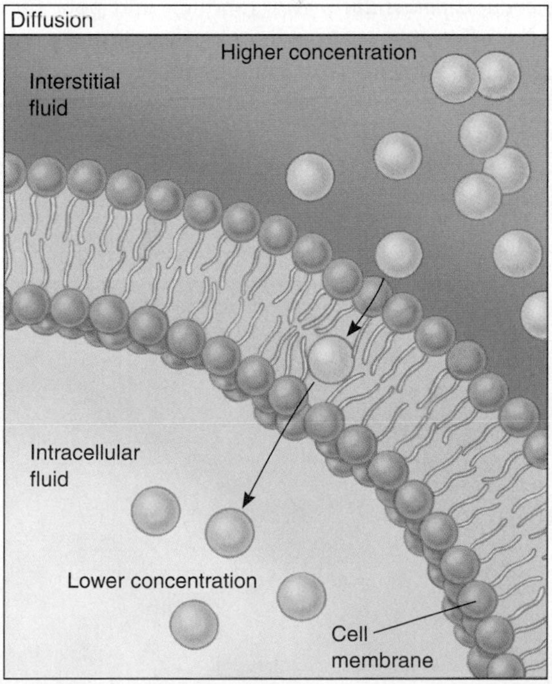

CONTENT REVIEW

▶ Factors That May Cause Dehydration

- Gastrointestinal losses (vomiting, diarrhea, malabsorption)
- Increased insensible loss (perspiration, water vapor, saliva)
- Increased sweating (diaphoresis)
- Internal losses ("third-space" losses to the interstitial space)
- Plasma losses (from burns, drains, fistulas, open wounds)

● **Figure 1-47**   Diffusion is the movement of a substance from an area of great concentration to an area of lesser concentration.

concentration to the area of lower concentration continues until balance is attained. This movement from an area of higher concentration to an area of lower concentration is termed a movement *with the osmotic gradient*.

Water also moves across the cell membrane so as to dilute the area of increased electrolyte concentration. The movement of water is more rapid than the movement of electrolytes. This form of diffusion (the passage of any solvent, usually water, through a membrane) is referred to as *osmosis* (Figure 1-48 ●). It occurs in the direction opposite to the direction of solute movement. For example, if a semipermeable membrane separates solutions of water and sodium, and if the concentration of sodium is two times higher on one side of the membrane than on the other, then two things will occur. Sodium will diffuse from the area of higher concentration (the hypertonic side) to the area of lesser concentration (the hypotonic side). Concurrently, water will diffuse in the opposite direction. That is, water will leave the hypotonic side and diffuse across the membrane to the hypertonic side. These actions will continue until the concentration of water and sodium on both sides has equalized.

In addition to diffusion, two other mechanisms—active transport and facilitated diffusion—can transport substances across cell membranes. *Active transport* is the movement of a substance across the cell membrane *against the osmotic gradient* (that is, toward the side that already has more of the substance). For example, the body requires cells of the myocardium to be negatively charged on the inside of the cells as compared to the outside. However, sodium, with its positive charge, tends to diffuse passively into the cell. This would destroy the negative charge inside the cell. In order to maintain the desired negative charge, sodium ions are actively pumped out of the cell, while potassium ions are pumped into the cell, by a mechanism known as the *sodium-potassium pump*. (Sodium and potassium ions are both positive, but more sodium ions are pumped out of the cell than potassium ions are pumped in, creating the desired negative charge inside the cell.) Active transport is faster than diffusion, but it requires the expenditure of energy, which diffusion does not. Proteins are moved across the cell membrane in a similar fashion.

Certain molecules can move across the cell membrane by another process known as *facilitated diffusion*. Glucose is an example of such a molecule. Facilitated diffusion requires the assistance of "helper proteins," parts of a membrane transport system that exist on the surface of the cell membrane. These proteins, once activated, bind to the glucose molecule. Following binding, the protein changes its configuration and transports the glucose molecule to the inside of the cell, where it is released. Depending on the substance that is being transported, facilitated diffusion may or may not require energy.

Water Movement between Intracellular and Extracellular Compartments

The mechanisms by which water and solutes move across cell membranes ensure that the *osmolality* of body water (the concentration of particles within the water) inside and outside the cells is normally in equilibrium. Sodium, the most abundant ion in the extracellular fluid, is responsible for the osmotic balance of the extracellular space. Potassium plays the same role in the intracellular space.

Generally, the osmolality of intracellular fluid does not change very rapidly. However, when there is a change in the osmolality of extracellular fluid, water will move from the intracellular to the extracellular compartment, or vice versa, until osmotic equilibrium is regained.

Water Movement between Intravascular and Interstitial Compartments

Within the extracellular compartment, movement of water between the plasma in the intravascular space and the interstitial space is primarily a function of forces at play in the capillary beds.

In general, the movement of water and solutes across a cell membrane is governed by *osmotic pressure*. Osmotic pressure is the pressure exerted by the concentration of solutes on one side of a semipermeable membrane, such as a cell membrane or the thin wall of a capillary. Osmotic pressure can be thought of as a "pull" rather than a "push," because a hypertonic concentration of solutes tends to pull water from the other side of the membrane until the osmotic pressure on both sides is equal.

Generally, as already described, this is a two-way street as solutes move out of a space while water moves into the space to balance the concentration of solutes and the osmotic pressure on both sides of the membrane. However, there is a somewhat different osmotic mechanism that operates between the plasma inside a capillary and the interstitial space outside the capillary. Blood plasma generates **oncotic force**, which is sometimes called *colloid osmotic pressure*. Plasma

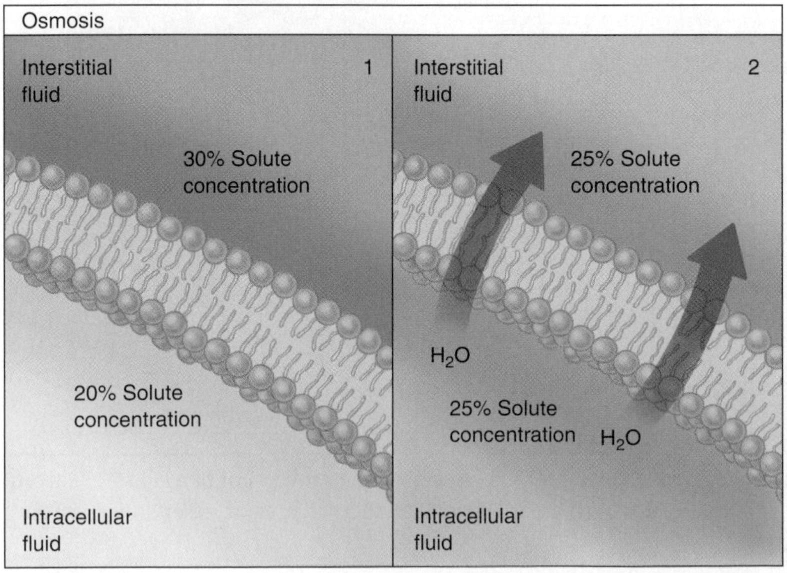

Osmosis

Interstitial fluid — 1

30% Solute concentration

20% Solute concentration

Intracellular fluid

Interstitial fluid — 2

25% Solute concentration

H_2O

25% Solute concentration H_2O

Intracellular fluid

● **Figure 1-48**   Osmosis is the movement of water from an area of higher water concentration to an area of lesser water concentration. Because water is a solvent, it moves from an area of lower solute concentration to an area of higher solute concentration.

proteins are colloids, large particles that do not readily move across the capillary membrane. They tend to remain within the capillary. At the same time, there is very little water in the interstitial space. The small amount of water that does get into the interstitial space is usually taken up by the lymphatic system. Therefore, since there is little water outside the capillary, and because plasma proteins do not readily move outside the capillary, the forces governing movement of water between the capillary and the interstitial space are almost all on one side, governed by the plasma on the inside of the capillary.

Another force inside the capillaries is **hydrostatic pressure**, which is the blood pressure, or force against the vessel walls, created by contractions of the heart. Hydrostatic pressure does tend to force some water out of the plasma and across the capillary wall into the interstitial space, a process that is called **filtration**. Hydrostatic pressure (a force that favors filtration, pushing water out of the capillary) and oncotic force (a force opposing filtration, pulling water into the capillary) together are responsible for **net filtration**, which is described in *Starling's hypothesis:*

Net filtration = (Forces favoring filtration) − (Forces opposing filtration)

Net filtration in a capillary is normally zero. It works this way: As plasma enters the capillary at the arterial end, hydrostatic pressure forces water to cross the capillary membrane into the interstitial space. This loss of water increases the relative concentration of plasma proteins. By the time the plasma reaches the venous end of the capillary, the oncotic force exerted by the increased concentration of plasma proteins is great enough to pull the water from the interstitial space back into the capillary. The outcome is that water is retained in the intravascular space and does not remain in the interstitial space.

Edema

Edema is the accumulation of water in the interstitial space. It occurs when there is a disruption in the forces and mechanisms that normally keep net filtration at zero (retaining water in the vascular system as plasma flows through the capillaries, according to Starling's hypothesis, previously described) or a disruption in the forces that would normally remove water from the interstitial space.

The mechanisms that most commonly result in accumulation of water in the interstitial space are a decrease in plasma oncotic force, an increase in hydrostatic pressure, increased permeability of the capillary membrane, and lymphatic obstruction.

- *A decrease in plasma oncotic force* may result from a loss or decrease in production of plasma proteins (albumins, globulins, and clotting factors). Plasma proteins are synthesized in the liver, so a liver disorder may be responsible for decreased production. Plasma loss from open wounds, hemorrhage, and burns may also cause a loss of plasma proteins. The result is that oncotic force is reduced to the point that some of the water lost through hydrostatic pressure is not regained.

- *An increase in hydrostatic pressure* can result from venous obstruction, salt and water retention, thrombophlebitis,

liver obstruction, tight clothing at the extremities, or prolonged standing. The increase in hydrostatic pressure forces more water into the interstitial space than the oncotic force can recover.

- *Increased capillary permeability* generally results from the mechanisms of inflammation and immune response. These can result from allergic reactions, burns, trauma, or cancer. The greater permeability allows plasma proteins to escape from the capillaries, permitting water to remain in the interstitial space through the osmotic pressure of increased interstitial proteins and the reduction of oncotic force within the capillaries.

- *Lymphatic channel obstruction* can result from infection. Lymphatic channels are also sometimes removed through surgery. The loss of lymphatic channels interferes with the normal absorption of interstitial fluid by the lymphatic system. For example, removal of axillary lymph nodes in the treatment of breast cancer can result in edema of the arm.

Edema can be localized or generalized. Local swelling may appear at the site of an injury (e.g., a sprained ankle) or within a certain organ system such as the brain (cerebral edema), lungs (pulmonary edema), heart (pericardial effusion), or abdomen (ascites). A generalized edema may present as dependent edema, in which gravity pulls water to the lowest areas (e.g., in the feet and ankles when standing or in the sacral area when supine). You can identify dependent edema by pressing a finger over a bony prominence. A pit may remain after you remove your finger (*pitting edema*).

Edema is not only a sign of an underlying disease or problem; edema itself causes problems. It interferes with the movement of nutrients and wastes between tissues and capillaries. It may diminish capillary blood flow, depriving tissues of oxygen. In turn, this may slow the healing of wounds, promote infection, and facilitate formation of pressure sores. Edema affecting organs such as the brain, lung, heart, or larynx may be life threatening.

Body water that is retained in the interstitial spaces is body water that is not available for metabolic processes in the cells. Therefore, even though the total body water is normal, edema can cause a relative condition of dehydration.

The body has regulatory mechanisms that help to maintain homeostasis by controlling total body water and water distribution. Antidiuretic hormone (ADH), also known as *vasopressin*, is the chief regulator of water retention and distribution. Throughout the body, a network of sensors detects fluctuations in fluid and changes in the osmolar concentration of plasma. Osmoreceptors are located in the anterior hypothalamus. If there is an increase of 1 to 2 percent in osmolality—that is, if there is relatively less fluid in the plasma—the osmoreceptors will stimulate the release of ADH in an attempt to retain more fluid. Another type of receptor, baroreceptors, will detect both high and low pressure levels. Baroreceptors located in the carotid sinus, aortic arch, and kidney detect increases and decreases in pressure. Signals from the baroreceptors are relayed to the hypothalamus which, again, will stimulate release of ADH as needed.

Definitive treatment of edema requires treatment of the underlying cause. Supportive care may include applying compression stockings, restricting salt intake, improving nutritional status, avoiding prolonged standing, and taking *diuretic* medications. Little can be done in the prehospital setting except elevation of edematous limbs.

Intravenous Therapy

Intravenous (IV) therapy is the introduction of fluids and other substances into the venous side of the circulatory system. It is used to replace blood lost through hemorrhage, for electrolyte or fluid replacement, and for introduction of medications directly into the vascular system.

Blood and Blood Components

To understand IV therapy, it is necessary to understand the function of blood and its components. The blood is the fluid of the cardiovascular system. An adequate amount of blood is required for the transport of nutrients, oxygen, hormones, and heat. Blood consists of the liquid portion, or plasma, and the formed elements, or blood cells (Figure 1-49 ●).

Plasma **Plasma** is made up of approximately 92 percent water, 6 to 7 percent proteins, and a small portion consisting of electrolytes, lipids, enzymes, clotting factors, glucose, and other dissolved substances.

Formed Elements The formed elements include the red blood cells, or **erythrocytes**; the white blood cells, or **leukocytes**; and the platelets, or **thrombocytes**. More than 99 percent of the blood cells are erythrocytes. Erythrocytes contain hemoglobin and are responsible for transporting oxygen to the body's peripheral cells. **Hemoglobin** is an iron-based compound that binds with oxygen in the pulmonary (lung) capillaries and transports the oxygen to the peripheral tissues where it can be unloaded and taken into the cells. Factors such as pH (to be discussed later in this chapter) and oxygen concentration affect the amount of oxygen that can be transported by hemoglobin.

The leukocytes are responsible for immunity and fighting infection. The thrombocytes play a major role in blood clotting. The viscosity (thickness) of the blood is determined by the ratio of plasma to formed elements. The greater the proportion of formed elements within the plasma, the greater the viscosity.

The plasma can be separated from the formed elements by centrifugation. That is, blood can be placed in a test tube inside a centrifuge and spun at high speed. The heavier cells, the erythrocytes, will be forced to the bottom of the tube, leaving the plasma portion at the top. Usually, the erythrocytes will account for approximately 45 percent of the blood volume. The percentage of blood occupied by erythrocytes is referred to as the **hematocrit** (Figure 1-50 ●).

Fluid Replacement

The most desirable fluid for blood loss replacement is whole blood. There are several reasons for this. First, blood contains hemoglobin, which can transport oxygen. In addition, it is the most natural replacement. However, even in the hospital setting, the routine use of whole blood is not practical (Table 1–9). Blood is a precious commodity, and it must be conserved so that it can benefit the most people. Because of this, blood is often

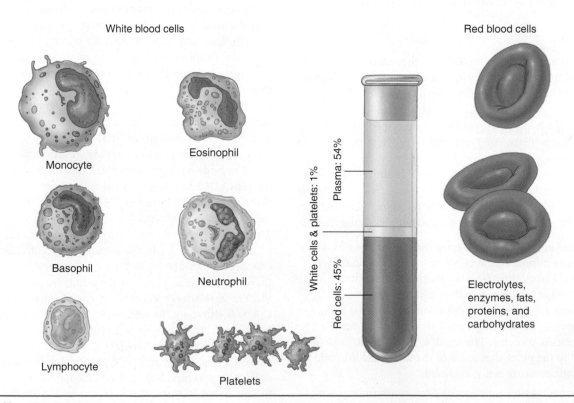

White blood cells

Red blood cells

Monocyte

Eosinophil

Basophil

Neutrophil

Lymphocyte

Platelets

Plasma: 54%

White cells & platelets: 1%

Red cells: 45%

Electrolytes, enzymes, fats, proteins, and carbohydrates

● **Figure 1-49** Blood components.

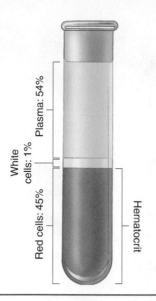

● **Figure 1-50** The percentage of the blood occupied by the red blood cells is termed the hematocrit.

fractionated, or separated into parts. The red cells are packaged separately as packed red blood cells. The white cells are used for other purposes. Plasma is packaged as fresh frozen plasma for use when plasma or clotting factors are needed. Thus, with the exception of true hemorrhagic shock (resulting from blood loss), where whole blood is the fluid of first choice, packed red blood cells are now more frequently used than whole blood.

Before blood, or blood products, can be administered to a patient, they must be typed and cross-matched to prevent a severe allergic reaction. The exception to this is fresh frozen plasma, which does not require cross-matching. If there is not adequate time for typing and cross-matching, O-negative blood (type O, Rh negative), the universal donor, can be administered.

Transfusion Reaction

Blood and blood products are rarely used in the field. However, on occasion, you may be called on to transport a patient with blood infusing. Because of this, you must be able to recognize the signs and symptoms of a transfusion reaction. Transfusion reactions occur when there is a discrepancy between the blood type of the patient and the blood type of the blood being transfused. In addition to the ABO and Rh types, there are many minor types that can cause a transfusion reaction. Common signs and symptoms of a transfusion reaction include fever, chills, hives, hypotension, palpitations, tachycardia, flushing of the skin, headaches, loss of consciousness, nausea, vomiting, or shortness of breath.

Intravenous Fluids

Intravenous fluids are the most common products used in prehospital care for fluid and electrolyte therapy. Intravenous fluids occur in two standard forms—colloids and crystalloids.

Colloids A **colloid** contains proteins, or other high-molecular-weight molecules, that tend to remain in the intravascular space for an extended period of time. In addition, as described earlier, colloids have oncotic force (colloid osmotic pressure), which means they tend to attract water into the intravascular space from the interstitial space and the intracellular space. Thus, a small amount of a colloid can be administered to a patient with a greater-than-expected increase in intravascular volume. The following are examples of colloids:

● *Plasma protein fraction (Plasmanate)* is a protein-containing colloid. The principal protein present is **albumin**, which is suspended along with other proteins in a saline solvent.

● *Salt-poor albumin* contains only human albumin. Each gram of albumin holds approximately 18 milliliters of water in the bloodstream.

● *Dextran* is not a protein, but a large sugar molecule with osmotic properties similar to albumin. It comes in two molecular weights: 40,000 and 70,000 Daltons. Dextran 40 has 2 to 2.5 times the colloid osmotic pressure of albumin.

● *Hetastarch (Hespan)*, like dextran, is a sugar molecule with osmotic properties similar to protein. It does not appear to share many of dextran's side effects. Colloid replacement therapy, at present, does not have a significant role in prehospital care except under rare circumstances. The colloid products are expensive and have a short shelf life.

Crystalloids **Crystalloids** are the primary compounds used in prehospital intravenous fluid therapy. There are multiple

TABLE 1–9 | Resuscitation Fluids				
	Resuscitation Fluid Used			
Diagnosis	**1st Choice**	**2nd Choice**	**3rd Choice**	**4th Choice**
Hemorrhagic Shock	Whole blood	Packed RBCs	Plasma or plasma substitute	Lactated Ringer's or normal saline
Shock Due to Plasma Loss (Burns)	Plasma	Plasma substitute	Lactated Ringer's or normal saline	—
Dehydration	Lactated Ringer's or normal saline	—	—	—

fluid preparations. It is often helpful to classify them according to their **tonicity** relative to plasma:

- *Isotonic solutions* have electrolyte composition similar to the blood plasma. When placed into a normally hydrated patient, they will not cause a significant fluid or electrolyte shift. Examples include normal saline (0.9 percent sodium chloride, also written as 0.9 percent NaCl) and lactated Ringer's.

- *Hypertonic solutions* have a higher solute concentration than the cells. These fluids will tend to cause a fluid shift out of the interstitial space and intracellular compartment into the intravascular space when administered to a normally hydrated patient. Later, there will be a diffusion of solute in the opposite direction. An example is 7.5 sodium chloride solution.

- *Hypotonic solutions* have a lower solute concentration than the cells. When administered to a normally hydrated patient, they will cause a movement of fluid from the intravascular space into the interstitial space and intracellular compartment. Later, solutes will move in an opposite direction. An example is 5 percent dextrose in water (D_5W).

Intravenous replacement fluids should be chosen based on the needs of the patient and the patient's underlying problem. This is typically guided by laboratory studies obtained in the hospital. However, these studies are not available in the prehospital setting. Hemorrhage occurs so fast that there is usually not time for a significant fluid shift to occur between the intravascular space and interstitial/intracellular spaces. Because of this, isotonic replacement fluids, such as lactated Ringer's and normal saline, should be used (Figure 1-51 ●).

Certain conditions, such as gastroenteritis (characterized by diarrhea, vomiting, and fever), can cause a patient to lose water more rapidly than sodium. These patients will have a deficit in total body water (TBW) due to reduced water intake, excessive water loss, or a combination of both. When water is lost in this manner, the level of sodium in the serum can increase, resulting in hypernatremia (elevated sodium levels). Patients with hypernatremia primarily need water. Because of this, hypotonic intravenous solutions, such as 0.45 percent sodium chloride (half-normal saline), are often chosen, because they provide the needed water with less sodium. However, it is important to point out that, even in cases of hypernatremia, initial fluid replacement therapy should consist of an isotonic solution until adequate blood pressure and adequate tissue perfusion have been restored.

Some replacement fluids contain a single element, such as sodium chloride or dextrose, while others contain multiple elements. Solutions such as lactated Ringer's are designed so that the concentration of electrolytes is very similar to that of the plasma. As a result, these solutions are referred to as balanced salt solutions.

The most commonly used solutions in prehospital care are lactated Ringer's solution, 0.9 percent sodium chloride (normal saline), and 5 percent dextrose in water (D_5W).

- *Lactated Ringer's* is an isotonic electrolyte solution of sodium chloride, potassium chloride, calcium chloride, and sodium lactate in water.

- *Normal saline* is an electrolyte solution of sodium chloride in water. It is isotonic with the extracellular fluid.

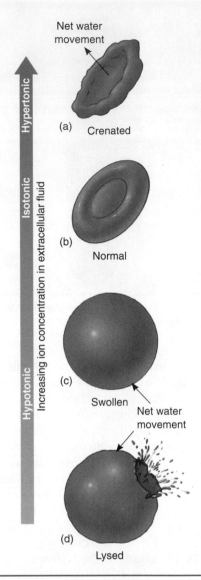

● **Figure 1-51** The effects of hypertonic, isotonic, and hypotonic solutions on red blood cells.

- D_5W is a hypotonic glucose solution used to keep a vein open and to supply calories necessary for cell metabolism. While it will have an initial effect of increasing the circulatory volume, glucose molecules rapidly diffuse across the vascular membrane. Water follows the glucose into the interstitial space, resulting in an increase in interstitial water.

Both lactated Ringer's solution and normal saline are used for fluid replacement, because their administration causes an immediate expansion of the circulatory volume. However, as was noted earlier, due to the movement of electrolytes and water, two-thirds of either of these solutions is lost into the interstitial space within 1 hour.

The Internal Cell

Earlier in this chapter we discussed the basic structure of the cell, its plasma membrane, and cytoplasm. Within the cell are numerous specialized structures called organelles as well as a permeating structure called the cytoskeleton that will be described next.

● **Figure 1-52** Diagram of the nucleus. *(Goodenough, Judith and Betty A. McGuire, Biology of Humans: Concepts, Applications, and Issues, 3rd Edition, © 2010. Reprinted and electronically reproduced by permission of Pearson Education, Inc. Upper Saddle River, NJ)*

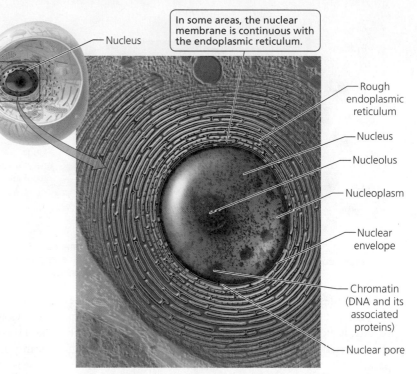

In some areas, the nuclear membrane is continuous with the endoplasmic reticulum.

— Nucleus

— Rough endoplasmic reticulum

— Nucleus

— Nucleolus

— Nucleoplasm

— Nuclear envelope

— Chromatin (DNA and its associated proteins)

— Nuclear pore

Diagram of the nucleus.

Organelles and Their Functions

As discussed previously, eukaryotic cells contain specialized internal compartments, enclosed by membranes, called organelles. Various biochemical processes that are necessary to cell survival and reproduction occur within the organelles. This is a much more efficient system than that seen in prokaryotic cells, because, in eukaryotic cells, molecules that perform a similar task are situated together for efficiency.

The roles and functions of the organelles are diverse. The following sections describe the major intracellular organelles and their functions.

Nucleus

The *nucleus* is among the largest organelles and contains all of the cell's genetic information (Figure 1-52 ●). Genetic information is encoded by base sequences on the DNA molecule. DNA controls cell functions and the production of specific proteins. All cells in an organism contain precisely the same information. However, some cells will express certain parts of the genetic information while others express other parts.

The genetic information is carried on threadlike structures called **chromosomes** made up of DNA and other proteins (Figure 1-53 ●). The number of chromosomes varies from species to species. Humans have 46 chromosomes (23 pairs), with one pair being the chromosomes that determine sex. Typically, chromosomes are only visible (with a light microscope) during the phase when cell division is occurring. During the process of division, chromosomes shorten and condense. The remainder of the time they are extended and are not visible. During this extended phase, before shortening and condensation, the genetic material is called **chromatin**.

Chromosomes

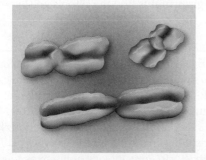

● **Figure 1-53** Chromosomes are composed of DNA and associated proteins. During cell division, as shown here, chromosomes shorten and condense.

A double membrane encases the nucleus and is referred to as the **nuclear envelope**. The nuclear envelope contains the chromatin and the other materials inside the nucleus that are collectively referred to as **nucleoplasm**. Communications between the inside of the nucleus and the surrounding cytoplasm occurs through openings in the nuclear envelope called **nuclear pores**.

There is a specialized region within the nucleus referred to as the **nucleolus**. As with the chromosomes, the nucleolus is only visible during certain cell phases. The nucleolus is not surrounded by a membrane. The nucleolus is a region of the DNA that is active in the production of a specialized type of RNA called ribosomal RNA (rRNA). The rRNA leaves the nucleus of the cell and joins with messenger RNA (mRNA) to form a ribosome. Ribosomes then manufacture the protein coded for by the RNA.

Ribosomes

Ribosomes are spherical structures that can account for up to 25 percent of the dry weight of a cell (Figure 1-54 ●). The primary role of the ribosomes is the synthesis of polypeptides and proteins. The ribosome consists of two subunits, each consisting of rRNA and protein. These subunits leave the cell nucleus, bind with mRNA, and become a functional ribosome in the cytoplasm. The ribosomes interpret the information from mRNA and translate it into an amino acid sequence until the desired protein is formed. The necessary conformational changes will occur (bending, folding) to make the protein fully functional.

Endoplasmic Reticulum

The **endoplasmic reticulum** is a network of tubules, vesicles, and sacs that interconnect with the plasma membrane, nuclear envelope, and many of the other organelles in the cell. Certain parts of the endoplasmic reticulum contain ribosomes during

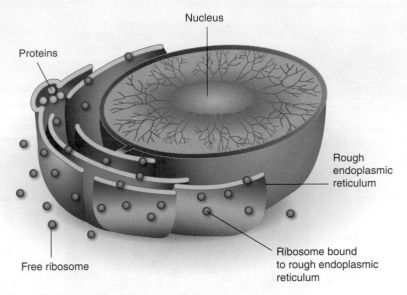

Nucleus

Proteins

Rough endoplasmic reticulum

Free ribosome

Ribosome bound to rough endoplasmic reticulum

protein synthesis and are referred to as **rough endoplasmic reticulum (RER)**. The RER sends the proteins to the Golgi apparatus in vesicles called cisternae or, if they are membrane proteins, insert them into the plasma membrane. (The Golgi apparatus and cisternae will be described next.)

The portion of the endoplasmic reticulum without ribosomes is called **smooth endoplasmic reticulum (SER)**. SER has multiple functions, depending on the cell type. The vast network of SER provides an increased surface area for the action or storage of key enzymes and the products of these enzymes. For example, SER in muscle cells serves as a store of calcium that is released as one step in the contraction process. Calcium pumps move the calcium.

Endoplasmic reticulum

Nucleus

Rough endoplasmic reticulum (RER) has ribosomes attached to its surface and is involved in modifying proteins made by the ribosomes.

Smooth endoplasmic reticulum (SER) lacks ribosomes and is involved in detoxifying certain drugs and in producing phospholipids for incorporation into membranes.

● **Figure 1-54** Ribosomes are spherical structures within the cell that function in the synthesis of polypeptides and proteins. Some ribosomes are suspended in the cytoplasm (free ribosomes); other ribosomes are attached to endoplasmic reticulum (bound ribosomes).

The endoplasmic reticulum also plays a major role in replenishment and maintenance of the plasma membrane. The protein components of the plasma membrane come from the RER, while the lipid components come from the SER (Figure 1-55 ●).

Golgi Apparatus

The **Golgi apparatus**, also called the *Golgi complex*, is an important organelle whose function is to process proteins for the cell membrane and other cell organelles. The Golgi apparatus serves as a sort of "post office" for the cell, as it is essentially a protein-processing and packaging center. The transport vesicles (**cisternae**) from the endoplasmic reticulum fuse with the face of the Golgi apparatus and empty their protein content into the lumen of the Golgi apparatus. The proteins are then transported to the opposite side of the Golgi apparatus and are modified along the way. They are labeled with a sequence of molecules according to their final destination. Some proteins, such as those bound for the plasma membrane, are packaged in vesicles (Figure 1-56 ●). Other proteins are packaged in lysosomes (described next).

Lysosomes

Lysosomes serve as the "garbage disposal system" of the cells. That is, they degrade and remove products of ingestion (the process called phagocytosis) and worn out parts from the cell. They also play a role in converting complex nutritional molecules to simple nutritional molecules. Lysosomes are spherical in shape and surrounded by a single membrane. Each lysosome can contain up to 40 digestive enzymes and has an extremely low pH (pH 4.8). The enzymes and membranes of lysosomes are manufactured by the RER and sent to the Golgi apparatus for packaging. Ultimately, a lysosome that contains all the necessary digestive enzymes surrounded by a plasma membrane will bud from the Golgi apparatus into the cytoplasm (Figure 1-57 ●).

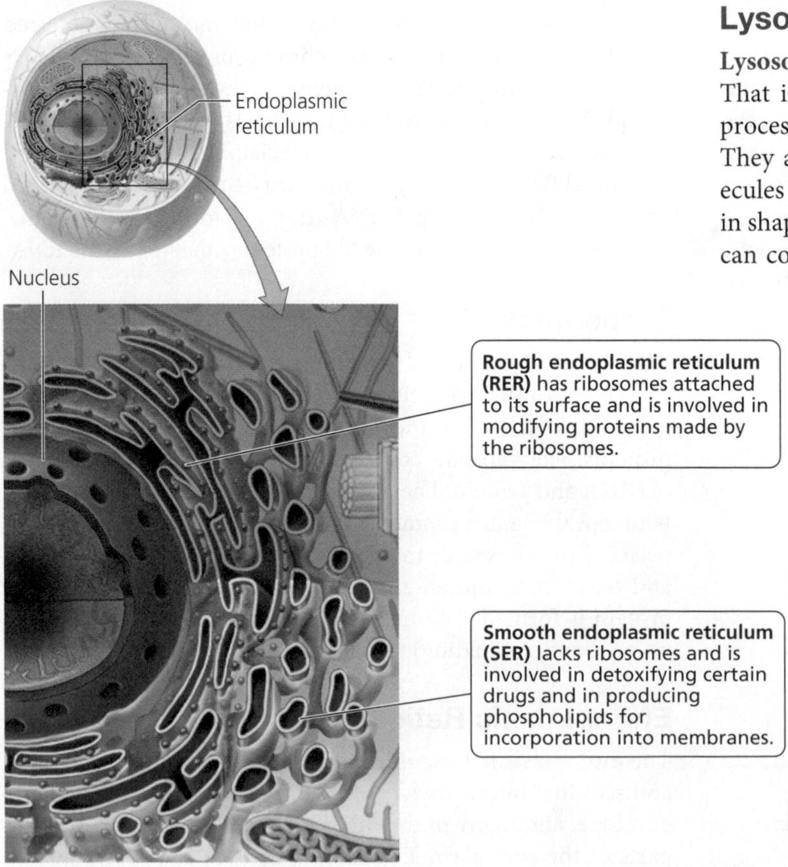

● **Figure 1-55** The endoplasmic reticulum has rough and smooth portions. Rough endoplasmic reticulum (RER) has ribosomes attached during protein synthesis. Smooth endoplasmic reticulum (SER) has no attached ribosomes and serves various functions, depending on the cell type. *(Goodenough, Judith and Betty A. McGuire,* Biology of Humans: Concepts, Applications, and Issues, *3rd Edition, © 2010. Reprinted and electronically reproduced by permission of Pearson Education, Inc. Upper Saddle River, NJ)*

● Figure 1-56 The route by which protein-filled vesicles from the rough endoplasmic reticulum travel to the Golgi complex for processing and then move on to the plasma membrane for release. *(Goodenough, Judith and Betty A. McGuire*, Biology of Humans: Concepts, Applications, and Issues, *3rd Edition, © 2010. Reprinted and electronically reproduced by permission of Pearson Education, Inc. Upper Saddle River, NJ)*

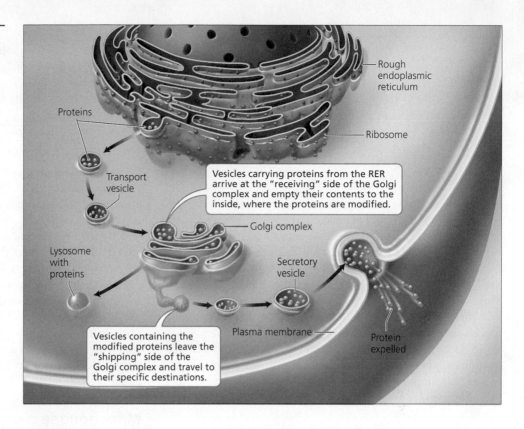

Proteins

Transport vesicle

Lysosome with proteins

Golgi complex

Secretory vesicle

Plasma membrane

Rough endoplasmic reticulum

Ribosome

Vesicles carrying proteins from the RER arrive at the "receiving" side of the Golgi complex and empty their contents to the inside, where the proteins are modified.

Vesicles containing the modified proteins leave the "shipping" side of the Golgi complex and travel to their specific destinations.

Protein expelled

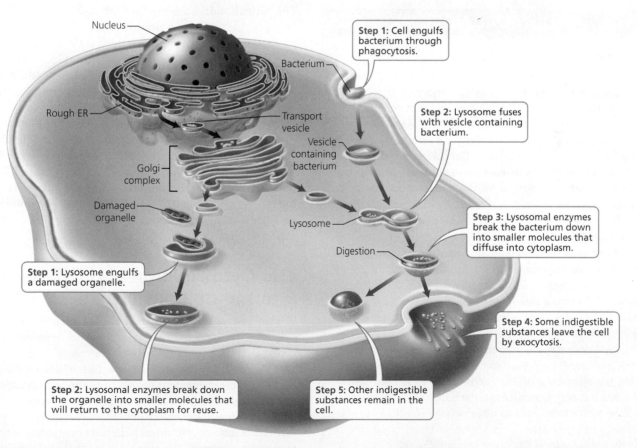

Nucleus

Bacterium

Step 1: Cell engulfs bacterium through phagocytosis.

Rough ER

Transport vesicle

Vesicle containing bacterium

Step 2: Lysosome fuses with vesicle containing bacterium.

Golgi complex

Damaged organelle

Lysosome

Step 3: Lysosomal enzymes break the bacterium down into smaller molecules that diffuse into cytoplasm.

Digestion

Step 1: Lysosome engulfs a damaged organelle.

Step 4: Some indigestible substances leave the cell by exocytosis.

Step 2: Lysosomal enzymes break down the organelle into smaller molecules that will return to the cytoplasm for reuse.

Step 5: Other indigestible substances remain in the cell.

● Figure 1-57 Lysosome formation and function in intracellular digestion. Lysosomes released from the Golgi complex digest a bacterium engulfed by the cell (pathway shown on right). Lysosomes also digest obsolete parts of the cell itself (pathway shown on left). *(Goodenough, Judith and Betty A. McGuire*, Biology of Humans: Concepts, Applications, and Issues, *3rd Edition, © 2010. Reprinted and electronically reproduced by permission of Pearson Education, Inc. Upper Saddle River, NJ)*

CONTENT REVIEW

► Organelles within Cells

- Nucleus
- Ribosomes
- Endoplasmic reticulum
- Golgi apparatus
- Lysosomes
- Vacuoles
- Peroxisomes
- Mitochondria

One of the major functions of lysosomes is to break down foreign substances and invaders, such as a bacterium. Once a bacterium is isolated through the process of phagocytosis, it is enclosed in a large vesicle called a vacuole. (Vacuoles will be described next.) Soon, vesicles containing lysosomal enzymes (primary lysosomes) will fuse with the vesicle. The pH of the newly formed complex then becomes more acidic, and this activates the digestive enzymes. The vacuole thus becomes a secondary lysosome and degrades the bacterium. Lysosomes also degrade worn out organelles such as mitochondria. The remnants of the process are either reprocessed for use again or released from the cell through exocytosis.

Lysosomes also process the macromolecule products needed for cell energy production. The macromolecule ultimately winds up in food vacuoles. These vacuoles then fuse with primary lysosomes, where digestive enzymes break down the macromolecules into simple molecules that diffuse out of the vesicle into the cytoplasm for use as energy substrates for the cell.

CLINICAL NOTE

Pediatric

Tay-Sachs disease (pronounced tay-SACKS) is a genetic disorder that can result in paralysis, blindness, convulsions, mental retardation, and death. It was first described in 1881, and in 1887 found to be more prevalent in Ashkenazi Jews (Jews of Central European descent). It is also seen, although on a more limited basis, in French Canadians of southeastern Quebec and in Cajuns of southern Louisiana. These populations all tend to marry within their population, leading to less genetic diversity and increased expression of mutations. Tay-Sachs disease is quite rare in families of other ethnic backgrounds.

It has been determined that a mutation on chromosome 15 causes the absence of the lysosomal enzyme hexosamidase (Hex A) which is responsible for breaking down lipids in nerve cells. Without Hex A, nerve cells swell with undigested lipids which ultimately causes a progressive and irreversible deterioration in nervous system functioning.

Tay-Sachs disease is normally noticeable around the age of six months. Prior to that, the baby acts normally. However, once the symptoms of Tay-Sachs begin to appear, several noticeable changes occur. First, the baby will become listless and will stop interacting with other people. The baby will often develop a staring gaze. Even normal levels of noise tend to startle the baby to an abnormal degree. Eventually, the baby will develop dementia, mental retardation, decreased muscle tone, seizures, and death. There is no treatment, and the disease is 100 percent fatal—usually by age 4 to 5.

Vacuoles

Vacuoles are membrane-bound organelles used for temporary storage or transport of substances such as food sources. The lysosome can fuse with the vacuole membrane and place digestive enzymes into the food vacuole to break down the food source within.

Peroxisomes

Peroxisomes are similar to lysosomes in size and the lack of obvious internal structure. Peroxisomes have the ability to generate and degrade hydrogen peroxide (H_2O_2). Hydrogen peroxide is highly toxic to cells. However, it can be degraded to water and oxygen by the enzyme catalase. Because of its toxicity, eukaryotic cells protect themselves by placing the biochemical pathways that generate and degrade H_2O_2 into the isolated compartment called a peroxisome.

Peroxisomes are found in virtually all cell types but are more prevalent in the liver and kidneys. They play an important role in detoxifying harmful substances such as alcohols and formaldehyde. Peroxisomes are also important in the breakdown of fatty acids. Because they can produce oxygen, peroxisomes play a role in the regulation of oxygen tension within the cell.

Mitochondria

The **mitochondria** are the "powerhouses" of the cells in that they provide the energy needed for all of a cell's biochemical processes. Cellular respiration, which is the conversion of food to energy, primarily occurs in the mitochondria. Cellular respiration is a three-phase process that first begins in the cytoplasm and continues in the mitochondria. (Cellular respiration will be described in more detail later.)

The number of mitochondria present varies from cell to cell, depending on the specialized function of the cell. Mitochondria, like the nucleus, are surrounded by a double membrane forming two separate compartments. The inner membrane folds form shelves within the mitochondria, referred to as **cristae**, where the last phases of cellular respiration occur. The mitochondria also can contain some ribosomes and some of the cell's genetic material (Figure 1-58 ●).

The Cytoskeleton and Other Internal Cell Structures

Within eukaryotic cells is a complex system of filaments, microtubules, and intermediate filaments referred to as the **cytoskeleton**.

Microtubules are long, hollow rods made of the protein tubulin. Microfilaments are made from the protein actin. Intermediate filaments are made up of different proteins, depending on the cell type. Near the cell nucleus are two structures called **centrioles** that are cylindrical structures composed of groups of microtubules arranged in a ring pattern that are thought to play an important role in cell division (Figure 1-59 ●).

The cytoskeleton forms a dynamic three-dimensional structure that fills the cytoplasm and serves as a skeleton for cell stability and as a muscle for cell movement. In addition to stability,

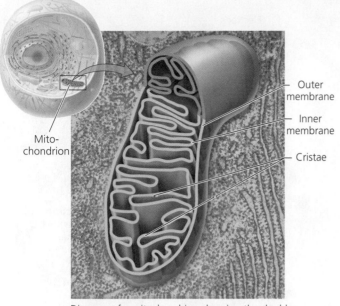

Mito-
chondrion

Outer
membrane

Inner
membrane

Cristae

Diagram of a mitochondrion showing the double
membrane that creates two compartments.

● **Figure 1-58**   Mitochondria are sites of energy conversion
in the cell. *(Goodenough, Judith and Betty A. McGuire,* Biology
of Humans: Concepts, Applications, and Issues, *3rd Edition,*
© 2010. Reprinted and electronically reproduced by permission
of Pearson Education, Inc. Upper Saddle River, NJ)

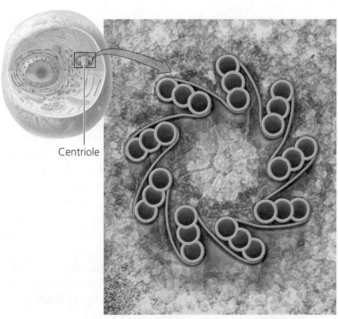

Centriole

Diagram of a centriole. Each centriole is
composed of nine sets of triplet microtubules
arranged in a ring.

● **Figure 1-59**   Centrioles are thought to play an important
role in cell division. *(Goodenough, Judith and Betty A. McGuire,*
Biology of Humans: Concepts, Applications, and Issues,
3rd Edition, © 2010. Reprinted and electronically reproduced by
permission of Pearson Education, Inc. Upper Saddle River, NJ)

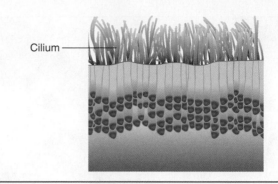

Cilium

● **Figure 1-60**   Cilia are short hairlike structures on the
surfaces of cells such as those that line the respiratory tract,
where they sweep away debris trapped in mucus.

the cytoskeleton plays an important role in both intracellular
transport and cellular division.

Two structures important in cell movement, cilia and flagella, are made up of microtubules. **Cilia** are numerous hairlike
structures that move in a back-and-forth motion. This motion
can sweep debris away from the cell and play an important role
in protection of the respiratory system and in the reproductive
system (Figure 1-60 ●). **Flagella** are much longer than cilia and
move in an undulating, wavelike manner. Human sperm move
through the undulations of flagella.

CELLULAR RESPIRATION AND ENERGY PRODUCTION

The cell needs a constant supply of energy. We get the energy
our body needs through nutrients in our diet. Our digestive
system breaks down the three major classes of nutrients—
carbohydrates, proteins, and lipids—into simpler compounds,
typically simple sugars and amino acids, that can enter the cell
and be converted to energy. Some of the energy is used to manufacture ATP while some is given off as heat. Once nutrients
reach the cells, they will enter a metabolic pathway—either cellular respiration or fermentation. Cellular respiration is aerobic
and requires oxygen. Fermentation is anaerobic and does not
require oxygen.

When nutrients are converted to energy by the cells, there
is a transport of electrons from one molecule to another. The
loss of electrons from one atom to another is called **oxidation**.
The gain of electrons by one atom from another is called **reduction**. In cellular respiration, glucose is oxidized to simpler
compounds, producing energy in the process.

Cellular Respiration

There are three distinct biochemical processes through which
a glucose molecule must pass to produce energy through
cellular respiration: glycolysis, the citric acid cycle, and
electron transport (Figure 1-61 ●). Glycolysis occurs in the
cytoplasm, while the citric acid cycle and electron transport occur in the mitochondria. The complete breakdown
of glucose yields water, carbon dioxide, and energy in the

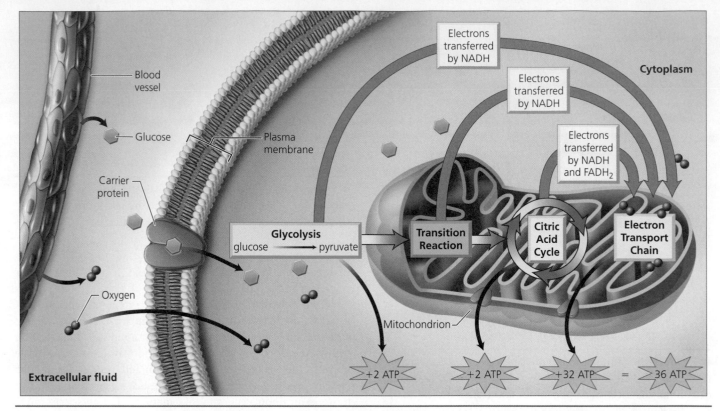

● **Figure 1-61** Summary of cellular respiration in which a glucose molecule undergoes glycolysis, the citric acid cycle, and transport to produce energy. (*Goodenough, Judith and Betty A. McGuire,* Biology of Humans: Concepts, Applications, and Issues, *3rd Edition, © 2010. Reprinted and electronically reproduced by permission of Pearson Education, Inc. Upper Saddle River, NJ*)

form of ATP. This relationship is illustrated by the following equation:

$$C_6H_{12}O_6 \ + \ 6O_2 \ \rightarrow \ 6CO_2 \ + 6H_2O \ + \approx 36ATP$$

Glucose	*Oxygen*	*Carbon Dixoide*	*Water*	*Energy*

Glycolysis

The first step in the breakdown of the six-carbon sugar glucose is called **glycolysis** and occurs in the cytoplasm. In glycolysis one molecule of glucose is oxidized through several steps to two molecules of pyruvic acid. The process of glycolysis is anaerobic—that is, it does not require oxygen.

There are two phases of glycolysis: the energy-using phase and the energy-yielding phase. During the first phase two molecules of ATP are used to prepare the glucose molecule for splitting into two 3-carbon subunits. During the second phase, the two 3-carbon molecules are broken down to pyruvic acid (the anion of pyruvic acid is pyruvate). During this phase four molecules of ATP are produced, giving a net yield of two molecules of ATP per molecule of glucose. The two molecules of pyruvic acid then move from the cytoplasm into the liquid matrix of the mitochondria where the citric acid cycle occurs. Glycolysis also produces two molecules of *nicotine adenine dinucleotide (NADH)*, which carry energy to the electron transport chain (Figure 1-62 ●).

Citric Acid Cycle

Once the two molecules of pyruvic acid have entered the mitochondria, they enter the second phase of glucose metabolism called the **citric acid cycle**. The citric acid cycle, also called *Kreb's cycle* or the *tricarboxylic acid (TCA) cycle*, requires oxygen. In the first step, called the transition reaction, the pyruvic acid molecule reacts with a substance called coenzyme A (CoA) (Figure 1-63 ●). This removes a carbon atom (in the form of carbon dioxide) from the pyruvic acid molecule. The resulting two-carbon molecule (called an acetyl group) binds to the CoA molecule and becomes acetyl CoA. Acetyl CoA then formally enters the citric acid cycle. In an eight-step process, the citric acid cycle completely oxidizes the remainder of the glucose molecule. On the completion of glucose oxidation, the citric acid cycle yields two molecules of ATP and releases carbon dioxide as waste (Figure 1-64 ●). It also yields several molecules of two other compounds: NADH and flavin adenine nucleotide (FADH$_2$). NADH and FADH$_2$ carry high-energy electrons into the final part of cellular metabolism—the electron transport chain.

Electron Transport

NADH and FADH$_2$ derived from glycolysis and the citric acid cycle donate their electrons to carrier proteins known as the electron transport chain. The **electron transport chain** consists of five types of carriers. (All the carriers except one are proteins.) These proteins are embedded on the cristae in the inner membrane of the mitochondria. When electrons are transferred from one molecule to the next, energy is released. This energy is then

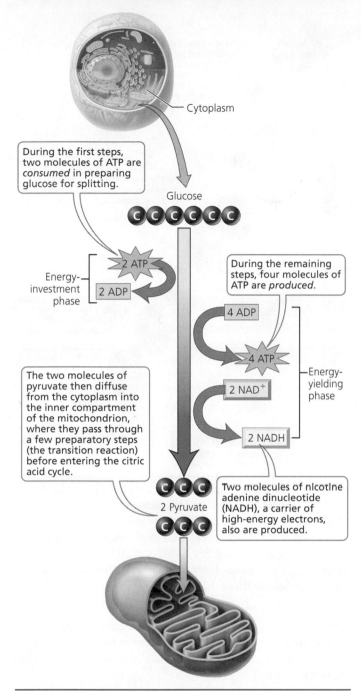

● **Figure 1-62** Glycolysis is a sequence of reactions in the cytoplasm in which glucose, a six-carbon sugar, is split into two 3-carbon molecules of pyruvate. *(Goodenough, Judith and Betty A. McGuire,* Biology of Humans: Concepts, Applications, and Issues, *3rd Edition, © 2010. Reprinted and electronically reproduced by permission of Pearson Education, Inc. Upper Saddle River, NJ)*

used to create ATP for use as an energy source by the cells. The electrons are ultimately passed to oxygen, which is the ultimate *electron acceptor*. On accepting the electron, oxygen combines with two molecules of hydrogen to form a molecule of water. If there is insufficient oxygen, electrons begin to accumulate on the carrier proteins, and this will ultimately stop the citric acid cycle.

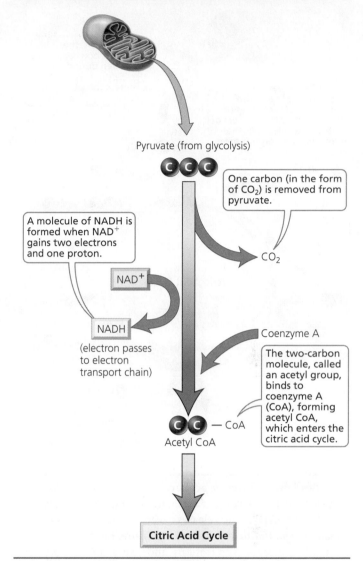

● **Figure 1-63** The transition reaction is the link between glycolysis and the citric acid cycle. *(Goodenough, Judith and Betty A. McGuire,* Biology of Humans: Concepts, Applications, and Issues, *3rd Edition, © 2010. Reprinted and electronically reproduced by permission of Pearson Education, Inc. Upper Saddle River, NJ)*

The electron transport chain, when functioning optimally, can produce 32 molecules of ATP. Together, cellular respiration produces approximately 36 molecules of ATP (2 ATP from glycolysis, 2 ATP from the citric acid cycle, and 32 ATP from electron transport). The actual number produced at any given time varies and is dependent on numerous factors (Figure 1-65 ●).

Fermentation

An alternative pathway to energy production is available during times when oxygen is unavailable. The breakdown of glucose without oxygen is called **fermentation**.

With fermentation, the glucose molecule proceeds through glycolysis as it does in cellular respiration, as glycolysis does not require oxygen. This results in the creation of two molecules

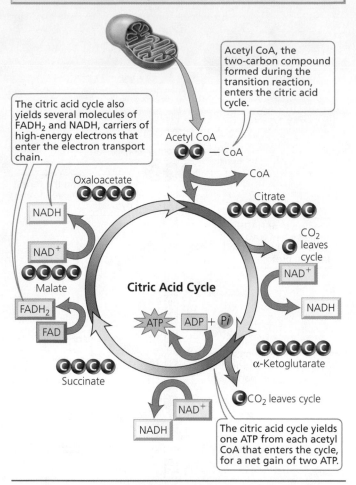

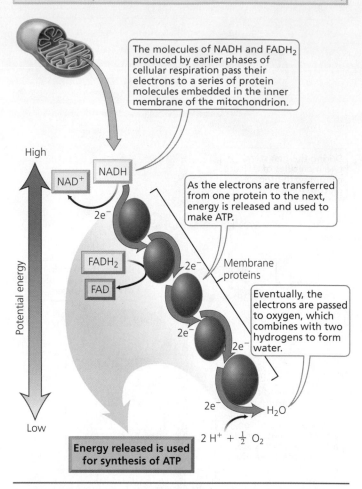

● **Figure 1-64** The citric acid cycle is a series of reactions that yields two molecules of ATP and several molecules of NADH and FADH$_2$ and releases carbon dioxide as waste. *(Goodenough, Judith and Betty A. McGuire,* Biology of Humans: Concepts, Applications, and Issues, *3rd Edition, © 2010. Reprinted and electronically reproduced by permission of Pearson Education, Inc. Upper Saddle River, NJ)*

● **Figure 1-65** The electron transport chain is the final phase of cellular respiration. This phase releases up to 32 molecules of ATP per molecule of glucose. *(Goodenough, Judith and Betty A. McGuire,* Biology of Humans: Concepts, Applications, and Issues, *3rd Edition, © 2010. Reprinted and electronically reproduced by permission of Pearson Education, Inc. Upper Saddle River, NJ)*

of pyruvate, NADH, and ATP. With fermentation, the chemical reactions continue in the cytoplasm instead of entering the mitochondria. In fermentation, the final electron acceptor is pyruvate, not oxygen. Electrons are transferred from the NADH molecule to pyruvate, which generates NAD$^+$. This helps generate ATP through glycolysis. Fermentation is very inefficient and produces only 2 ATP compared to 36 ATP from cellular respiration.

There are two types of fermentation that can occur in humans: lactic acid fermentation and alcohol fermentation. As just discussed, NADH passes electrons directly to pyruvate. Pyruvate is converted by an enzyme called lactate dehydrogenase (LDH) into the waste product known as lactate or lactic acid (lactate is the anion of lactic acid). During periods of extreme stress or exercise, oxygen levels in muscle tissue become low. In this case, muscle tissues may use lactic acid fermentation to generate ATP (Figure 1-66 ●).

Alcohol fermentation is more complex. With alcohol fermentation, a molecule of carbon dioxide is removed from

pyruvate leaving a two-carbon molecule called acetaldehyde. With alcohol fermentation, electrons are not passed to pyruvate. Instead, NADH passes electrons to acetaldehyde forming ethanol (ethyl alcohol).

CELLULAR RESPONSE TO STRESS

The cell normally functions within a stable environment. It can react to changes in its environment through homeostasis, the tendency of the body to initiate whatever processes are necessary to restore stability when it is disrupted. Severe stresses and pathological conditions may require the cell itself to change. Such physiologic and structural changes to the cell, in response to change or stress, are referred to as **cellular adaptation**.

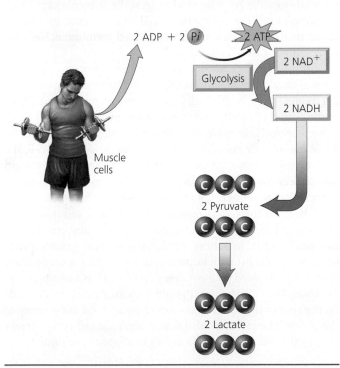

● **Figure 1-66** Lactic acid fermentation does not require oxygen and yields two molecules of ATP per molecule of glucose. *(Goodenough, Judith and Betty A. McGuire,* Biology of Humans: Concepts, Applications, and Issues, *3rd Edition, © 2010. Reprinted and electronically reproduced by permission of Pearson Education, Inc. Upper Saddle River, NJ)*

Cellular Adaptation

There are several possible cellular responses to an increase in stress. Some cellular responses can come in the form of normal growth while others involve abnormal changes in size or function. There are two types of normal-growth responses to cellular stress: an increase in the number of cells (hyperplasia) and an increase in the size of the cells (hypertrophy). Other types of responses to stress may involve a decrease in the size and function of the cell (atrophy) or a change from one cell type to another (metaplasia) (Figure 1-67 ●).

Hyperplasia

An increase in the number of cells in a tissue or organ is termed **hyperplasia**. This usually results in the tissue or organ in question increasing in size. Hyperplasia can be divided into two functional categories: hormonal hyperplasia and compensatory hyperplasia. Hormonal hyperplasia results from stimulation by hormones. Examples of hormonal hyperplasia are the development of the breasts during puberty and enlargement of the breasts during pregnancy. Compensatory hyperplasia is an increase in tissue mass following tissue injury or loss. An example of compensatory hyperplasia is regeneration of the liver following partial hepatic lobectomy.

Sometimes hyperplasia is pathological. That is, if the hyperplasia is not compensatory and is not due to hormonal stimulation (or does not revert to normal after hormonal stimulation is removed), the process may be pathological and a possible precursor of cancer.

Hypertrophy

An increase in the size of cells in a tissue or organ is referred to as **hypertrophy**. Hypertrophy is not due to the cells swelling. Instead, it is due to the creation of more structural components (i.e., organelles) within the cell. An organ that is hypertrophied does not contain more cells (as would be the case with hyperplasia). Instead, the cells that are present have simply enlarged. If the cell is capable of dividing in response to stress, both hyperplasia and hypertrophy may develop. Some cells, such as cardiac muscle cells, do not divide and simply hypertrophy in response to stress.

Hypertrophy can be classified as physiologic or pathologic. Physiologic hypertrophy usually results from increased physical demand. For example, a person begins a vigorous exercise program. Since the cells of the heart cannot increase in number, the cells that are there increase in size to handle the added demand. Enlargement of the uterus during pregnancy is due to both physiologic hypertrophy and hormonal hyperplasia. It returns to normal once the stress of pregnancy and the hormonal influence are removed.

Pathological hypertrophy results from abnormal stress, in contrast to physiologic hypertrophy that is associated with pregnancy or exercise. There is an observable difference in the two types of cardiac hypertrophy. With physiologic hypertrophy, the

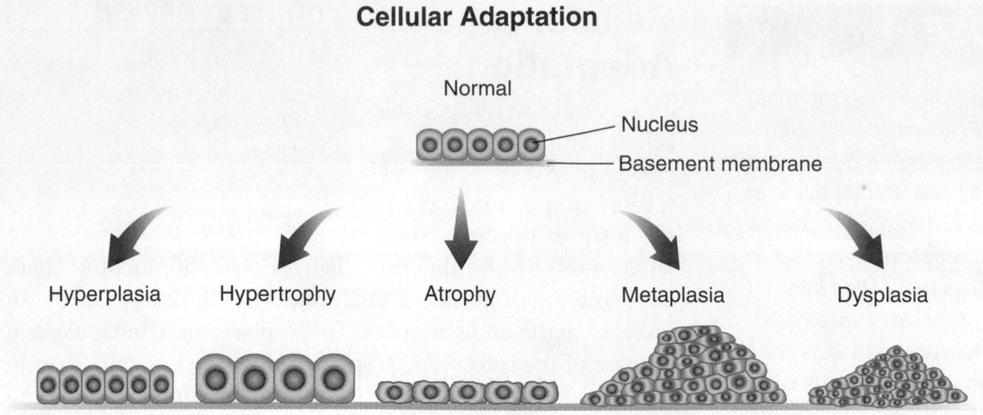

Cellular Adaptation

● **Figure 1-67** Abnormal cell responses to stress include hypertrophy, hyperplasia, atrophy, metaplasia, and dysplasia.

cardiac septum (vertical wall between halves of the heart) enlarges and so do the sizes of the cardiac chambers. With pathological hypertrophy, the septum thickens while the chambers decrease in size.

Atrophy

A decrease in the size of a cell is termed **atrophy**. Atrophy can result from several factors, including a decreased workload, decreased blood supply, loss of nervous control, inadequate nutritional intake, lack of endocrine stimulation, and aging. As with hypertrophy, atrophy may be either physiologic or pathological. For example, during the reproductive years, the vagina is soft and well-lubricated. This is principally due to the effect of hormones (primarily estrogen), an excellent blood supply, and periodic use. As a woman ages, the vagina atrophies. The tissues of the vagina become thin and friable, and the overall size decreases. This is due primarily to a combination of the loss of hormonal stimulation, aging, and decreased use. Some of the effects of vaginal atrophy can be delayed through the use of hormonal therapy (topical and oral estrogen). Vaginal atrophy with aging is an example of physiologic atrophy.

Pathological atrophy is a result of disease or injury. For example, a person who has sustained a spinal cord injury will eventually develop atrophy in the muscles affected by the injury. This results from a combination of the loss of nervous control, a decreased workload, and in some instances a change in blood supply.

Metaplasia

In certain situations, a cell can change from one adult cell type to another adult cell type. This process is called **metaplasia** and is reversible. Metaplasia is an adaptive response that serves to protect the organism from stress. For example, portions of the respiratory tract are lined with columnar epithelial cells. These cells contain cilia that help to move mucus and foreign materials up the airway to the pharynx from which they can be swallowed or expelled by sneezing or coughing. This action serves to protect the airway. With exposure to a chronic irritant, such as cigarette smoke, the ciliated columnar epithelial cells can transition to stratified squamous epithelial cells, thereby replacing delicate cells with hardier ones better able to withstand the irritant. When this occurs, the benefits of ciliary motion are lost.

By itself, metaplasia is not harmful and does not lead to cancer. When the irritant is removed (e.g., the person stops smoking), the cells return to their normal state as ciliated columnar epithelial cells. However, when the irritant continues to be present, the metaplastic cells may eventually become cancerous. Thus, while metaplasia can be beneficial and protective for the organism, the precursors that cause metaplasia, if not corrected, can induce malignant cell transformation.

Cell Injury and Cell Death

When cells are stressed to the point that they can no longer adapt, or when they are exposed to toxic agents, cell injury can result. If cell injury is persistent or severe, cell death may ultimately occur.

Cell injury may be classified as reversible or irreversible. If the cell injury is irreversible, cell death will occur. Irreversibly damaged cells will undergo either necrosis or apoptosis. If there is damage to the plasma membranes of the cell, enzymes released from the lysosomes will digest the contents of the cell, resulting in cellular **necrosis**, or cell death caused by outside forces such as infection that attack the cell membrane. Necrosis is sometimes called "cell murder."

However, cell death occurs as a normal process of keeping the body healthy by sloughing off old or damaged cells and making room for new, healthy cells. This preprogrammed form of cell death occurs normally and is called **apoptosis**. To distinguish it from necrosis, apoptosis is sometimes called "cell suicide." In apoptosis, if toxic substances damage the DNA of the cell, the nucleus will dissolve, yet the membranes of the cell will remain intact. Necrosis is always a pathological process, while apoptosis is normally physiologic but may also have a pathological cause.

There are numerous factors that can cause cell injury and possibly cell death. These include hypoxia, physical agents, chemical agents, infection, immune reactions, genetic problems, and problems with nutrition. In some cases, a single agent is all that is involved. In most cases, cell death has a combination of causes. Overall, the way the cell responds to injury depends on the type of injury, the duration of injury, and the severity of the injury. The response also depends on the cell type, current state of the cell, and the cell's ability to adapt to the injury.

Ischemic and Hypoxic Injury

The most common type of cellular injury is that due to ischemia and hypoxia. **Ischemia** results from diminished blood flow, while **hypoxia** is due to decreased availability of oxygen. When cells face ischemia or hypoxia, cellular respiration is usually impaired, and energy production is usually limited to glycolysis.

The beneficial effects of glycolysis stop after all the pyruvate stores have been depleted, ATP is unavailable for the first step, or metabolic products that would normally be removed begin to accumulate. Because of this, ischemia tends to injure cells and tissues faster than does hypoxia (Figure 1-68 ●).

The extent of injury resulting from ischemia depends on several factors. First, up to a certain point, cellular injury from ischemia is reversible if the cell has not been significantly damaged before blood flow is restored. However, if not reversed, the cell eventually reaches a point of no return where cellular damage is so massive that the cell cannot overcome it and survive. With ischemic cell injury, the oxygen concentration of the blood falls. Since oxygen is the ultimate electron acceptor, this stops the action of the electron transport chain and that, in turn, stops the citric acid cycle. This causes a markedly decreased supply of ATP. The lack of ATP causes failure of the sodium-potassium pump. This allows sodium to diffuse into the cell and potassium to diffuse out. Since water follows sodium readily across the plasma membrane, the cell will begin to swell until it lyses (splits open), causing cell death.

Oxidative Stress

Even when the blood supply and oxygen are restored to cells previously inadequately perfused, these cells still may die. Generally, cells that are reversibly injured may survive, while those that are irreversibly injured will not. However, some cells that are reversibly injured will die even after blood flow resumes—either by necrosis or by apoptosis. With the introduction of reperfusion, some tissues that were reversibly damaged may become irreversibly damaged. This can be the result of new damage from oxygen free radicals, increased permeability of the mitochondria, and inflammation.

Oxygen free radicals (oxygen atoms with unpaired electrons in the outer shell) steal electrons from other compounds and generate new species of free radicals. This process can continue until the components of the cell are used up. Increased mitochondrial permeability results in the entry of macromolecules into the mitochondria, resulting in mitochondrial swelling and

rupture, eventually leading to cell death. The infiltration of cells of the immune system, in the process of inflammation, also can cause secondary ischemic injury and cell death.

Chemical Injury

Various chemicals, including drugs, can cause injury to a cell. This occurs through two mechanisms: direct action on cells or through the creation of chemical precursors that are converted to a **cytotoxic** metabolite. (*Cytotoxic* means "poisonous to cells.") Numerous toxins are capable of cellular injury. Also, some substances used routinely in medicine, such as acetaminophen, can cause cellular toxicity (mainly to the liver) if an overdose occurs.

Apoptosis

Apoptosis occurs when a cellular program is activated that causes the release of enzymes that destroy the genetic material within the nucleus of the cell and selected proteins in the cytoplasm. Fragments of the dead cell (apoptotic bodies) are then cleared by scavenger cells before the toxic contents leak out and cause inflammation (Figure 1-69 ●).

Apoptosis can be physiologic or pathological. Causes of physiologic apoptosis include the programmed destruction of the cell just described, involution of the cell following removal of a hormonal stimulus, normal cell deletion in areas where there is a proliferating cell population, cells that have served their purpose, elimination of cells that are potentially harmful to the organism, and through a defensive mechanism where cytotoxic cells of the immune system cause the cell death.

Pathological apoptosis results from cell death secondary to cell injury, cell death from viral infections, cell death from atrophy after destruction or blockage of a duct, and cell death in tumors. Even in cells that die by necrosis, there may be a component of apoptosis present to help minimize the possibility of an inflammatory response.

Dysplasia

Abnormal or disordered growth in a cell is referred to as **dysplasia**. Dysplasia is more common in cells that reproduce rapidly, such as epithelial cells, and is often a

CONTENT REVIEW

► Cellular Injury

• Ischemic and hypoxic injury
• Oxidative stress
• Chemical injury
• Apoptosis
• Dysplasia

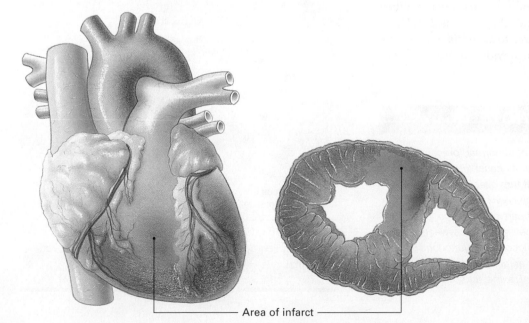

— Area of infarct —

● **Figure 1-68** Prolonged ischemia resulting from reduced flow of arterial blood to the heart muscle is the chief cause of myocardial infarction (death of heart muscle).

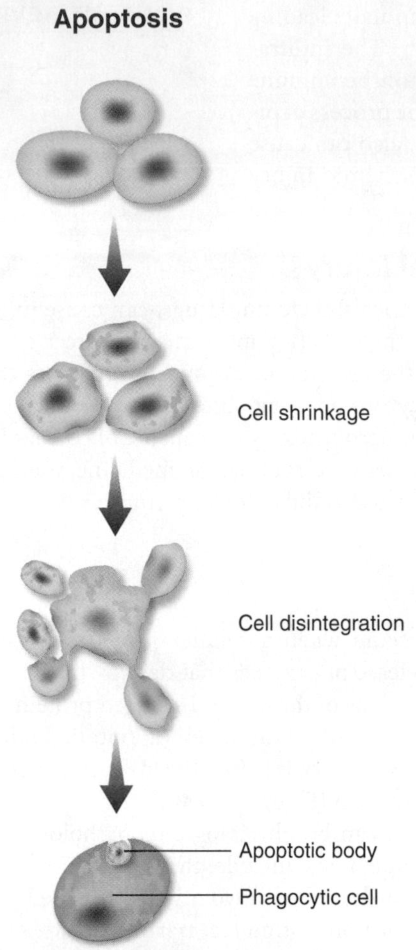

Apoptosis

Cell shrinkage

Cell disintegration

Apoptotic body

Phagocytic cell

● **Figure 1-69**   The process of apoptosis. Once the cell is dead, fragments called apoptotic bodies are cleared by scavenger cells (phagocytosis).

precursor to the development of cancer. With dysplasia there is a loss in the uniformity of the cells present as well as in their architectural orientation. In addition, the nucleus of dysplastic cells tends to be abnormally large and abnormally dense. When an entire cell layer contains dysplastic cells, it is considered to be a preinvasive neoplasm and is referred to as ***carcinoma-in-situ***. Although dysplasia is often associated with cancer, it does not necessarily progress to cancer.

CLINICAL NOTE

Cervical dysplasia is the presence of abnormal, precancerous cells on the surface of the cervix or its canal (Figure 1-70 ●). Cervical cells are epithelial cells that turn over fairly rapidly and thus grow rapidly. The interior of the cervix consists of columnar epithelial cells, while the outer part of the cervix consists of squamous epithelial cells. The demarcation between these two cell types is called the squamocolumnar junction. Distal to the squamocolumnar junction is an area of immature squamous metaplastic epithelial cells. Trauma, chronic irritation,

and cervical infections play a role in the development and maturation of the squamous epithelium of the cervix. The squamocolumnar junction is the point at which cervical dysplasia often arises and should be monitored yearly through a sampling called a Pap smear (more frequently if there is a history of cervical dysplasia).

It has been established that there is a relationship between the human papilloma virus (HPV) and cervical dysplasia and cancer. In fact, over 90 percent of women with cervical cancer carry HPV. HPV is the virus that causes genital warts and is quite common, affecting more than 24 million Americans. The warts are sometimes hard to detect, as they can be skin colored or occur only in the vagina.

The risk of cervical dysplasia is increased in women who have multiple sex partners, who had unprotected sex at a young age (under 18) or with partners who have had multiple partners, who have a history of sexually transmitted diseases, or who smoke cigarettes.

Cervical dysplasia, carcinoma-in-situ, and cervical cancer can be successfully treated if detected early enough. A vaccine is now available that can protect women against HPV infection, which helps to mitigate the chances of cervical cancer.

Cervical Dysplasia

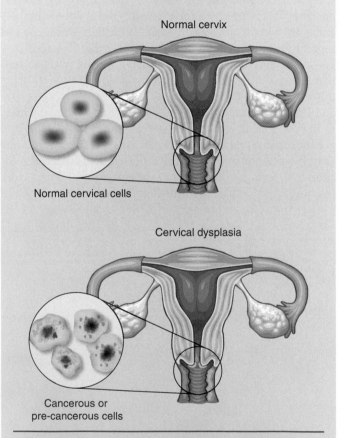

Normal cervix

Normal cervical cells

Cervical dysplasia

Cancerous or pre-cancerous cells

● **Figure 1-70**   Cervical dysplasia is the presence of abnormal, precancerous cells on the surface of the cervix or its canal.

PART 4: Disease at the Tissue Level

TISSUES

A group of cells that serve a common purpose are called a **tissue**. There are four general categories of tissue: epithelial, connective, muscle, and nervous. The study of tissues is called **histology**. The study of abnormal or diseased tissue is called **histopathology**.

In this section we will describe the types of tissue as they apply to emergency care. In addition, we will discuss the development of cancerous tissues and factors that contribute to the process.

Origin of Body Tissues

All the tissues of the body are derived from three distinct cell lines seen during early embryonic development. About two weeks after conception, the cells of the embryo start to differentiate into three layers (Figure 1-71 ●). These cell layers are referred to as **germ layers** and consist of primitive cell types that differentiate into the various tissues and organs of the body. There are three germ layers (Figure 1-72 ●):

● *Endoderm.* The **endoderm** is the innermost germ cell layer and gives rise to epithelial tissue, most of which is glandular epithelium. The endoderm is the first germ layer to develop. Cells from the endoderm eventually form the entire epithelial lining of the digestive tract with the exception of a portion of the mouth and a portion of the rectum. In addition to the digestive tract, the endoderm gives rise to the epithelial cells that line all the exocrine glands and structures that open into the digestive tract. These include:

○ Liver and associated ducts
○ Pancreas
○ Epithelium of the auditory tube and tympanic cavity
○ Trachea, bronchi, and alveoli (except the nasal cavity)
○ Urinary bladder and part of the urethra
○ Lining of follicles in the thyroid and thymus glands

● *Mesoderm.* The middle germ layer, or **mesoderm**, gives rise to numerous body tissues. These include:

○ Skeletal muscle
○ Cardiac muscle
○ Smooth muscle

Germ Cell Theory

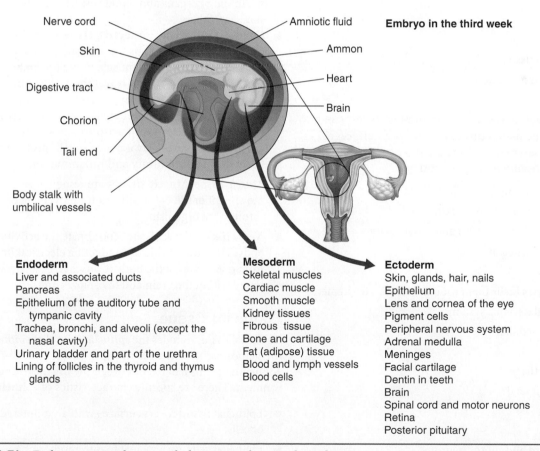

Nerve cord
Skin
Digestive tract
Chorion
Tail end
Body stalk with umbilical vessels

Amniotic fluid
Ammon
Heart
Brain

Embryo in the third week

Endoderm
Liver and associated ducts
Pancreas
Epithelium of the auditory tube and tympanic cavity
Trachea, bronchi, and alveoli (except the nasal cavity)
Urinary bladder and part of the urethra
Lining of follicles in the thyroid and thymus glands

Mesoderm
Skeletal muscles
Cardiac muscle
Smooth muscle
Kidney tissues
Fibrous tissue
Bone and cartilage
Fat (adipose) tissue
Blood and lymph vessels
Blood cells

Ectoderm
Skin, glands, hair, nails
Epithelium
Lens and cornea of the eye
Pigment cells
Peripheral nervous system
Adrenal medulla
Meninges
Facial cartilage
Dentin in teeth
Brain
Spinal cord and motor neurons
Retina
Posterior pituitary

● **Figure 1-71**   Embryonic germ layers: endoderm, mesoderm, and ectoderm.

Germ Cell Differentiation

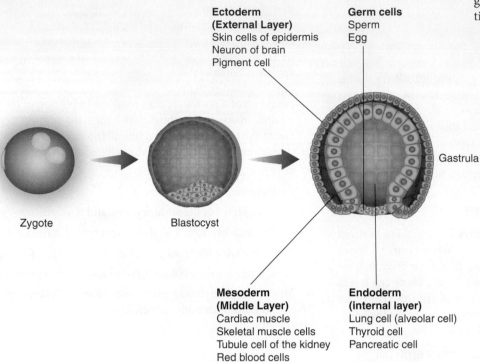

**Ectoderm
(External Layer)**
Skin cells of epidermis
Neuron of brain
Pigment cell

Germ cells
Sperm
Egg

Gastrula

Zygote

Blastocyst

**Mesoderm
(Middle Layer)**
Cardiac muscle
Skeletal muscle cells
Tubule cell of the kidney
Red blood cells
Smooth muscle (in gut)

**Endoderm
(internal layer)**
Lung cell (alveolar cell)
Thyroid cell
Pancreatic cell

● **Figure 1-72**   The germ layers give rise to the various differentiated tissues of the body.

Epithelium is derived from all three germ layers. In summary, cells from the endoderm form the epithelial lining inside viscera, cells from the mesoderm form the lining outside viscera, and cells from the ectoderm become the epithelium in skin.

Tissue Types

The germ layers just described ultimately differentiate into four primary tissue types:

● *Epithelial tissue.* **Epithelial tissues** cover the body surfaces. In addition, they line all passageways that communicate with the outside. Distribution of the epithelial tissues includes the interior of body cavities, the lining of organs and blood vessels, the outer layers of skin, and others.

● *Connective tissue.* **Connective tissues** provide a framework on which epithelial tissue rests and within which nerve tissue and muscle tissue are embedded. Blood vessels and nerves travel through connective tissue. Connective tissue not only functions as a mechanical support for other tissues but also provides an avenue for communication and transport among other tissues. Connective tissues play a major role in protecting the body through immunity and inflammation.

● *Muscle tissue.* **Muscle tissues** are responsible for the movement of the organism and for movement of substances through the organism.

● *Nerve tissue.* **Nerve tissues** coordinate the activities of the body. They are capable of conducting electrical impulses from one region of the body to another. Most nerve tissue is found within the brain and the spinal cord.

Epithelial Tissue

Epithelial tissue includes the *epithelia* (plural of *epithelium*) and the glands associated with the epithelia (Figure 1-73 ●). The epithelium forms a barrier between the organism and the environment. There are specific characteristics of epithelial tissues:

● Epithelial tissue covers surfaces with an uninterrupted layer of cells.

● Epithelial cells are attached to one another.

● Intercellular spaces in epithelia are small.

● Epithelial cells are polarized.

○ Kidney tissue

○ Fibrous tissue

○ Bone and cartilage

○ Fat (adipose) tissue

○ Blood and lymph vessels

○ Blood cells

● *Ectoderm.* The **ectoderm** is the outermost germ layer and gives rise to all the tissues that cover the body surfaces as well as the nervous system. There are three parts of the ectoderm, each resulting in different tissues:

○ External Ectoderm

■ Skin (along with glands, hair, nails)

■ Epithelium of the mouth and nasal cavity

■ Lens and cornea of the eye

○ Neural Crest

■ Melanocytes (cells that produce melanin, or pigment)

■ Peripheral nervous system

■ Adrenal medulla

■ Meninges

■ Facial cartilage

■ Dentin (in teeth)

○ Neural Tube

■ Brain

■ Spinal cord and motor neurons

■ Retina

■ Posterior pituitary

● Figure 1-73 Types and locations of epithelial tissue. *(Bledsoe, Bryan E.; Colbert, Bruce J.; Ankney, Jeff E., Essentials of Anatomy & Physiology for Emergency Care, 1st Ed., © 2011. Reprinted and electronically reproduced by permission of Pearson Education, Inc. Upper Saddle River, NJ)*

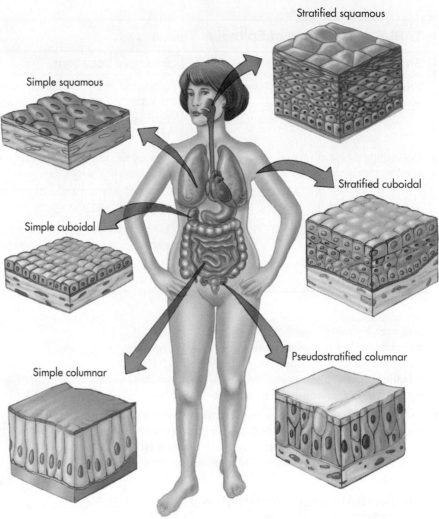

- Epithelial cells are separated from the underlying tissue by a **basement membrane**.
- There is an absence of blood vessels within epithelial tissue.

Epithelial tissue covers both external and internal body surfaces and lines any passageways that communicate with the outside. The functions of epithelial tissue are either protective or metabolic in nature. Specifically they include the following:

- *Provides physical protection.* Epithelial tissue efficiently protects both the external and internal surfaces from injury, infection, and water loss.
- *Controls permeability.* Epithelial tissue is a selective barrier in that it allows the passage of certain substances, such as proteins, but is impermeable to other substances.
- *Provides special senses.* Specialized epithelial cells provide information to the nervous system regarding changes in the environment.
- *Produces specialized secretions.* Some types of epithelial tissue contain glands that produce secretions. These secretions are classified by the mode of secretion: exocrine or endocrine. **Exocrine secretions** are deposited on the surface of the skin or another epithelial surface through ducts. There are three types of exocrine secretions:
  - ○ *Serous*—watery secretions that contain enzymes (e.g., digestive secretions)
  - ○ *Mucous*—thick, slippery secretions (e.g., nasal mucus)
  - ○ *Mixed*—contains secretions from more than one type of cell (e.g., salivary glands)

  Endocrine secretions are released into the bloodstream or surrounding tissues and occur without the aid of ducts.

Classes of Epithelium   As epithelial tissue arises from embryonic germ layers, it becomes differentiated and specialized. Each type of epithelium has a special purpose in the organism. Epithelial tissues are usually classified according to the number of cell layers present and the shape of the exposed cells.

Epithelial tissues can be classified as *simple epithelium* or *stratified epithelium*. Simple epithelium is a single cell layer thick and provides limited protection. Thus, it is primarily found in internal body surfaces. Stratified epithelium is several layers thick and provides a greater degree of protection.

The shape of the cell is also used to describe and classify epithelial tissues. Tissues with thin and flat cells are called *squamous epithelium*. Cells that have a cube-like or square shape are called *cuboidal epithelium*. Finally, cells that are tall and more slender are called *columnar epithelium*.

Using this classification system, there are several types of epithelial tissue, each with a different appearance and function. These include (Table 1–10):

- *Simple squamous epithelia*—found in areas where absorption occurs or when friction reduction is necessary, such as the renal tubules, the alveoli, the lining of body cavities, the lining of blood vessels, and the lining of the heart.
- *Simple cuboidal epithelia*—found in areas where secretion or absorption is occurring. Simple cuboidal epithelium secretes enzymes and buffers in the pancreas and salivary glands and lines the ducts of these glands. It is also found in portions of the kidney tubules.
- *Simple columnar epithelia*—found in areas where secretion and absorption occur—but where additional protection is needed such as the lining of the stomach and digestive tract as well as in many excretory ducts.
- *Pseudostratified epithelia*—found in areas where there is a mixture of cell types. Pseudostratified epithelium

TABLE 1–10 | Types of Epithelial Tissue

Shape	Number of Layers	Example Locations	Functions
Squamous (flat, scale-like cells)	Simple (single layer)	Linings of heart and blood vessels; air sacs of lungs	Allows passage of materials by diffusion
	Striated (multi layers)	Linings of mouth, esophagus, vagina; outer layer of skin	Protects underlying areas
Cuboidal (cube-shaped cells)	Simple	Kidney tubules; secretary portions of glands and ducts	Secretion; absorption
	Striated	Ducts of sweat glands, mammary glands, salivary glands	Protects underlying areas
Columnar	Simple	Most of digestive tract; bronchi; excretory ducts of some glands; uterus	Absorbs; secretes mucus, enzymes, and other substances
	Striated	Rare: urethra; junction of esophagus and stomach	Protects underlying areas; secretes mucus

is not really stratified, although it appears to be. In pseudostratified epithelia all cells are in contact with the basement membrane. This tissue type will often have cilia. It is found in the respiratory tract (nasal cavity, trachea, bronchi) and portions of the male reproductive tract.

- *Transitional epithelia*—found in areas where there is a need for protection and where there are significant changes in volume that can give rise to changes in physical factors such as pressure. Transitional cells are found in the ureters and urinary bladder.

- *Stratified squamous epithelia*—found in areas where mechanical stresses are severe. These include the surface of the skin and the lining of the mouth, tongue, esophagus, vagina, and anus.

- *Glandular epithelia*—selected types of epithelia produce exocrine secretions. These are secreted by one of three methods (Figure 1-74 ●):

  ○ *Merocrine secretion*—the secretion is released through exocytosis (the most common method)

  ○ *Apocrine secretion*—the part of the cell containing the secretion "pinches" off and then releases the secretion

  ○ *Holocrine secretion*—the entire cell is packed with secretions and then bursts apart and dies in the process

Connective Tissue

Connective tissues are deep tissues that are never exposed to the external environment (Figure 1-75 ●). They bind together and support the tissues of the body. Unlike epithelial tissue, which consists primarily of cells, connective tissue consists primarily of a substance called the *extracellular matrix*. Specific characteristics of connective tissue include the following:

- Connective tissue consists of individual cells scattered within an extracellular matrix consisting of protein fiber and a noncellular material called *ground substance*. There are three types of protein fibers:

  ○ *Collagen fibers* are strong and have great tensile strength such as seen in ligaments and tendons.

Exocrine Secretions

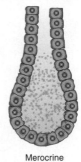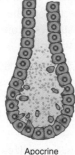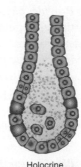

Merocrine Apocrine Holocrine

Multicellular exocrine gland	Method of Secretion	Examples
1. Merocrine	Watery serous fluid or mucus secreted through the cell membrane.	• salivary glands • pancreatic glands • some sweat glands
2. Apocrine	The part of the cell containing the secretion "pinches" off and then releases its contents.	• some sweat glands • mammary glands
3. Holocrine	Cells fill up with secretion and then burst, releasing their product.	• sebaceous glands

● **Figure 1-74** Multicellular exocrine glands and their methods of secretion.

  ○ *Elastic fibers* are randomly coiled and thus capable of stretch. They are common in the skin, lungs, and blood vessels.

  ○ *Reticular fibers* are thin strands of **collagen** that form interconnective networks that help support other tissues.

Ground substance can be solid (as in bone), liquid (as in blood), or flexible (as in cartilage). In ordinary connective tissue, the ground substance consists of water stabilized by proteins and glycoproteins. In bone, the ground substance includes minerals. In blood, the ground substance is liquid (plasma).

- Cells of connective tissue are not directly attached to one another (unlike epithelial cells).

- Individual connective tissue cells are normally separated from one another by varying amounts of extracellular matrix.

- Connective tissue is derived from the embryonic mesoderm (unlike most epithelial tissue, which is derived from ectoderm and endoderm).

There are several cell types found in connective tissues. These include:

- *Fibroblasts.* **Fibroblasts** are the most abundant cell type found in connective tissue and are responsible for the production of connective tissue fibers and ground substance.

- *Macrophages.* **Macrophages** are scattered throughout the connective tissues and engulf damaged cells or pathogens.

- *Adipocytes.* **Adipocytes**, or fat cells, contain large amounts of lipids and serve as energy stores.

- *Mast cells.* **Mast cells** are small mobile cells that are found in the connective tissues—often near blood vessels. They release chemicals as part of the body's defense system.

- *Other cells.* Occasionally other cells can be found in connective tissue such as white blood cells reacting to injury or infection.

Classes of Connective Tissue Connective tissue is classified by the physical properties of the ground substance. It is often classified as connective tissue proper and specialized connective tissue.

Connective tissue proper includes (Table 1–11):

- *Loose connective tissue.* Loose connective tissue, also called *areolar tissue*, contains more cells and fewer fibers than dense connective tissue. Loose connective tissue forms the layer that separates the skin from underlying muscle.

  ○ *Adipose tissue.* **Adipose tissue**, or fat, is a form of loose connective tissue that contains a large number of fat cells (adipocytes).

- *Dense connective tissue.* Dense connective tissue, also called *fibrous tissue*, consists mainly of collagen fibers. They include:

  ○ *Cartilage.* **Cartilage** provides a cushion between bones and helps maintain the structure of certain body parts (ear, nose). Cartilage contains specialized cells called *chondrocytes* that reside in pockets of cells in the matrix called *lacunae*. These are suspended in a firm gel extracellular matrix that contains protein fibers for strength and ground substance for resilience. Cartilage does not contain blood vessels, so the tissue obtains nutrients and removes wastes through diffusion. There are three types of cartilage:

    ■ *Hyaline*—found at the end of long bones, provides support and flexibility, and reduces friction. It is the most abundant form of cartilage.

● **Figure 1-75** Types and locations of connective tissues. *(Bledsoe, Bryan E.; Colbert, Bruce J.; Ankney, Jeff E., Essentials of Anatomy & Physiology for Emergency Care, 1st Ed., © 2011. Reprinted and electronically reproduced by permission of Pearson Education, Inc. Upper Saddle River, NJ)*

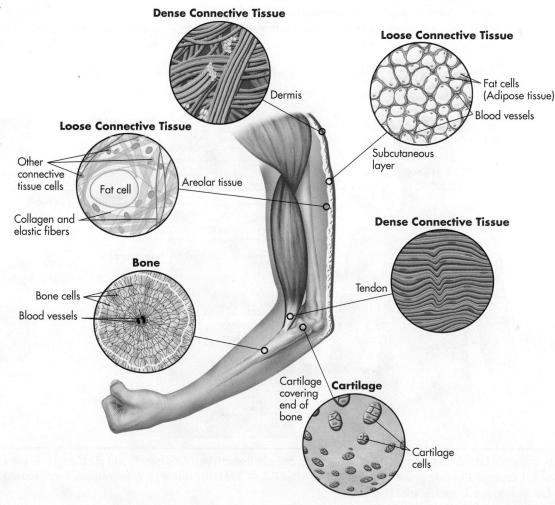

TABLE 1–11 | Types of Connective Tissue

Type	Example Locations	Functions
Connective Tissue Proper		
Loose, areolar	Between muscles, surround glands, wrapping small blood vessels and nerves	Wraps and cushions organs
Loose, adipose (fat)	Under skin, around kidneys and heart	Stores energy, insulates, cushions organs
Dense	Tendons, ligaments	Attaches bone to bone (ligaments) or bone to muscle (tendons)
Specialized Connective Tissue		
Cartilage (semisolid)	Nose (tip); rings in respiratory air tubules; external ear	Provides support and protection (by enclosing) and levers for muscles to act on
Bone (solid)	Skeleton	Provides support and protection (by enclosing) and serves as lever for muscles to act on
Blood (fluid)	Within blood vessels	Transports oxygen and carbon dioxide, nutrients, hormones, and wastes; helps fight infections

■ *Elastic*—more flexible than hyaline cartilage, elastic cartilage is found in the pinna of the ear.

■ *Fibrocartilage*—forms the outer part of the intervertebral disks that cushion the vertebral bodies. Fibrocartilage is also found between the bones of the pelvis and in selected joints. It contains fewer cells than hyaline or elastic cartilage.

○ *Bone.* Bone provides protection and support for the organism. Bone contains specialized cells called **osteocytes** situated in lacunae. Bone, along with cartilage and joints, makes up the bulk of the skeletal system. The matrix in bones contains calcium that gives the bones strength.

○ *Ligaments.* Ligaments hold bone together and contain both elastic and collagen fibers.

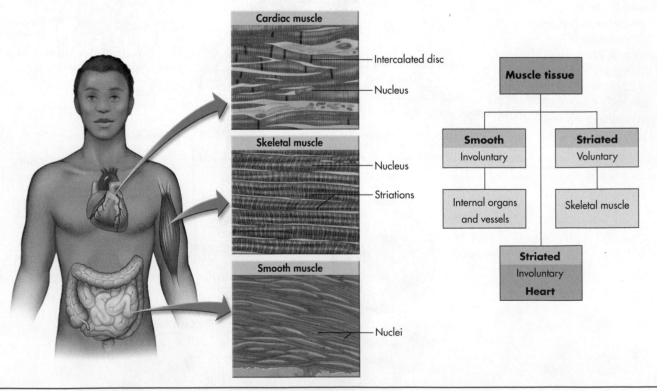

● **Figure 1-76**   Diagram and chart of the three muscle tissue types. *(Bledsoe, Bryan E.; Colbert, Bruce J.; Ankney, Jeff E., Essentials of Anatomy & Physiology for Emergency Care, 1st Ed., © 2011. Reprinted and electronically reproduced by permission of Pearson Education, Inc. Upper Saddle River, NJ)*

TABLE 1–12 | Types of Muscle Tissue

Type	Description	Example Locations	Functions
Skeletal	Long, cylindrical cells; multiple nuclei per cell; obvious striations	Muscles attached to bones	Provides voluntary movement
Cardiac	Branching, striated cells; one nucleus; specialized junctions between cells	Wall of heart	Contracts and propels blood through the circulatory system
Smooth	Cells taper at each end; single nucleus; arranged in sheets; no striations	Walls of digestive system, blood vessels, and tubules of urinary system	Propels substances or objects through internal passageways

○ *Tendons.* Tendons connect muscle to bone and allow for movement of the organism. Collagen fibers run the length of tendons, giving them strength.

Specialized connective tissues include:

● *Blood.* Blood is a collection of cells in a liquid matrix. The proteins in blood, under normal conditions, do not form fibers. Approximately half of the cells in blood are red blood cells. The remaining cells are white blood cells and platelets.

● *Lymph.* Lymph is the fluid within the lymphatic system. The lymphatic system is a network of organs, lymph nodes, lymph ducts, and lymph vessels that produce and transport lymph from tissues to the bloodstream. The lymphatic system is a major component of the body's immune system.

Muscle Tissue

Muscle tissues are specialized for contraction. They contain muscle cells that contract when stimulated. This allows for movement of the organism and for movement of substances through the organism. There are three types of muscle tissue (Figure 1-76 ● and Table 1–12):

● *Skeletal muscle.* Skeletal muscle is usually attached to bones, hence the name. When skeletal muscle contracts, bones are moved. Skeletal muscles are under voluntary control. Skeletal muscle contains striations (alternating dark and light bands) that give them a characteristic appearance under the microscope.

● *Smooth muscle.* Smooth muscle does not contain the striations seen in skeletal muscle, hence the name. Smooth muscle is under involuntary control and found in internal organs such as the digestive system, blood vessels, and bladder. Smooth muscle plays a major role in moving food through the digestive tract and removing waste. It is also important in the control of blood pressure and perfusion.

● *Cardiac muscle.* Cardiac muscle is found only in the heart and contains striations. Cardiac muscle cells are tightly connected to other cardiac muscle cells by special junctions at the plasma membranes called *intercalated discs*. These discs allow the rapid transmission of electrical impulses from one cell to another. Cardiac muscle cells are almost totally dependent on aerobic metabolism to obtain the energy needed to continue contracting. Because of this, cardiac muscle cells contain large numbers of mitochondria and abundant reserves of oxygen stores in myoglobin. Energy reserves are maintained in the form of glycogen and lipid inclusions.

Nervous Tissue

The last type of tissue is nervous tissue, is found in the brain, spinal cord, and peripheral nerves. Approximately 98 percent of nervous tissue is located in the brain and spinal cord. Nervous tissue conducts electrical impulses from one part of the body to another and controls numerous body functions.

There are two types of cells found in nervous tissue: **neurons** and **neuroglia**. Neurons are responsible for transmitting electrical impulses (Figure 1-77a ●). The neuroglia, often simply called *glial cells*, support, insulate, and protect neurons (Figure 1-77b ●).

Neoplasia

Neoplasia is an abnormal type of tissue growth where the cells grow and multiply in an uncontrolled fashion. In neoplasia, the factors that normally control cell and tissue growth are

Neuron

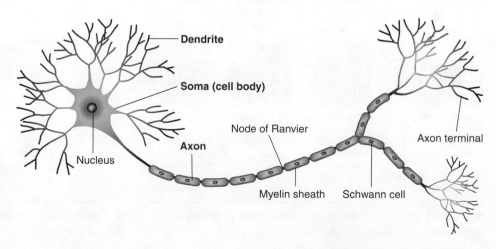

● **Figure 1-77a** Neuron.

Neuroglia

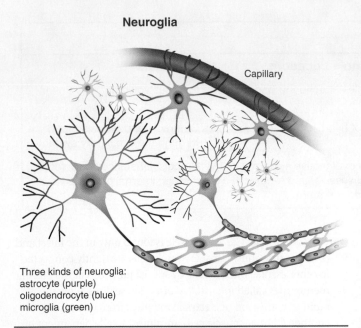

Capillary

Three kinds of neuroglia:
astrocyte (purple)
oligodendrocyte (blue)
microglia (green)

● **Figure 1-77b** Neuroglia.

lost, resulting in a continuing increase in the number of dividing cells. This mass of uncontrolled cell growth is referred to as a **tumor**.

All cell lines go through the process of differentiation. That is, primitive nonspecialized cells called **stem cells** mature into specific cell types, depending on function. Some stem cells will mature to muscle cells, others will become connective tissue cells, and so on. Cells that have not differentiated are those that have either remained in an early stage or regressed to an early stage in a process called *anaplasia*. Neoplastic cells are often less differentiated than normal cells from the same tissue or are totally undifferentiated.

As discussed before, all cells go through differentiation and adaptation. The processes of hypertrophy, hyperplasia, atrophy, and metaplasia can all occur in response to stress. However, some

Differentiation

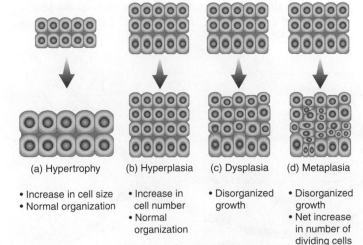

| (a) Hypertrophy | (b) Hyperplasia | (c) Dysplasia | (d) Metaplasia |

- Increase in cell size
- Normal organization

- Increase in cell number
- Normal organization

- Disorganized growth

- Disorganized growth
- Net increase in number of dividing cells

● **Figure 1-78** Processes of cell differentiation: hypertrophy, hyperplasia, dysplasia, neoplasia.

cells will develop abnormal growth patterns. When these cells are examined under a microscope, some of the cells may look abnormal. Such cells are called **dysplastic** or *atypical*. Most often the abnormalities are seen in the nucleus of the cell. A common example of dysplasia is abnormal cervical cells found on a Pap smear. These vary in their level of dysplasia with the highest level being considered cancerous (*carcinoma-in-situ*) (Figure 1-78 ●).

Neoplasia, by definition, means new growth. The tumors may be benign or malignant. Benign and malignant tumors have different characteristics. For example, benign neoplastic lesions are slow growing, usually encased by cells that are adherent, do not invade local tissue, do not spread to other body areas, and do not recur once removed. Cancerous tumors have the opposite characteristics. They grow fast and are not encapsulated, thus making removal more difficult. Malignant cells do not adhere together well, thus allowing cancerous cells to shed to other areas of the body—often through the bloodstream in a process called **metastasis**. Cancer is locally invasive (Figure 1-79 ●), and recurrence is common.

Cancer Development

Cell with genetic mutation

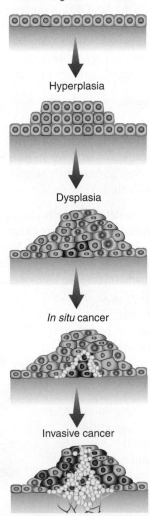

Hyperplasia

Dysplasia

In situ cancer

Invasive cancer

● **Figure 1-79** Abnormal cell development, progressing to invasive cancer.

TABLE 1–13 | Tumor Origins and Names

Origin/Prefix	Cell Type	Benign Tumor	Malignant Tumor
Epithelial			
Adeno-	Gland	Adenoma	Adenocarcinoma
Basal cell	Basal cell	Basal cell adenoma	Basal cell carcinoma
Squamous cell	Squamous cell	Keratoacanthoma	Squamous cell carcinoma
Melano-	Pigmented cell	Mole	Melanoma
Terato-	Multipotential cell	Teratoma	Teratocarcinoma
Supporting/Connective			
Chandro-	Cartilage	Chondroma	Chondrosarcoma
Fibro-	Fibroblast	Fibroma	Fibrosarcoma
Hemangio-	Blood vessel	Hemangioma	Hemangiosarcoma
Leiomyo-	Smooth muscle	Leiomyoma	Leiomyosarcoma
Lipo-	Fat	Lipoma	Liposarcoma
Meningio-	Meninges	Meningioma	Meningiosarcoma
Myo-	Muscle	Myoma	Myosarcoma
Osteo-	Bone	Osteoma	Osteosarcoma
Rhabdomyo-	Striated muscle	Rhabdomyoma	Rhabdomyosarcoma
Blood/Lymphatic			
Lympho-	Lymphocyte		Lymphoma or lymphocytic leukemia
Erythro-	Erythrocyte		Erythrocytic leukemia
Myelo-	Bone marrow		Myeloma or myelogenous leukemia

Most cancers are either of epithelial origin or connective tissue origin. Some tumors contain cells that are so undifferentiated that the cell of origin cannot be determined (Table 1–13).

Various factors have been associated with the development of cancer, termed *oncogenesis.* Among these oncogenic factors are carcinogens and radiation (Figure 1-80 ●). Carcinogens are chemicals capable of causing cancer. Radiation is also capable of causing cancer—most often tumors of the skin, internal organs, and leukemia. Radiation can result from several sources and damages the genetic material in the cell, possibly resulting in a mutation. Some mutations repair themselves, while others remain but do not cause adverse effects, and yet others result in the development of cancer. While carcinogens and radiation have been proven to cause cancer, there are several factors that remain highly suspect. These include such possible causes of cancer as viruses, genetics, environmental factors, hormones, and perhaps chronic infection or irritation.

Viruses that produce cancers are called *oncogenic viruses.* That is, genetic material within the virus (either RNA or DNA), called an *oncogene,* can cause malignant transformation of host cells when they are incorporated into the host cell DNA. The link between certain viruses and cancer is pretty strong. As already noted, human papilloma virus (HPV) has been found to be a cause of cervical cancer in women. Chronic infections with hepatitis B virus (HBV) and hepatitis C virus (HCV) have been associated with the development of hepatocellular carcinoma. Whether this results from the virus itself or the resultant infection and inflammation caused by the virus remains unclear.

Genetics is thought to be responsible for some cancers. While the link between genetics and cancer has not been definitively made, it is clear that some families tend to develop cancers while others do not. In these cases, the environment may be a confounding variable. A number of genes have been identified that play a role in the development of some cancers. Persons born with one of these genes may be more prone to cancer yet may not ultimately develop cancer.

The environment is a definite risk factor for the development of cancer. Some environmental factors have been documented to be carcinogenic. Asbestos exposure, for example,

Oncogenesis

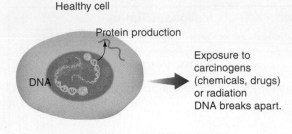

Healthy cell

Protein production

DNA

Exposure to carcinogens (chemicals, drugs) or radiation DNA breaks apart.

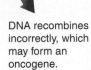

DNA recombines incorrectly, which may form an oncogene.

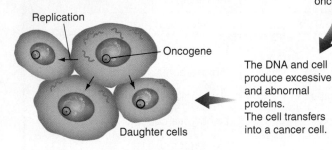

Replication

Oncogene

Daughter cells

The DNA and cell produce excessive and abnormal proteins.
The cell transfers into a cancer cell.

The cancer cell replicates its DNA and divides, forming daughter cells with an identical oncogene. Replication continues, causing the cancer to grow and spread.

● **Figure 1-80** Oncogenesis (development of cancer).

has been linked to a rare form of cancer called a mesothelioma. These tumors are more common in people who have a history of significant exposures to asbestos. Bladder cancer was noted to be more common in printing press operators. The cause was later linked to a chemical (benzidine) in the ink. Again, in these cases there is an identified carcinogen.

Our environment is so diverse and there are so many possible carcinogens present that many have not been clearly linked to the development of cancers. Radiation is also present in the environment. For example, the incidence of thyroid cancers was markedly increased in Japan after the United States dropped atomic bombs on the cities of Nagasaki and Hiroshima in 1945. When the nuclear reactor at the Chernobyl nuclear plant in the Ukraine exploded in 1986, over five million people were exposed to the resulting radiation. Subsequently, that nuclear disaster has produced the biggest group of cancers ever from a single incident with almost 2,000 cases of thyroid cancer being documented since the reactor explosion. Consequences of the disruptions to nuclear power plants in Japan resulting from a severe earthquake and tidal wave in 2011 are yet to develop and be analyzed.

Hormones are thought to play a role in the development of certain cancers. Some tumors, especially tumors of the breast, have been found to have receptors for the female hormone estrogen. Breast cancers with estrogen receptors have increased growth while estrogen is present and decreased growth or even tumor regression when estrogen is removed. The administration of estrogen to men with prostate cancer sometimes inhibits cancer growth.

The process of developing a malignant neoplasia is called **carcinogenesis** and occurs in three stages: initiation, promotion,

and progression (Figure 1-81 ●). *Initiation* is the event that begins the transformation from normal tissue to cancer. As just discussed, the factor may be a carcinogen, radiation, or a combination of factors. Initiation does not mean that malignancy will ultimately develop, just that the process has started. For example, a carcinogen such as tar from tobacco will bind to the DNA in the susceptible cells, causing errors in replication and the subsequent formation of dysplastic daughter cells. Dysplasia can result in anaplasia.

The second phase is *promotion*. A promoter can be a carcinogen or any of the factors discussed earlier that are associated with cancer development. Promotion is necessary for the continued development of the tumor and speeds up the process. The growth rate increases because the cells divide more rapidly. During promotion, cells begin to change from dysplasia to anaplasia. However, the promotion stage is still considered precancerous.

The last stage in carcinogenesis is *progression*. At this point, a malignancy exists and the cells are anaplastic in appearance. The more poorly differentiated and primitive the cells are in appearance, the faster will be the growth of the tumor. Progression is followed by growth and, subsequently, local tissue invasion and possible metastasis. Unfortunately, in many cases, cancer is not diagnosed until this stage of carcinogenesis.

Once cancer develops, it becomes invasive. If the affected tissue is a squamous epithelium, and the tumor has not extended past the basement membrane, it is considered *carcinoma-in-situ*. Cancer spreads along tissue planes and attaches to various tissues. Sometimes, individual cells or clumps of cells will be shed from the primary tumor and travel through a blood vessel or lymphatic channel to another part of the body, where they will begin to develop a secondary tumor (metastasis). The distal spread of tumor cells makes treatment difficult and often causes death.

Cancer cells are usually graded by the degree of cell differentiation present. The grade impacts the prognosis (likely outcome). The grading system is as follows:

- *Grade X.* The grade cannot be assessed. (Undetermined Grade) Prognosis: Undetermined

- *Grade 1.* The cells are well-differentiated and closely resemble the cells of the tissue of origin. Few mitotic figures (cells undergoing division) are seen. (Low-Grade) Prognosis: Good

- *Grade 2.* The cells are moderately differentiated with some structural similarity to the tissue of origin. Moderate mitotic figures seen. (Intermediate Grade) Prognosis: Fair

- *Grade 3.* The cells are poorly differentiated with little resemblance to the tissue of origin. Many mitotic figures seen. (High Grade) Prognosis: Fair to Poor

● Figure 1-81 Carcinogenesis (development of a malignant neoplasia).

● *Grade 4.* The cells are undifferentiated or dedifferentiated, appear bizarre and primitive, and do not resemble the tissue of origin. Many mitotic figures seen. (High Grade) Prognosis: Poor

Carcinogenesis

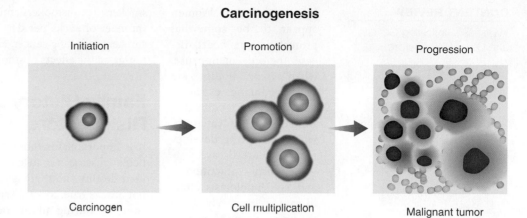

Initiation — Carcinogen

Promotion — Cell multiplication

Progression — Malignant tumor

Grading is somewhat subjective. Nevertheless, the higher the grade, the more the cells are undifferentiated and the worse the prognosis.

Often cancer is *staged* based on numerous findings but primarily indicating the degree to which the cancer is spread. Stages 1 to 4 are usually described, with stage 1 being the least advanced stage of the cancer's progression and stage 4 being the most advanced. Staging is usually based on the size of the tumor, whether lymph nodes contain cancer, and whether the cancer has spread from the original site to other parts of the body. Staging is particularly important in planning treatment strategies and in determining the prognosis.

PART 5: Disease at the Organ Level

GENETIC AND OTHER CAUSES OF DISEASE

When we think of disease at the **organ** level, at the level of **organ systems**, and at the level of the total human **organism**, we are likely to think first of infections caused by pathogens, including bacteria, viruses, fungi, and parasites. In recent years, great strides have been made in the medical treatment of infectious diseases, but—as we have been discussing throughout this chapter—many diseases result from genetic causes, which have been far more difficult to identify and treat. The picture is additionally complicated by the fact that many diseases result from a combination of genetic and environmental factors (including lifestyle factors) as well as factors such as age and gender.

Even a family history of a particular disease does not necessarily mean that the disease has a purely genetic origin, because families also share environmental and lifestyle factors that may cause or contribute to the family disease. While family history points to the possibility of genetic causes, these cannot be confirmed, much less treated, until scientists are able to make definitive identifications of the defective genes or chromosomes that cause or contribute to particular diseases.

At present, there is increasing progress in identifying and understanding genetic and other noninfectious causes of disease. Many promising advances toward gene therapies (the replacement of defective genes with normal genes) and other therapies for diseases have been made.

Genetics, Environment, Lifestyle, Age, and Gender

As noted earlier, our inherited traits are determined by molecules of deoxyribonucleic acid, or DNA, which form structures called genes that reside on larger structures called chromosomes within the nuclei of all our cells. We inherit our genetic structure from our parents. Every one of a person's somatic cells (all the cells except the sex cells) contains 46 chromosomes. The sex cells, however, contain only 23 chromosomes each. The sex cells contribute these 23 chromosomes to the offspring. Thus, the offspring receives 23 chromosomes from the father and 23 chromosomes from the mother, resulting in a total of 46 chromosomes. Occasionally one or more of a person's genes or chromosomes is abnormal, and this may cause a congenital disease (one we are born with) or a propensity toward acquiring a disease later in life.

Some diseases are thought to be purely genetic. For example, cystic fibrosis, which affects mainly people of European origin, and sickle cell disease, which affects mainly people of African origin, are known to be caused by disorders of single genes. They affect different populations to a different degree because of the evolutionary history of those populations. A genetic disease may be caused by a single defective gene or by several defective genes or chromosomes. Single-gene causes are, obviously, easier for medical researchers to identify and potentially devise treatments for than are other, more complex genetic causes of disease.

Other diseases are caused by a combination of genetic and environmental factors and are called *multifactorial disorders.* For example, Type II (adult-onset) diabetes has a very high correlation with family history of the disease. However, it is also affected by environmental and lifestyle factors such as a high-fat or high-carbohydrate diet and lack of exercise, which results in obesity, and with age. (There is a higher incidence of Type II diabetes in overweight people, and the disease tends to appear in middle age or later.) Heart disease, which is highly correlated with family history and age, also has a gender/

CONTENT REVIEW

▶ Diseases Involving Genetic
and Other Risk Factors

- Immunologic disorders
- Cancer
- Endocrine disorders
- Hematologic disorders
- Cardiovascular disorders
- Renal disorders
- Rheumatic disorders
- Gastrointestinal disorders
- Neuromuscular disorders
- Psychiatric disorders

hormonal factor: Women appear to be somewhat protected from heart disease before menopause, when their bodies are still producing estrogen. Following menopause, women quickly "catch up" with men in the development of heart disease.

Clinical practitioners and epidemiologists study disease, respectively, from the point of view of their effects on individuals and from the point of view of their effects on populations as a whole.

- *Effects on individuals.* Physicians and other clinical practitioners study the effects of diseases on individuals, and find it instructive to view the development of diseases as products of the interactions among three factors: *host, agent,* and *environment.* This establishes a framework for determining how one, or a combination, of these factors may precipitate a disease state. Genetic predisposition, gender, and ethnic origin are determinants related to the host. These may interact with a specific agent, in a specific type of environment, to cause illness. The agent may be a bacterium, toxin, gunshot, or other pathophysiologic process. The environment may be defined by the local climate, socioeconomic or demographic features, culture, religion, and associated factors. Determination of how the host, agent, and environment interact may yield solutions to curing a disease process. Injury and trauma are now being viewed as "diseases," in the sense of how the interaction of host, agent, and environment may contribute to an understanding of what, heretofore, have been perceived as social problems.

- *Effects on populations.* Epidemiologists, who study the effects of diseases on populations, generally report disease data with three basic measures: *incidence, prevalence,* and *mortality. Morbidity,* a term commonly used in discussing disease statistics, can be more precisely reported as incidence and prevalence. Incidence is the number of new cases of the disease that are reported in a given period of time, usually 1 year. Prevalence is the proportion of the total population who are affected by the disease at a given point in time. (Prevalence is higher than incidence, as those who acquire the disease each year are added to those who already have the disease.) *Mortality* is the rate of death from the disease.

Epidemiologists and clinical practitioners are now collaborating to study risk factors, such as the relationship between smoking and lung cancer. Risk factor analysis is both statistical and complex. Although the correlation of smoking to lung cancer is extremely high, not everyone who smokes develops lung cancer, and not everyone who develops lung cancer has been a smoker. Risk factor analysis would compare the number of smokers to nonsmokers among lung cancer cases, the pack/year (number of packs per day = number of years) history of the smokers with lung cancer, factors that might have aggravated or mitigated the effects of smoking, and so on.

Family History and Associated Risk Factors

It is important for those who have a family history of a particular disease not to conclude that acquiring the disease is their destiny and there is nothing they can do about it. This is not always true. Most diseases with a genetic component that come on during adulthood also have associated risk factors that can be modified to prevent, delay, or reduce the impact of the disease.

Consider the variety of possible risk factors for disease: People who live in less-developed countries are often at higher risk for disease from microorganisms flourishing in their water supply and disease transmission caused by poor sanitation. Physical conditions commonly seen in larger U.S. cities as well as rural areas, such as inadequate housing, poor nutrition, and little or no medical attention, potentiate disease transmission. Chemical factors such as smoke, smog, illicit drug use, occupational chemical exposure, and additives in our food are causative agents for a variety of diseases.

Personal habit is among the most publicized—and controllable—causes of disease in our society. For example, predisposing factors for cardiovascular disease include smoking, excessive alcohol consumption, inactivity, and obesity. Unfortunately, changes in individual lifestyle often occur only after a disease has already manifested itself. As we age, the predisposing factors and causative agents take their toll. The body's ability to defend itself against disease decreases due to the effects of aging on our immunologic system and other compensatory mechanisms.

Following is a discussion of some of the most common diseases in which both genetics and other risk factors play a role. You will notice, as you read, that the causation of various diseases varies widely, and that while the causes are known for some diseases, the causes of other diseases are still not clearly understood.

Immunologic Disorders

A number of immunologic disorders, such as rheumatic fever, allergies, and asthma, are more prevalent among those with a family history of the disorder but also involve other risk factors.

Rheumatic fever is an inflammatory reaction to an infection but is not an infection itself. There seems to be a hereditary factor, but inadequate nutrition and crowded living conditions are contributing factors.

Allergies often have a family history factor (and some allergies can be passed from the mother to the fetus during pregnancy). However, allergic reactions are triggered by exposure to allergens and can usually be controlled by avoiding or reducing the presence of allergens as well as with medication.

Asthma sufferers may inherit the propensity for airway-narrowing in response to various stimuli, but other triggering factors may be identified and, perhaps, controlled, including stress, overexertion, exposure to cold air, and stimuli such as pollens, dust mites, cockroach detritus, and smoke.

Cancer

A wide variety of family history and environmental factors are included among the risk factors for cancer. Some kinds of cancer, such as breast and colorectal cancer, tend to cluster in families and seem to have a combination of genetic and environmental causes. Others, such as lung cancer, are more strongly identified with environmental causes.

For *breast cancer*, the greatest risk factor is female gender. The second highest risk factor is age. Approximately two out of three women with invasive breast cancer are diagnosed after age 55. A history of breast cancer in a first-degree relative (mother, sister, or daughter) increases the risk by two or three times. Some progress has been made in identifying genes for certain breast cancers. Lifestyle factors such as lack of exercise and obesity may contribute slightly to the incidence of breast cancer, but this has not been proven.

As with breast cancer, *colorectal cancer* risk factors include age (with the incidence rising after age 40 and peaking between 60 and 75) and family history (incidence in a first-degree relative increases the risk by two or three times). There are gender factors, with rectal cancer being more common in men and colon cancer more common in women. Diet may also be a risk factor, although recent studies have failed to confirm a link between a high-fat, low-fiber diet and colorectal cancer. (However, a high-fat, low-fiber diet has been positively linked to heart disease and other health problems.)

The causes of *lung cancer* are overwhelmingly environmental. Smoking has been identified as the main cause of 90 percent of lung cancers in men and 70 percent of lung cancers in women. Lung cancer can also be caused by inhaling substances such as asbestos, arsenic, and nickel, usually in the workplace.

Endocrine Disorders

The most common endocrine disorder is *diabetes mellitus,* which is a leading cause of blindness, heart disease, kidney failure, and premature death. The causes of diabetes are complex and still not well understood.

There are two major types of diabetes: type I and type II. Type I diabetes usually occurs before age 40, sometimes in childhood. Although it is less prevalent than type II diabetes (accounting for about 20 percent of diabetes cases), it is more severe. In the type I diabetic, the pancreas produces no or almost no insulin, which is required for the cellular utilization of glucose, the body's chief source of energy. Type I diabetics must take insulin daily. There is some association of type I diabetes with family history (siblings of type I diabetics have a 6 percent risk compared to 0.3 percent in the general population), and medical researchers have pinpointed some possible genetic factors. Other causative factors may include autoimmunity disorders and viral infections that invade the pancreas and destroy the insulin-producing cells.

Type II diabetes accounts for about 80 percent of all diabetes cases. It usually occurs after age 40 and the incidence increases with age. It clusters much more strongly in families than does type I diabetes (siblings have a 10 to 15 percent risk). In contrast to type I diabetes, in which there is a total lack of insulin, type II diabetes is associated with a decreased insulin receptor response or a decrease in insulin production. Diet and exercise may also be factors, since the majority of type II diabetics are obese. Type II diabetes can often be controlled with diet and exercise or with oral medications.

Hematologic Disorders

Hereditary coagulation disorders have been studied by geneticists and physicians in great detail. There are many causes of hereditary hematologic disorders such as gene alteration and histocompatibility (tissue interaction) dysfunctions.

Hemophilia is a bleeding disorder that is caused by a genetic clotting factor deficiency. It can be mild, but if severe it can cause not only serious bruising but also bleeding into the joints, which can lead to crippling deformities. A slight bump on the head can cause bleeding within the skull, often resulting in brain damage and death. The heredity is sex-linked (associated with the sex chromosomes), inherited through the mother, and affects male children almost exclusively. There is no cure, but administration of concentrated clotting factors can improve the condition.

Hemochromatosis is another genetic disorder, but this time caused by a histocompatibility complex dysfunction. It is marked by an excessive absorption and accumulation of iron in the body, causing weight loss, joint pain, abdominal pain, palpitations, and testicular atrophy in males. It is treated by removing blood from the body at intervals.

Not all blood disorders are genetic. Environmental factors, for example, can cause *anemia* (reduction in circulating red blood cells). For example, some antihypertensive medications and other drugs may cause a drug-induced hemolytic (red-blood-cell-destroying) anemia.

Cardiovascular Disorders

The cardiovascular system can be greatly affected by genetic disorders. Disorders such as *prolongation of the QT interval* (a delay between depolarization and repolarization of the ventricles as revealed in an electrocardiogram) and *mitral-valve prolapse* (an upward ballooning of the valve between the left ventricle and atrium that allows blood to regurgitate back into the atrium when the ventricle contracts) tend to cluster in families.

The American Heart Association lists heredity as a major risk factor for cardiovascular disease. Those with parents who have *coronary artery disease* (deposits on the walls of the coronary arteries that reduce blood flow to the heart muscle) have an approximately fivefold risk of developing the disease. This is why it is important to ask about family history of congenital heart disease (CHD), hypertension, and stroke when assessing patients with possible cardiovascular disease. However, environmental factors, such as a diet high in saturated fats and cholesterol (or a diet high in carbohydrates) and lack of exercise, also play a large role in cardiovascular disease.

Hypertension (high blood pressure) is a major risk factor, not only for cardiac disease but also for stroke and kidney disease.

Studies of family history show that approximately 20 to 40 percent of the causation of hypertension is genetic. The remaining causative factors, then, are environmental, and may include high sodium ingestion, lack of physical activity, stress, and obesity.

Not all cardiac disorders have a genetic component. For example, *cardiomyopathy* (disease affecting the heart muscle) is thought to occur secondarily to other causes such as infectious disease, toxin exposure, connective tissue disease, or nutritional deficiencies, which may be partially or totally environmental.

Renal Disorders

Renal (kidney) failure is caused by a variety of factors (primarily hypertension) that may eventually require a patient to receive dialysis treatment several times a week. As the location of dialysis treatment shifts from medical centers to homes and community satellite centers, EMS personnel are increasingly being called to deal with the complications of dialysis. These include problems with vascular access devices (shunts, fistulas), localized infection and sepsis, and electrolyte abnormalities (hyperkalemia), which can result in cardiac arrest.

Rheumatic Disorders

Gout is a condition that may have both genetic and environmental causes. It is characterized by severe arthritic pain caused by deposit of crystals in the joints, most commonly the great toe. The crystals form as the result of an abnormally high level of uric acid in the blood that may be caused when the kidneys do not excrete enough uric acid or by high production of uric acid. High production of uric acid may be caused by a hereditary metabolic abnormality. Although the underlying cause may be genetic, attacks of gout can be triggered by environmental factors such as trauma, alcohol consumption, ingestion of certain foods, stress, or other illnesses. Patients with gout also have a tendency to develop *kidney stones.*

Gastrointestinal Disorders

Gastrointestinal disorders have a variety of causes, and the causes of some are not known. *Lactose intolerance,* for example, is usually identified by the inability of the patient to tolerate milk and some other dairy products. The patient lacks lactase, the enzyme that usually breaks down lactose in the digestive tract. This enzyme deficiency may be congenital (inborn) or may develop later on. It is more common in those of Asian, African, Native American, or Mediterranean ancestry than it is among northern and western Europeans.

Crohn's disease is a chronic inflammation of the wall of the digestive tract that usually affects the small intestine, the large intestine, or both. The cause is not known, but medical researchers have focused on immune system dysfunction, infection, and diet as the major probabilities. A similar disorder is ulcerative colitis, in which the large intestine becomes inflamed and develops ulcers. As with Crohn's disease, the cause is not known, but an overactive immune response is suspected, and heredity seems to play a role.

Peptic ulcers develop when the normal protective structures and mechanisms, such as mucous production, break down and areas in the lining of the stomach or duodenum are inflamed by stomach acid and digestive juices. Environmental factors, bacterial infection (by *Helicobacter pylori*), diet, stress, and alcohol consumption are thought to play roles in the development of peptic ulcers. Many medications, particularly nonsteroidal anti-inflammatory medications, are associated with ulcer formation.

Cholecystitis is an inflammation of the gallbladder that usually results from blockage by a gallstone. There may be a genetic predisposition for gallstone formation. Gallstones are more prevalent in women and in some groups such as Native Americans and Mexican Americans. Other risk factors include age, a high-fat diet, and obesity.

Obesity can be defined as being more than 20 percent over the ideal body weight. Obesity has both an environmental and familial risk transmission. Research has shown that children whose parents are obese have a much-increased chance of developing obesity. Environmental factors such as proper nutrition and exercise may not be modeled or taught by obese parents, but there also seems to be a genetic factor to many cases of obesity. Obesity has been linked to, or defined as a cause for, diseases such as hypertension, heart disease, and vascular diseases.

Neuromuscular Disorders

Diseases of the nervous and muscular systems also have a variety of causes. *Huntington's disease* (which results in uncontrollable jerking and writhing movements) and muscular dystrophy (which results in progressive muscle weakness) are both known to be caused by genetic defects.

Multiple sclerosis (which affects the nerves of the eye, brain, and spinal cord) seems to have some hereditary factor with clustering among close relatives. Its exact cause is unknown, but it seems to result when the virus-triggered autoimmune response begins to attack the myelin sheath that protects the nerves.

Alzheimer's disease is thought to cause about 50 percent of dementias, or progressive mental deterioration. Its cause is unknown, but it does cluster strongly in families and appears to be either caused or influenced by specific gene abnormalities.

Psychiatric Disorders

Genetic and biological causes of psychiatric disorders are being studied and increasingly understood. An example is *schizophrenia,* which affects about 1 percent of the population worldwide and is more prevalent than Alzheimer's disease, diabetes, or multiple sclerosis. The schizophrenic loses contact with reality and suffers from hallucinations, delusions, abnormal thinking, and disrupted social functioning. People who develop schizophrenia are now thought to be "biologically vulnerable" to the disease, but what makes them vulnerable is not fully understood. The cause may be a genetic predisposition or some problem that occurs before, during, or after birth or a viral infection of the brain.

Another common psychiatric disorder is *manic-depressive illness,* also called *bipolar disorder,* in which the person experiences alternating periods of depression and mania or excitement. It can be mild or severe enough to interfere with the patient's ability to work or function socially. Manic-depressive illness affects about twice as many people as schizophrenia. It is believed to be hereditary, but the exact gene deficit has not yet been discovered.

HYPOPERFUSION

Hypoperfusion (shock) is a condition that is progressive (that is, it triggers a self-worsening cycle of pathophysiologic events) and fatal if not corrected. It can occur for many reasons such as trauma, fluid loss, myocardial infarction, infection, allergic reaction, spinal cord injury, and other causes. Although causes differ, all forms of shock have the same underlying pathophysiology at the cellular and tissue levels.

The Physiology of Perfusion

As discussed earlier, all body cells require a constant supply of oxygen and other essential nutrients (primarily glucose), while waste products, such as carbon dioxide, must be constantly removed. It is the circulatory system, in conjunction with the respiratory and gastrointestinal systems, that provides the body's cells with these essential nutrients and removal of wastes. This is accomplished by the passage of blood through the capillaries, the small vessels that interface with body cells, while oxygen, carbon dioxide, nutrients, and wastes are exchanged by movement across the capillary walls and cell membranes. This constant and necessary passage of blood through the body's tissues is called **perfusion**.

Inadequate perfusion of body tissues is **hypoperfusion**, which is commonly called **shock**. Shock occurs first at a cellular level. If allowed to progress, the tissues, organs, organ systems, and ultimately the entire organism are affected.

Components of the Circulatory System

Perfusion is dependent on a functioning and intact circulatory system. The three components of the circulatory system are listed below. A derangement in any one of these can adversely affect perfusion (Figure 1-82 ●).

- The pump (heart)
- The fluid (blood)
- The container (blood vessels)

The Pump   The heart is the pump of the cardiovascular system. It receives blood from the venous system, pumps it to the lungs for oxygenation, and then pumps it to the peripheral tissues. The amount of blood ejected by the heart in one contraction is referred to as the **stroke volume**. Factors affecting stroke volume include:

- Preload
- Cardiac contractile force
- Afterload

Preload is the amount of blood delivered to the heart during diastole (when the heart fills with blood between contractions). Preload depends on venous return. The venous system is a capacitance, or storage, system. That is, it can be contracted or expanded, to some extent, as needed to meet the physiologic demands of the body. When additional oxygenated blood is required, the venous capacitance is reduced, thus increasing the amount of blood delivered to the heart. The greater the preload, the greater the stroke volume.

Preload also affects **cardiac contractile force**. The greater the volume of preload, the more the ventricles are stretched. The greater the stretch, up to a certain point, the greater will be the subsequent cardiac contraction. This is referred to as the *Frank Starling mechanism* and can be illustrated through the example of a rubber band. The more the rubber band is stretched, the greater will be its velocity when released.

In addition, cardiac contractile strength is affected by circulating hormones called **catecholamines** (epinephrine and norepinephrine) controlled by the sympathetic nervous system. Catecholamines enhance cardiac contractile strength by action on the beta-adrenergic receptors on the surface of the cells.

Finally, stroke volume is affected by **afterload**. Afterload is the resistance against which the ventricle must contract. This resistance must be overcome before ventricular contraction can result in ejection of blood. Afterload is determined by the degree of peripheral vascular resistance (defined later). This, in effect, is due to the amount of vasoconstriction present. The arterial system can be expanded and contracted to meet the metabolic demands of the body. The greater the resistance offered by the arterial system, the less the stroke volume.

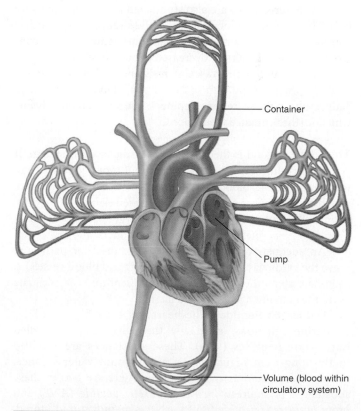

Container

Pump

Volume (blood within circulatory system)

● **Figure 1-82**   Components of the circulatory system.

The amount of blood pumped by the heart in 1 minute is referred to as the **cardiac output**. It is a function of stroke volume (milliliters per beat) and heart rate (beats per minute). Cardiac output is usually expressed in liters per minute. It can be defined by this equation:

$$\text{Stroke volume} \times \text{Heart rate} = \text{Cardiac output}$$

The foregoing equation illustrates the factors that can affect cardiac output. An increase in stroke volume or an increase in heart rate can increase cardiac output. Conversely, a decrease in stroke volume or a decrease in heart rate can decrease cardiac output. The blood pressure is dependent on both cardiac output and peripheral vascular resistance.

$$\text{Cardiac output} \times \text{Peripheral vascular resistance} = \text{Blood pressure}$$

Peripheral vascular resistance is the pressure against which the heart must pump. Since the circulatory system is a closed system, increasing either cardiac output or peripheral vascular resistance will increase blood pressure. Likewise, a decrease in cardiac output or a decrease in peripheral vascular resistance will decrease blood pressure.

The body strives to keep the blood pressure relatively constant by employing *compensatory mechanisms* and **negative feedback loops**. As noted earlier, baroreceptors in the carotid sinuses and in the arch of the aorta closely monitor blood pressure. If blood pressure increases, the baroreceptors send signals to the brain that cause the blood pressure to return to its normal values. This is accomplished by decreasing the heart rate, decreasing the preload, or decreasing peripheral vascular resistance.

The baroreceptors are also stimulated if the blood pressure falls. The heart rate is increased, as is the strength of the cardiac contractions. There is also arteriolar constriction, venous constriction (which results in decreased container size), and overall increased peripheral vascular resistance. Also, the adrenal medulla (the inner portion of the adrenal gland) is stimulated. This results in the secretion of epinephrine and norepinephrine, which further enhance the response.

The Fluid   Blood is the fluid of the cardiovascular system. It is a viscous fluid; that is, it is thicker and more adhesive than water. As a result, blood flows more slowly than water. Blood, which consists of the plasma and the formed elements (red cells, white cells, and platelets), transports oxygen, carbon dioxide, nutrients, hormones, metabolic waste products, and heat.

An adequate amount of blood is required for perfusion. Since the cardiovascular system (the heart and blood vessels) is a closed system, the volume of blood present must be adequate to fill the container, as described later.

Natriuretic Peptides   The heart has been found to have endocrine functions, especially through substances called **natriuretic peptides (NPs)**. These substances are involved in the long-term regulation of sodium and water balance, blood volume, and arterial pressure. There are two of these substances of interest: *atrial natriuretic peptide (ANP)* and *brain natriuretic peptide (BNP)*. ANP is manufactured, stored, and released by the heart's atrial muscle cells in response to such things as atrial distension and sympathetic stimulation.

BNP is manufactured, stored, and released by the heart's ventricular muscle cells in response to ventricular dilation and sympathetic stimulation. BNP was first identified in the brains of rats, which is why it was named brain natriuretic peptide, although it was later found to be manufactured in both the brain and in the ventricles.

Natriuretic peptides serve as a sort of counterregulatory system to the renin-angiotensin system. They are involved in the long-term regulation of sodium and water balance, blood volume, and arterial blood pressure. These hormones decrease aldosterone release from the adrenal cortex, which increases the glomerular filtration rate (GFR) and produces natriuresis (sodium loss) and diuresis (water loss). It also decreases renin release by decreasing angiotensin II. This results in a reduction in blood volume and thus a reduction in central venous pressure (CVP), cardiac output (CO), and arterial blood pressure. Chronic elevation of natriuretic peptides appears to decrease arterial blood pressure primarily by decreasing peripheral vascular resistance (Figure 1-83 ●).

BNP levels are elevated in congestive heart failure (CHF) and have become a marker for the presence of CHF. BNP (marketed as nesiritide) can be administered as a treatment for acute decompensated CHF.

The Container   Blood vessels (arteries, arterioles, capillaries, venules, and veins) serve as the container of the cardiovascular system. The blood vessels can be thought of as a continuous, closed, and pressurized pipeline by which blood moves throughout the body. While the heart functions as the pump of the circulatory system, the blood vessels—under the control of the autonomic nervous system—can regulate blood flow to different areas of the body by adjusting their size as well as by selectively rerouting blood through the microcirculation.

While the arteries and veins, like the heart, are subject to direct stimulation from sympathetic portions of the autonomic

Physiology of the Natriuretic Peptides

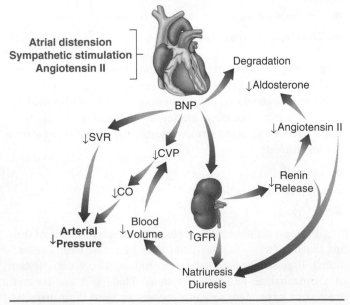

● **Figure 1-83**   Physiology of the natriuretic peptides.

nervous system, the *microcirculation* (comprised of the small vessels: the arterioles, capillaries, and venules) is primarily responsive to local tissue needs. The capability of some vessels in the capillary network to adjust their diameter permits the microcirculation to selectively supply undernourished tissue, while temporarily bypassing tissues with no immediate need. Capillaries have a sphincter at the origin of the capillary (between arteriole and capillary), called the *precapillary sphincter,* and another at the end of the capillary (between capillary and venule), called the *postcapillary sphincter.* The precapillary sphincter responds to local tissue conditions, such as acidosis and hypoxia, and opens as more arterial blood is needed. The postcapillary sphincter opens when blood is to be emptied into the venous system.

Blood flow through the vessels is regulated by two factors: peripheral vascular resistance and pressure within the system. Peripheral vascular resistance, as noted earlier, is the resistance to blood flow. Vessels with larger inside diameters offer less resistance, while vessels with smaller inside diameters offer greater resistance. Peripheral vascular resistance is governed by three factors—the length of the vessel, the diameter of the vessel, and blood viscosity.

There is very little resistance to blood flow through the aorta and arteries, but a significant change in peripheral resistance occurs at the arterioles and precapillary sphincters. This is because the inside diameter of the arteriole is much smaller, as compared to that of the aorta and arteries. Additionally, the arteriole has the ability to make a pronounced change in its diameter, as much as fivefold. It tends to do this in response to local tissue needs and autonomic nervous signals.

Contraction of the venous side of the vascular system results in decreased capacitance and increased cardiac preload. The arterial system, however, provides systemic vascular resistance. An increase in arterial tone increases resistance, which increases blood pressure.

Oxygen Transport

Oxygen is brought into the body via the respiratory system. During inspiration, approximately 500 to 800 mL of atmospheric air is taken in through the upper and lower airways, coming to rest in the alveoli of the lungs.

Surrounding the alveoli are capillaries that are perfused by the pulmonary circulation. The blood that comes into the pulmonary capillaries is oxygen-depleted blood that was returned from the body to the right atrium of the heart, then pumped by the right ventricle of the heart into the pulmonary arteries and thence into the pulmonary capillaries.

The air in the alveoli contains a concentration of about 13.6 percent oxygen. This is less than the 21 percent concentration of oxygen in atmospheric air because of various factors, including the fact that some air always remains in the alveoli from earlier respirations and oxygen is constantly being absorbed from this air. Nevertheless, alveolar air is far richer in oxygen than blood that enters the pulmonary capillaries.

Another way of stating this is that the *partial pressure of oxygen* present in air in the alveoli of the lungs is greater than the partial pressure of oxygen in the blood within the pulmonary circulation. (In a mix of gases, the portion of the total pressure

exerted by each component of the mix is known as the *partial pressure* of that component.) For this reason, oxygen from the alveoli diffuses across the alveolar-capillary membrane and into the bloodstream—from the area of greater partial pressure to the area of lower partial pressure.

The red blood cells "pick up" this oxygen while passing through the pulmonary capillary bed. Oxygen binds to the hemoglobin molecules of the red blood cells, which serve as the primary carriers of oxygen within the bloodstream. Normally, between 95 and 100 percent of the hemoglobin is saturated with oxygen. Approximately 97 percent of oxygen is transported reversibly bound to hemoglobin while the remaining 3 percent is transported as a gas dissolved in the plasma. The oxygen-enriched blood then circulates back to the heart through the venous side of the pulmonary circulation. Passing through the left atrium and into the left ventricle, the oxygen-enriched blood is pumped throughout the body via the systemic circulation.

On reaching capillaries throughout the body, the oxygen-rich blood interfaces with the tissues. The tissues contain cells that are oxygen-deficient as a result of normal metabolic activity. Since the partial pressure of oxygen is greater in the bloodstream than in the cells, oxygen will diffuse from the red blood cells across the capillary wall-cell membrane barrier, into the cells and tissues.

Overall, the movement and utilization of oxygen in the body is dependent on the following conditions:

- Adequate concentration of inspired oxygen
- Appropriate movement of oxygen across the alveolar-capillary membrane into the arterial bloodstream
- Adequate number of red blood cells to carry the oxygen
- Proper tissue perfusion
- Efficient off-loading of oxygen at the tissue level

The dependence on this set of conditions for oxygen movement and utilization is known as the **Fick principle**.

Waste Removal

The waste products of cellular metabolism are expelled from the cells and carried away by the blood. Carbon dioxide leaves the bloodstream during the oxygen-carbon dioxide exchange, which occurs through the alveolar-capillary membranes. The majority of carbon dioxide (approximately 70 percent) is transported in the form of bicarbonate ion (HCO_3^-). Only 23 percent is reversibly bound to hemoglobin (carbon dioxide binds to a different site on hemoglobin than oxygen). Only 7 percent of carbon dioxide is transported as a gas dissolved in the plasma. Carbon dioxide is ultimately eliminated by exhalation from the lungs.

CONTENT REVIEW

► Causes of Hypoperfusion
(Shock)

• Inadequate pump (heart
malfunction)
• Inadequate fluid
(hypovolemia)
• Inadequate container
(dilated or leaking blood
vessels)

Some cellular waste products are expelled into the interstitial fluid and picked up by the lymphatic system. These ultimately flow through the lymph channels into the thoracic duct. The thoracic duct empties the waste products into the venous side of the circulatory system. Other wastes are cleansed from the blood by the kidneys and excreted as urine. Finally, some cellular waste products are emptied into the gastrointestinal system and expelled in the feces.

There is some local control of both tissue perfusion and waste removal. When the amounts of metabolic waste products (such as lactic acid) increase, the tissues subsequently become acidotic. This local acidosis causes nearby precapillary sphincters to relax, thus opening the capillaries and increasing perfusion of the affected tissues. This provides increased capacity for waste elimination and response to local metabolic demands.

The Pathophysiology of Hypoperfusion

Causes of Hypoperfusion

Hypoperfusion (shock) is almost always a result of inadequate cardiac output. A number of factors can decrease effective cardiac output. These include:

- Inadequate pump
  - Inadequate preload
  - Inadequate cardiac contractile strength
  - Inadequate heart rate
  - Excessive afterload
- Inadequate fluid
  - Hypovolemia (abnormally low circulating blood volume)
- Inadequate container
  - Dilated container without change in fluid volume (inadequate systemic vascular resistance)
  - Leak in container

Occasionally, hypoperfusion can develop even when cardiac output is adequate. This can happen when cell metabolism is so excessive that the body cannot increase perfusion enough to meet the cells' metabolic requirements. It can also happen when abnormal circulatory patterns develop, so that circulating blood is bypassing critical tissues.

As mentioned earlier, the conditions that lead to hypoperfusion can result from a number of underlying causes, such as infection, trauma and hemorrhage, loss of plasma through burns, severe cardiac arrhythmia, central nervous system dysfunction, and many others. But the outcome is always the same: inadequate delivery of oxygen and essential nutrients to, and removal of wastes from, all the tissues of the body, especially the critical tissues (brain, heart, kidneys).

Shock at the Cellular Level

Shock is a complex phenomenon. The causes vary. The signs and symptoms vary. At the simplest level, however, shock is inadequate tissue perfusion. Additionally, all types of shock have this in common: The ultimate outcome is impairment of cellular metabolism. Two characteristics of impaired cellular metabolism in any type of shock are impaired oxygen use and impaired glucose use.

Impaired Use of Oxygen One characteristic of any type of shock is that the cells are either not receiving enough oxygen or are unable to use it effectively. This may be caused by hypoperfusion resulting from reduced cardiac function, inadequate blood volume, or vasodilation (pump, fluid, or container problems). It may result from insufficient red cells to carry the oxygen, from fever that increases cellular oxygen demand, or chemical disruption of cellular metabolism.

When the cells don't receive enough oxygen or cannot use it effectively, they change from **aerobic metabolism** to **anaerobic metabolism**, a far less efficient means of producing energy—as explained in the following text.

The primary energy source for the cells is glucose, taken into the cell with the aid of insulin. Glucose does not provide energy until it is broken down inside the cell. The first stage of glucose breakdown, called glycolysis, is anaerobic (does not require oxygen). Glycolysis produces pyruvic acid as an end-product but yields very little energy. Thus, by itself, glycolysis is an inefficient utilization of glucose. Therefore, in a normal state of metabolism, a second stage of glucose breakdown is required. During this second stage, which is aerobic (requires oxygen), pyruvic acid is further degraded into carbon dioxide, water, and energy in a process termed the Krebs or citric acid cycle. The energy yield of this second-stage aerobic process is much higher than from the first-stage anaerobic process (Figure 1-84 ●).

During shock, or any condition in which the cells do not receive adequate oxygen or cannot use it effectively, glucose breakdown can only complete the first-stage, anaerobic process of glycolysis and cannot enter into the second-stage, aerobic, citric acid cycle. This causes an accumulation of the end product of glycolysis, pyruvic acid. In these cases, pyruvic acid is quickly degraded to lactic acid. If oxygen is promptly restored to the cells, lactic acid will be reconverted to pyruvic acid. However, if time elapses and the cellular hypoxia is not corrected, lactic acid and other metabolic acids will accumulate. One outcome is that the acidic condition of the blood reduces the ability of hemoglobin in red blood cells to bind with and carry oxygen, which compounds the problem of cellular oxygen deprivation.

The energy that is produced during glucose breakdown is in the form of the chemical adenosine triphosphate (ATP), which is essential to all the metabolic processes in the cells. As just noted, the amount of energy, or ATP, produced during first-stage, anaerobic glycolysis is very small. Without oxygen, when the process of glucose breakdown stops after glycolysis (during which very little energy has been produced), cellular stores of ATP are used up much faster than they can be replaced, so that all the processes of cellular metabolism are gravely impaired.

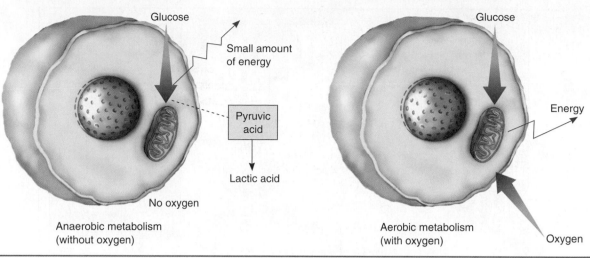

(a) Stage one: Anaerobic metabolism

Glucose

Small amount
of energy

Pyruvic
acid

Lactic acid

No oxygen

Anaerobic metabolism
(without oxygen)

(b) Stage two: Aerobic metabolism

Glucose

Energy

Aerobic metabolism
(with oxygen)

Oxygen

● **Figure 1-84**   Glucose breakdown. (a) Stage one, glycolysis, is anaerobic (does not require oxygen). It yields pyruvic acid, with toxic by-products such as lactic acid, and very little energy. (b) Stage two is aerobic (requires oxygen). In a process called the Krebs or citric acid cycle, pyruvic acid is degraded into carbon dioxide and water, which produces a much higher yield of energy.

Because of changes to the internal cell and because blood flow has been slowed by the decreased pumping action and vasodilation, sludging of the blood occurs. This further impedes blood flow. Thus, the normal diffusion of nutrients and wastes in and out of the cells is disrupted and the balance of the cellular electrolytes is altered. Lysosomes, the organelles that assist in digestion of nutrients, are normally enclosed by a membrane that prevents the digestive enzymes from damaging other cell components. Now the lysosomes rupture, releasing the lysosomal enzymes into the cell. The sodium-potassium pumping mechanism fails, changing the electrical charge of the cells' internal environment. There is an increase in sodium and water (since water follows sodium) inside the cells, causing cellular edema. The cell membrane then ruptures, allowing lysosomal enzymes and other cellular contents to leak into the interstitial spaces. Cellular death soon follows.

Impaired Use of Glucose   The same factors that reduce delivery of oxygen to the cells also reduce delivery of glucose to the cells. In addition, uptake of glucose by the cells may be disrupted by fever, cell damage, or the presence of bacteria, toxins, histamine, or other substances produced or activated by the body's immune and inflammatory responses to disease or injury. Compensatory mechanisms activated by shock may also be responsible for substances that inhibit glucose uptake, including catecholamines and the hormones cortisol and growth hormone.

Glucose that is prevented from entering the cells remains in the blood, resulting in a condition of high serum glucose, or hyperglycemia. Since glucose is the substance from which cells produce energy, the consequences of reduced glucose delivery and uptake are critical.

In the absence of an adequate supply of glucose, certain body cells can create fuel for energy production by converting other substances to glucose. One source is glycogen, the form of glucose that cells store and hold in reserve. Cells convert glycogen to glucose in a process called *glycogenolysis.* However, there is very little stored glycogen in cells other than the liver, kidneys, and muscles. When glycogen reserves are depleted, which typically

occurs in 4 to 8 hours, the cells will then derive energy from the breakdown of fats (*lipolysis*) and from the conversion of noncarbohydrate substrates, such as amino acids from proteins, to glucose (*gluconeogenesis*). The energy costs of glycogenolysis and lipolysis are high and contribute to the failure of cells. But the depletion of proteins in gluconeogenesis will ultimately cause organ failure (Figure 1-85 ●).

In addition, the anaerobic breakdown of proteins produces ammonia, which is toxic to the cells, and urea, which leads to uric acid, which is also toxic to cells. Finally, when cellular metabolism is impaired, the waste products of metabolism build up in the cells, further impairing cell function and damaging cell membranes.

Impaired use of oxygen and glucose soon leads to cellular death. Cellular death will ultimately lead to tissue death, tissue death will lead to organ failure, and organ failure will lead to death of the individual.

Compensation and Decompensation

Usually, the body is able to compensate for any of the changes previously described. However, when the compensatory mechanisms fail, shock develops and may progress.

Compensation   In shock, the fall in cardiac output, detected as a decrease in arterial blood pressure by the baroreceptors, activates several body systems that attempt to reestablish a normal blood pressure—a process known as *compensation.* The sympathetic nervous system stimulates the adrenal gland of the endocrine system to secrete the catecholamines epinephrine and norepinephrine. These chemicals profoundly affect the cardiovascular system, causing an increased heart rate, increased cardiac contractile strength, and arteriolar constriction—all of which serve to elevate the blood pressure.

Another compensatory mechanism, the *renin-angiotensin system,* aids the body in maintaining an adequate blood pressure. When the renin-angiotensin system is activated by a fall in blood pressure, the enzyme *renin* is released from the kidneys into the systemic circulation. Renin acts on a specialized

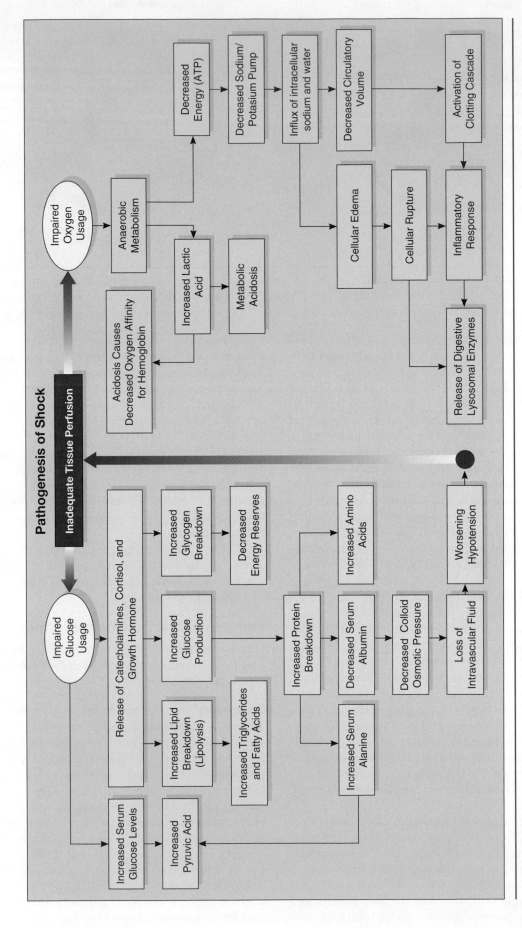

● **Figure 1-85**   The pathogenesis of shock in the human.

plasma protein called *angiotensin* to produce a substance called *angiotensin I*. Angiotensin I is converted to *angiotensin II* by an enzyme found in the lungs called *angiotensin converting enzyme (ACE)*. Angiotensin II is a potent vasoconstrictor. As angiotensin II causes the diameter of the vascular container to decrease, the blood pressure increases. Angiotensin II also stimulates the production of aldosterone, a hormone secreted by the adrenal cortex (outer layer of the adrenal gland) that, in turn, stimulates the kidneys to reabsorb sodium, and, subsequently, water (as noted earlier, "water follows sodium") into peritubular capillaries. The intravascular volume is maintained, and elimination of water by the kidneys is reduced.

Another endocrine response by the pituitary gland results in the secretion of antidiuretic hormone (ADH), which also causes the kidneys to reabsorb water, creating an additive effect to that of aldosterone.

The spleen, capable of storing over 300 mL of blood, can expel up to 200 mL of blood into the venous circulation and can contract, consequently increasing blood volume, preload, cardiac output, and blood pressure in response to a sudden drop in blood pressure.

Some passive compensatory responses also occur, with beneficial fluid shifts taking place as a result of simple diffusion. With volume loss, the hydrostatic pressure in capillary beds is reduced, and water from the interstitial spaces diffuses into the capillaries.

All the aforementioned mechanisms work to compensate for the shock state, and may be able to restore normal circulatory volume—if excessive bleeding is managed and the shock state has not progressed too far. In this case, the patient is said to be in **compensated shock**.

Once normal circulatory function and blood pressure are reestablished, the blood pressure will "feed back" on all the compensatory mechanisms so that all systems can return to normal. In this way, negative feedback loops work to maintain stability by "signaling" the systems to cease the compensatory responses. In this way, stability and homeostasis are maintained.

Decompensation If the conditions causing shock are too serious, or progress too rapidly, compensatory mechanisms may not be able to restore normal function. In those cases, *decompensation* is said to occur, and the patient is in a state of **decompensated shock**, also called *progressive shock*. During decompensated or progressive shock, medical intervention may still be able to correct the condition.

Since all the "responding" systems have a point at which they can no longer sustain their action (i.e., a limited duration of action), the shock state may progress to a condition where correction, either by the body's own compensatory mechanisms or through medical intervention, is no longer possible. This condition is known as **irreversible shock**.

A critical factor in the downward spiral of decompensation is cardiac depression. The compensatory mechanisms that increase heart rate and contractile strength create a greatly increased demand for oxygen by the myocardium. When arterial blood pressure has fallen sufficiently, however, coronary blood flow is reduced below the level necessary to adequately perfuse the myocardium. The heart is weakened and cardiac output falls even further.

Depression of the vasomotor center of the brain is another consequence of reduced blood pressure. In early shock, as previously discussed, the sympathetic nervous system is stimulated to cause release of catecholamines that support the function of the circulatory system. But when blood pressure falls to a certain point, in the late stages of shock, reduced blood supply to the vasomotor center results in a slowing, then stoppage, of sympathetic activity.

Metabolic wastes, products of anaerobic metabolism, are released into the slower-flowing blood. The blood in the capillary beds becomes acidic, causing formation of minute blood clots ("sludged" blood), which further slows the flow of blood. And a more generalized, systemic acidosis develops, causing further deterioration of cells and tissues, including the capillary walls.

Capillary cells, like other cells, suffer from lack of oxygen and other nutrients, as well as from the ravages of acidosis. This begins to cause permeability of the capillaries and leakage of fluid into the interstitial spaces. This is another self-perpetuating process, as the decreased circulating volume and anaerobic metabolism cause further cell hypoxia and increased permeability.

Cellular deterioration progresses to tissue deterioration, which progresses to organ failure. (See Multiple Organ Dysfunction Syndrome, later in the chapter.) Medical intervention may save the patient if initiated early enough, but when enough damage has been done to cells, tissues, and organs, no known treatment can help the patient to recover. Medical therapies may support function for a while, but death becomes inevitable.

Types of Shock

Shock is usually classified according to the cause. Some newer terminology classifies shock as *cardiogenic* (caused by impaired pumping power of the heart), *hypovolemic* (caused by decreased blood or water volume), *obstructive* (caused by an obstruction that interferes with return of blood to the heart, such as a pulmonary embolism, cardiac tamponade, or tension pneumothorax), and *distributive* (caused by abnormal distribution and return of blood resulting from vasodilation, vasopermeability, or both, as in neurogenic, anaphylactic, or septic shock).

Another, more familiar terminology classifies shock as *cardiogenic, hypovolemic, neurogenic, anaphylactic,* and *septic.* The following discussion of types of shock uses these classifications.

Although all types of shock ultimately have the same effects on the body's cells, tissues, and organs, it is important to try to identify the underlying cause, because correcting the cause is the most important element in reversing the condition and saving the patient's life. Many of the treatments that you, as a paramedic, will provide for the shock patient will be the same, no matter what the cause or type of shock is, but some differ in important ways. For example, providing IV fluid boluses, which may be appropriate to support circulating volume in the hypovolemic patient, would not be indicated for the patient in cardiogenic shock with pulmonary edema.

CONTENT REVIEW

▶ Two Classifications of Shock

Classification #1

• Cardiogenic shock
• Hypovolemic shock
• Obstructive shock
• Distributive shock

Classification #2

• Cardiogenic shock
• Hypovolemic shock
• Neurogenic shock
• Anaphylactic shock
• Septic shock

Cardiogenic Shock

An inability of the heart to pump enough blood to supply all body parts is referred to as **cardiogenic shock**. Cardiogenic shock is usually the result of severe left ventricular failure secondary to acute myocardial infarction or congestive heart failure. The reduced blood pressure that accompanies this form of shock aggravates the situation by decreasing coronary artery perfusion. With decreased coronary perfusion, the heart muscle becomes even more damaged, thus establishing a vicious cycle that ultimately results in complete pump failure.

During cardiogenic shock, as noted earlier, the activation of compensatory mechanisms can actually worsen the situation. When the peripheral resistance increases in an attempt to maintain blood pressure, the myocardial workload increases. This, in turn, increases the myocardial oxygen demand, further aggravating myocardial ischemia and infarction. Cardiac output is further depressed and ejection fraction (the percentage of blood in the ventricle that is ejected with each beat) is decreased (Figure 1-86 ●).

While the most common cause of cardiogenic shock is severe left ventricular failure, a number of other factors can have the same result. These include chronic progressive heart disease such as cardiomyopathy, rupture of the papillary heart muscles or intraventricular septum, and end-stage valvular disease (mitral stenosis or aortic regurgitation).

Most patients who experience cardiogenic shock will have normal blood volume. However, some patients will be hypovolemic from an excessive use of prescribed diuretics or the

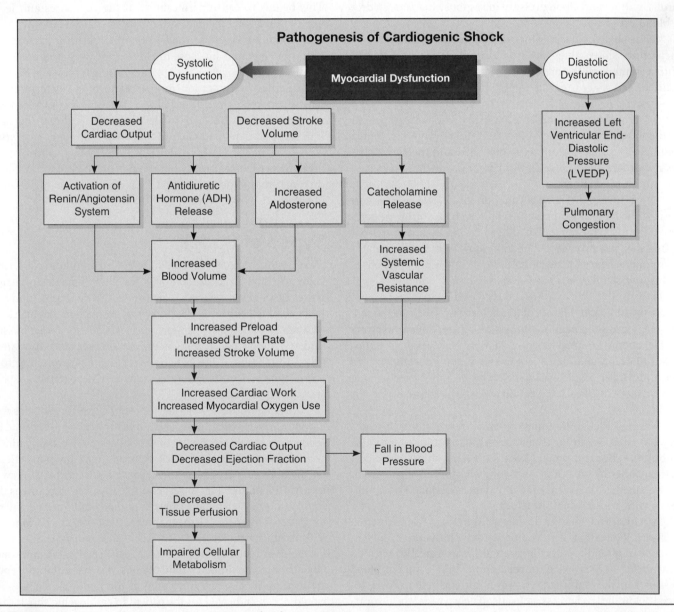

● **Figure 1-86**   The pathogenesis of cardiogenic shock.

severe diaphoresis that accompanies some acute cardiac events. Patients may also experience relative hypovolemia (neurogenic shock) from the vasodilatory (vessel dilation) effects of drugs such as nitroglycerin.

Evaluation and Treatment A major difference between cardiogenic and other types of shock is the presence of pulmonary edema (excess fluid in the lungs), which will probably result in a complaint of difficulty breathing. There may be diminished lung sounds as fluid enters the interstitial spaces of the lungs. As fluid levels rise, wheezes, crackles, or rales may be heard. A productive cough may develop, characterized by white- or pink-tinged foamy sputum. Cyanosis (a dusky blue-gray skin color) is typical, resulting from the decreased diffusion of oxygen across the alveolar-capillary interface, decreasing oxygen delivery to cells that are already hypoxic because of decreased blood pressure and perfusion. Other signs of shock include altered mentation (resulting from reduced perfusion of the brain) and oliguria (diminished urination resulting from compensatory mechanisms that stimulate reabsorption of water by the kidneys to enhance circulating volume).

Treatment of cardiogenic shock includes the supportive measures that should be provided for shock of any origin: Ensure an open airway, administer supplemental oxygen if the patient is hypoxic and assist ventilations if necessary (to support oxygenation of myocardial and other body cells), and keep the patient warm (because impaired cellular metabolism is no longer producing enough energy to keep body temperature normal).

Hypovolemic Shock

Shock due to a loss of intravascular fluid volume is referred to as **hypovolemic shock**. Possible causes of hypovolemic shock include:

- Internal or external hemorrhage (This type of hypovolemic shock is also known as hemorrhagic shock.)
- Traumatic injury
- Long bone or open fractures
- Severe dehydration from vomiting or diarrhea
- Plasma loss from burns

● **Figure 1-87** The pathogenesis of hypovolemic shock.

- Excessive sweating
- Diabetic ketoacidosis with resultant **osmotic diuresis**

Hypovolemic shock can also be due to internal third-space loss (loss from intracellular or, more commonly, from intravascular spaces into the interstitial spaces). Such a condition can occur with bowel obstruction, peritonitis, pancreatitis, or liver failure resulting in ascites (accumulation of fluid within the abdominal cavity) (Figure 1-87 ●).

Evaluation and Treatment The signs of hypovolemic shock are considered the "classic" signs of shock. The mental status becomes altered, progressing from anxiety to lethargy or combativeness to unresponsiveness. The skin becomes pale,

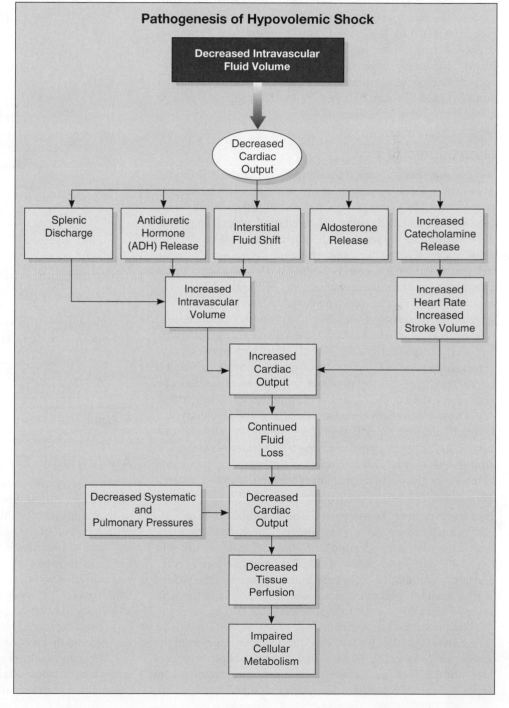

cool, and clammy (sweaty). The blood pressure may be normal during compensated shock, but then begins to fall. The pulse may be normal in the beginning, then become rapid, finally slowing and disappearing. As the kidneys continue to reabsorb water, urination decreases. Cardiac arrhythmias may develop in late shock, deteriorating to asystole (absence of heartbeat).

While it is accepted practice to administer crystalloid or colloid solutions to replace fluids lost through vomiting, diarrhea, burns, excessive sweating, or osmotic diuresis, the replacement of fluids in trauma patients is quite controversial. It has been demonstrated that the body provides a natural compensation for low-flow states when the systolic pressure is maintained between 70 and 85 mmHg. In a few studies, elevating the systolic blood pressure to greater than 85 mmHg has been associated with worsened outcomes. The worsened outcomes are attributed to the fact that aggressive fluid resuscitation, before the source of bleeding is repaired, causes progressive dilution of the blood, which decreases the oxygen-carrying capacity of the blood. Thus, many surgeons and EMS medical directors are now recommending administering only enough fluid to maintain a systolic blood pressure between 70 and 85 mmHg—a process called "permissive hypotension."

Neurogenic Shock

Neurogenic shock results from injury to either the brain or the spinal cord. Spinal cord injuries can result in an imbalance between sympathetic and parasympathetic tone depending on the level of the spinal cord injured. This can result in an interruption of nerve impulses to the arteries. The arteries lose tone and dilate, causing a relative hypovolemia. There has been no loss of fluid, but the container has been enlarged. With this inappropriate vasodilation, a disproportionate amount of blood collects in the capillary bed. This reduces venous return, cardiac output, and arterial blood pressure. Sympathetic nerve impulses to the adrenal glands are lost, which prevents the release of catecholamines and their compensatory effects. With injury high in the cervical spine, there may be interruption of impulses to the peripheral nervous system, causing paralysis and loss of sensation. The respiratory and cardiac centers of the brain may also be affected.

The usual cause of neurogenic shock is central nervous system injury. Neurogenic shock is most commonly due to an injury that has resulted in severe spinal cord injury or total transection of the cord (which may be called *spinal shock*) or injury or deprivation of oxygen or glucose to the medulla of the brain (Figure 1-88 ●).

Evaluation and Treatment   The vasodilation in neurogenic shock causes warm, red skin, and sweat gland malfunction causes dry skin—in contrast to the cool, pale, sweaty skin associated with hypovolemic shock. Because of the lack of compensatory stimulation from catecholamine release, the patient will have a low blood pressure and a slow pulse even in the early stages—again, in contrast to hypovolemic shock.

Treatment for neurogenic shock or spinal shock is similar to treatment for other types of shock and includes support of the airway, oxygenation, ventilation, maintenance of body temperature, and intravenous access. Spinal shock is characterized by hypotension, reflex bradycardia, and warm, dry skin.

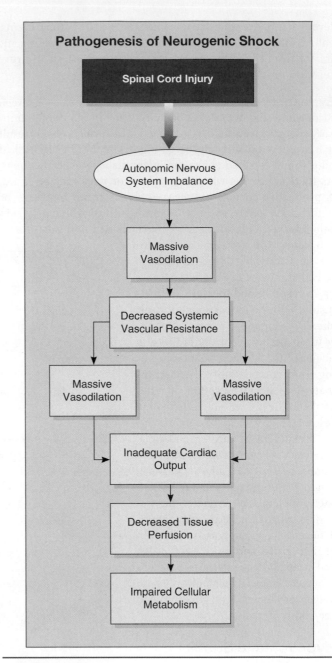

● **Figure 1-88**   The pathogenesis of neurogenic shock.

Anaphylactic Shock

When a foreign substance enters the body, the immune system responds to rid the body of the invader. (See the discussion of immunity later in this chapter.) This usually happens with no noticeable effects, and the person is not even aware that an immune response is taking place. Some foreign substances (antigens) provoke an exaggerated immune response (allergic response) that will cause noticeable symptoms such as a rash (as from contact with poison ivy) or swollen, irritated airway passages (as with hay fever). In rare cases, an allergic response is very severe and life threatening. This kind of severe allergic response is called **anaphylaxis**, or *anaphylactic shock* (Figure 1-89 ●).

An anaphylactic reaction usually occurs very rapidly. Signs and symptoms most often appear within a minute or less, but occasionally may appear an hour or more after exposure. Generally,

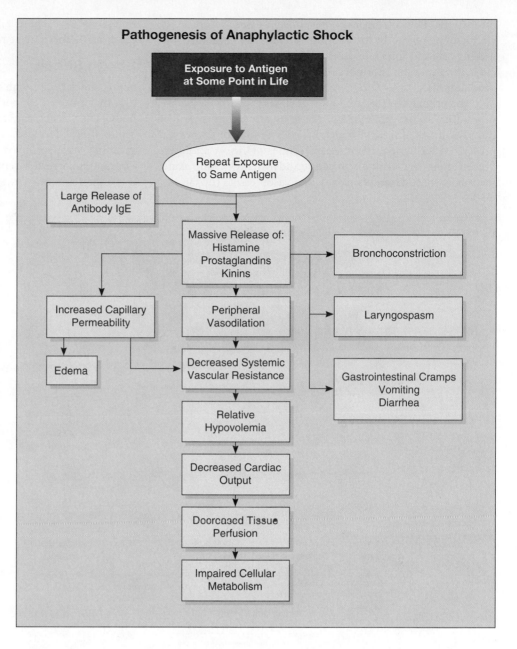

Pathogenesis of Anaphylactic Shock

Exposure to Antigen at Some Point in Life

Repeat Exposure to Same Antigen

Large Release of Antibody IgE

Massive Release of: Histamine Prostaglandins Kinins

Bronchoconstriction

Increased Capillary Permeability

Peripheral Vasodilation

Laryngospasm

Edema

Decreased Systemic Vascular Resistance

Gastrointestinal Cramps Vomiting Diarrhea

Relative Hypovolemia

Decreased Cardiac Output

Decreased Tissue Perfusion

Impaired Cellular Metabolism

the faster the reaction develops, the more severe it is likely to be. Death can occur before the patient can get to a hospital, so prompt intervention is critical. This is a situation when the paramedic at the scene can make the difference between life and death.

Anaphylactic reactions can be triggered by a variety of substances, including foods (especially nuts, eggs, and shellfish), venoms, aspirin or nonsteroidal anti-inflammatory drugs (NSAIDs), hormones (animal-derived insulin), preservatives, and others. The most rapid and severe reactions are usually caused by substances injected directly into the bloodstream, which is one reason that penicillin injections and hymenoptera stings (e.g., from bees, wasps, hornets) are the most common causes of fatal anaphylactic reactions.

Evaluation and Treatment Because the immune responses involved in anaphylaxis can affect different body systems, the signs and symptoms can vary widely. For example:

- Skin
  - Flushing
  - Itching
  - Hives
  - Swelling
  - Cyanosis
- Respiratory system
  - Breathing difficulty
  - Sneezing, coughing
  - Wheezing, stridor
  - Laryngeal edema
  - Laryngospasm
- Cardiovascular system
  - Vasodilation
  - Increased heart rate
  - Decreased blood pressure
- Gastrointestinal system
  - Nausea, vomiting
  - Abdominal cramping
  - Diarrhea

- Nervous system
  - Altered mental status
  - Dizziness
  - Headache
  - Seizures
  - Tearing

The patient may present with an altered mental status that can progress to unresponsiveness, so gather a brief history as soon as possible, including previous allergic reactions and any information about what the patient may have ingested or been exposed to that could have caused the present reaction. Be sure the patient is no longer in contact with the allergen; if a stinger is in the skin, scrape it away with a fingernail or scalpel blade.

Since laryngeal edema is often a problem, protecting the patient's airway will be your first concern. Administer oxygen by nonrebreather mask or, as necessary, by endotracheal intubation. The anaphylactic response causes depletion of circulatory volume by promoting capillary permeability and leaking of fluid into interstitial spaces, so establish an IV of crystalloid solution (normal saline or lactated Ringer's) for volume support.

The primary treatment for anaphylaxis is pharmacological. In addition to oxygen, epinephrine is usually administered (if the patient has a history of anaphylaxis, he may be carrying a prescribed spring-loaded epinephrine injector), as are antihistamines (diphenhydramine), corticosteroids (methylprednisolone, hydrocortisone, dexamethasone), and vasopressors (dopamine, norepinephrine, epinephrine). Occasionally an inhaled beta agonist (albuterol) may be required. Follow local protocols.

Septic Shock

Septic shock begins with *septicemia* (also called *sepsis*), an infection that enters the bloodstream and is carried throughout the body. The person may have septicemia for some time before septic shock develops, but eventually toxins released by the invading organism overcome the compensatory mechanisms. Unless it is corrected, septic shock will cause the dysfunction of more than one organ system, resulting in multiple organ dysfunction syndrome (discussed in the next section) (Figure 1-90 ●).

Evaluation and Treatment The signs and symptoms of septic shock are progressive. In the beginning, cardiac output is increased, but toxins causing vasodilation may prevent an increase in blood pressure. The person may seem to be sick, but not alarmingly so. By the last stages, toxins have increased permeability of the blood vessels to the point where great amounts of fluid are lost from the vasculature and blood pressure falls drastically.

Signs and symptoms can vary widely as the patient progresses from early to late stages of septic shock. Some patients may have a high fever, but others, especially the elderly or the very young, may have no fever or may even be hypothermic. The skin can be flushed, if fever is present, or very pale and cyanotic in the late stages.

The most susceptible organ system is the lungs and respiratory system, so the patient may present with breathing difficulty and altered lung sounds. The brain may be infected, resulting in altered mental status. Suspicion of septic shock is usually based on a history of recent infection or illness.

Multiple Organ Dysfunction Syndrome

In the 1970s, a syndrome of multiple organ failure began to be noticed in hospital intensive care units. Medical advances were allowing patients to

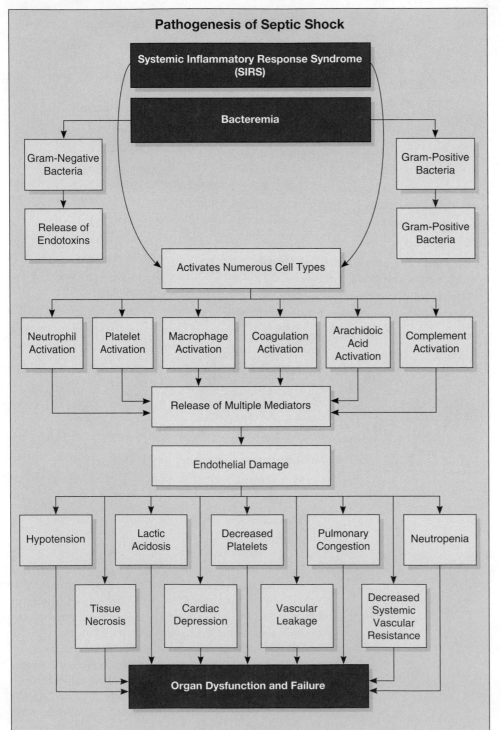

● **Figure 1-90** The pathogenesis of septic shock.

survive serious illness and trauma—only to die later of complications of the original disease or injury. The syndrome was described in 1975 as *multisystem organ failure*. In 1991, the American College of Chest Physicians and the Society of Critical Care Medicine named it **multiple organ dysfunction syndrome (MODS)**.

MODS is the progressive impairment of two or more organ systems resulting from an uncontrolled inflammatory response to a severe illness or injury. Sepsis and septic shock are the most common causes of MODS, with MODS being the end stage. (The progression from infection to sepsis to septic shock to MODS is known as systemic inflammatory response syndrome, or SIRS).

Actually, MODS can result from any severe disease or injury that triggers a massive systemic inflammatory response—including trauma, burns, surgery, circulatory shock, acute pancreatitis, acute renal failure, and others. Risk factors include age (>65), malnutrition, and preexisting chronic disease such as cancer or diabetes. With a mortality rate of 60 to 90 percent, MODS is the major cause of death following sepsis, trauma, and burn injuries.

Pathophysiology of MODS

MODS occurs in two stages. In primary MODS, organ damage results directly from a specific cause such as ischemia or inadequate perfusion resulting from an episode of shock, trauma, or major surgery. There are stress and inflammatory responses (discussed in detail later in this chapter) to this initial injury, but they may be mild and not readily detectable. However, during this response, neutrophils and macrophages (cells that attack and destroy bacteria, protozoa, foreign cells, and cell debris) as well as mast cells (cells that produce histamine and other components of allergic response) are thought to be "primed" by cytokines (proteins released during an inflammatory or immune response).

The next time there is an insult, such as an additional injury or ischemia or infection—even though the insult may be mild—the primed cells are activated, producing an exaggerated inflammatory response, known as secondary MODS.

Now the inflammatory response enters a self-perpetuating cycle. As inflammatory mediators are released by the injured organ, they enter the circulation, activating inflammatory responses in organ systems throughout the body. These mediators, especially cytokines such as tumor necrosis factor (TNF) and interleukin 1 (IL-1), damage the endothelium (cells that line the blood vessels, the heart, and body cavities). Gram-negative bacteria, if present, release endotoxins that also damage endothelial cells. The injured endothelial cells release factors that aggravate the inflammation and cause vasodilation. The injured epithelium becomes permeable, allowing leakage of fluid into interstitial spaces, and loses much of its anticoagulation function, which allows formation of tiny blood clots (thrombi) in the microvasculature.

The secondary insult also triggers an exaggerated neuroendocrine response. Catecholamine release causes many of the manifestations of MODS, including tachycardia, increased metabolic rates, and increased oxygen consumption. Release of a variety of hormones contributes to the hypermetabolism, and release of endorphins contributes to vasodilation. Additionally, plasma protein systems are activated: specifically, the complement system, the coagulation system, and the kallikrein-kinin system. Plasma proteins are key mediators of the inflammatory response. When activated, each of these systems triggers a cascade of responses with the overall result of increased vasodilation, vasopermeability, cardiovascular instability, endothelial damage, and clotting abnormalities.

As a result of the release of the inflammatory mediators and toxins and the plasma protein cascades, a massive immune/inflammatory and coagulation response develops. Vascular changes (vasodilation, increased capillary permeability, selective vasoconstriction, and microvascular thrombi) continue and worsen. Two metabolites that are released have opposing vascular effects: Prostacyclin, also called prostaglandin I_2 (PGI_2), is a vasodilator, while thromboxane A_2 (TXA_2) is a vasoconstrictor. They are released in differing amounts within different organ tissues, contributing to a maldistribution of blood flow to organs and organ systems.

As noted earlier, the release of catecholamines stimulates hypermetabolism within the body cells, which in turn creates a greatly increased oxygen demand. Because of lung damage, **hypoxemia** and hypoperfusion, a severe oxygen supply/demand imbalance, develop. As the cells switch from aerobic to anaerobic metabolism, fuel supplies within the cells (ATP and glucose) are used up faster than they can be replenished. Without adequate ATP, the cells lose their ability to operate the sodium-potassium pump, which is essential to cardiac function. The myocardium is profoundly weakened. Cellular lysosomes begin to break down, releasing lysosomal enzymes that damage the cell membrane and the surrounding cells. Large amounts of lactic acid are released, contributing to acidosis, which further damages the cells. The overall response is similar to that seen in septic and anaphylactic shock, except on a larger scale.

Clinical Presentation of MODS

The cumulative effects of MODS at the cellular and tissue levels begin to cause the breakdown of organ systems: The organs that fail first are not necessarily the organs where the initial insult occurred, and there is a lag time between the initial insult and the onset of organ failure. Dysfunction may develop in the pulmonary, gastrointestinal, hepatic, renal, cardiovascular, hematologic, and immune systems. There is decreased cardiac function and myocardial depression, caused by the factors discussed earlier, possibly abetted by release of myocardial depressant factor (MDF) and a decrease in beta-adrenergic receptors in the heart. The smooth muscle of the vascular system fails with consequent release of capillary sphincters and increased vasodilation.

MODS does not occur in one intense crisis. It will usually develop over a period of two, three, or more weeks. There is no specific therapy for MODS, and the only chance of rescuing the patient from its self-perpetuating spiral toward death is early recognition and initiation of supportive measures. For this reason, it is important to understand how MODS usually presents in the first 24 hours after initial resuscitation.

CONTENT REVIEW

► Infectious Agents

• Bacteria
• Viruses
• Fungi
• Parasites
• Prions

Although MODS will usually be detected in the hospital rather than the prehospital setting, there may be occasions when a patient who has not been hospitalized or has returned home from the hospital is the subject of a call to EMS, or when a patient being transported by EMS from one facility to another is suffering from MODS.

The most common presentation of MODS over time is as follows:

24 Hours after Resuscitation

● Low-grade fever
● Tachycardia (rapid heart rate)
● Dyspnea (breathing difficulty)
● Altered mental status
● General hypermetabolic, hyperdynamic state

Within 24 to 72 Hours

● Pulmonary (lung) failure begins

Within 7 to 10 Days

● Hepatic (liver) failure begins
● Intestinal failure begins
● Renal (kidney) failure begins

Within 14 to 21 Days

● Renal and hepatic failure intensify
● Gastrointestinal collapse
● Immune system collapse

After 21 Days

● Hematologic (blood system) failure begins
● Myocardial (heart muscle) failure begins
● Altered mental status resulting from encephalopathy (brain infection)
● Death

PART 6: The Body's Defenses Against Disease and Injury

SELF-DEFENSE MECHANISMS

So far in this chapter, we have discussed normal body conditions (the normal cell and its environment: fluids and electrolytes, the acid-base balance) and how the body may be attacked or injured (cellular injury, infection, genetic and other causes of disease, hypoperfusion, and multiple organ dysfunction syndrome). In the remainder of the chapter, we will discuss how the body defends itself from infection and injury.

It is important to keep in mind that the body has powerful ways of defending and healing itself (restoring homeostasis) and that medical intervention is needed only when, on occasion, these natural defense mechanisms are unequal to the task and become overwhelmed.

Infectious Agents
Bacteria

Bacteria are single-cell organisms that consist of internal cytoplasm surrounded by a rigid cell wall. Bacteria are prokaryotic cells that, unlike the eukaryotic cells of the human body, lack an organized nucleus and other intracellular organelles. Bacteria can reproduce independently, but they need a host to supply food and other support. Inside the body, they achieve this by binding to host cells.

Bacteria can be cultured and identified readily in most hospital laboratories. Many bacteria are categorized according to their appearance under the microscope after staining with several dyes referred to as *Gram stains*. Some bacteria stain blue, while others stain red. Bacteria that stain blue are referred to as *Gram-positive* bacteria. They are somewhat similar to each other in their structure. Bacteria that stain red are referred to as *Gram-negative* bacteria. They are also somewhat similar to each other in their structure.

Bacteria can cause many of the common infections in medicine, including middle ear infections in children, many cases of tonsillitis, and meningitis. (These kinds of infections can also be caused by viruses, which are discussed in the next section.) Most bacterial infections respond to treatment with drugs called **antibiotics**. Once administered, antibiotics kill or inhibit the growth of invading bacteria. As mentioned earlier, the bacterial cell membrane is the site of action for many antibiotics. Once the cell membrane is broken down, phagocytes (cells that ingest and destroy pathogens and other foreign and abnormal substances) can begin to destroy the bacterium. A variety of antibiotic drugs have been developed with mechanisms of action tailored to different types of bacteria. However, the broad variety of infectious bacteria, and their ability to develop resistance to drugs, makes developing antibiotics to battle them a difficult job.

Some bacteria protect themselves by forming a capsule outside the cell wall that protects the organism from digestion by phagocytes. Some bacteria, such as *Mycoplasmic* bacteria, have no protective capsule but rely on other mechanisms to survive and attack the body. *Mycobacterium tuberculosis*, which has no protective capsule, can actually survive and be transported by phagocytes. Other bacteria simply multiply faster than the body's defense systems can respond. Still others overpower the body's defenses by producing enzymes and toxins that attack and injure cells and produce hypersensitivity reactions.

Simple infection is not the only consequence of a bacterial invasion. Many bacteria release poisonous chemicals, or *toxins*. There are two types of toxins produced by bacteria: exotoxins and endotoxins. **Exotoxins** are proteins secreted and released by the bacterial cell during its growth. They travel throughout the body via the blood or lymph, ultimately causing problems. For example, botulism toxin, released by the bacterium *Clostridium botulinum,* blocks the release of cholinergic neurotransmitters at neuromuscular junctions and elsewhere in the autonomic nervous system, causing systemic paralysis. Another example is tetanus, which is caused by the bacterium *Clostridium tetani.* The actual infection by the bacteria themselves is mild and may be limited, for example, to the site of a puncture wound in the foot. Yet, on entering the body, the bacteria release their toxin, *tetanospasmin.* This toxin then travels through the blood to the skeletal muscles, causing the spastic rigidity classically seen in tetanus.

Endotoxins are complex molecules that are contained in the cell walls of certain Gram-negative bacteria. Endotoxins can be released during the destruction of the bacterial cell by phagocytes or even when the bacterial cell is attacked by an antibiotic, so that antibiotics cannot control the endotoxic effects of bacteria. When released, endotoxins trigger the inflammatory process and produce fever. In the bloodstream, they can cause widespread clotting within the blood vessels, capillary damage, and hypotension, as well as respiratory distress and fever—a condition known as endotoxin shock. Endotoxins can survive even when the cell that produced them is dead.

Depending on their amount and site of release, the effects of toxins can be local or systemic. When a bacterial organism enters the circulatory system, its released toxins can spread throughout the body. The systemic spread of toxins through the bloodstream is known as **septicemia,** or *sepsis,* and is a grave medical illness.

The body counters the bacterial invasion and release of enzymes and toxins through activation of the immune system. The immune system will mobilize foreign-cell-destroying macrophages (a type of white blood cell) to the site of infection in an attempt to rid the body of the foreign pathogen. As the macrophages attempt to destroy the bacteria, they release substances known as pyrogens. Pyrogens are responsible for causing the increase in temperature known as fever. Pyrogens act on the thermoregulation center in the hypothalamus to cause the increased body temperature, which is thought to aid in the destruction of pathogens.

Viruses

Most infections are caused by **viruses.** Viruses are much smaller than bacteria and can only be seen with an electron microscope. In addition, they cannot grow without the assistance of another organism. In fact, viruses are referred to as *intracellular parasites,* since they must invade the cells of the organism they infect.

A virus has no organized cellular structure except a protein coat (capsid) surrounding the internal genetic material, deoxyribonucleic acid (DNA) or ribonucleic acid (RNA). With no organized cellular structure or cellular organelles, viruses are incapable of metabolism. Once inside a cell, they take over, using the cellular enzymes to replicate and produce more viruses, which decreases synthesis of macromolecules vital to the host cell.

Some viruses develop a coating in addition to the capsid, called an envelope. The envelope and the protein capsid allow the virus to resist destruction by the phagocytes of the immune system. However, since viruses cannot reproduce outside a host cell, if the virus does not find a host cell, it will die.

The symptoms of a virus may not be readily apparent because it is hidden within the host cell. After replication is complete, the virus will sometimes destroy the host cell. In other cases, a virus will remain dormant within a cell for months or years. An example is the *varicella zoster virus,* which causes childhood chicken pox and may then remain dormant, only to cause shingles in the adult decades later. Some viruses form a long-term symbiotic (living in close association) relationship with the host cell, resulting in a persistent but unapparent infection.

Viruses do not produce toxins, but they can still cause very serious illnesses. Some viruses are capable of altering the host cell to induce a malignancy (cancer). Others, such as the *human immunodeficiency virus (HIV),* which causes AIDS, can proliferate, attacking cells of the immune system and destroying its ability to ward off infections of all types.

Unlike bacteria, viruses are very difficult to treat. Once a virus infects a cell, it can only be killed by destroying the infected cell. Drugs have not yet been developed that can selectively destroy cells infected by viruses while leaving uninfected cells unharmed. This partially explains the dilemma facing researchers trying to find a cure for AIDS. An additional problem is that some viruses mutate (change) frequently, which is why a new flu vaccine must be developed for every flu season. Fortunately, most viral illnesses are mild and fairly self-limiting. (Because viral agents must spread from cell to cell, the immune system is eventually able to "catch" them outside a host cell and destroy them.) Even so, at present, viruses usually cannot be treated with more than symptomatic care.

Other Agents of Infection

Other biological agents that cause human infection include *fungi* (the plural of *fungus*) and parasites.

Fungi, which includes yeasts and molds, are more like plants than animals. Fungi rarely cause human disease other than minor skin infections such as athlete's foot and some common vaginal infections. Fungus infections are called *mycoses.* Patients with an impaired immune system, such as HIV patients or patients with organ transplants, suffer fungal infection more commonly than healthy people. In such patients, the fungi can invade the lungs, blood, and several organs. Treatment of complicated, deep fungal infections has proven difficult, even in the hospital setting.

Parasites range in size from protozoa (single-cell animals not much larger than bacteria) to large intestinal worms. Parasites tend to be more common in developing nations than in the United States. Treatment depends on the organism and the location.

Prions are the most recently recognized classification of infectious agents. Initially thought to be slow-acting viruses, prions differ from viruses in that they are smaller, are made entirely of proteins, and do not have protective capsids.

For more about infectious diseases, see Volume 4, Chapter 10.

Three Lines of Defense

There are three chief lines of self-defense against infection and injury. One involves anatomic barriers. The other two—the inflammatory response and the immune response—rely on actions of the leukocytes (white blood cells). Each line of defense can be characterized as external or internal, nonspecific or specific (Table 1–14)—characterizations you may want to keep in mind as you read the following sections and compare the ways these defenses protect the body.

Before an infectious agent can attack the body, it has to get past the body's natural anatomic barrier, the epithelium (the skin and the mucous membranes that line the respiratory, gastrointestinal, and genitourinary tracts). The epithelium is more than just a physical barrier; it also provides a chemical defense against infection. The sebaceous glands of the skin secrete fatty and lactic acids, which attack bacteria and fungi. Sweat, tears, and saliva secreted by other glands contain bacteria-attacking enzymes. Various mechanical responses also work to get rid of invading substances. For example, the invader may be coughed or sneezed out of the respiratory tract, flushed out of the urinary tract, or eliminated from the gastrointestinal tract by vomiting or diarrhea.

The anatomic defenses are *external* and *nonspecific.* They are considered external because they prevent substances from penetrating the skin or the coverings of internal passageways. They are nonspecific because they defend against all invaders, such as foreign bodies, chemicals, or microorganisms, without targeting any specific type of invader.

If an invading foreign body, chemical, or microorganism penetrates the anatomic barriers and begins to attack internal cells and tissues, two other lines of defense are triggered: the inflammatory response and the immune response. These twin responses of the immune system have contrasting characteristics of speed, specificity, duration (memory), and of the plasma systems and cell types that are involved in the response (Table 1–15).

The *inflammatory response,* or *inflammation,* begins within seconds of injury or invasion by a pathogen. As noted earlier, it is nonspecific, attacking any invader by surrounding it with cells and fluids to isolate, destroy, and eliminate it. Inflammation is mediated by multiple plasma protein systems, especially the complement system, the coagulation system, and the kinin

system (which will be explained later) and involves a variety of cell types as it attacks the invader.

The *immune response* develops more slowly (one type of response requires a second exposure after priming by the first exposure to the invader). The immune response is specific, in that it will develop a specialized response for each different invader. It is mediated by just one plasma protein system (immunoglobulin) and attacks the invader mainly with a single cell type (lymphocytes, which are one type of leukocyte, or white blood cell).

Inflammation and the immune response interact in many ways. We will discuss the immune response first, because understanding the immune response is necessary for understanding some parts of the inflammatory response.

THE IMMUNE RESPONSE

How the Immune Response Works: An Overview

Most viruses, bacteria, fungi, and parasites—as well as noninfectious substances such as pollens, foods, venoms, drugs, and others that may enter the body—have proteins on their surface called **antigens**. The immune system detects these antigens as being foreign, or "non-self," and responds to produce substances called **antibodies** that combine with antigens to control or destroy them. This is known as the **immune response**. As part of this process, *memory cells* "remember" the antigen and will trigger an even faster and more effective response to destroy the same antigen if it enters the body again. Such long-term protection against specific foreign substances is known as **immunity**.

Characteristics of the Immune Response and Immunity

The immune response and immunity can be classified in various ways: natural versus acquired immunity, primary versus secondary immune responses, and humoral versus cell-mediated immunity.

Natural versus Acquired Immunity

Natural immunity is not generated by the immune response. It is inborn, part of the genetic makeup of the individual or of the species in general. For example, the measles virus cannot reproduce in canine cells, so dogs are naturally immune to measles. Conversely, canine distemper cannot thrive within human cells, so humans are naturally immune to that disease. (Some diseases such as leukemia, however, can affect more than one species.)

Acquired immunity develops as an outcome of the immune response. Acquired immunity can be either active or passive.

TABLE 1–14	Three Lines of Defense Against Infection and Injury				
	External	**Internal**	**Nonspecific**	**Specific**
Anatomic Barriers	✓		✓	
Inflammatory Response		✓	✓	
Immune Response		✓		✓

TABLE 1–15	Characteristics of the Inflammatory and Immune Responses	
	Inflammatory Response	**Immune Response**
Speed	Fast	Slow
Specificity	Nonspecific	Specific
Duration (Memory)	Transient (no memory)	Long-term (memory)
Involving Which Plasma Systems	Multiple plasma protein (complement, coagulation, kinin systems)	One plasma protein (immunoglobulin)
Involving Which Cell Type	Multiple cell types (granulocytes, monocytes, macrophages)	One blood cell type (lymphocytes)

Active acquired immunity is generated by the host's (infected person's) immune system after exposure to an antigen. *Passive acquired immunity* is transferred to a person from an outside source. For example, a mother may transfer antibodies through the placenta to the fetus. Or antibodies may be administered to a patient as an immune serum to aid the body's response to a dangerous invader such as rabies, tetanus, or snake venom. Active acquired immunity is long-lasting. Passive acquired immunity is temporary.

Primary versus Secondary Immune Responses

There are two phases to the immune response to an antigen, the primary immune response and the secondary immune response.

On exposure to an antigen, B lymphocyte cells (explained in the next section) produce antibodies to attack the antigen. These antibodies are called **immunoglobulins**, which are proteins present in the plasma portion of the blood. There are five classes of immunoglobulins—IgM, IgG, IgA, IgE, and IgD.

On first exposure to an antigen, after a lag-time of five to seven days, the presence of IgM antibodies can be detected in the blood, with a lesser presence of IgG antibodies. This constitutes the **primary immune response**, also called the *initial immune response*. If there is no further exposure to the antigen, the antibodies are catabolized (broken down)—but the immune system has been "primed." If there is a second exposure to the antigen, the body responds much faster, and a far greater quantity of IgG antibodies is produced. The level of IgG antibodies, with their memory for the specific antigen, will remain elevated for many years. This constitutes the **secondary immune response**, also called the *anamnestic* (or memory-assisting) *immune response*.

The primary and secondary immune responses together create active acquired immunity to the specific antigen.

Humoral versus Cell-Mediated Immunity

A special type of leukocyte (white blood cell) is the **lymphocyte**. Lymphocytes (which constitute about 20 to 35 percent of all leukocytes) are responsible for several critical functions of the immune response, including recognizing foreign antigens, producing antibodies (the immunoglobulins such as IgM and IgG, previously mentioned), and developing memory (Figure 1-91 ●).

As lymphocytes mature, they become one of several types, including B lymphocytes and T lymphocytes. **B lymphocytes** do not attack antigens directly. Instead, they produce the antibodies (immunoglobulins) that attack antigens. B lymphocytes also develop memory, and confer long-term immunity to specific antigens. This type of immunity is called **humoral immunity** (Figure 1-92 ●). (*Humor* refers to the blood and other fluids of the body; *humoral immunity* refers to the long-lasting antibodies and memory cells present in the blood and lymph.)

T lymphocytes do not produce antibodies. Instead, they recognize the presence of a foreign antigen and attack it directly. This type of immunity is called **cell-mediated immunity** (Figure 1-93 ●).

Lymphocytes and the Lymphatic System Lymphocytes—including B lymphocytes, T lymphocytes, and secretory lymphocytes (discussed later)—are circulated through the body as part of the lymphatic system. Lymph (the fluid of the lymphatic system) consists primarily of interstitial fluid carrying proteins, bacteria, and other substances. (As discussed earlier in the chapter, most interstitial fluid reenters the bloodstream via the capillaries, but the small amount that does not reenter the capillaries is carried away by the lymphatic system.)

Lymph is carried through the lymphatic vessels, which are parallel to but separate from the blood vessels, and is filtered through *lymph nodes* in various parts of the body. Eventually, the lymph empties into one of two lymphatic ducts in the thorax. The smaller of the two is the *right lymphatic duct,* which drains lymph from the right arm, the right side of the head, and the right side of the thorax. The larger is the *thoracic duct,* which is located in the left thorax and receives lymph from the rest of the body. These ducts drain the lymph into the right and left subclavian veins, respectively, and the lymph then travels through the bloodstream. The cycle is completed as the lymph is returned from the blood to the tissues to the lymphatic system. In this way, lymph, and the lymphocytes it carries, are circulated through the blood and lymphatic system again and again.

The B lymphocytes and T lymphocytes carried by the blood and the lymphatic system are the key elements in humoral and cell-mediated immunity, which will be discussed in more detail in the next sections.

CONTENT REVIEW

► Classifications of the Immune Response
- Natural versus acquired immunity
- Primary versus secondary immune responses
- Humoral versus cell-mediated immunity

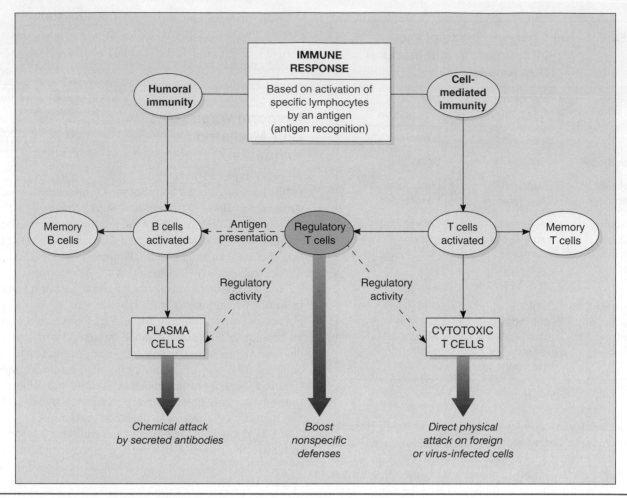

● **Figure 1-91**   Humoral and cell-mediated immunity—an overview.

Induction of the Immune Response

The immune response must be triggered, or induced. The following sections discuss the role of antigens and immunogens, histocompatibility, and blood groups in induction of the immune response.

Antigens and Immunogens

Antigens that can trigger the immune response are called **immunogens**. Not every antigen is an immunogen. In other words, not every antigen is capable of triggering the immune response. As an example, antigens are present on various helpful bacteria that reside within our bodies, but the immune response is not triggered by these antigens.

What makes a molecule an antigen is a chemical structure that is capable of reacting with existing components of the immune system, such as antibodies and T lymphocytes. However, having this chemical structure, the ability to *react* once the immune system has been triggered, is not enough to *trigger* the immune system in the first place. In order to be immunogenic—able to trigger an immune response—an antigen must have certain additional characteristics.

Characteristics of Antigenic Immunogenicity

● Sufficient foreignness

● Sufficient size

● Sufficient complexity

● Presence in sufficient amounts

As mentioned earlier, the body can distinguish between self and non-self, or foreign, antigens. Normally, the immune system is not triggered by self-antigens. In fact, the immune system does not just "tolerate" self-antigens, it actively protects them through suppression of the immune system by T lymphocytes and a special antibody called antiidiopathic antibody.

Large molecules, such as proteins, polysaccharides, and nucleic acids, are the most likely to trigger the immune response. Smaller molecules, such as amino acids, monosaccharides, and fatty acids, are less likely to induce the immune response. Some small molecules, however, can function as **haptens**, meaning that they can become immunogenic when combined with larger molecules.

More complex molecules, and molecules that are present in sufficient numbers, are more likely to trigger an immune response. Additionally, different routes of entry can stimulate different types of cell-mediated or humoral immune response (which dictates the route by which serum antigens may be administered, such as intravenous, subcutaneously, orally, intraperitoneally, intranasally). Other substances present in the

● **Figure 1-92**   Humoral immune response.

body can help to stimulate the immune response. Also, as noted earlier, the person's genetic makeup can affect the ability to respond to antigens.

Histocompatibility Locus Antigens

The body recognizes whether a substance is self or non-self as a result of certain antigens that are present on almost all cells of the body, except the red blood cells. These antigens are called **HLA antigens** (for *histocompatibility locus antigens—* or *human leukocyte antigens,* because these antigens were originally found on leukocytes). HLA antigens are the antigens that the body recognizes as self or foreign. The chief genetic source of HLA antigens has been identified as genes located at several sites (loci) on chromosome 6 that are known as the **major histocompatibility complex (MHC)**.

HLA antigens determine the suitability, or compatibility, of tissues and organs that will be grafted or transplanted from a donor. The more closely related the donor and recipient are, the more likely the recipient's body is to accept the graft or transplant. Why? Every person receives half of his genetic inheritance from each parent.

Like all genes, the genes that produce HLA antigens occur as pairs (alleles) on corresponding loci on chromosome 6. A group of alleles on one chromosome is called a haplotype. Every person has two HLA haplotypes, one on each of the pair of chromosomes. Of each pair of chromosomes (and the HLA haplotypes they carry), the person inherits one from his father and one from his mother.

Since each parent has two haplotypes, but only one gets passed along to each child (to pair up with one from the other parent), various combinations of inherited haplotypes are possible among the children of those parents. In general, each child will share one haplotype with half their siblings, both haplotypes with a quarter of their siblings, and no haplotypes with a quarter of their siblings.

Siblings and other close relatives are generally considered first as donors of tissues and organs because they have the highest likelihood of histocompatibility, hence the least likelihood of the immune system's rejecting the graft or transplant. (Identical twins, who come from the same egg fertilized by the same sperm, have identical genetic makeups and identical haplotypes. Therefore, they are the most reliable match for grafts and transplants.)

Other factors besides HLA makeup can affect the success of a graft or transplant, so they sometimes fail, even when from a histocompatible donor. However, histocompatibility is the most important factor in graft and transplant success.

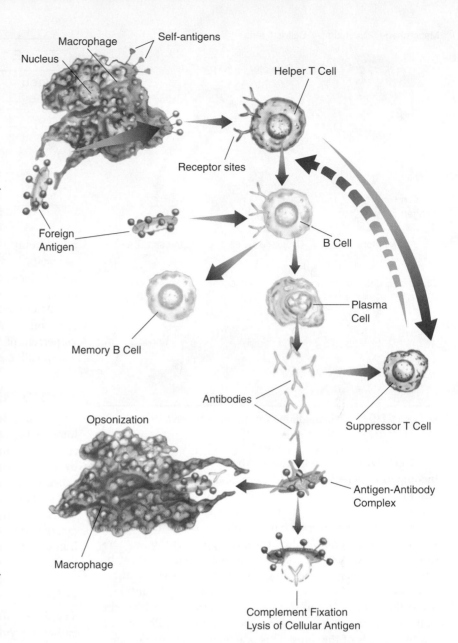

Blood Group Antigens

HLA antigens do not exist on the surface of erythrocytes (red blood cells), but other antigens, known as the blood group antigens, do. There are more than 80 of these red cell antigens that have been grouped into a number of different blood group systems. The two groups that trigger the strongest immune response are the Rh system and the ABO system.

The Rh System   The **Rh blood group** is named for the rhesus monkey in which it was first identified. One of several antigens in this group is known as Rh antigen D, or the **Rh factor**. Rh factor is present in about 85 percent of North Americans (Rh positive), but absent in about 15 percent (Rh negative).

Incompatibility between Rh positive and Rh negative blood can cause harmful immune responses. For example, if a patient with Rh negative blood receives a transplant of Rh positive blood, a primary immune response is triggered. If there is a second transfusion of Rh positive blood, a severe transfusion reaction may result.

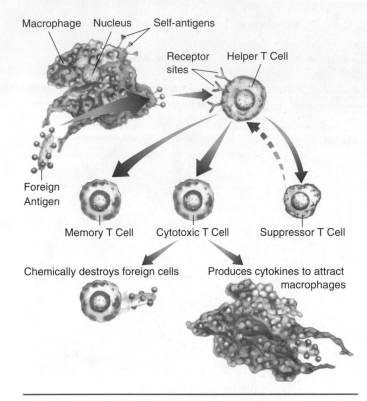

Macrophage   Nucleus   Self-antigens

Receptor sites   Helper T Cell

Foreign Antigen

Memory T Cell   Cytotoxic T Cell   Suppressor T Cell

Chemically destroys foreign cells

Produces cytokines to attract macrophages

● **Figure 1-93**   Cell-mediated immune response.

Hemolytic disease of the newborn may result from Rh incompatibility between mother and fetus. Problems will usually not occur in a first pregnancy where the mother is Rh negative and the fetus is Rh positive, because few fetal erythrocytes cross the placental barrier to the mother. However, a significant number of fetal erythrocytes do enter the mother's bloodstream at birth when the placenta separates from the uterus. These may (depending on several factors) activate a primary immune response and development of Rh antibodies. If the fetus in her next pregnancy is also Rh positive, the mother's Rh antibodies can cross the placenta and destroy the red blood cells of the fetus. This is actually a rare occurrence. Rh incompatibility occurs in only about 10 percent of pregnancies, and because not all such incompatibilities actually produce Rh antibodies in the mother, only about 5 percent of women ever have babies with hemolytic disease, even after numerous pregnancies.

The ABO System   The **ABO blood groups** are formed because there are two types of antigens that may be present on the surface of red blood cells. These antigens are named A and B. Persons with blood type A carry only A antigens on their red blood cells. Those with blood type B carry only B antigens. Those with blood type AB carry both, and those with blood type O carry neither (Table 1–16).

An immune response will be activated in a person with type A blood who receives a transfusion of type B blood, which is recognized as non-self. The same will happen when a person with type B blood receives type A blood. People with type O blood are known as *universal donors,* because type O blood has no antigens that will trigger an immune response in any

other group. Those with type AB blood are known as *universal recipients,* because they have both types of antigens and will not produce antibodies in response to any other blood groups (Table 1–17).

ABO incompatibility between mother and fetus is more common than Rh incompatibility, occurring in about 20 to 25 percent of pregnancies. However, only 10 percent of ABO incompatibilities will result in hemolytic disease of the infant.

Humoral Immune Response

Earlier, we identified the humoral immune response as the long-lasting response provided by production in the bloodstream of antibodies (immunoglobulins) and memory cells by B lymphocytes (review Figure 1-92). This is sometimes called the *internal* or *systemic immune system.* Another kind of humoral immunity is provided by secretions at the body surfaces, such as sweat and saliva, and is sometimes called the *external, mucosal,* or *secretory immune system.* These types of humoral immune responses will be discussed in the following sections.

B Lymphocytes

The blood cells that are involved in immune response, as noted earlier, are lymphocytes, which are one type of white blood cell. Lymphocytes are generated from *stem cells* in the bone marrow, from which all blood cells are generated. Lymphocytes

TABLE 1–16 | Blood Groups—ABO System		
Blood Type	**Antigen Present on Erythrocyte**	**Antibody Present in Serum**
O	None	Anti-A, Anti-B
AB	A and B	None
B	B	Anti-A
A	A	Anti-B

TABLE 1–17 | Compatibility among ABO Blood Groups				
Reaction with Serum of Recipient				
Cells of Donor	**AB**	**B**	**A**	**O**
AB	−	+	+	+
B	−	−	+	+
A	−	+	−	+
O	−	−	−	−
− = NO REACTION				
+ = REACTION				

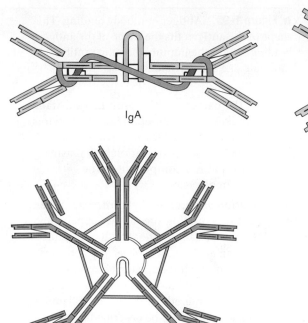

IgA

IgG

IgM

then take one of two paths as they mature. In one path, lymphocytes that travel through the thymus gland mature into T lymphocytes, which are involved in cell-mediated immunity and will be discussed in detail later. On the other path, lymphocytes that travel through a set of lymphoid tissues, including the spleen and lymph nodes, mature into B lymphocytes, which are involved in humoral immunity.

Each mature B cell recognizes, through an antigen receptor on its surface, a single type of antigen and then produces antibodies to that antigen. But since there are many, many kinds of antigens—and since exactly which foreign antigens may ever invade the body cannot be anticipated—how does a B cell develop a receptor that is specialized to a specific antigen?

It is thought that this specialization of B cells takes place through the processes of clonal diversity and clonal selection. **Clonal diversity** is generated as the precursors of mature B cells develop in the bone marrow. During this process, a B cell precursor develops receptors for every possible kind of antigen it may ever encounter. Later, after the immature B cells have migrated into the peripheral lymphoid organs, primarily the spleen and the lymph nodes, antigen that is present in the system reacts with the appropriate receptors on the surfaces of B cell clones, which is the process of **clonal selection**.

Clonal selection activates the immature B cell, prompting it to proliferate and differentiate, the end result being the mature B cell that produces plasma cells that secrete immunoglobulin antibodies into the blood and secondary lymphoid organs. The mature B cell also produces **memory cells** that will trigger a swifter and stronger immune response if they encounter the same antigen again (the secondary immune response). The process of clonal selection is probably responsible (during the primary immune response) for the lag time of five to seven days between introduction of an antigen and the first detectable appearance of antibodies in the blood.

Immunoglobulins

Immunoglobulins and Antibodies   Antibodies are proteins secreted by plasma cells that are produced by B cells in response to an antigen. All antibodies are immunoglobulins, but researchers have not yet determined whether all immunoglobulins function as antibodies.

The Structure of Immunoglobulins   The structure of immunoglobulin molecules consists of Y-shaped chains, arranged somewhat differently in the different immunoglobulin classes (Figure 1-94 ●). At the two "upper" tips of the Y are the *antigen-binding sites*. The interaction of amino acids with parts of the chain determines the shape of the immunoglobulin molecule's antigen-binding site. The shape of the antigen-binding site determines which antigen the immunoglobulin molecule will bind to—because there is an area on the antigen (the antigenic determinant) that will fit the shape of the antigen-binding site like a key in a lock (Figure 1-95 ●). In some cases, substitution of a single amino acid changes the conformation of the antigen-binding site and, therefore, the antigen it will combine with.

The Functions of Antibodies   An antibody circulates in the blood or is suspended in body secretions until it meets and binds to its specific antigen. The antibody can then have either a direct or an indirect effect on the target antigen that results in inactivation or destruction of the antigen. Both direct and indirect effects result from the binding of antibodies and antigens, forming **antigen-antibody complexes**, also called *immune complexes*.

Direct Effects of Antibodies on Antigens

- *Agglutination*—A soluble antibody combines with a solid antigen, causing it to clump together.
- *Precipitation*—The antigen-antibody complex precipitates out of the blood and is carried away by body fluids.
- *Neutralization*—The antibody, in combining with the antigen, inactivates the antigen by preventing it from binding to receptors on the surface of body cells.

Indirect Effects of Antibodies on Antigens

- *Enhancement of phagocytosis*—Phagocytosis is one of the chief processes of inflammation (described later in the chapter) in which certain types of white blood cells (neutrophils and macrophages) ingest and digest foreign substances. The actions of antibodies can encourage phagocytosis.

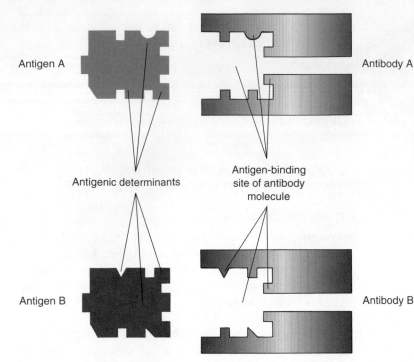

Antigen A

Antibody A

Antigenic determinants

Antigen-binding
site of antibody
molecule

Antigen B

Antibody B

● **Figure 1-95** Antigen-antibody binding. The shape of the antigen fits the shape of the antigen-binding site on the immunoglobulin (antibody) molecule like a key in a lock.

coats the bacteria with opsonin, a substance that makes them vulnerable to phagocytosis. Antibodies themselves are opsonins, and they also cause opsonization by a plasma protein that is a component of the complement system.

● *Activation of inflammatory processes.* When the antigen-binding sites at the "upper" tips of the Y-shaped immunoglobulin molecule bind to an antigen, the "lower" tip activates elements of the inflammatory response, transmitting the information that a foreign invader has entered the body. The inflammatory response (which will be described later) enhances the attack by the immune system against the invader.

● *Activation of plasma proteins*—Antibodies can activate plasma proteins of the complement system (described later) that, in turn, attack and destroy antigens.

Through the direct and indirect effects previously described, antibodies serve four main functions: neutralizing bacterial toxins, neutralizing viruses, opsonizing bacteria, and activating portions of the inflammatory response.

● *Neutralization of bacterial toxins.* As noted earlier, many bacteria produce harmful toxins that increase their pathogenic effect. However, bacterial toxins sow the seeds of their own destruction by triggering the humoral immune response. In this case the antigen-antibody complex is a *toxin-antitoxin complex.* Antibodies neutralize the bacterial toxins by occupying their antigenic determinant sites, which prevents them from binding to and harming tissue cells. Detection of specific antitoxins aids in the diagnosis of disease. Vaccines against diseases such as diphtheria and tetanus work by injecting a form of the bacterial toxin, which is altered to greatly reduce its toxic effects but to retain its immugenicity.

● *Neutralization of viruses.* Antibodies can prevent some viruses from attaching to and entering body cells. The antibodies attach to the viruses, causing agglutination or fostering phagocytosis. The effectiveness of antibodies against viruses depends on whether the virus circulates in the bloodstream (as with polio and flu) or spreads by direct cell-to-cell contact (as with measles and herpes). Antibodies against the latter may help prevent the initial infection but cannot prevent the spread or recurrence of an established infection. Vaccines are effective against some viral infections such as influenza, rubella, and polio.

● *Opsonization of bacteria.* Many bacteria have an outer capsule that is resistant to phagocytosis. Opsonization

Classes of Immunoglobulins   As noted earlier there are five classes of immunoglobulins. They are:

IgM—the antibody that is produced first during the primary immune response. It is the largest immunoglobulin.

IgG—the antibody that has "memory" and recognizes repeated invasions of an antigen. IgG comprises 80 to 85 percent of immunoglobulins in the blood. It is the major class of immunoglobulin in the immune response and has four subclasses. IgG is responsible for antibody functions such as agglutination, precipitation, and complement activation.

IgA—the antibody present in mucous membranes. One subclass of IgA is the predominant immunoglobulin in body secretions. The other subclass of IgA is present mostly in the blood.

IgE—the least-concentrated immunoglobulin in the circulation. It is the principal antibody that contributes to allergic and anaphylactic reactions and to the prevention of parasitic infections.

IgD—an antibody that is present in very low concentrations; little is known about its role. It is present principally on the surfaces of developing B cells.

Antibodies as Antigens   A molecule that functions as an antibody in the human body can function as an antigen if it enters the body of another person or a member of another species. To function in the role of antigens, antibody molecules usually contain antigenic determinants with which the antigen-binding sites on other antibodies can combine.

The antigenic determinants on human antibody molecules are classified into three groups:

● *Isotypic antigens* are species-specific. That is, they are the same within a given species but differ from those within other species. For example, isotypic antigens in human serum would function as antigens if injected into a rabbit.

- *Allotypic antigens* can differ between members of the same species. The serum from a person with one form of allotype might function as an antigen in another person.
- *Idiotypic antigenic determinants* can differ within the same individual. For example, IgG subclass 3 molecules produced against mumps and those produced against tetanus in the same person will differ from each other.

Monoclonal Antibodies Most antigens have multiple antigenic determinants, which stimulate a response from multiple clones of B lymphocytes. This is known as a *poly clonal response*. Each B cell clone secretes antibody that is slightly different from that of the other clones. Recently, researchers have been working with monoclonal antibodies. A **monoclonal antibody**, produced in the laboratory, is very pure and specific to a single antigen. Monoclonal antibodies are being put to a variety of cutting-edge and experimental uses, including identification of infectious organisms, blood and tissue typing, and treatment of autoimmune diseases and some cancers.

The Secretory Immune System

The **secretory immune system** (also known as the *external* or *mucosal immune system*) consists of lymphoid tissues beneath the mucosal endothelium. These tissues secrete substances such as sweat, tears, saliva, mucus, and breast milk. Some antibodies are present in these secretions (mostly IgA, with some IgM and IgG) and can help defend the body (or the nursing baby) against antigens that have not yet penetrated the skin or the mucous membranes.

The secretory immune system's primary function is to protect the body from pathogens that are inhaled or ingested. Other mechanisms must be functioning adequately to complete that task. For example, gastric acid helps destroy pathogens, and mechanisms such as blinking, sneezing, coughing, and peristalsis (the wavelike muscle contractions that move substances through the passageways of the digestive system) help move pathogens out of the system.

The lymphocytes of the secretory immune system follow a different developmental path after leaving the bone marrow than do the lymphocytes of the systemic immune system. As they mature, systemic lymphocytes migrate through the spleen and lymph nodes, whereas lymphocytes of the secretory system travel through the lacrimal (tear-producing) and salivary glands and through mucosal-associated lymphoid tissues in the bronchi, breasts, intestines, and genitourinary tract.

Secretory lymphocytes circulate through the lymphatic system and bloodstream in a pattern that is different from the circulatory pattern of the systemic lymphocytes. Secretory lymphocytes are returned from the blood through the tissues to the mucosal-associated lymphoid tissues, rather than to the lymphoid tissues of the systemic immune system.

The secretory immune system is the body's first line of defense against pathogens, whereas the systemic immune system is the body's last line of defense.

Cell-Mediated Immune Response

Some lymphocytes develop into B cells, which are responsible for *humoral immunity,* which we have discussed in the prior sections. Other lymphocytes develop into T cells, which are responsible for *cell-mediated immunity,* the subject of this section (review Figure 1-93).

A key difference between the two is that B cells do not attack pathogens directly. Instead, they produce antibodies that combine with antigens on the surfaces of pathogenic cells. The antibodies remain in the bloodstream for a long time and will attack the antigen again on any subsequent exposure. Thus, the humoral immunity created by B cells is long-lasting. T cells, however, do not produce antibodies. Rather, they attack pathogens directly, and the immunity they create, called cell-mediated immunity, is temporary.

Another key distinction is that one kind of T cell (helper T cells) is responsible for activating both T cells (in cell-mediated immune response) and B cells (in humoral immune response). (To compare humoral and cell-mediated responses, review Figure 1-91 as well as Figures 1-92 and 1-93.)

T Lymphocytes and Their Major Effects

In contrast to B lymphocytes, which travel through the spleen and lymph nodes as they mature, T cells travel through the thymus gland (hence the name *T cell*).

T cells become specialized through processes that are similar to the processes described earlier for B cells: clonal diversity and clonal selection. After generation by stem cells in the bone marrow, lymphocytes destined to become T cells travel to the thymus. There, through the process of *clonal diversity,* maturing T cells develop the capacity to recognize all the antigens they will ever encounter. Later, after the T cells have migrated into the peripheral lymphoid organs, they undergo the process of *clonal selection.* In this process, the immature T cells encounter antigens that react with appropriate receptors on the surfaces of the T cells, causing them to proliferate and differentiate into five different types of mature T cells, each with distinct functions.

Five Types of Mature T Cells

- *Memory cells* induce secondary immune responses.
- *Td cells* transfer delayed hypersensitivity (allergic responses) and secrete proteins called lymphokines that activate other cells such as macrophages.
- *Tc cells* are cytotoxic cells that directly attack and destroy cells that bear foreign antigens.
- *Th cells* are *helper cells* that facilitate both cell-mediated and humoral immune processes.
- *Ts cells* are *suppressor cells* that inhibit both cell-mediated and humoral immune processes.

As a result of this specialization, T cells are capable of attacking an antigen in a variety of ways. The major effects of cell-mediated immune response result from the specialized functions of the four types of T cells: memory, delayed hypersensitivity, cytotoxicity, and control.

Memory   Memory cells "remember" an antigen and trigger the immune response to any repeated exposure to that antigen.

Delayed Hypersensitivity   Td cells (delayed hypersensitivity cells) are involved in allergic reactions and the inflammatory response. They produce substances (lymphokines) that communicate with and influence the behavior of other cells.

Cytotoxicity   Tc cells (cytotoxic cells) mediate the direct killing of target cells, such as cells that have been infected by a virus, tumor cells, or cells in transplanted organs (Figure 1-96 ●).

Control   Th (helper) cells and Ts (suppressor) cells effect control of both humoral and cell-mediated immune responses. Th cells facilitate the response; Ts cells inhibit the response.

Cellular Interactions in Immune Response

The immune and inflammatory responses are interacting, not separate. For example:

Sequence of Events	Interaction
Macrophages released during an inflammatory response activate the helper T cells (Th cells).	Inflammatory response interacting with cell-mediated immune response
The helper T cells (Th cells) then activate other T cells, and they also activate B cells.	Cell-mediated immune response interacting with humoral immune response
Delayed hypersensitivity T cells (Td cells) stimulate the production of more macrophages.	Cell-mediated immune response interacting with inflammatory response

The three key interactions that occur during an immune response (review Figures 1-92 and 1-93) are:

1. Antigen-presenting cells (macrophages) interact with Th (helper) cells.

2. Th (helper) cells interact with B cells.

3. Th (helper) cells interact with Tc (cytotoxic) cells.

Cytokines

Cytokines, proteins produced by white blood cells, are the "messengers" of the immune response. When released by one cell, they can bind with nearby cells, affecting their function. They can also bind with the same cell that produced them and alter the function of that cell. They help to regulate cell functions during both inflammatory and immune responses. For example, a cytokine must be released by a macrophage to facilitate activation of a helper T cell.

A cytokine that is released by a macrophage is called a **monokine** ("mono" because a macrophage is a kind of monocyte, a single-nucleus white blood cell). A cytokine that is released by a lymphocyte (a T cell or B cell) is called a **lymphokine**. Types of cytokines include proteins known as *interleukins, interferon,* and *tumor necrosis factor.*

Antigen Processing, Presentation, and Recognition

A sequence of three processes is necessary before an immune response can begin:

1. Antigen processing (by macrophages)

2. Antigen presentation (by macrophages)

3. Antigen recognition (by T cells or B cells)

More will be said later in the chapter about how macrophages are released during the inflammatory response. For now, keep in mind that a *macrophage* is a large cell (a type of white blood cell) that will ingest and destroy or partially destroy an invading organism. As it does so, the invader's antigens are released into the cytosol (fluid interior) of the macrophage cell. The ingestion of an invading organism and breakdown of its antigens is the beginning of **antigen processing**.

Once the macrophage has broken down the antigens, it then expresses these antigen fragments and "presents" them on its own surface, along with its own self-antigens. When these

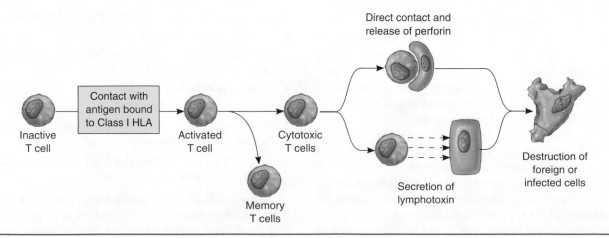

● **Figure 1-96**   The physiology of cytotoxic T cells.

two markers on the surface of the macrophage—the foreign antigens and the self-antigens—are recognized by helper T cells, the helper T cells are activated.

Because macrophages (and other macrophagelike cells) present portions of antigen on their surfaces, they are called **antigen-presenting cells (APCs)**.

The helper T cells recognize the presented antigen through receptors on their surfaces. There are two types of receptors. One type, called a **T cell receptor (TCR)**, is antigen-specific; that is, it will respond only to one specific antigen. The other type, CD4 or CD8 receptors, will respond no matter what antigen is presented.

As discussed earlier, the body recognizes whether an antigen is self or non-self as a result of HLA antigens. For presentation of an antigen to be effective, the antigen must be in a complex with either class I or class II HLA antigens. The HLA class determines which cells will respond. Th (helper) cells respond only to class II HLA antigens. Tc (cytotoxic) cells and Ts (suppressor) cells respond only to class I HLA antigens.

In addition to the antigen-receptor interaction, another requirement for intercellular communication between the macrophage cell and the T cell is an interaction between *self-adhesion molecules* on the surface of the macrophage and the T cell. These molecules, in connecting, strengthen the interactions between the cells.

The macrophage also produces the cytokine interleukin-1 (IL-1) that helps the T cell respond to the presented antigens.

T Cell and B Cell Differentiation

T cells and B cells are not differentiated until antigens present in the system react with the appropriate receptors on the cell surfaces. As previously described, this reaction occurs as a result of antigen processing and presentation by macrophages and antigen recognition by the T or B cell. The presence of secreted cytokines is also usually necessary to facilitate the antigen-receptor reaction.

Once a reaction between antigen and T cell receptor takes place, the immature T cells proliferate and differentiate, depending on the specific receptors and antigens involved, into Th, Tc, Td, Ts, and memory cells.

After stimulation by Th cells or direct recognition of antigen, B cells will proliferate and produce antibodies differentiated as IgM, IgG, IgA, IgE, and IgD immunoglobulins.

Control of T Cell and B Cell Development

There are several parameters that control immune responses, activating them when needed but stopping or inhibiting them when not needed, thus preventing them from destroying the body's own tissues. As noted earlier, Ts (suppressor) cells help suppress immune responses; so do some macrophages and other monocytes.

The exact function of suppressor cells is still not fully understood. Some suppressor cells seem to affect antigen recognition, while others seem to suppress the proliferation that follows antigen recognition. Tolerance of self-antigens seems to be another function of suppressor cells.

Fetal and Neonatal Immune Function

The human infant develops some immune response capabilities, even *in utero*, but the immune response system is normally not fully mature when the infant is born. For example, in the last trimester, the fetus can produce a primary immune response involving mostly IgM antibody to some infections. The ability to produce IgG and IgA antibodies is underdeveloped.

To protect the child *in utero* and during the first few months after birth, maternal antibodies cross the placenta into the fetal circulation. In the placenta, specialized cells called *trophoblasts* separate maternal from fetal blood. The trophoblastic cells actively transport the large immunoglobulin cells from maternal to fetal circulation. This transport is so effective that the level of antibodies in the umbilical cord is sometimes higher than in the mother's blood.

After birth, when antibodies can no longer be transported from the mother's blood, the levels of antibodies in the newborn's blood begin to drop as the immunoglobulins present at birth are catabolized, while the infant's ability to produce immunoglobulins on its own is still not fully developed. The levels are generally at their lowest at about five or six months of age (when many infants experience recurrent respiratory tract infections). Then, as the immune system matures, the levels of immunoglobulin begin to rise.

Aging and the Immune Response

As the human body ages, immune function begins to deteriorate. B cell antibody production is affected, but the primary assault is on T cell function. The thymus, which is the organ responsible for T cell development, reaches its maximum size at sexual maturity and then decreases in size until, in middle age, it has shrunk by 65 percent. Circulating T cells do not decrease, but T cell function may diminish. Men and women over age 60 generally have decreased hypersensitivity (allergic) responses and decreased T cell response to infections.

For a summary of the immune response, see Figure 1-97 ●.

INFLAMMATION

Inflammation Contrasted to the Immune Response

Inflammation, also called the *inflammatory response*, is the body's response to cellular injury. It differs from the immune response in many ways. As you read the following sections, keep in mind that:

● The immune response develops *slowly;* inflammation develops *swiftly.*

● The immune response is *specific* (targets specific antigens); inflammation is *nonspecific* (it attacks all unwanted substances in the same way). In fact, inflammation is sometimes called "the nonspecific immune response."

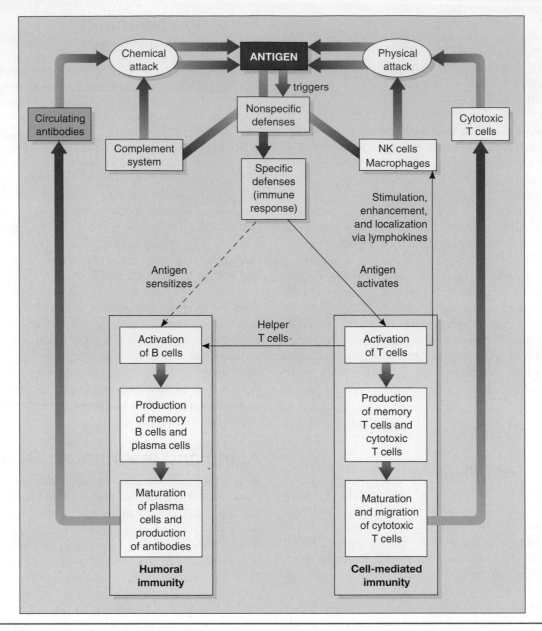

● **Figure 1-97**   The immune response.

- The immune response is *long-lasting* (memory cells will remember an antigen and trigger a swift response on reexposure, even years later); inflammation is *temporary,* lasting only until the immediate threat is conquered— usually only a few days to two weeks.

- The immune response involves *one type of white blood cell* (lymphocytes); inflammation involves *platelets and many types of white blood cells* (the granulatory cells called neutrophils, basophils, and eosinophils; and the monocytes that mature into macrophages).

- The immune response involves *one type of plasma protein* (immunoglobulins, also called antibodies); inflammation involves *several plasma protein systems* (complement, coagulation, and kinin).

However, the immune response and inflammation are interdependent. For example, macrophages that are developed during the inflammatory response must ingest antigens before helper T cells can recognize them and trigger the immune response. Conversely, IgE antibody produced by B cells during an immune response can stimulate mast cells to activate inflammation.

Although inflammation differs from the immune response in many ways, inflammation and the immune response are both considered to be part of the body's immune system.

How Inflammation Works: An Overview

Inflammation is somewhat easier to understand than the immune response, because we have all observed it. The immune response is often hidden; your body's immune system may be knocking out an infectious antigen without your ever being aware of it. However, if you cut your finger, you will probably be acutely aware of the inflammatory process. You will actually see the redness and swelling and feel the pain. You may observe the formation of pus. As days go by, you will see the progress of wound healing and, perhaps, scar formation.

This is not to say that inflammation is simple; in its way, it is as complex as the immune response. There are several phases to inflammation. After each phase, healing may take place, and that will be the end of it. If healing doesn't take place, inflammation moves into its next phase. However, healing is the goal of all the phases.

Phases of Inflammation

Phase 1: Acute inflammation

(If healing doesn't take place, moves to phase 2)

Phase 2: Chronic inflammation

(If healing doesn't take place, moves to phase 3)

Phase 3: Granuloma formation

Phase 4: Healing

During each phase, the components of inflammation work together to perform four functions.

The Four Functions of Inflammation (during All Phases)

- Destroy and remove unwanted substances
- Wall off the infected and inflamed area
- Stimulate the immune response
- Promote healing

Acute Inflammatory Response

Acute inflammation is triggered by any injury, whether lethal or nonlethal, to the body's cells. As discussed earlier in this chapter, cell injury can result from causes such as hypoxia, chemicals, infectious agents (bacteria, viruses, fungi, parasites), trauma, heat extremes, radiation, nutritional imbalances, genetic factors, and even the injurious effects of the immune and inflammatory responses themselves. When cells are injured, the acute inflammatory response begins within seconds (Figure 1-98 ●).

The basic mechanics are always the same: (1) Blood vessels contract and dilate to move additional blood to the site. Then, (2) vascular permeability increases so that (3) white cells and plasma proteins can move through the capillary walls and into the tissues to begin the tasks of destroying the invader and healing the injury site (Figure 1-99 ●).

Mast Cells

Mast cells, which resemble bags of granules, are the chief activators of the inflammatory response. They are not blood cells. Instead, they reside in connective tissues just outside the blood vessels.

Mast cells activate the inflammatory response through two functions: *degranulation* and *synthesis* (Figure 1-100 ●).

Degranulation

Degranulation is the process by which mast cells empty granules from their interior into the extracellular environment. This occurs when the mast cell is stimulated by one of the following events:

- *Physical injury,* such as trauma, radiation, or temperature extremes
- *Chemical agents,* such as toxins, venoms, enzymes, or a protein released by neutrophils (the latter an example of inflammatory response causing further cellular injury)
- *Immunologic and direct processes,* such as hypersensitivity (allergic) reactions involving release of IgE antibody or activation of complement components (discussed later)

During degranulation, biochemical agents in the mast cell granules are released, notably vasoactive amines and chemotactic factors.

Vasoactive Amines **Histamine** is a vasoactive amine (organic compound) released during degranulation of mast cells. The effect of vasoactive amines is the constriction of the smooth muscle of large vessel walls and dilation of the postcapillary sphincter, resulting in increased blood flow at the injury site.

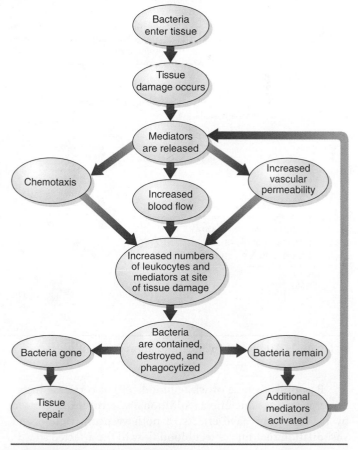

● **Figure 1-98** The inflammatory response.

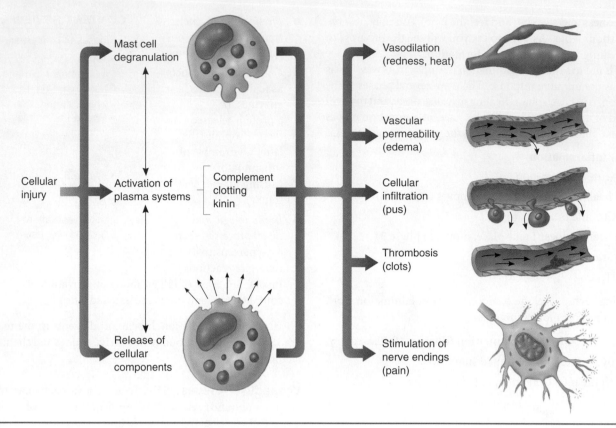

● **Figure 1-99**   The acute inflammatory response.

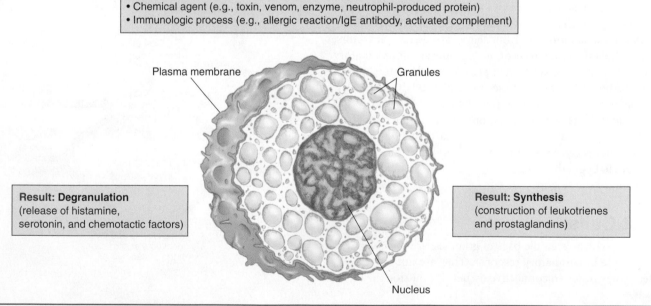

● **Figure 1-100**   Mast cell degranulation and synthesis.

Basophils (a type of white blood cell) also release histamine, with the same effect. Additionally, **serotonin**, released by platelets, can have effects of both vasoconstriction and vasodilation that may affect blood flow to the affected site.

Chemotactic Factors   Another consequence of degranulation of mast cells is the release of **chemotactic factors**. Chemotactic factors are chemicals that attract white cells to the site of inflammation. This attraction of white cells is called **chemotaxis**.

Synthesis

When stimulated, mast cells synthesize, or construct, two substances that play important roles in inflammation: leukotrienes and prostaglandins.

Leukotrienes Leukotrienes are also known as *slow-reacting substances of anaphylaxis (SRS-A)*. They have actions similar to those of histamines—vasoconstriction, vasodilation, and increased permeability—as well as chemotaxis. However, they are more important in the later stages of inflammation, because they promote slower and longer-lasting effects than histamines.

Prostaglandins Like leukotrienes, **prostaglandins** cause increased vasodilation, vascular permeability, and chemotaxis. They are also the substances that cause pain. In addition, prostaglandins act to control some inflammation by suppressing release of histamine from mast cells and suppressing release of lysosomal enzymes from some white cells.

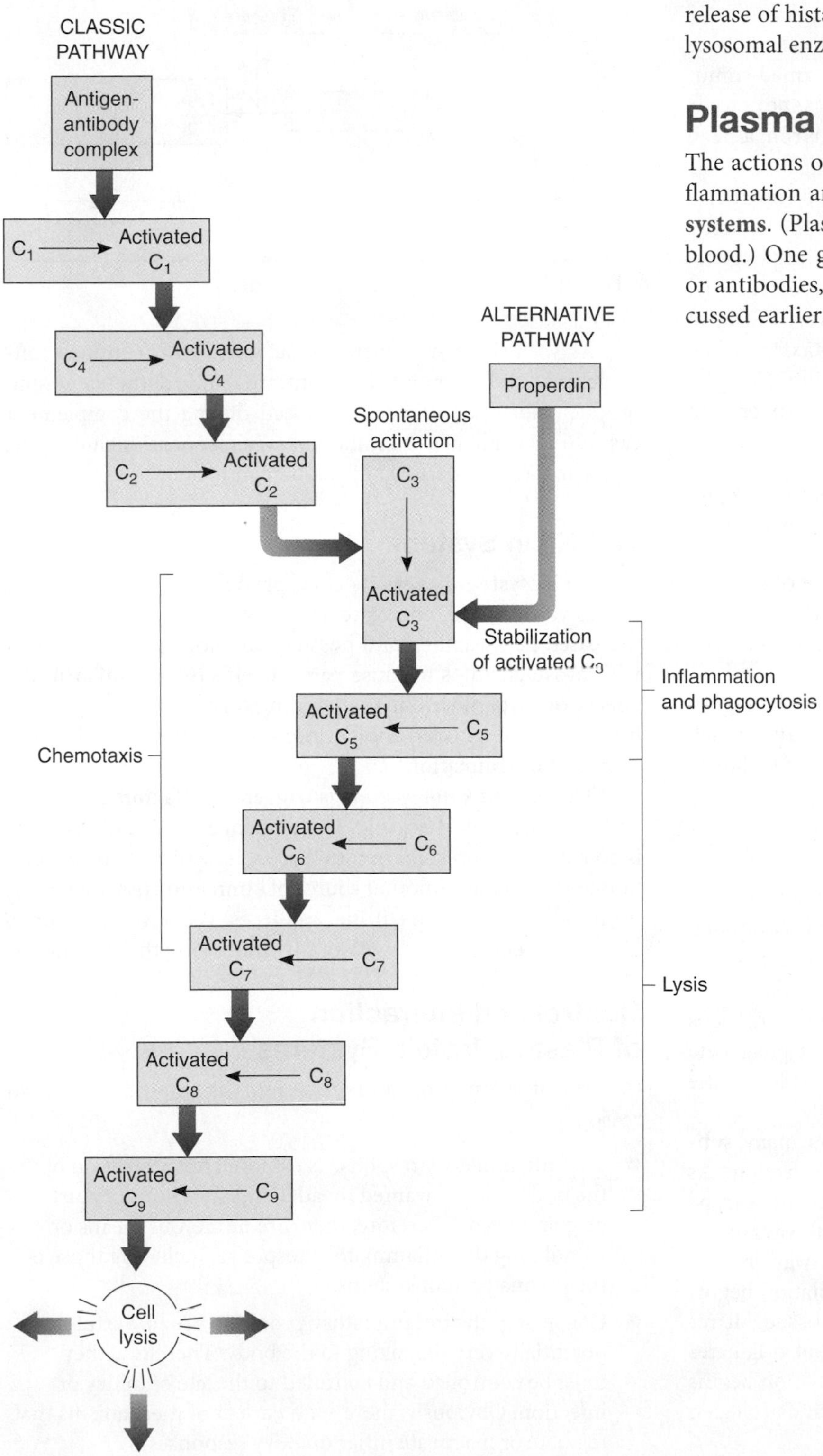

Plasma Protein Systems

The actions of white blood cells and other components of inflammation are mediated by three important **plasma protein systems**. (Plasma proteins are proteins that are present in the blood.) One group of plasma proteins, the immunoglobulins, or antibodies, are key factors in the immune response, as discussed earlier. Three other plasma protein systems are critical to inflammation: the complement system, the coagulation system, and the kinin system.

Important to an understanding of these plasma protein systems is the concept of **cascade**. In a cascade, a first action is stimulated, that action causes the next action, which causes the next action, and so on until a final action has been completed.

The Complement System

The **complement system** consists of 11 proteins (numbered C_1 through C_9 plus factors B and D) and comprises about 10 percent of all the proteins that circulate in the blood. The complement proteins lie inactive in the blood until they are activated. The complement system can be activated by formation of antigen-antibody complexes, by products released by invading bacteria, or by components of other plasma protein systems.

Once the C_1 complement is activated, the *complement cascade* proceeds through the rest of the sequence of proteins. When activated, the complement system takes part in almost all the events of the inflammatory response. The last few complements in the cascade have the ability to directly kill microorganisms.

There are two chief pathways by which the complement cascade is activated and proceeds: the classic pathway and the alternative pathway (Figure 1-101 ●).

● **Figure 1-101** The complement cascade. The classic pathway is activated at C_1 while the alternative pathway is activated at C_3.

CONTENT REVIEW

► Plasma Protein Functions

In immune response:

• Immunoglobulins

In inflammatory response:

• Complement system
• Coagulation system
• Kinin system

The Classic Pathway

In the classic pathway, the complement system is activated by formation of an antigen-antibody complex during the immune response. Complement factor C_1 is activated, and the cascade proceeds through complement factor C_9. Only a few antigen-antibody complexes are required to activate the complement cascade. The enzymes that are formed stimulate formation of increasing numbers of enzymes as the cascade proceeds, so that a very large response ensues, even from a small initial stimulus.

A number of effects that result from the complement cascade assist in destroying or limiting the damage of the invading organism. These include opsonization (coating) and phagocytosis (ingesting) of the organism, lysis (rupturing of bacterial cell membranes), agglutination (causing invading organisms to clump together), neutralization of viruses, chemotaxis of white cells, increased blood flow, and increased permeability. Complement proteins also lodge in the tissues and help to prevent spread of the infection.

The Alternative Pathway In some instances, the complement cascade can be activated without an intervening antigen-antibody complex formed by the immune response. Substances produced by some invading organisms are capable of reacting with complement factors B and D, which produce a substance that activates complement factor C_3, and the complement cascade then proceeds to its end.

Because the alternative pathway begins without waiting for the development of an antigen-antibody complex, it is much faster than the classic pathway and acts as part of the first line of inflammatory defense.

The Coagulation System

The **coagulation system**, also called the *clotting system,* forms a network at the site of inflammation. The network is composed primarily of a protein called *fibrin,* which is the end product of the coagulation cascade. The fibrinous network stops the spread of infectious agents and products of inflammation, keeps microorganisms "corralled" in the area of greatest phagocyte concentration, forms a clot that stops bleeding, and forms the foundation for repair and healing (Figure 1-102 ●).

The *coagulation cascade* can be activated by many substances released during tissue destruction and infection. As with the complement cascade, the coagulation cascade can be activated through either of two pathways. The pathways of coagulation cascade activation are the extrinsic pathway and the intrinsic pathway. The *extrinsic pathway* of coagulation begins with injury to the vascular wall or surrounding tissues. It requires exposure of the blood to a tissue factor that originates outside the blood. The *intrinsic pathway* of coagulation begins with exposure to elements in the blood itself, such as collagen from a traumatized vessel wall.

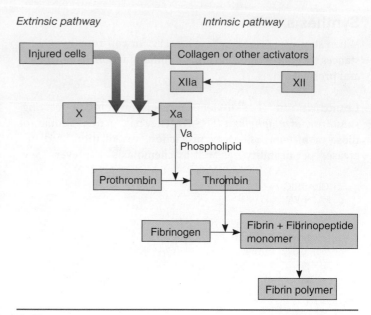

● **Figure 1-102** The coagulation cascade.

As with the complement cascade, the two pathways converge at a certain point and continue toward the same end product, fibrin. Substances produced during the complement cascade also enhance the inflammatory response, including increase of vascular permeability and chemotaxis.

The Kinin System

The **kinin system** has, as its chief product, *bradykinin,* which causes vasodilation, extravascular smooth muscle contraction, increased permeability, and possibly chemotaxis. It also works with prostaglandins to cause pain. Its effects are similar to the effects of histamine, but bradykinin works more slowly than histamine and so is probably more important during the later phases of inflammation.

The *plasma kinin cascade* is triggered by factors associated with the coagulation cascade. The sequence of the kinin cascade is conversion of prekallikrein to kallikrein, which then converts kininogen to kinin. Another source of kinin is the tissue kallikreins in saliva, sweat, tears, urine, and feces. Whatever the source, kinin is the end product, with bradykinin being the chief kinin.

Control and Interaction of Plasma Protein Systems

Control of the plasma protein systems is important for two reasons:

● The inflammatory response is essential for protection of the body from unwanted invaders. Its functioning must be guaranteed. Therefore, there are numerous means of stimulating the inflammatory response, including those of the plasma protein systems.

● Conversely, the inflammatory processes are powerful and potentially very damaging to the body. Therefore, they must be controlled and confined to the site of injury or infection. Obviously, there are a variety of mechanisms that regulate or inactivate inflammatory responses.

The inflammatory response is controlled at a number of levels and by a variety of mechanisms. For example, many components of inflammation are destroyed within seconds by enzymes from the blood plasma. Antagonists (substances or actions that counteract other substances or actions) exist for histamine, kinins, complement components, and other components of the inflammatory response.

An example of antagonistic control of inflammation is the function of histamine receptors. Histamine works by attaching itself to two types of receptors on the surface of target cells, H1 and H2 receptors. H1 receptors, when contacted by histamine, promote inflammation. H2 receptors are antagonistic to H1 receptors; when contacted by histamine, H2 receptors inhibit inflammation, mainly by suppressing leukocyte function and mast cell degranulation. In this way, the inflammatory action of histamine is triggered when needed, yet kept within bounds.

Most of the inflammatory processes interact; a substance or action that activates one element tends to activate others as well. For example, plasmin, an important factor in clot formation in the coagulation cascade, also has a role in activating the complement and kinin cascades. Conversely, controls on inflammatory processes also tend to interact. For example, a substance known as C1 esterase inhibitor inhibits plasmin activation that, in turn, tends to inhibit the coagulation, complement, and kinin cascades.

An example of what happens when interacting controls fail is the genetic deficiency of C1 esterase inhibitor. Its absence seems to permit uncontrolled activation of plasmin and triggering of the three plasma protein cascades when the patient undergoes emotional distress. This results in out-of-control effects typical of inflammation, including extreme edema of the gastrointestinal and respiratory tracts and the skin. The patient may die as a result of laryngeal swelling.

In other words, inflammatory processes have to be both reliably started and reliably stopped. Normally, this is ensured by the interacting processes of activation and control.

Cellular Components of Inflammation

An important term to remember in connection with inflammation is **exudate**, a collective term for all the helpful substances, including white cells and plasma, that move out of the capillaries into the tissues to attack unwanted substances and promote healing. This occurs in the sequence outlined below.

Sequence of Events in Inflammation

1. *Vascular response.* The first response of inflammation is vascular. First, arterioles near the site constrict; then there is vasodilation of the postcapillary venules. The result is an increase in blood flow to the injury site. One result is increased pressure within the microcirculation (arterioles, capillaries, and venules), which helps to exude plasma and blood cells into the tissues.

   When plasma and blood cells move out of the microcirculation, pressure is decreased, and blood moves more sluggishly, thickening and becoming sticky. White cells migrate to the vessel walls and adhere to them—a phenomenon known as **margination** that is important in the next two events.

2. *Increased permeability.* At the same time, chemical substances cause the endothelial cells of the vessel walls to constrict, creating openings between the cells in the vessel walls.

3. *Exudation of white cells.* The white cells adhering to the vessel walls now squeeze out through the openings and into the tissues. Note that, ordinarily, white cells are too large to move through vessel walls. The inflammation-caused constriction of vessel-wall cells that creates openings between them and allows white cells to squeeze through is known as **diapedesis**.

Earlier, we discussed lymphocytes, which are the category of white cells involved in the immune response. The inflammatory response involves two other categories of white cells: granulocytes and monocytes (Table 1–18). **Granulocytes** (like mast cells, discussed earlier) have the appearance of a bag of granules, hence their name. They are also called *polymorphonuclear cells* because they have multiple nuclei. There are three types of granulocytes: *neutrophils, eosinophils,* and *basophils.* **Monocytes,** so-named because they have a single nucleus, change and mature when they become involved in inflammation. Monocytes are the largest normal blood cell. During inflammation, they grow to several times their original size, becoming *macrophages.*

All the granulocytes and monocytes are **phagocytes**, blood cells that have the ability to ingest other cells and substances such as bacteria and cell debris. (The word comes from the Greek *phagein*, meaning "to eat," and *cyte,* for "cell"—so a phagocyte is a cell that eats.) A phagocyte behaves something like a Pac-Man® in the video game, destroying its "enemies" by swallowing them up. The most important

TABLE 1–18 | Types of White Blood Cells (Leukocytes)
Lymphocytes (25–30 percent of all white blood cells)*
T cells B cells
Granulocytes**
Neutrophils (55–70 percent of all white blood cells) Basophils Eosinophils
Monocytes**
Monocytes (immature) become macrophages (mature)**
*Involved in the immune response. **Involved in inflammation.

phagocytes involved in inflammation are the neutrophils and the macrophages.

Neutrophils are the first phagocytes to reach the inflamed site. They ingest bacteria, dead cells, and cell debris, and then they die. Neutrophils can begin phagocytosis quickly because they are already mature cells. *Macrophages* come along later, because they first have to go through the process of maturing from their parent monocytes.

Eosinophils, basophils, and platelets also migrate to the site to join the inflammatory response. These cells function with assistance from plasma proteins of the complement, coagulation, and kinin systems, acting to kill microorganisms, remove the dead cells and debris, and prepare the site for healing.

Eosinophils are the primary defense against parasites. They contain large numbers of lysosomes. The eosinophils attach themselves to parasites and degranulate, depositing the caustic lysosomes, and killing the parasites by damaging their surfaces. Eosinophils also release chemicals that control the vascular effects of serotonin and histamine. Additionally, eosinophils help to control the inflammatory response, preventing it from spreading beyond the area where it is needed by degrading vasoactive amines, thereby limiting their effects.

Basophils are thought to function in the same way within the blood as mast cells do outside the blood, releasing histamines and other chemicals that control constriction and dilation of vessels.

Platelets, another cellular component of the inflammatory response, are fragments of cytoplasm that circulate in the blood. When cellular injury occurs, platelets act with components of the coagulation cascade to promote blood clotting. Platelets also release serotonin, a substance with effects similar to those of histamine.

Cellular Products

As mentioned earlier, *cytokines* are proteins produced by white blood cells that act as "messengers" between cells. They are important in mediating both immune and inflammatory responses. Cytokines produced by lymphocytes are called *lymphokines*. Cytokines produced by macrophages and monocytes are called *monokines*.

Actually, cytokines are produced by a wide variety of cells, including some that are not part of the immune system. They play a wide variety of roles. Cytokines can interact in a synergistic manner (so that their combined effect is greater than the sum of their individual contributions) or they can interact in an antagonistic manner (so that they inhibit or cancel out each other's actions). Examples of the variety of sources and activities of cytokines can be found among the interleukins, lymphokines, and interferon.

Interleukins (ILs) are an important group of cytokines. They are produced by both lymphocytes and macrophages. Interleukin-1 is a lymphocyte-stimulating factor. As noted earlier, during the immune response macrophages that ingest antigens release IL-1, which assists helper T cells to respond to the antigens. It also enhances production of IL-2 by the helper T cells, which encourages antibody production. As part of the inflammatory process, IL-1 produced by macrophages induces neutrophilia, the proliferation of neutrophils.

Lymphokines are produced by T cells as a result of antigen stimulation during the immune response. In turn, these lymphokines stimulate monocytes to develop into macrophages, a critical phase of the inflammatory response. Different kinds of lymphokines have different effects. One type, called *migration-inhibitory factor (MIF)*, inhibits macrophages from migrating away from the site of inflammation. Another type, called *macrophage-activating factor (MAF)*, enhances the phagocytic activities of macrophages.

Interferon is a cytokine that is critical in the body's defense against viral infection. It is a small, low-molecular-weight protein produced and released by cells that have been invaded by viruses. It doesn't kill viruses, nor does it have any effect on a cell that is already infected by a virus. However, interferon prevents viruses from migrating to and infecting healthy cells.

Systemic Responses of Acute Inflammation

The three chief manifestations of acute inflammation are fever, leukocytosis (proliferation of circulating white cells), and an increase in circulating plasma proteins.

Endogenous pyrogen is a fever-causing chemical that is identical to IL-1 and is released by neutrophils and macrophages. It is released after the cell engages in phagocytosis or is exposed to a bacterial endotoxin or to an antigen-antibody complex. Fever can have both beneficial and harmful effects. On the one hand, an increase in temperature can create an environment that is inhospitable to some invading microorganisms. On the other hand, fever may increase susceptibility of the infected person to the effects of endotoxins associated with some Gram-negative bacterial infections.

In some infections, the number of circulating leukocytes, especially neutrophils, increases. Several components of the inflammatory response stimulate production of neutrophils, including a component of the complement system. Phagocytes produce a factor that induces production of granulocytes, including neutrophils, eosinophils, and basophils.

Plasma proteins called *acute phase reactants,* mostly produced in the liver, increase during inflammation. Their synthesis is stimulated by interleukins. Many of these act to inhibit and control the inflammatory response.

Chronic Inflammatory Responses

Defined simply, chronic inflammation is any inflammation that lasts longer than two weeks. It may be caused by a foreign object or substance that persists in the wound—for example, a splinter, glass, or dirt. Or it may accompany a persistent bacterial infection. This can occur because some microorganisms have cell walls with a high lipid or wax content that resist phagocytosis. Other microorganisms can survive inside a macrophage. Still others produce toxins that persist even after the bacterium is dead, continuing to incite inflammatory responses.

Inflammation can also be prolonged by the presence of chemicals and other irritants.

During chronic inflammation, large numbers of neutrophils—the phagocytes that were first on the scene during acute inflammation—degranulate and die. Now, the neutrophils are replaced by components that have taken longer to develop, and there is a large infiltration of lymphocytes from the immune response and of macrophages that have matured from monocytes. In addition to attacking foreign invaders, macrophages produce a factor that stimulates *fibroblasts*, cells that secrete collagen, a critical factor in wound healing.

As neutrophils, lymphocytes, and macrophages die, they infiltrate the tissues, sometimes forming a cavity that contains these dead cells, bits of dead tissue, and tissue fluid, a mixture called **pus**. Enzymes present in pus eventually cause it to self-digest, and it is removed through the epithelium or the lymphatic system.

Occasionally, when macrophages are unable to destroy the foreign invader, a **granuloma** will form to wall off the infection from the rest of the body. The granuloma is formed as large numbers of macrophages, other white cells, and fibroblasts are drawn to the site and surround it. Cells decay within the granuloma, and the released acids and lysosomes break the cellular debris down to basic components and fluid. The fluid eventually diffuses out of the granuloma, leaving a hollow, hard-walled structure buried in the tissues. Some granulomas persist for the life of the individual. Granuloma formation is common in leprosy and tuberculosis, which are caused by mycobacteria, bacteria that resist destruction by phagocytes.

Tissue repair and possible scar formation are the final stages of inflammation and will be discussed in more detail later.

Local Inflammatory Responses

All the manifestations observed at the local inflammation site result from (1) vascular changes and (2) exudation. Redness and heat result from vascular dilation and increased blood flow to the area. Swelling and pain result from the vascular permeability that permits infiltration of exudate into the tissues.

Exudate has three functions:

- To dilute toxins released by bacteria and the toxic products of dying cells

- To bring plasma proteins and leukocytes to the site to attack the invaders

- To carry away the products of inflammation (e.g., toxins, dead cells, pus)

The composition of exudate varies with the stage of inflammation and the type of injury or infection. Early exudate (serous exudate) is watery with few plasma proteins or leukocytes, as in a blister. In a severe or advanced inflammation, the exudate may be thick and clotted (fibrinous exudate) as in lobar pneumonia. In persistent bacterial infections, the exudate contains pus (purulent, or suppurative, exudate), as with cysts and abscesses. If bleeding is present, the exudate contains blood (hemorrhagic exudate).

The lesions (infected areas or wounds) that result from inflammation vary, depending on the organ affected. In myocardial infarction, cellular death results in the replacement of dead tissue by scar tissue. An infarction of brain tissue may result in liquefactive necrosis, in which the dead cells liquefy and are contained in walled cysts. In the liver, destroyed cells result in the regeneration of liver cells.

Keep in mind that inflammation can only occur in vascularized tissues (tissues to which blood can flow). When perfusion is cut off, as in a gangrenous limb or a limb distal to a tourniquet, inflammation cannot take place—and without inflammation, healing cannot take place.

Resolution and Repair

Healing begins during acute inflammation and may continue for as long as two years. The best outcome is **resolution**, the complete restoration of normal structure and function. This can happen if the damage was minor, there are no complications, and the tissues are capable of **regeneration** through the proliferation of the remaining cells. If resolution is not possible, then **repair** takes place with scarring being the end result. This happens if the wound is large, an abscess or granuloma has formed, or fibrin remains in the damaged tissues.

Both resolution and repair begin in the same way, with the **debridement** ("cleaning up") of the site of inflammation. Debridement involves the phagocytosis of dead cells and debris and the dissolution of fibrin cells (scabs). After debridement, there is a draining away of exudate, toxins, and particles from the site, and vascular dilation and permeability are reversed. At this point, either regeneration and resolution or repair and scar formation will take place.

Minor wounds with little tissue loss, like paper cuts, close and heal easily. They are said to heal by **primary intention**. More extensive wounds require more complex processes of sealing the wound, filling the wound, and contracting the wound and are said to heal by **secondary intention**.

Both resolution and repair proceed in two overlapping phases: reconstruction and maturation. Reconstruction begins three or four days after injury or infection and takes about two weeks. Maturation begins several days after injury or infection and can take up to two years.

Reconstruction

Reconstruction of a wound proceeds through four steps: initial wound response, granulation, epithelialization, and contraction.

Initial Response   The first step of healing is the sealing off of the wound by a clot (scab) that contains a mesh of fibrin and trapped red and white blood cells. The fibrin mesh is formed as a result of activation of the coagulation cascade. The fibrin traps platelets, which enhance the seal. The fibrin seal creates a barrier to bacterial invasion and a framework for collagen to fill the wound.

Eventually the fibrin clot is dissolved by enzymes and cleared away through debridement by macrophages and any remaining neutrophils. The clot will then be replaced by normal tissue (in the case of resolution) or by scar tissue (in the case of repair).

Granulation   Repair begins with **granulation**. Granulation tissues grow inward from the healthy connective tissues surrounding the wound. The granulation tissues are filled with capillaries. Some capillaries differentiate into venules and arterioles. Similarly, new lymph channels develop in the granulation tissues.

The granulation tissues are surrounded by macrophages. The macrophages secrete fibroblast-activating factor, which stimulates fibroblasts to enter the tissues and secrete collagen. The macrophages also secrete angiogenesis factor, which causes formation of the capillary buds, and an unidentified factor that stimulates epithelial factors to grow over the wound.

Epithelialization   While granulation is taking place and the original clot, or scab, is being dissolved, **epithelialization** takes place. Epithelial cells move in under the scab, separating it from the wound surface, and providing a protective covering for the healing wound.

Contraction   Six to twelve days after the injury, **contraction** begins as the wound edges begin to move inward. Contraction is caused by myofibroblasts in the granulation tissues. These are similar to the collagen-secreting fibroblasts, but myofibroblasts contain parallel fiber bundles in their cytoplasm similar to those in smooth muscle cells. They exert a contractile force as they connect to neighboring cells, slowly bringing the wound edges together.

Maturation

At the end of the reconstructive phase, collagen deposition, tissue regeneration, and wound contraction are seldom completed. These processes may continue into the maturation phase, possibly for years. During **maturation**, scar tissue is remodeled; blood vessels disappear, leaving an avascular scar; and the scar tissue becomes stronger.

Only epithelial, hepatic (liver), and bone marrow cells are capable of the total regeneration by mitosis known as hyperplasia (discussed earlier in the chapter). In most wounds, healing produces new tissues that are not structured exactly like the original tissues. Typically, repaired tissues regain about 80 percent of their original strength.

Dysfunctional Wound Healing

Dysfunctional healing can result in an insufficient repair, an excessive repair, or a new infection. Causes of dysfunctional healing vary, including disease states such as diabetes, hypoxemia, nutritional deficiencies, and the use of certain drugs. Dysfunctional healing can occur during the inflammatory response or during reconstruction.

Dysfunctional Healing during Inflammation   During inflammation, several factors can disrupt healing. If bleeding hasn't stopped, healing can be delayed by clotting that takes up space and inhibits granulation and by blood-cell debridement from the site. Blood is also a hospitable medium for infection, which in turn exacerbates inflammation and delays healing.

If there is excess fibrin in the wound, this, too, must be cleared away so as not to delay healing. Sometimes excess fibrin causes *adhesions,* fibrous bands that bind organs together and pose a significant problem if they occur in the abdominal, pleural, or pericardial cavities.

Other problems that can arise during inflammation include hypovolemia, which inhibits inflammation (remember that perfusion is necessary to inflammation), and anti-inflammatory steroid drugs that inhibit macrophage and fibroblast migration.

Dysfunctional Healing during Reconstruction   A number of factors can disrupt the phases of reconstruction. For example, various nutritional deficiencies can inhibit collagen synthesis. Collagen synthesis can also become excessive, causing the formation of raised scars. Steroid drugs can suppress epithelialization.

Wounds can also be disrupted by pulling apart. Surgical wounds are sometimes disrupted as a result of strain or obesity. In some cases, frequently with burns, wound contraction is excessive, resulting in a deformity called *contracture.* Internal contractures may occur in cirrhosis of the liver, duodenal strictures caused by improper healing of an ulcer, or esophageal strictures from lye burns.

Positioning, exercises, surgery, and administration of drugs can sometimes help to prevent or correct the results of dysfunctional wound healing.

Age and the Mechanisms of Self Defense

Newborns and the elderly are particularly susceptible to problems of insufficient immune and inflammatory responses.

As noted earlier in the chapter, neonates generally go through a phase at about five or six months of age when immune system protection received from their mother is depleted and their own immune system is still immature, making them particularly susceptible to respiratory tract infections. Inflammatory responses are similarly immature in the neonate. For example, neutrophils and monocytes may not be capable of chemotaxis, the release of ctors that attract other white cells to the site of infection. This makes newborns prone to infections such as cutaneous abscesses and cutaneous candidiasis. As another example, the deficiency of a component of the complement cascade in infants can cause a severe, overwhelming sepsis or meningitis when infants are infected by bacteria for which they do not have transferred maternal antibody.

The elderly also have difficulties with both the immune and the inflammatory responses. As discussed earlier in the chapter, B cell and especially T cell functions of the immune system decrease markedly after age 60. The elderly are also prone to impaired wound healing. This is thought not to be due to the normal processes of aging but rather to the higher incidence of chronic diseases such as diabetes and cardiovascular disease in the elderly. Also, many elderly persons take prescribed anti-inflammatory steroids for conditions such as arthritis, and these inhibit inflammation. Decreased perfusion contributes to hypoxia in the wound bed, inhibiting inflammation and healing. Unfortunately, the elderly are also more prone to wounding as the protective fat layer diminishes and skin loses its elasticity and becomes more vulnerable to tearing. Diminished sensitivity, mobility, and balance also lead to falls and wounds.

VARIANCES IN IMMUNITY AND INFLAMMATION

Sometimes the immune and inflammatory systems work "too well" and sometimes not well enough. Hypersensitivity reactions are an example of the former, while immune deficiency diseases are an example of the latter.

Hypersensitivity: Allergy, Autoimmunity, and Isoimmunity

Immune responses are normally protective and helpful. **Hypersensitivity**, however, is an exaggerated and harmful immune response. The word *hypersensitivity* is often used as a synonym for *allergy*. However, *hypersensitivity* is also used as an umbrella term for allergy and two other categories of harmful immune response, which are defined as follows:

Three Types of Hypersensitivity

- **Allergy**—an exaggerated immune response to an environmental antigen, such as pollen or bee venom.

- **Autoimmunity**—a disturbance in the body's normal tolerance for self-antigens, as in hyperthyroidism or rheumatic fever.

- **Isoimmunity** (also called *alloimmunity*)—an immune reaction between members of the same species, commonly of one person against the antigens of another person, as in the reaction of a mother to her infant's Rh negative factor or in transplant rejections.

The exact cause of such pathological immune responses is not known, but at least three factors seem to be involved: (1) the original insult (exposure to the antigen); (2) the person's genetic makeup, which determines susceptibility to the insult; and (3) an immunologic process that boosts the response beyond normal bounds.

Hypersensitivity reactions are classified as **immediate hypersensitivity reactions** or **delayed hypersensitivity reactions**, depending on how long it takes the secondary reaction to appear after reexposure to an antigen. The swiftest immediate hypersensitivity reaction is *anaphylaxis,* a severe allergic response that usually develops within minutes of reexposure. (Review anaphylactic shock earlier in this chapter. Also see Volume 3, Chapter 6 on allergies and anaphylaxis.)

Mechanisms of Hypersensitivity

Usually, when a hypersensitivity reaction takes place, inflammation is triggered that results in destruction of healthy tissues. Four mechanisms, or types, of hypersensitivity that cause this destructive reaction have been identified.

Mechanisms of Hypersensitivity Reaction

- Type I—IgE-mediated allergen reactions
- Type II—tissue-specific reactions
- Type III—immune-complex-mediated reactions
- Type IV—cell-mediated reactions

In reality, hypersensitivity reactions are not so easy to categorize. Most involve more than one type of mechanism.

Type I—IgE Reactions As noted earlier in the chapter, IgE is the type of immunoglobulin (antibody) that contributes most to allergic and anaphylactic reactions. The first exposure to the allergen (antigen that causes allergic reaction) stimulates B lymphocytes to produce IgE antibodies. These bind to receptors on mast cells in the tissues near blood vessels. On reexposure (or after several reexposures), the allergen binds to the IgE on the mast cell, which causes degranulation of the mast cell, release of histamine, and triggering of the inflammatory process.

The potency of the inflammatory response is controlled in two ways. As discussed earlier, H1 receptors on target cells promote inflammation when contacted by histamine, while H2 receptors inhibit inflammation when contacted by histamine. Another control mechanism is the autonomic nervous system, which stimulates production of chemical mediators (epinephrine, acetylcholine) that govern release of inflammatory mediators from the mast cells and the degree to which target cells will respond to inflammatory processes.

The clinical indications of type I IgE-mediated responses are the familiar signs and symptoms of allergic and anaphylactic response.

Clinical Indications of IgE-Mediated Responses

- *Skin*—flushing, itching, urticaria (hives), edema
- *Respiratory system*—breathing difficulty, laryngeal edema, laryngospasm, bronchospasm
- *Cardiovascular system*—vasodilation and permeability, increased heart rate, increased blood pressure
- *Gastrointestinal system*—nausea, vomiting, cramping, diarrhea
- *Nervous system*—dizziness, headache, convulsions, tearing

CONTENT REVIEW

▶ Four Types of Hypersensitivity Reactions

- *Type I*—IgE reactions
- *Type II*—Tissue-specific reactions
- *Type III*—Immune-complex-mediated reactions
- *Type IV*—Cell-mediated reactions

There is a genetic component to Type I, IgE-mediated responses. Some individuals suffer from *atopia,* in which higher amounts of IgE are produced, and there are more receptors for IgE on the mast cells. In families where one parent has an allergy, approximately 40 percent of the offspring will also have allergies. If both parents are atopic, approximately 80 percent of their off-spring will also be atopic.

Anaphylactic reactions are life threatening. Therefore, people who have reason to believe they are susceptible need to find out what specific allergens they are sensitized to so they can avoid them. A number of tests have been developed that are successful in making these identifications. Additionally, there has been some success in desensitizing some individuals by injecting small but increasing doses of the offending allergen over a long period of time. Research in desensitization techniques is ongoing.

Type II—Tissue-Specific Reactions Most cells of the body present HLA antigens, the antigens that the body recognizes as self or non-self. In addition to HLA antigens, most tissues have other antigens, but these are not the same in all tissues. They are called *tissue-specific antigens* because they exist on the cells of only some body tissues. An immune response against one of these antigens will affect only the organs or tissues that present that particular antigen; this is called a *tissue-specific reaction.*

There are four mechanisms by which Type II tissue-specific reactions attack cells. The first involves the complement system. Antibody bound to the antigen of the target cell initiates the complement cascade, which causes lysis (dissolving) of the cell's plasma membrane. The second mechanism is clearance of the target cells by macrophages. In the third mechanism, antibody bound to the antigen on the target cell also binds to cytotoxic cells, which release toxins that destroy the target cell. In the fourth mechanism, the antibody disables the target cell by occupying receptor sites on the cell, preventing them from binding to molecules that are needed for normal cell functioning.

Type III—Immune-Complex-Mediated Reactions Type III immune-complex-mediated reactions result from antigen-antibody complexes (also called *immune complexes*) that, as discussed earlier, are formed when antibody circulating in the blood or suspended in body secretions meets and binds to a specific antigen. The immune complexes generally circulate for a time before finally being deposited in vessel walls or other tissues. For this reason, which organs are affected may have very little connection with where or how the antigen or the immune complex originated.

The harmful effects of the immune complex result from the activation of the complement system. Some complement fragments are chemotactic for (attract) neutrophils. The neutrophils attempt to ingest the immune complexes but frequently fail because the complexes are bound to the tissues. During this attempt, the neutrophils release large quantities of damaging lysosomal enzymes into the tissues.

The nature and course of immune complex diseases vary tremendously. This results from the fact that immune complex formation is dynamic and constantly changing. There can be variations in the quantity and quality of circulating antigen and the antigen-antibody ratio. Also, many immune complexes bind complement components effectively, which causes complement levels in the blood to fluctuate. In some cases, the interaction between complement and the immune complexes results in dissolving the complex and mitigating its effects. As a result of these factors, immune complex diseases are characterized by tremendous variability in symptoms and periods of alternating remission and exacerbation.

Some immune complex diseases are systemic and some are localized. Systemic immune complex diseases are called *serum sickness.* They typically present with fever, enlarged lymph nodes, rash, and pain, commonly affecting the blood vessels, joints, and kidneys. *Raynaud's phenomenon* is a form of serum sickness in which temperature governs deposition of immune complexes in the peripheral circulation. Typical presentations include numbness in the fingers and toes, followed by cyanosis and gangrene or redness and pain.

Arthrus reaction is an example of a localized immune complex disease. It results from the interaction of an environmental antigen with preformed antibody lodged in the walls of blood vessels. A typical inflammatory response follows, resulting in edema, hemorrhage, clotting, and tissue damage. The antigen can enter the body through injection, ingestion, or inhalation. Examples of arthrus reactions are skin reactions following inoculations, gastrointestinal reactions to ingestion of wheat products, or hemorrhagic inflammation of the alveoli following inhalation of fungus from a source such as moldy hay.

Type IV—Cell-Mediated Tissue Reactions Types I, II, and III hypersensitivity reactions are mediated by antibody. Type IV reactions are activated directly by T cells and do not involve antibody. There are two cell-mediated mechanisms. One involves lymphokine-producing T cells (Td cells). The other involves cytotoxic T cells (Tc cells). The lymphokine produced by Td cells activates other cells such as macrophages. The Tc cells attack antigen-bearing cells directly and destroy them with the toxins they produce.

Graft rejection and contact allergic reactions such as poison ivy are examples of Type IV reactions. There may also be Type IV components to autoimmune diseases such as rheumatoid arthritis, where the self-antigen is a protein present in joint tissues, and insulin-dependent diabetes, where the self-antigen is a protein on the cell of the pancreas that produces insulin.

Targets of Hypersensitivity

Antigens, the proteins or "markers" on the surface of cells, are the targets of the immune response and of the exaggerated immune response called hypersensitivity. As noted earlier, cells bearing these antigens can come from one of three sources: the environment, the person's own body, or another person.

The source of the target antigen is what defines the type of hypersensitivity, as follows:

Type of Hypersensitivity	Targeted Antigen
Allergy	Environmental antigens
Autoimmunity	Self-antigens
Isoimmunity	Other person's antigens

In Allergy The antigens that are the targets of allergic reaction are called *allergens*. Allergens typically occur on cells from such environmental sources as ragweed, molds, certain foods such as shellfish or peanuts, animal sources such as cat dander, cigarette smoke, and components of house dust. Often, an allergen is contained in a capsule that is too large to be phagocytosed or is surrounded by a nonallergenic coating. The actual allergen is not released until the capsule or coating is broken down by enzymes. Most allergens are low-molecular weight immunogens or haptens (which are too small to cause an immune response unless they bind with larger molecules).

In some situations, an allergen combines with components of the host tissue (tissues of the person's body) to form a new substance, called a *neoantigen,* which in its turn induces an allergic response. For example, a drug such as penicillin, which causes an allergic reaction in some people, is a hapten. It does not cause an allergic reaction until it binds to proteins on the plasma membranes of host cells. The immune system attacks the neoantigen and destroys the cell it is bound to as well. In the case of penicillin, which attaches to red blood cells, the immune response kills the red cells and causes anemia.

In Autoimmunity The immune system normally recognizes the person's own tissues as self and tolerates the self-antigens presented by the body's own cells. If the body generated an immune response to its own tissues, it would destroy itself. Autoimmunity is a form of exactly this undesirable situation: There is a breakdown in the body's tolerance for self-antigens, and the immune system begins to attack the body's own cells.

Tolerance for self-antigens begins in the embryo when any lymphocytes that react to self-antigens are eliminated or suppressed. Several causes of a later breakdown in tolerance have been identified.

For example, some cells are *sequestered* (hidden) from the immune system by existing in areas of the body that are not drained by lymph (for example, the cornea and the testicles). If these cells become exposed to the immune system (e.g., during trauma), the body may recognize them as foreign and initiate an autoimmune response.

A neoantigen can trigger an immune response to the cells it is bound to. Infectious diseases can also trigger autoimmune responses in one of two ways. A foreign infectious antigen, in binding with an antibody, can form an immune complex that lodges in host tissues and causes an autoimmune response to the cells of those tissues. Additionally, a foreign antigen may resemble a self-antigen to such a degree that the antibody to the foreign antigen also attacks the self-antigen.

Suppressor T cell dysfunction is another cause of autoimmune disorders. In normal immune function, some T cells develop clones that attack self-antigens. Suppressor T cells are thought to have the function of suppressing these autoimmune responses. However, if the suppressor T cells dysfunction, the autoimmune response caused by T cell clones is able to develop.

The original insult that causes the autoimmune response is usually easy to identify; for instance, an administered drug causing autoimmune anemia or a recent infection such as rubella causing autoimmune encephalitis. In other cases, the causative insult cannot be identified. In these cases, the autoimmune disease is thought to have resulted from a prior infection that is no longer traceable.

Genetic causes are actually easier to identify than pathological causes. Most autoimmune diseases are familial. All affected family members may not have the same disorder, but each may have a different autoimmune disorder or a disorder characterized by hypersensitivity responses.

In Isoimmunity In isoimmunity, one member of a species has an immune reaction to cells from another member of the same species. In humans, two types of isoimmune disorders are most common, as discussed earlier in this chapter. One type consists of transient neonatal diseases, in which the mother becomes sensitized to fetal antigens, as in Rh negative sensitivity. The other type is encountered in the rejection of grafts or transplants from one person to another.

Autoimmune and Isoimmune Diseases

A number of diseases are recognized or suspected to have an autoimmune or isoimmune basis. Some examples are noted below.

- *Graves' disease* is thought to be caused by an antibody that stimulates overproduction of thyroid hormone. People with Graves' disease have the symptoms of hyperthyroidism (e.g., elevated heart rate and blood pressure, increased appetite, increased activity level) plus a visibly enlarged thyroid gland (goiter), bulging eyes, and sometimes raised areas of skin over the shins. A pregnant woman with Graves' disease can pass the antibody and the disease along to the newborn.

- *Rheumatoid arthritis* is a disease that causes inflammation of the joints and eventual destruction of the interior of the joint. Its exact cause is not known, but it is recognized as an autoimmune disorder, probably involving antibody reactions to self-antigen in the collagen of the joints.

• *Myasthenia gravis* is a disease caused by antibody response to self-antigens on acetylcholine receptors and the striations of skeletal and cardiac muscle. It is characterized by abnormal function of the neuromuscular junction, resulting in episodes of muscular weakness. Like Graves' disease, the mother's antibody can bind with receptors on the infant's muscle cells, causing neonatal muscle weakness.

• *Immune thrombocytopenic purpura (ITP)* presents with pinhead-sized red spots on the skin, unexplained bruises, and bleeding from the gums and nose and into the stool. It is characterized by a low platelet count. The exact cause is not known, but an autoimmune disorder in which antibodies destroy the person's own platelets appears to be involved. Maternal antibodies can also destroy platelets in the neonate.

• *Isoimmune neutropenia* occurs when a mother has developed antibodies that attack and severely reduce the level of neutrophils in her blood. The antibody in the maternal blood can also attack and destroy neutrophils in the blood of the neonate.

• *Systemic lupus erythematosus (SLE),* also called simply *lupus,* is an autoimmune disease in which a variety of antibodies to self-antigens are developed that then attack nucleic acids, red blood cells, coagulation proteins, lymphocytes, platelets, and many other targets within the person's own body. The disease causes episodal inflammations of joints, tendons, and other connective tissues and organs. The diversity of antibodies in maternal blood can cause a variety of problems, such as congenital heart defects, in the infant.

• *Rh and ABO isoimmunization,* or hemolytic disease of the newborn, was discussed earlier in the chapter. It is an isoimmune disease that causes severe anemia in the neonate. Immune problems occur if antigens on fetal red blood cells are different from antigens on maternal red blood cells.

Deficiencies in Immunity and Inflammation

Immune deficiency disorders result from impaired function of some component of the immune system, including phagocytes, complement, and lymphocytes (T cells and B cells), with lymphocyte dysfunction being the primary cause. Immune deficiency can be congenital (inborn) or acquired (after birth). The most common manifestations of immune deficiency are recurrent infections, because the body's ability to ward off invaders has been damaged.

Congenital Immune Deficiencies

Congenital, or primary, immune deficiency develops if the development of lymphocytes in the fetus or embryo is impaired or halted. Different immune-deficiency diseases may develop, depending on whether the T cells, the B cells, or both have been affected.

In the *DiGeorge syndrome,* there is a lack or partial lack of thymus development, resulting in a severe decrease in T cell production and function. *Bruton agammaglobulinemia* is caused by impaired development of B cell precursors, resulting in B cells that cannot produce IgM or IgD antibodies. In *bare lymphocyte syndrome,* lymphocytes and macrophages are unable to produce Class I or Class II HLA antigens, which disrupts the ability of cells to recognize self or non-self substances, resulting in severe infections that are usually fatal before age 5.

Sometimes there is a defect that depresses the function of just a small portion of the immune system. For example, in *Wiskott-Aldrich syndrome,* IgM antibody production is reduced. *Selective IgA deficiency* is the most common immune deficiency. IgA is the antibody present in mucous membranes. People with IgA deficiency frequently suffer from sinus, lung, and gastrointestinal infections.

Some immune system deficiencies cause a decreased ability to respond to one particular antigen. For example, in *chronic mucocutaneous candidiasis,* the T lymphocytes are unable to respond against candida infections.

Acquired Immune Deficiencies

Acquired, or secondary, immune deficiencies develop after birth and do not result from genetic factors. They can be caused by or associated with pregnancy, infections, and diseases such as diabetes or cirrhosis. The elderly are more prone to acquired immune deficiencies than the young. Among the factors that can severely affect immune function are nutritional deficiencies, medical treatment, trauma, and stress. Of special interest is the fatal acquired immune disorder AIDS.

Nutritional Deficiencies   Critical deficits in calorie or protein ingestion can lead to depression of T cell production and function. Complement activity, neutrophil chemotaxis, and the ability of neutrophils to kill bacteria are also seriously affected by starvation. Zinc deficiencies and vitamin deficiencies can affect both B cell and T cell function.

Iatrogenic Deficiencies   Iatrogenic deficiencies are those that are caused by medical treatment. Some drugs depress blood cell formation in the bone marrow. Others trigger immune responses that destroy granulocytes. Immunosuppressive drugs administered in the treatment for transplants, cancer, or autoimmune diseases suppress B and T cell function and antibody production. Radiation treatment for cancer exacerbates this effect. Surgery and anesthesia also can suppress B and T cell function, with severely depressed white cell levels persisting for several weeks after surgery. Surgical removal of the spleen depresses humor response against encapsulated bacteria, depresses IgM levels, and decreases the levels of opsonins.

Deficiencies Caused by Trauma   Burn victims are especially susceptible to bacterial infection. Not only has the normal barrier presented by the skin been disrupted, but thermal burns also appear to decrease neutrophil function, complement levels, and other immune functions while increasing immunosuppressive functions, which further depress immune function.

Deficiencies Caused by Stress It has long been suggested that persons undergoing emotional stress (major stresses such as divorce, but also minor stresses such as studying for final exams) are more prone to illness. The speculation was that stress has deleterious effects on immune function. Research into the possible mechanisms of stress-induced immune deficiency are just getting under way. (Stress and susceptibility to disease will be discussed later in the chapter.)

AIDS AIDS is an acronym for *acquired immunodeficiency syndrome,* which has become the best known acquired immune deficiency disorder. AIDS is a syndrome of disorders that develop from infection with **HIV**, the *human immunodeficiency virus.*

HIV is a retrovirus; that is, it carries its genetic information in RNA rather than DNA molecules. As a retrovirus, HIV infects target cells by binding to receptors on their surfaces, then inserting the HIV RNA into the cell. There, the RNA is converted into DNA and becomes part of the infected cell's genetic material. HIV can remain dormant inside the host cell for years; however, once the cell is activated (and the mechanism by which this occurs is not fully understood), HIV proliferates, kills the host cell, and can then infect other cells. The result is a pervasive breakdown of the immune defenses, making the body vulnerable to a wide variety of infections and disorders.

HIV can infect anybody, male or female, homosexual or heterosexual, mostly through the exchange of body fluids during sexual intercourse or through injection. In the United States, most cases to date have involved homosexual men and intravenous drug users. However, preventive measures (safe sex practices, including use of condoms, and clean-needle programs) have reduced the incidence of HIV/AIDS among homosexual populations and drug users. An increasing proportion of new patients are females who have acquired the infection during heterosexual intercourse. In other parts of the world, HIV/AIDS occurs equally among men and women.

The possibility of acquiring HIV/AIDS by contact with patients or accidental needlesticks fostered something of a panic among health care workers when AIDS first spread so alarmingly in the United States in the 1970s. Following recommendations by OSHA, universal precautions (Standard Precautions) have been widely adopted—including the use of disposable gloves, protective eyewear, masks, and gowns, as appropriate, to avoid contact with any body fluids, along with improved techniques for handling needles and other sharps. These measures have proved effective in reducing the fear of HIV/AIDS infection and also in making such infections very rare among health care workers.

Until recently, more than 90 percent of those with AIDS have died within five years of the development of severe symptoms. This picture has improved somewhat in developed nations with the initiation of treatments involving multiple chemotherapies (treatment "cocktails") that have shown success in prolonging life, greatly improving feelings of health and well-being, and suppressing measurable blood levels of HIV.

It is not yet known if such treatments can eradicate HIV and cure AIDS. One fear is that the treatments suppress but do not totally destroy the HIV virus, which "hides" somewhere in the body, waiting to proliferate at some later date. Another fear is that HIV will develop strains that are resistant to the treatments that appear to be successful in the short term. Nevertheless, the success of these treatments has caused the first feelings of optimism since AIDS was identified. Preventive measures have also helped to greatly reduce the number of new cases reported in the United States. In some parts of the world, however, including Africa and Asia, HIV/AIDS is still spreading at an extremely alarming rate, with seriously inadequate reporting, prevention, and treatment.

Replacement Therapies for Immune Deficiencies

Advances have been made in the treatment of immune deficiencies through the use of replacement therapies, such as those listed below.

Replacement Therapies

Gamma globulin therapy. Gamma globulin is administered to individuals with B cell deficiencies that cause immunoglobulin (antibody) deficiencies.

Transplantation and transfusion. HLA-matched bone marrow is transplanted into patients suffering *severe combined immune deficiencies (SCID),* which is caused by a lack of the stem cells from which T cells and B cells develop. In patients who lack a thymus or have a defective thymus, fetal thymus tissue may be transplanted. Enzyme deficiencies that cause SCID have been treated with transfusions of red blood cells that contain the needed enzyme. Other substances have been transfused into individuals to help restore T cell function and reactivity against certain antigens.

Gene therapy. Therapies involving identification of defective genes that are responsible for immune disorders, and replacement of these defective genes with cloned normal genes, are in the early stages of development and use.

STRESS AND DISEASE

Stress is a word that is used a lot in modern life. You might have a stressful job, or feel stressed out by too many demands on your job, or be going through a lot of emotional stress in connection with a personal relationship. In some situations, you may be acutely aware of some of the physiologic components of stress—for example, sweaty palms and a pounding heart just before you have to get up and give a speech. If so, you already have a basic understanding of stress that can help you grasp the physiologic and medical concepts of stress and how stress is related to disease.

CONTENT REVIEW

▶ General Adaptation
Syndrome (GAS)

• *Stage I*—Alarm
• *Stage II*—Resistance,
or adaptation
• *Stage III*—Exhaustion

Concepts of Stress

Today, it is commonly understood that mind and body interact. It was not always so. In fact, the concept that psychological states influence physiologic states—and particularly that there is a cause-effect relationship between stress and disease—date primarily from the work of Hans Selye, an Austrian-born Canadian physician and educator, in the 1940s.

General Adaptation Syndrome

Dr. Selye was not studying stress when he made his discovery. Instead, he was trying to identify a new sex hormone. He was injecting ovarian extracts into laboratory rats when he discovered the following triad of physiologic effects:

Triad of Stress Effects

- Enlargement of the cortex (outer portion) of the adrenal gland
- Atrophy of the thymus gland and other lymphatic structures
- Development of bleeding ulcers of the stomach and duodenum

Dr. Selye soon discovered that this triad of effects was not a response only to the ovarian extracts. The same effects occurred when he subjected the rats to other stimuli, such as cold, surgical injury, and restraint. He concluded that the triad of effects was not specific to any particular stimulus but comprised a nonspecific response to any noxious stimulus, or stressor. (**Stress** is generally defined as a state of physical and/or psychological arousal to a stimulus. Dr. Selye originally intended to use the word *stress* for the stimulus, or cause, but through a mistranslation of his work, *stress* came to mean the arousal, or effect. Dr. Selye then coined the word **stressor** for the stimulus/cause.)

Because the same responses occurred to a wide array of stimuli, Dr. Selye named it the **general adaptation syndrome (GAS)**. Later, he identified three stages in the development of GAS:

Stages of GAS

- *Stage I, Alarm.* The sympathetic nervous system is aroused and mobilized in the "fight-or-flight" response syndrome. Pupils dilate, heart rate increases, and bronchial passages dilate. In addition, blood glucose levels rise, digestion slows, blood pressure rises, and the flow of blood to the skeletal muscles increases. At the same time, the endocrine system is aroused, resulting in secretion of hormones by the pituitary and adrenal glands that enhance the body's readiness to meet the challenge.
- *Stage II, Resistance, or Adaptation.* The person begins to cope with the situation. Sympathetic nervous system

responses and circulating hormones return to normal. In most situations, this is the last stage; the stress is resolved. If the stress is very severe or prolonged, however, stress is not resolved and stage III occurs.

- *Stage III, Exhaustion.* This is the stage sometimes known as "burnout." During this stage, the triad of physiologic effects described by Dr. Selye occurs. The person can no longer cope with or resolve the stress, and physical illness may ensue.

The stages of GAS begin with **physiologic stress**, defined by Dr. Selye as a chemical or physical disturbance in the cells or tissue fluid produced by a change, either in the external environment or within the body itself, that requires a response to counteract the disturbance. Selye identified three components of physiologic stress: (1) the stressor that initiates the disturbance, (2) the chemical or physical disturbance the stressor produces, and (3) the body's counteracting (adaptational) response.

Psychological Mediators and Specificity

Since Dr. Selye defined GAS, others who have studied adaptation to stress have refined the concept. For example, more attention has been paid to the psychological mediators of stress. Experiments have shown that there isn't a direct correlation between stressor and response. People react differently to the same stressor. One person may take in stride the same situation that greatly upsets another person, and the degree of physiologic response may be governed more by the psychological, emotional, or social response to the stressor than to the stressor itself. In particular, research has demonstrated pituitary gland and adrenal cortex sensitivity to emotional/psychological/social influences.

Another way in which recent research has diverged from Dr. Selye's original hypotheses regards specificity. Dr. Selye postulated that the triad of physiologic responses he identified were nonspecific, or the same for any stressor. It is now thought that, while the triad of responses he identified may occur in response to a wide variety of stressors, the total body response to different stressors must be specific—that is, targeted toward correction of the specific disturbance. For example, the body reacts to cold by shivering, and to heat through vasodilation and sweating.

Homeostasis as a Dynamic Steady State

An older definition of homeostasis states that the body maintains itself at a "constant" composition. More recently, homeostasis has been described as a **dynamic steady state**. This takes into account the concept of **turnover**, the continual synthesis and breakdown of all body substances (e.g., fats, proteins). Thus, the internal environment of the body is always changing, not constant, but the net effect of all the changes is the dynamic (always changing), yet steady (tending always toward normal balance) state.

Stressors cause a series of reactions that alter the dynamic steady state. Usually, there is a return to normal, which may be rapid or slow. If a disturbance in the dynamic steady state—for example, a high blood glucose level—is prolonged and a causative stressor is no longer present, it is considered a sign of disease.

Stress Responses

Alteration of the immune system is the ultimate outcome of a stress response that resists quick and successful adaptation. The interactions of psychological, neurologic/endocrine, and immunologic factors that lead to this outcome are known as **psychoneuroimmunologic regulation**.

The **stress response** is initiated by a stressor. The input of the stressor into the central nervous system, as mediated by the person's psychological response, leads to production of corticotropin-releasing factor (CRF) from the hypothalamus, which in turn stimulates responses by the sympathetic nervous system and the endocrine system (neuroendocrine regulation), which then affect the immune system. This chain of events is outlined in Figure 1-103 ● and described in the next sections.

Neuroendocrine Regulation

As previously mentioned, when a person encounters a stressor and has a psychological response to the stressor, the sympathetic nervous system is stimulated by *corticotropin-releasing factor (CRF).* In turn this stimulates release of catecholamines, cortisol, and other hormones.

Catecholamines Sympathetic nervous system stimulation results in the release of norepinephrine (noradrenalin) and epinephrine (adrenalin), which constitute the category of hormones called *catecholamines.* The nerves of the sympathetic nervous system exit the spine at the thoracic and lumbar levels, and norepinephrine is released into the synaptic spaces (the spaces between the presynaptic ganglia and the postsynaptic nerves).

Additionally, sympathetic nervous system stimulation results in direct stimulation of the adrenal medulla, the inner portion of the adrenal gland. The adrenal medulla, in turn, releases the norepinephrine and epinephrine into the circulatory system. Approximately 80 percent of the hormones released by the adrenal medulla are epinephrine, while norepinephrine accounts for the remaining 20 percent. Once

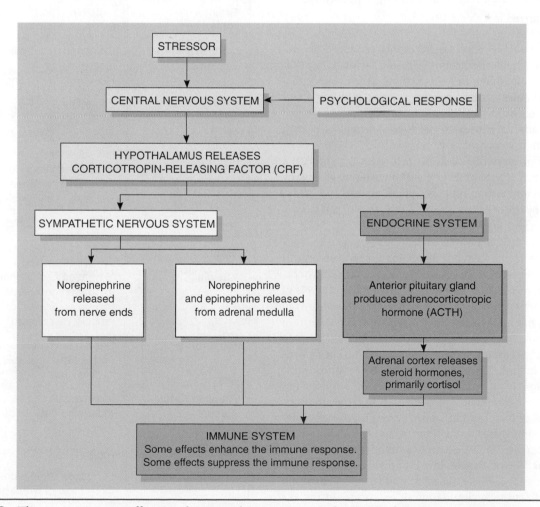

● **Figure 1-103**   The stress response: effects on the sympathetic nervous, endocrine, and immune systems.

released, these hormones are carried throughout the body where their effects (preparing the body to deal with stressful situations) act on hormone receptors.

Both epinephrine and norepinephrine interact with specialized adrenergic receptors on the membranes of target organs. These receptors are located throughout the body. Once stimulated by the appropriate hormone, they cause a response in the organ or organs they control.

The adrenergic receptors are generally divided into five types, designated alpha 1 (α_1), alpha 2 (α_2), beta 1 (β_1), beta 2 (β_2), and beta 3 (β_3). The α_1 receptors cause peripheral vasoconstriction, mild bronchoconstriction, and stimulation of metabolism. The α_2 receptors are found on the presynaptic surfaces of sympathetic neuroeffector junctions. Stimulation of α_2 receptors is inhibitory. These receptors serve to prevent over-release of norepinephrine in the synapse. When the level of norepinephrine in the synapse gets high enough, the α_2 receptors are stimulated and norepinephrine release is inhibited. Stimulation of β_1 receptors causes increases in heart rate, cardiac contractile force, and cardiac automaticity and conduction. Stimulation of β_2 receptors causes vasodilation and bronchodilation. Stimulation of β_3 receptors causes fat to be broken down in adipose tissues and heat production in muscle tissue.

All the effects of the catecholamines prepare the body to "fight-or-flight" in response to a stressor. Their physiologic effects are summarized in Table 1–19.

Cortisol Cortisol is another hormone produced in response to stress. The corticotropin-releasing factor (CRF) that stimulates the sympathetic nervous system, as previously discussed, simultaneously stimulates the anterior pituitary gland to produce *adrenocorticotropic hormone (ACTH),* which in turn stimulates the adrenal cortex to produce a variety of steroid hormones, primarily cortisol.

One of the primary functions of cortisol is the stimulation of gluconeogenesis. It enhances the elevation of blood glucose by other hormones and also inhibits peripheral uptake and oxidation of glucose by the cells. Because of these functions, it has the overall effect of elevating blood glucose.

Cortisol also affects protein metabolism—increasing synthesis of proteins in the liver but increasing breakdown of proteins in the muscle, lymphoid tissue, fatty tissues, skin, and bone. The breakdown of proteins results in increased blood levels of amino acids. Cortisol also promotes lipolysis (fat breakdown) in the extremities and lipogenesis (fat synthesis and deposition) in the face and trunk.

Cortisol acts as an immunosuppressant by inhibiting protein synthesis, including synthesis of immunoglobulins (antibodies). Additionally, it reduces the numbers of lymphocytes, eosinophils, and macrophages in the blood. In large amounts, cortisol can cause lymphoid atrophy. Through a series of actions, cortisol diminishes the actions of helper T cells, which results in a decrease in B cells and antibody production. It inhibits production of interleukin-1 and interleukin-2 and, consequently, blocks cell-mediated immunity and generation of fever. It inhibits the accumulation of leukocytes at the site of inflammation and inhibits release of substances that are critical in the inflammatory response, including kinins, prostaglandins, and histamine. Cortisol also inhibits fibroblast proliferation during inflammatory response, which in turn causes poor wound healing and increased susceptibility to wound infection.

In the gastrointestinal tract, cortisol increases gastric secretions, occasionally enough to cause ulcer formation. Cortisol also suppresses the release of sex hormones, including testosterone and estradiol.

The immunosuppressive actions of cortisol seem clearly harmful, yet its production in response to stress indicates that it is beneficial in protecting against stress. Its beneficial effects in stress, however, are not well understood. It has been suggested that its promotion of gluconeogenesis helps ensure an adequate source of glucose as energy for body tissues, especially nerve tissues. Pooled amino acids from protein breakdown may promote protein synthesis in some cells. Its depressive influence on inflammatory responses may play a role in decreasing

TABLE 1–19 | Physiologic Effects of Catecholamines

Organ	Effects
Brain	Increased blood flow Increased glucose metabolism
Cardiovascular System	Increased contractile force and rate Peripheral vasoconstriction
Pulmonary System	Increased ventilation Bronchodilation Increased oxygen supply
Liver	Increased glucose production Increased gluconeogenesis Increased glycogenolysis Decreased glycogen synthesis
Gastrointestinal and Genitourinary Tracts	Decreased protein synthesis
Muscle	Increased glycogenolysis Increased contraction Increased dilation of skeletal muscle vasculature
Skeleton	Decreased glucose uptake and utilization (insulin release decreased)
Adipose (fatty) Tissue	Increased lipolysis Increased fatty acids and glycerol
Skin	Decreased blood flow
Lymphoid Tissue	Increased protein breakdown (shrinkage of lymphoid tissue)

peripheral blood flow and redirecting blood to critical organs or sites of injury. Suppression of immune function may also help prevent tissue damage that results from prolonged immune responses. The physiologic effects of cortisol are summarized in Table 1–20.

Other Hormones In addition to the catecholamines and cortisol, other hormones are associated with stress response. For example, *beta-endorphins* (endogenous opiates) are released into the blood from the pituitary gland, or possibly the central nervous system, in response to CRF stimulation. They may play a part in regulating ACTH secretion and inhibiting CRF secretion, which means that beta-endorphins may exercise a control over the stress response. The beta-endorphins also are associated with decreased pain sensitivity and increased feelings of well-being, which may help to moderate the psychological response to a stressor.

Growth hormone (GH) is released by the anterior pituitary gland. GH affects protein, lipid, and carbohydrate metabolism and immune function. Its levels have been noted to increase after stressful experiences such as electroshock, cardiac catheterization, and surgery. However, the levels of GH become depressed with prolonged stress. *Prolactin* is released by the anterior pituitary gland and is necessary for breast development and lactation. Levels of prolactin have been noted to rise after a variety of stressful stimuli. *Testosterone* is a hormone produced in the testicles and also by the adrenal cortex in both males and females. It is necessary for development of male sexual characteristics and also affects many metabolic activities. Many stressful activities lead to a decrease in testosterone, which is thought to be a result of increased cortisol levels. Some competitive sports activities, however, appear to increase testosterone levels.

Role of the Immune System in Stress

During a stress response, as noted earlier, there is a complex interaction among the nervous and endocrine systems and the immune system. As a consequence, a variety of immune-related disorders are associated with stress.

The specific mechanisms by which stress leads to immune-related disorders is the subject of ongoing research but is not yet well understood. However, research points to the substances that serve as communicators between the cells of the nervous system, the endocrine system, and the immune system—including hormones, neurotransmitters, neuropeptides, and cytokines—as the pathways of cause and effect.

The pathway is not a straight line. The directional arrows of cause and effect move forward, backward, and in circles. Many components of the immune system can be affected by the factors produced by the neuroendocrine system. Conversely, immune system products can affect components of the neuroendocrine system. Here are two examples (Figure 1-104 ●):

● *Pathway 1: Central nervous system to immune system.*
  The central nervous system *stimulates* the hypothalamus

TABLE 1–20 | Physiologic Effects of Cortisol

Function	Effects
Carbohydrate Metabolism	Diminished peripheral uptake/use of glucose; promotes gluconeogenesis; elevates blood glucose levels
Protein Metabolism	Increases protein synthesis in liver; depresses protein synthesis in other tissues; depresses immunoglobulin production
Inflammatory Effects	Decreases blood levels of lymphocytes, macrophages, eosinophils; decreases leukocytes at inflammation site; delays healing/promotes wound infection
Lipid Metabolism	Increases lipolysis in extremities, lipogenesis in face and trunk
Immune Reserves	Decreases lymphoid tissue mass; decreases circulation white cells; inhibits production of interleukin-1 and interleukin-2; blocks cell-mediated immunity and generation of fever
Digestive Function	Promotes gastric secretions; at high levels causes ulceration
Urinary Function	Enhances production of urine
Connective Tissue Function	Decreases proliferation of fibroblasts (delays healing)
Muscle Function	Maintains normal contractility and work output for skeletal and cardiac muscle
Bone Function	Decreases bone formation
Cardiovascular Function	Maintains normal blood pressure; assists arteriole constriction; supports myocardial function
Central Nervous System Function	Modulates perceptual/emotional functioning and daytime arousal

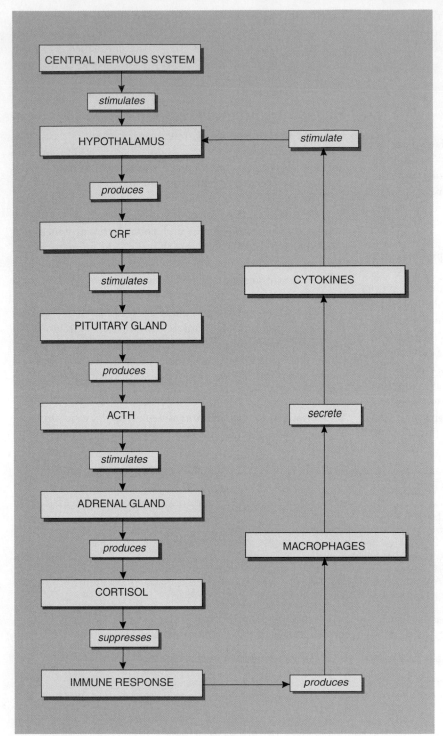

These are only two examples of the many pathways and interactions that take place among the nervous, endocrine, and immune systems.

The suppression of immune system function that is caused by stress-related products of the sympathetic nervous and endocrine systems—especially catecholamines and cortisol—has been linked to a number of immune-mediated diseases, as listed in Table 1–21.

Stress, Coping, and Illness Interrelationships

Research has shown that the ability to cope with stress has significant effects on associated illnesses. Those who cope positively with stress have a reduced chance of becoming ill in the first place and a better chance of getting better or getting better faster if they do become ill. Conversely, those who don't cope as well with stress have a greater chance of becoming ill or of prolonging the course of illness or of not surviving an illness.

Physiologic stress is caused by events that directly affect the body, such as a burn, extreme cold, or starvation. *Psychological stress* consists of the unpleasant emotions caused by life events, such as taking exams or a divorce. The effects that these stresses will have on the body depend on the individual's ability to cope with them. Some people are "thrown" by events others would perceive as relatively minor, such as a traffic jam or a sprained ankle. Others can take in stride events that others would find very difficult, such as loss of a job or a long-term disability.

The effects of stress, including the degree to which stress causes or affects illness, are moderated by the type, duration, and severity of the stressor in combination with the individual's perception and ability to cope with it. Stressors that are the most likely to have a negative effect on immunity and disease have been characterized as those that are not only undesirable but also are uncontrollable and that overtax the person's ability to cope.

Effective and ineffective coping has been seen to have potentially different effects in healthy persons, symptomatic persons (those who already have some manifestations of disease), and persons who are undergoing medical treatment.

to produce CRF which *stimulates* the pituitary gland to produce ACTH, which *stimulates* the adrenal gland to secrete cortisol, which *suppresses* the development of macrophages, T cells, B cells, and natural killer (NK) cells, a lymphocyte specially adapted to recognize and kill virally infected cells and malignant cells.

● *Pathway 2: Immune system to central nervous system.* During immune system response, macrophages secrete cytokines which stimulate the hypothalamus to secrete CRF (which begins Pathway 1 again).

TABLE 1–21 | Stress- and Immune-Related Diseases and Conditions	
Target Organ	**Diseases and Conditions**
Cardiovascular System	Coronary artery disease Hypertension Stroke Arrhythmias
Muscles	Tension headaches Muscle-related backaches
Connective Tissues	Rheumatoid arthritis
Pulmonary System	Asthma Hay fever
Immune System	Immunosuppression or immune deficiency
Gastrointestinal System	Ulcer Irritable bowel syndrome Ulcerative colitis
Genitourinary System	Diuresis Impotence
Skin	Eczema Acne
Endocrine System	Diabetes mellitus
Central Nervous System	Fatigue Depression Insomnia

Potential Effects of Stress Based on Effectiveness of Coping

- *In a healthy person:*

  Effective coping → Transient effects, return to normal function

  Ineffective coping → Significant stress effects, illness

- *In a symptomatic person:*

  Effective coping → Little or no effect on symptoms

  Ineffective coping → Exacerbation of symptoms, illness

- *In a person undergoing medical treatment:*

  Effective coping → Person does not perceive the treatment itself as stressful → Treatment is more likely to have a positive effect on symptoms and the course of illness

  Ineffective coping → Person perceives the treatment itself as stressful → Treatment is more likely to have a negative effect on symptoms and the course of illness

Because of the importance of coping ability in the interplay between stress and illness, attention is increasingly being paid to providing counseling and support systems—including family members, friends, and other support networks—to assist persons who are ill or in stressful life situations. There is recognition that supporting the patient's ability to cope is a critical adjunct to medical treatment itself.

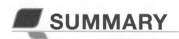

SUMMARY

The cell is the basic unit of life. It contains all the components needed to turn nutrients into energy, remove waste products, reproduce, and carry on other essential life functions. The body's cells interact via electrochemical substances including hormones, neurotransmitters, neuropeptides, and cytokines. The cells exist in an environment of fluids and electrolytes. When something interferes with normal cell function, the normal cell environment, or normal cell intercommunication, disease can begin or advance.

Groups of cells that perform similar functions form tissues. A group of tissues functioning together is an organ. A group of organs that work together is an organ system.

Perfusion of the tissues is necessary to provide essential nutrients to the cells (especially oxygen and glucose) and to remove wastes. Inadequate perfusion, called hypoperfusion or shock, can be caused by a problem in any of the three parts of the cardiovascular system (the heart, the blood vessels, or the blood), sometimes abetted by problems with the respiratory or gastrointestinal system in which the normal intake and transfer of oxygen and glucose may be interrupted. If not corrected, positive feedback mechanisms can enhance the process of shock, creating a downward spiral toward irreversible shock, possible multiple organ dysfunction syndrome (MODS), and death.

Cells can be injured in a variety of ways, including hypoxia, chemicals, infectious agents, immunologic/inflammatory injuries, and others. Diseases can be caused by genetic factors, environmental factors, or a combination of factors (multifactorial diseases).

The body responds to cellular injury in a variety of ways to restore homeostasis, the body's normal dynamic steady state. Cells can adapt through atrophy, hypertrophy, hyperplasia, metaplasia, and dysplasia. Negative feedback mechanisms work to correct, or compensate for, shock—if shock has not progressed too far.

The body's chief means of self-defense is the immune system and the immune and inflammatory responses, which work to attack and destroy infectious agents and other unwanted invaders. Occasionally, the immune response system works "too well," as in hypersensitivity reactions, or not well enough, as in immune deficiency disorders. Stress can also contribute to disease through the interactions of the nervous, endocrine, and immune systems.

Keep in mind that an understanding of the cell is essential to an understanding of all of these physiologic and pathophysiologic systems and processes. The more you understand what is happening at the cellular level, the better you will be able to understand the disease/injury process. This will help you make better decisions for treatment and transport of your patient.

YOU MAKE THE CALL

You have volunteered to work at a high school rodeo for your fire department. You and another paramedic take the backup EMS unit to the arena. This event brings in participants from several states. Over 300 people are expected to attend. Upon arrival at the arena, you park the unit at the designated spot and move your equipment to the "first-aid room."

Shortly after the rodeo is under way, an elderly gentleman stumbles into the first-aid room and slumps onto the treatment table. He states that he feels very weak and wants to be "checked out." You perform a quick assessment. The patient is pale but dry. His pulse rate is 110 beats per minute, blood pressure is 110/60, and his respirations are 36 per minute. You notice the characteristic odor of ketones on his breath. You ask the patient if he is diabetic. He says he is, but has not had his insulin in two days as he ran out of syringes. A finger stick glucose reads "HIGH." On further exam you note that the patient's mucous membranes are very dry.

1. Explain the physiologic basis for the patient's apparent dehydration.

2. Describe the role of insulin in glucose transport into the cell.

3. Prepare a prehospital treatment plan given the information provided.

See Suggested Responses at the back of this book.

REVIEW QUESTIONS

1. The clear liquid portion of the cytoplasm in a cell is called:
   a. cytosol.
   b. cytoskeleton.
   c. monocyte.
   d. granulocytes.

2. The _____ are the energy factories, sometimes called the "powerhouses," of the cells.
   a. lysosomes
   b. mitochondria
   c. Golgi apparatus
   d. endoplasmic reticulum

3. _____ is the function of nerve cells that creates and transmits an electrical impulse in response to a stimulus.
   a. Movement
   b. Maturation
   c. Conductivity
   d. Metabolic absorption

4. _____ tissue has the capability of contraction when stimulated.
   a. Nerve
   b. Muscle
   c. Connective
   d. Epithelial

5. _____ is the term for the body's natural tendency to keep the internal environment and metabolism steady and normal.
   a. Anatomy
   b. Physiology
   c. Metabolism
   d. Homeostasis

6. _____ is the study of disease and its causes.
   a. Pathology
   b. Anatomy
   c. Physiology
   d. Pathophysiology

7. _____ is an increase in the number of cells through cell division.
   a. Multiplasia
   b. Metaplasia
   c. Dysplasia
   d. Hyperplasia

8. _____ is the constructive or "building up" phase of metabolism.
   a. Anabolism
   b. Apoptosis
   c. Catabolism
   d. Hyperplasia

9. Water accounts for approximately _____ percent of the total body weight.
   a. 40
   b. 50
   c. 60
   d. 70

10. The fluid found outside cells and within the circulatory system is the _____ fluid.
   a. synovial
   c. intravascular
   b. interstitial
   d. extracellular

11. The most frequently occurring anions include all of the following except:
   a. chloride.
   c. phosphate.
   b. calcium.
   d. bicarbonate.

12. The mechanisms that most commonly result in accumulation of water in the interstitial space include:
   a. lymphatic obstruction.
   b. an increase in hydrostatic pressure.
   c. increased permeability of the capillary membrane.
   d. all of the above.

13. _____ are secreted by plasma cells in response to antigenic stimulation.
   a. Antigens
   c. Antibiotics
   b. Antibodies
   d. Haptens

14. Progressive impairment of two or more organ systems resulting from an uncontrolled inflammatory response to a severe illness or injury is called:
   a. ALS.
   c. ARDS.
   b. MODS.
   d. AODS.

15. Advanced stages of shock when the body's compensatory mechanisms are no longer able to maintain normal perfusion are called:
   a. reversible shock.
   b. compensated shock.
   c. homeostatic shock.
   d. decompensated shock.

16. The most commonly used fluids in prehospital care are:
   a. D$_5$W.
   c. lactated Ringer's.
   b. normal saline.
   d. all of the above.

17. Every human somatic cell contains _____ chromosomes.
   a. 48
   c. 24
   b. 46
   d. 23

18. The amount of blood ejected by the heart in one contraction is referred to as the:
   a. preload.
   c. stroke volume.
   b. afterload.
   d. cardiac force.

19. The energy that is produced during glucose breakdown is in the form of the chemical:
   a. ATP.
   c. TAP.
   b. APT.
   d. PTA.

20. Obstructive shock is caused by an obstruction that interferes with the return of blood to the heart, such as:
   a. cardiac tamponade.
   b. pulmonary embolism.
   c. tension pneumothorax.
   d. all of the above.

21. Prehospital care for hypovolemic shock should include either lactated Ringer's or normal saline, administered in small boluses to maintain the systolic blood pressure between _____ and _____ mmHg.
   a. 70, 90
   c. 80, 90
   b. 70, 85
   d. 85, 95

22. With a mortality rate of _____ percent, MODS is the major cause of death following sepsis, trauma, and burn injuries.
   a. 40–50
   c. 60–90
   b. 50–60
   d. 80–90

23. People with type _____ blood are known as universal donors, because this type of blood has no antigens that will trigger an immune response in any other group.
   a. A
   c. O
   b. B
   d. AB

24. _____ cells are the chief activators of the inflammatory response.
   a. T
   c. Immune
   b. Mast
   d. Histamine

25. _____ occurs when a mother has developed antibodies that attack and severely reduce the level of neutrophils in her blood.
   a. Myasthenia gravis
   b. Rheumatoid arthritis
   c. Isoimmune neutropenia
   d. Systemic lupus erythematosus

See Answers to Review Questions at the back of this book.

REFERENCES

1. Behar, D. M., E. Metspala, T. Kivisild, et al. "The Matrilineal Ancestry of Ashkenazi Jewry: Portrait of a Recent Founder Event." *Am J Hum Genet* 78 (2006): 487–497.

2. Lotti, M., L. Bergamo, and B. Murer. "Occupational Toxicology of Asbestos-Related Malignancies." *Clin Toxicol (Phla)* 48 (2010): 485–496.

3. Hendricks, K. A., J. S. Simpson, and R. D. Larsen. "Neural Tube Defects along the Texas-Mexico Border, 1993–1995." *Am J Epidemiol* 15 (1999): 1119–1127.

4. Williams, D. "Radiation Carcinogenesis: Lessons from Chernobyl." *Oncogene* 27 (Suppl 2) (2008): S9–S18.

5. Harman, D. "Aging: A Theory Based upon Free Radical and Radiation Chemistry." *J Gerontol* 11 (1956): 298–300.

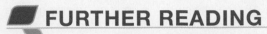
FURTHER READING

Bledsoe, B. E., F. H. Martini, E. F. Bartholomew, and W. C. Ober. *Anatomy and Physiology for Emergency Care,* 2nd ed. Upper Saddle River, NJ: Brady/Pearson/Prentice-Hall, 2008.

Bledsoe, B. E. and R. W. Benner. *Critical Care Paramedic*. Upper Saddle River, NJ: Brady/Pearson/Prentice-Hall, 2006.

Bledsoe, B. E., B. J. Colbert, and J. E. Ankney. *Essentials of A&P for Emergency Care*. Upper Saddle River, NJ: Brady/Pearson/Prentice-Hall, 2011.

Freeman, S. *Biological Science with Mastering Biology®,* 4th ed. Upper Saddle River, NJ: Pearson Education, 2011.

Goodenough, J. and B. A. McGuire. *Biology of Humans: Concepts, Applications, and Issues,* 3rd ed. Upper Saddle River, NJ: Pearson Education, 2010.

Hall, J. E. *Guyton and Hall Textbook of Medical Physiology,* 12th ed. St Louis, MO: Elsevier, 2011.

Zelman, M., E. Tompary, J. Raymond, and P. Holdaway. *Human Diseases: A Systemic Approach,* 7th ed. Upper Saddle River, NJ: Prentice-Hall/Pearson, 2010.

chapter

2

Human Life Span Development

Bryan Bledsoe, DO, FACEP, FAAEM, EMT-P

STANDARD
Life Span Development

COMPETENCY
Integrates comprehensive knowledge of life span development.

OBJECTIVES

Terminal Performance Objective
After reading this chapter you should be able to anticipate and respond to the physical, physiologic, and psychosocial needs of patients across the life span.

Enabling Objectives
To accomplish the terminal performance objective, you should be able to:

1. Define key terms introduced in this chapter.
2. Describe the physiologic characteristics of infants.
3. Describe the psychosocial characteristics of infants.
4. Discuss the impact of family processes on the psychosocial development of infants.
5. Describe the physiologic characteristics of toddlers and preschoolers.
6. Describe the psychosocial characteristics of toddlers and preschoolers.
7. Explain the impact of relationships with others, including parents, on toddlers and preschoolers.
8. Describe the impact of parenting styles, divorce, television and video games, and modeling on toddlers and preschoolers.
9. Describe the physiologic development of school-age children.
10. Describe the psychosocial characteristics of school-age children.
11. Describe the physiologic characteristics of adolescents.
12. Describe the psychosocial characteristics of adolescents.
13. Describe the physiologic and psychosocial characteristics of early adulthood and middle adulthood.
14. Describe the physiologic characteristics associated with aging and late adulthood.
15. Describe the psychosocial characteristics and concerns associated with aging and late adulthood.

KEY TERMS

CASE STUDY

You and your partner respond to an early morning call and find several people upset and milling around. As you announce yourselves as paramedics, a woman sticks her head out of a doorway down the hallway and beckons you into a room. There you find a woman in her early 20s. She's lying in bed and seems very uncomfortable. A young man, visibly pale, is sitting on the edge of the bed holding her hand.

The first woman tells you that the patient is in her final month of pregnancy and that she has been experiencing mild contractions for about 12 hours. She spoke with her doctor several hours ago and was told to go to the hospital when her contractions were approximately 5 minutes apart. "Unfortunately, her water broke, and since that time the contractions have been really close together; about 3 minutes apart," the woman tells you. They were afraid to attempt the drive to the hospital, so they decided to call the paramedics.

After asking some pertinent questions, you prepare to examine the patient for crowning. Having done so, you realize it will be necessary to allow the child to be delivered at home. Preparations are made, and within a short time, a beautiful little girl is wrapped in warm blankets and snuggled in her mother's arms. You explain that you will now prepare the mother and baby to be transported to the hospital where they can be examined to be sure there are no problems.

As you leave the room to get your stretcher, the first woman, who is the grandmother of the new baby, is spreading the happy news to the rest of the family. By the time you return to the room, several family members are gathered around a rocking chair where an elderly woman sits, holding her new great-grandchild in her arms. You think to yourself: "Four generations. Wow." Truly a beautiful family event, which you have been privileged to attend.

INTRODUCTION

Though human anatomy and physiology basically stay the same, people do change over the span of a lifetime (Figure 2-1 ●). Besides the obvious changes in size and appearance, there are also changes in vital signs, body systems, and psychosocial development. Some of those changes make it necessary for you to adjust your treatment of patients. For example, the amount of medication a patient receives is based on body size, weight, and the ability of the patient to process it. A child, therefore, usually requires a smaller dosage than a full-grown adult does. Many of the changes experienced over a lifetime can be identified in developmental stages. Those discussed in this chapter are:

- *Infancy*—birth to 12 months
- *Toddler*—12 to 36 months
- *Preschool age*—3 to 5 years
- *School age*—6 to 12 years
- *Adolescence*—13 to 18 years
- *Early adulthood*—19 to 40 years
- *Middle adulthood*—41 to 60 years
- *Late adulthood*—61 years and older

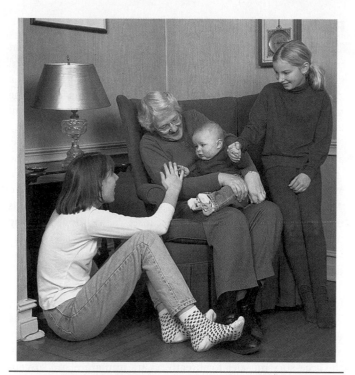

● **Figure 2-1** People change over the span of a lifetime.

INFANCY
Physiologic Development
Vital Signs

The greatest changes in the range of vital signs are in the pediatric patient (Table 2–1 ●). The younger the child, the more rapid are the pulse and respiratory rates. At birth, the heart rate ranges from 100 to 180 beats per minute during the first 30 minutes of life and usually settles to around 120 beats per minute after that. The initial respiratory rate is from 30 to 60 breaths per minute but tends to drop to 30 to 40 breaths per minute after the first few minutes of life. Tidal volume is 6 to 8 mL/kg initially and increases to 10 to 15 mL/kg by 12 months of age.

As with the other vital signs, the normal range for blood pressure is related to the age and weight of the infant, tending to increase with age. The average systolic blood pressure increases from a range of 60 to 90 at birth to a range of 87 to 105 at 12 months.

Weight

Normal birth weight of an infant usually is between 3.0 and 3.5 kg. Because of the excretion of extracellular fluid in the first

CONTENT REVIEW

► The younger the child, the more rapid are the pulse and respiratory rates.

TABLE 2–1 | Normal Vital Signs

	Pulse (Beats per Minute)	Respiration (Breaths per Minute)	Blood Pressure (Average mmHg)	Temperature (Fahrenheit)	Temperature (Celsius)
Infancy:					
At birth:	100–180	30–60	60–90 systolic	98–100°F	36.7–37.8°C
At 1 year:	100–160	30–60	87–105 systolic	98–100°F	36.7–37.8°C
Toddler (12 to 36 months)	80–110	24–40	95–105 systolic	96.8–99.6°F	36.0–37.6°C
Preschool age (3 to 5 years)	70–110	22–34	95–110 systolic	96.8–99.6°F	36.0–37.6°C
School-age (6 to 12 years)	65–110	18–30	97–112 systolic	98.6°F	37°C
Adolescence (13 to 18 years)	60–90	12–26	112–128 systolic	98.6°F	37°C
Early adulthood (19 to 40 years)	60–100	12–20	120/80	98.6°F	37°C
Middle adulthood (41 to 60 years)	60–100	12–20	120/80	98.6°F	37°C
Late adulthood (61 years and older)	*	*	*	98.6°F	37°C

* Depends on the individual's physical health status.

CONTENT REVIEW

▶ An infant's airway is shorter, narrower, less stable, and more easily obstructed than at any other stage in life.

week of life, the infant's weight usually drops by 5 to 10 percent; however, infants usually exceed their birth weight by the second week. During the first month, infants grow at approximately 30 grams per day, and they should double their birth weight by 4 to 6 months and triple it at 9 to 12 months (Figure 2-2 ●). The infant's head is equal to 25 percent of total body weight.

Growth charts are good for comparing physical development to the norm, but parents and health care providers should keep in mind that every child develops at his own rate.

Cardiovascular System

As newborns make the transition from fetal to pulmonary circulation in the first few days of life, several important changes occur. Shortly after birth, the *ductus venosus,* a blood vessel that connects the umbilical vein and the inferior vena cava in the fetus, constricts. As a result, blood pressure changes and the *foramen ovale,* an opening in the interatrial septum of the fetal heart, closes. The *ductus arteriosus,* a blood vessel that connects the pulmonary artery and the aorta in the fetus, also constricts after birth. Once it is closed, blood can no longer bypass the lungs by moving from the pulmonary trunk directly into the aorta.

These changes lead to an immediate increase in systemic vascular resistance and a decrease in pulmonary vascular resistance. Although the constriction of the ductus arteriosus may be functionally complete within 15 minutes, the permanent closure of the foramen ovale may take from 30 days to 1 year. The left ventricle of the heart will strengthen throughout the first year.

(You may wish to note that in an adult, the ductus venosus becomes a fibrous cord called the *ligamentum venosum,* which is superficially embedded in the wall of the liver. Also, in an adult, the site of the foramen ovale is marked by a depression called the *fossa ovalis,* and the ductus arteriosus is represented by a cord called the *ligamentum arteriosum.*)

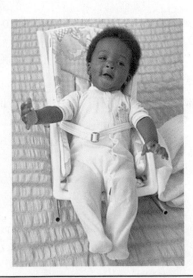

● **Figure 2-2**   Infants double their weight by 4 to 6 months old and triple it by 9 to 12 months. (© *Michal Heron*)

Pulmonary System

The first breath an infant takes must be forceful, because until that moment the lungs have been collapsed. Fortunately, the lungs of a full-term fetus continuously secrete surfactant. Surfactant is a chemical that reduces the surface tension that tends to hold the moist membranes of the lungs together. After the first powerful breath begins to expand the lungs, breathing becomes easier.

In general, an infant's airway is shorter, narrower, less stable, and more easily obstructed than at any other stage in life. The infant is primarily a "nose breather" until at least 4 weeks of age; therefore, it is important for the nasal passages to stay clear. A common complaint in infants less than 6 months of age is nasal congestion. This occurs because, as mentioned, young infants are obligate nasal breathers. Even a mild nasal obstruction, as occurs with a viral upper respiratory infection, can cause difficulty breathing, especially during feeding.

An infant's lung tissue is fragile and prone to *barotrauma* (an injury caused by a change in atmospheric pressure). Because of this, prehospital personnel must be careful when applying mechanical ventilation with a bag-valve-mask unit. There are fewer alveoli with decreased collateral ventilation. In addition, the accessory muscles for breathing are immature and susceptible to early fatigue, so they cannot sustain a rapid respiratory rate over a long period of time. Breathing becomes ineffective at rates higher than 60 breaths per minute because air moves only in the upper airway, never reaching the lungs. Rapid respiratory rates also lead to rapid heat and fluid loss.

The chest wall of the infant is less rigid than an adult's, and the ribs are positioned horizontally, causing diaphragmatic breathing. So when you assess respiratory rate and effort in an infant, it is important to observe the abdomen rise and fall. An infant needs less pressure and a lower volume of air for ventilation than an adult does, but the infant has a higher metabolic rate and a higher oxygen-consumption rate than an adult.

Renal System

Usually, the newborn's kidneys are not able to produce concentrated urine, so the baby excretes a relatively dilute fluid with a specific gravity that rarely exceeds 1.0. (Specific gravity is the weight of a substance compared to an equal amount of water. For comparisons, water is considered to have a specific gravity of 1.0.) For this reason, the newborn can easily become dehydrated and develop a water and electrolyte imbalance.

Immune System

During pregnancy, certain antibodies pass from the maternal blood into the fetal bloodstream. As a result, the fetus acquires some of the mother's active immunities against pathogens. Thus, the fetus is said to have naturally acquired passive immunities, which may remain effective for six months to a year after birth. A breast-fed baby also receives antibodies through the breast milk to many of the diseases the mother has had.

Nervous System

Sensation is present in all portions of the body at birth, so a young infant feels pain but lacks the ability to localize it and isolate a response to it. As nerve connections develop, the response to pain becomes much more localized. In addition, motor and sensory development are most advanced in the cranial nerves at birth, because of their life-sustaining function and protective reflexes. Since the cranial nerves control such things as blinking, sucking, and swallowing, the infant has strong, coordinated sucking and gag reflexes. The infant also will have well-flexed extremities, which move equally when the infant is stimulated.

Reflexes   The infant has several reflexes that disappear over time. These include the Moro, palmar, rooting, and sucking reflexes. The **Moro reflex**, which is sometimes referred to as the "startle reflex," is the characteristic reflex of newborns. When the baby is startled, he throws his arms wide, spreading his fingers and then grabbing instinctively with the arms and fingers. The reflex should be brisk and symmetrical. An asymmetric Moro reflex (in which one arm does not respond exactly like the other) may imply a paralysis or weakness on one side of the body.

The **palmar grasp** is a strong reflex in the full-term newborn. It is elicited by placing a finger firmly in the infant's palm. The palmar grasp weakens as the hand becomes less continuously fisted. Sometime after 2 months, it merges into the voluntary ability to release an object held in the hand.

The **rooting reflex** causes the hungry infant to turn his head to the right or left when a hand or cloth touches his cheek. If the mother's nipple touches either side of the infant's face, above or below the mouth, the infant's lips and tongue tend to follow in that direction. Stroking the infant's lips causes a sucking movement, or the **sucking reflex**, in the infant. Both the rooting and sucking reflexes should be present in all full-term babies and are most easily elicited before a feeding. They usually last until the infant is 3 or 4 months old; however, the rooting reflex may persist during sleep for seven or eight months.

Fontanelles   Fontanelles allow for compression of the head during childbirth and for rapid growth of the brain during early life. They are diamond-shaped soft spots of fibrous tissue at the top of the infant's skull where three or four bones will eventually fuse together. The fibrous tissue is strong and, generally, can protect the brain adequately from injury. The posterior fontanelle usually closes in two or three months, and the anterior one closes between 9 and 18 months. You may wish to note that the fontanelles, especially the anterior one, may be used to provide an indirect estimate of hydration. Normally, the anterior fontanelle is level with the surface of the skull, or slightly sunken. With dehydration, the anterior fontanelle may fall below the level of the skull and appear sunken.

Sleep   A newborn usually sleeps for 16 to 18 hours daily, with periods of sleep and wakefulness evenly distributed over a 24-hour period. Sleep time will gradually decrease to 14 to 16 hours per day, with a 9- to 10-hour period at night. Infants usually begin to sleep through the night within two to four months. The normal infant is easily aroused.

Musculoskeletal System

The developing infant's extremities grow in length from growth plates, which are located on each end of the long bones. The infant also has *epiphyseal plates,* or secondary bone-forming centers that are separated by cartilage from larger (or parent) bones. As each epiphysis grows, it becomes part of the larger bone. Bones grow in thickness by way of deposition of new bone on existing bone. Factors affecting bone development and growth include nutrition, exposure to sunlight, growth hormone, thyroid hormone, genetic factors, and general health. Muscle weight in infants is about 25 percent of the entire musculoskeletal system.

Other Developmental Characteristics

Expect rapid changes during an infant's first year of life. At about 2 months of age, he is able to track objects with his eyes and recognize familiar faces. At about 3 months of age, he can move objects to his mouth with his hands and display primary emotions with distinct facial expressions (such as a smile or a frown). At 4 months of age, he drools without swallowing and begins to reach out to people. By 5 months, he should be sleeping through the night without waking for a feeding, and he should be able to discriminate between family and strangers. Teeth begin to appear between 5 and 7 months of age.

At 6 months, the baby can sit upright in a high chair and begin to make one-syllable sounds, such as "ma," "mu," "da," and "di." At 7 months, he has a fear of strangers and his moods can quickly shift from crying to laughing. At 8 months, the infant begins to respond to the word "no," he can sit alone, and he can play "peek-a-boo." At 9 months, he responds to adult anger.

At about 9 months old, the baby begins to pull himself up to a standing position, and explores objects by mouthing, sucking, chewing, and biting them. At 10 months, he pays attention to his name and crawls well. At 11 months, he attempts to walk without assistance and begins to show frustration about restrictions. By 12 months, he can walk with help, and he knows his own name.

Psychosocial Development
Family Processes and Reciprocal Socialization

The psychosocial development of an individual begins at birth and develops as a result of instincts, drives, capacities, and interactions with the environment. A key component of that environment is the family. The interactions babies have with their families help them to grow and change and help their families do the same. This is called "reciprocal socialization," a model that recognizes the child's active role in its own development.

Raising a baby requires a lot of hard work, but studies show that healthy, happy, and self-reliant children are the products of stable homes in which parents give a great deal of time and attention to their children.

Crying   A newborn's only means of communication is through crying. While every cry may seem the same to a stranger, most mothers quickly learn to notice the differences in a basic cry, an anger cry, and a pain cry.

Attachment   Infants have their own unique timetables and paths to becoming attached to their parents. **Bonding** is initially based on **secure attachment**, or an infant's sense that his needs will be met by his caregivers. Secure attachment is consistent with healthy development, and leads to a child who is bold in his explorations of the world and competent in dealing with it. It is important for this sense of security to develop within the first six months of an infant's life.

When an infant is uncertain about whether or not his caregivers will be responsive or helpful when needed, another type of attachment develops. It is called **anxious resistant attachment**. It leads to a child who is always prone to separation anxiety, causing him to be clinging and anxious about exploring the world.

A third type of attachment is called **anxious avoidant attachment**. It occurs when the infant has no confidence that he will be responded to helpfully when he seeks care. In fact, the infant expects to be rebuffed. This causes him to attempt to live without the love and support of others. The most extreme cases result from repeated rejection or prolonged institutionalization and can lead to a variety of personality disorders from compulsive self-sufficiency to persistent delinquency.

Trust vs. Mistrust   Some psychologists believe that human life progresses through a series of stages, each marked by a crisis that needs to be resolved. Each of the crises involves a conflict between two opposing characteristics. From birth to approximately 1½ years of age, the infant goes through the stage called **trust vs. mistrust**. According to psychologists, the infant wants the world to be an orderly, predictable place where causes and effects can be anticipated. When this is true, the infant develops trust based on consistent parental care. When an infant begins life with irregular and inadequate care, he develops anxiety and insecurity, which have a negative effect on family and other relationships important to the development of trust. This may lead to feelings of mistrust and hostility, which may in turn develop into antisocial or even criminal behavior.

Scaffolding

Infants learn in many ways from their parents and others around them. One way they learn—from infancy and throughout their school years—is through **scaffolding**, or building on what they already know. For example, parents or caregivers usually talk to infants as a natural part of caring for them. With scaffolding, the dialogue is maintained just above the level where the child can perform activities independently. As the baby learns, the parent or caregiver changes the nature of the dialogues so that they continue to support the baby but also give him responsibility for the task. In this way, infants continue to build on what they know.

Temperament

An infant may be classified as an easy child, a difficult child, or a slow-to-warm-up child. An **easy child** is characterized by regularity of bodily functions, low or moderate intensity of reactions, and acceptance of new situations. A **difficult child** is characterized by irregularity of bodily functions, intense reactions, and withdrawal from new situations. A **slow-to-warm-up child** is characterized by a low intensity of reactions and a somewhat negative mood.

Situational Crisis and Parental-Separation Reactions

Infants who have good relationships with their parents usually follow a predictable sequence of behaviors when they experience a situational crisis (a crisis caused by a particular set of circumstances), such as being separated from parents. The first stage of parental-separation reaction is protest, the second stage is despair, and the last is detachment or withdrawal.

Protest may begin immediately upon separation and continue for about one week. Loud crying, restlessness, and rejection of all adults show how distressed the infant is. In the second stage, despair, the infant's behavior suggests growing hopelessness marked by monotonous crying, inactivity, and steady withdrawal. In the final stage, detachment or withdrawal, the infant displays renewed interest in its surroundings, even though it is usually a remote, distant kind of interest. This phase is apathetic and may persist even if the parent reappears.

TODDLER AND PRESCHOOL AGE

Physiologic Development

Vital signs for toddlers (12 to 36 months, Figure 2-3 ●) and preschool-age children (3 to 5 years old, Figure 2-4 ●) are not the same as an infant's. The heart rate for toddlers ranges from 80 to 110 beats per minute. Respiratory rate ranges from 24 to 40 breaths per minute. Systolic blood pressure ranges from 95 to 105 mmHg. For preschoolers, heart rate ranges from 70 to

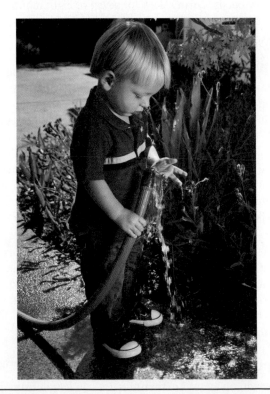

● **Figure 2-3**   A toddler beginning to stand and walk on his own.

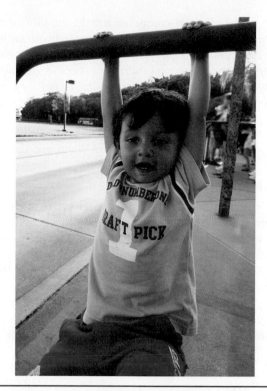

● **Figure 2-4** In the preschool-age child, exploratory behavior accelerates. (© Dr. Bryan E. Bledsoe)

110 beats per minute, respiratory rate from 22 to 34 breaths per minute, and systolic blood pressure from 95 to 110 mmHg. Normal temperature for both ranges from 96.8 to 99.6°F (36.0 to 37.6°C). In addition, the rate of weight gain is slowing dramatically. The average toddler or preschooler gains approximately 2.0 kg per year.

Changes in body systems include the following:

- *Cardiovascular system.* The capillary beds are now better developed and assist in thermoregulation of the body more efficiently. Hemoglobin levels approach normal adult levels at this point.

- *Pulmonary system.* The terminal airways continue to branch off from the bronchioles and alveoli increase in number, providing more surfaces for gas exchange to take place in the lungs. It is still important to remember that children have immature chest muscles and cannot sustain an excessively rapid respiratory rate for long. They will tire quickly and their respiratory rate will decrease, indicating the onset of ventilatory failure.

- *Renal system.* The kidneys are well-developed by the toddler years. Specific gravity and other characteristics of urine are similar to what would be found in an adult.

- *Immune system.* By this point in life, the passive immunity born with the infant is lost, and the child becomes more susceptible to minor respiratory and gastrointestinal infections. This occurs at the same time the child is being exposed to the infections of other children in child care and preschool. Fortunately, the toddler and preschooler will develop their own immunities to common pathogens as they are exposed to them.

- *Nervous system.* The brain is now at 90 percent of adult weight. Myelination (the development of the covering of nerves) has increased, which allows for effortless walking as well as other basic skills. Fine motor skills, including the use of hands and fingers in grasping and manipulating objects, begin developing at this stage.

- *Musculoskeletal system.* Both muscle mass and bone density increase during this period.

- *Dental system.* All the primary teeth have erupted by the age of 36 months.

- *Senses.* Visual acuity is at 20/30 during the toddler years. Hearing reaches maturity at 3 to 4 years old.

In addition, though children are physiologically capable of being toilet trained by the age of 12 to 15 months, they are not psychologically ready until 18 to 30 months of age. So, it is important not to rush toilet training. Children will let their parents know when they are ready. The average age for completion of toilet training is 28 months.

Psychosocial Development

Cognition

Children begin to use actual words at about 10 months, but they do not begin to grasp that words "mean" something until they are about 1 year of age. Usually, by the time they are 3 or 4 years old, they have mastered the basics of language, which they will continue to refine throughout their childhood. Between 18 and 24 months, they begin to understand cause and effect. Between the ages of 18 and 24 months, they develop separation anxiety, becoming clingy and crying when a parent leaves. Between 24 and 36 months, they begin to develop "magical thinking" and engage in play-acting, such as playing house and similar activities.

Play

Exploratory behavior accelerates at this stage. The child is able to play simple games and follow basic rules, and he begins to display signs of competitiveness. Play provides an emotional release for youngsters, because it lacks the right-or-wrong, life-and-death feelings that may accompany interactions with adults. Therefore, observations of children at play may uncover frustrations otherwise unexpressed.

Sibling Relationships

While there are many positive aspects to growing up with siblings, there also may be negative ones, which can lead to sibling rivalry. The first-born child often finds it very difficult to share the attention of his parents with a younger sibling. If the older child must also help care for the younger ones, he may become even more frustrated. While first-born children usually maintain a special relationship with parents, they also are expected to exercise more self-control and show more responsibility when

CONTENT REVIEW

▶ Vital signs in most children reach adult levels during the school-age years.

interacting with younger siblings. Younger children often see only the apparent privileges extended to the older children, such as later bedtimes and more freedom to come and go. Still, when asked if they would be happier if their siblings did not exist, most prefer to keep them around.

Peer-Group Functions

Peers, or youngsters who are similar in age (within 12 months of each other), are very important to the development of toddler and school-age children. In fact, peer groups actually become more important as childhood progresses. Peers provide a source of information about other families and the outside world. Interaction with peers offers opportunities for learning skills, comparing oneself to others, and feeling part of a group.

Parenting Styles and Their Effects

There are three basic styles of parenting: authoritarian, authoritative, and permissive.

- **Authoritarian** parents are demanding and desire instant obedience from a child. No consideration is given to the child's view, and no attempt is made to explain why. Frequently, the child is punished for even asking the reason for some decision or directive. This parenting style often leads to children with low self-esteem and low competence. Boys are often hostile, and girls are often shy.

- **Authoritative** parents respond to the needs and wishes of their children. While they believe in parental control, they attempt to explain their reasons to the child. They expect mature behavior and will enforce rules, but they still encourage independence and actualization of potential. These parents believe that both they and children have rights and try to maintain a happy balance between the two. This parenting style usually leads to children who are self-assertive, independent, friendly, and cooperative.

- **Permissive** parents take a tolerant, accepting view of their children's behavior, including aggressive behavior and sexual behavior. They rarely punish or make demands of their children, allowing them to make almost all of their own decisions. They may be either "permissive-indifferent" or "permissive-indulgent" parents, but it is very difficult to make the distinction. This parenting style may lead to impulsive, aggressive children who have low self-reliance, low self-control, low maturity, and lack responsible behavior.

Divorce and Child Development

Nearly half of today's marriages end in divorce. As a result of divorce, a child's physical way of life often changes (a new home, for example, or a reduced standard of living). The child's psychological life is also touched. The effects on the child's development, however, depend greatly on the child's age,

his cognitive and social competencies, the amount of dependency on his parents, how the parents interact with each other and the child, and even the type of child care. Toddlers and preschoolers commonly express feelings of shock, depression, and a fear that their parents no longer love them. They may feel they are being abandoned. They are unable to see the divorce from their parents' perspective, and therefore believe the divorce centers on them. The parent's ability to respond to a child's needs greatly influences the ultimate effects of divorce on the child.

Television and Video Games

Virtually every family has at least one television in the home, and many have video game players of one kind or another. Most children watch television and/or play video games for several hours each day, many with few, if any, parental restrictions. Television violence increases levels of aggression in toddlers and preschoolers, and it increases passive acceptance of the use of aggression by others. Parental screening of the television programs children watch may be effective in avoiding these outcomes. Some video games also feature violent scenarios that parents may do well to monitor.

Modeling

Toddlers and preschool-age children begin to recognize sexual differences, and, through **modeling**, they begin to incorporate gender-specific behaviors they observe in parents, siblings, and peers.[1, 2]

SCHOOL AGE

Physiologic Development

Between the ages of 6 and 12 years, a child's heart rate is between 65 and 110 beats per minute, respiratory rate is between 18 and 30 breaths per minute, and systolic blood pressure ranges from 97 to 112 mmHg. Body temperature is approximately 98.6°F (37°C). The average child of this age gains 3 kg per year and grows 6 cm per year. In most children, vital signs reach adult levels during this period of time, but their lymph tissues are proportionately larger than those of an adult. In addition, brain function increases in both hemispheres, and primary teeth are being replaced by permanent ones.

Psychosocial Development

School-age children (Figure 2-5 ●) have developed decision-making skills, and usually are allowed more self-regulation, with parents providing general supervision. Parents spend less time with school-age children than they did with toddlers and preschoolers.

The development of a self-concept occurs at this age. School-age children have more interaction with both adults and other children, and they tend to compare themselves to others. They are beginning to develop self-esteem, which tends to be higher during the early years of school than in the later years. Often self-esteem is based on external characteristics and may

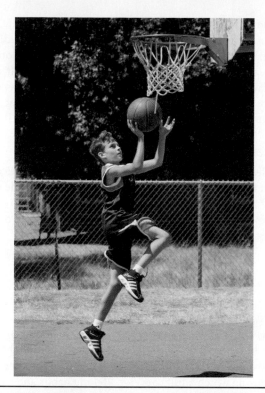

● **Figure 2-5** School-age children are allowed more self-regulation and independence as they grow older.

be affected by popularity with peers, rejection, emotional support, and neglect. Negative self-esteem can be very damaging to further development.

As children mature, moral development begins when they are rewarded for what their parents believe to be right and punished for what their parents believe to be wrong. With cognitive growth, moral reasoning appears and the control of the child's behavior gradually shifts from external sources to internal self-control. According to one theory, there are three levels of moral development: **preconventional reasoning**, **conventional reasoning**, and **postconventional reasoning**, with each level having two stages.

- *Preconventional reasoning.* Stage one is punishment and obedience; that is, children obey rules in order to avoid punishment. There is no concern about morals. Stage two is individualism and purpose; that is, children obey the rules but only for pure self-interest. They are aware of fairness to others but only as it pertains to their own satisfaction.

- *Conventional reasoning.* In stage three, children are concerned with interpersonal norms, seeking the approval of others and developing the "good boy" or "good girl" mentality. They begin to judge behavior by intention. In stage four, they develop the social system's morality, becoming concerned with authority and maintaining the social order. They realize that correct behavior is "doing one's duty."

- *Postconventional reasoning.* Stage five is concerned with community rights as opposed to individual rights. Children at this level believe that the best values

are those supported by law because they have been accepted by the whole society. They believe that if there is a conflict between human need and the law, individuals should work to change the law. Stage six is concerned with universal ethical principles, such as that an informed conscience defines what is right, or people act not because of fear, approval, or law, but from their own standards of what is right or wrong.

According to this theory, individuals will move through the levels and stages of moral development throughout school age and young adulthood at their own rates.

ADOLESCENCE

Physiologic Development

Vital signs in adolescents (13 to 18 years old) are as follows: heart rate is between 60 and 90 beats per minute, respiratory rate is between 12 and 26 breaths per minute, and systolic blood pressure is between 112 and 128 mmHg. Body temperature is approximately 98.6°F (37°C). In addition, the adolescent usually experiences a rapid 2- to 3-year growth spurt, beginning distally with enlargement of the feet and hands followed by enlargement of the arms and legs. The chest and trunk enlarge in the final stage of growth. Girls are usually finished growing by the age of 16 and boys by the age of 18. In late adolescence, the average male is taller and stronger than the average female. At this age, both males and females reach reproductive maturity (Figure 2-6 ●). Secondary sexual development occurs, with noticeable development of the

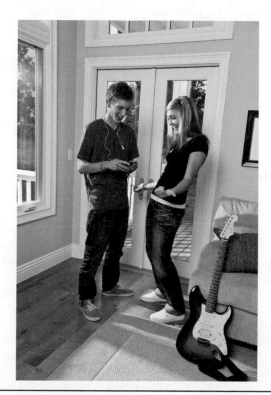

● **Figure 2-6** Children reach reproductive maturity during adolescence.

external sexual organs. Pubic and axillary hairs appear and, mostly in males, vocal quality changes. In females, menstruation has begun, breasts and the ductile system of the mammary glands develop, and there is increased deposition of adipose tissue in the subcutaneous layer of the breasts, thighs, and buttocks. In addition, in the female, endocrine system changes include the release of *follicle-stimulating hormone (FSH), luteinizing hormone (LH),* and *gonadotropin,* which promotes estrogen and progesterone production. In the male, gonadotropin promotes testosterone production.

Muscle mass and bone growth are nearly complete at this stage. Body fat decreases in early adolescence and increases later. Females require 18 to 20 percent body fat in order for menarche, or the first menstruation, to occur. Blood chemistry is nearly equal to that of an adult, and skin toughens through sebaceous gland activity. (You may wish to note that a disorder of the sebaceous glands is responsible for acne, which is common in adolescence. In acne, the glands become overactive and inflamed, ducts become plugged, and small red elevations containing blackheads or pimples appear.)

Psychosocial Development

Family

Adolescence can be a time of serious family conflicts as the adolescent strives for autonomy and parents strive for continued control. The many biological changes that occur at this stage cause inner conflict in both the adolescent and parents. Privacy becomes extremely important at this stage of life and, because of modesty, the adolescent prefers that parents not be present during physical examinations. It also is likely that when a patient history is being taken, questions asked in the presence of parents or guardians may not be answered honestly.

Children experience an increase in idealism during adolescence. They believe that adults should be able to live up to their expectations, which of course they cannot always do, which leads to disappointment.

Development of Identity

At this age, adolescents are trying to achieve more independence. They take "time out" to experiment with a variety of identities, knowing that they do not have to assume responsibility for the consequences of those identities. As they attempt to develop their own identity, self-consciousness and peer pressure increase. They become interested in the opposite sex, and they find this somewhat embarrassing. They really do not know how to handle this increased interest. They want to be treated like adults and do not know how to achieve this.

How well and how fast adolescents progress through the various stages of identity development depends on how well they are able to handle crises. Minority adolescents tend to have more identity crises than others. In general, antisocial behavior usually peaks at around the eighth or ninth grade.

Body image is a great concern at this point in life. Peers continually make comparisons, and certainly the media lead to unrealistic ideas of what the "perfect" body should look like. This is a time when eating disorders are common. It also is a time when self-destructive behaviors begin, such as use of tobacco, alcohol, and illicit drugs. Depression and suicide are more common at this age group than in any other.

Ethical Development

As adolescents develop their capacity for logical, analytical, and abstract thinking, they begin to develop a personal code of ethics. Just as they get disappointed when adults do not live up to their expectations, they tend to get disappointed in anyone who does not meet their personal code of ethics.

EARLY ADULTHOOD

Between the ages of 19 and 40 years, heart rate averages 70 beats per minute, respiratory rate averages between 12 and 20 breaths per minute, blood pressure averages 120/80 mmHg, and body temperature averages 98.6°F (37°C). This is the period of life during which adults develop lifelong habits and routines.

Peak physical condition occurs between the ages of 19 and 26 years of age, when all body systems are at optimal performance levels (Figure 2-7 ●). At the end of this period, the body begins its slowing process. Spinal disks settle, leading to a decrease in height. Fatty tissue increases, leading to weight gain. Muscle strength decreases, and reaction times level off and stabilize. Accidents are a leading cause of death in this age group.

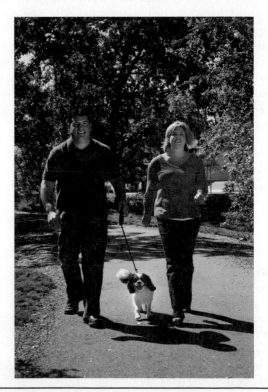

● **Figure 2-7** Peak physical conditions occur in early adulthood.

The highest levels of job stress occur at this point in life, the time in which the young adult strives to find his place in the world. Love develops, both romantic and affectionate. Childbirth is most common in this age group, with new families providing new challenges and stress. In spite of all this, this period is not associated with psychological problems related to well-being.

MIDDLE ADULTHOOD

Between the ages of 41 and 60 years, average vital signs are as follows: heart rate, 70 beats per minute; respiratory rate between 12 and 20 breaths per minute; blood pressure at 120/80 mmHg; and body temperature averages 98.6°F (37°C).

The body still functions at a high level with varying degrees of degradation based on the individual (Figure 2-8 ●). There are usually some vision and hearing changes during this period. Cardiovascular health becomes a concern, with cardiac output decreasing and cholesterol levels increasing. Cancer often strikes this age group, weight control becomes more difficult, and for women in the late 40s to early 50s, menopause commences.

Adults in this age group are more concerned with the "social clock" and become more task oriented as they see the time for accomplishing their lifetime goals recede. Still, they tend to approach problems more as challenges than as threats. This is also the time of life for "empty-nest syndrome," or the time after the last offspring has left home. Some women feel depression or a sense of loss and purposelessness at this time, feelings that are made worse by aging and menopause. Sometimes a father also becomes depressed, but the syndrome seems to affect mothers to a greater extent. Many parents, however, view the period after children have left home as a time of increased freedom and opportunity for self-fulfillment. Unfortunately, adults in this age group often find themselves burdened by financial commitments for elderly parents, as well as for young adult children.

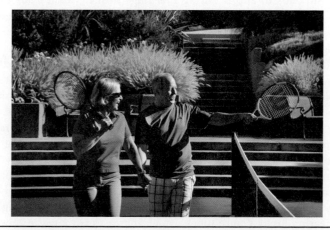

● **Figure 2-8**   People in middle adulthood still function at a high level.

LATE ADULTHOOD

Maximum life span is the theoretical, species-specific, longest duration of life, excluding premature or "unnatural" death. For human beings, maximum life span is approximately 120 years. **Life expectancy**, which is based on the year of birth, is defined as the average number of additional years of life expected for a member of a population. Human beings almost always die of disease or accident before they reach their biological limit.

Physiologic Development
Vital Signs

At 61 years of age and older, vital signs—heart rate, respiratory rate, and blood pressure—depend on the individual's physical health status. Body temperature still averages 98.6°F (37°C).

Cardiovascular System

During late adulthood, the cardiovascular system changes in ways that affect its overall function. The walls of the blood vessels thicken, causing increased peripheral vascular resistance and reduced blood flow to organs. There is decreased baroreceptor sensitivity and, by 80 years of age, there is approximately a 50 percent decrease in vessel elasticity.

In addition, the heart tends to show disease in the heart muscle, heart valves, and coronary arteries. Increased workload causes cardiomegaly (enlargement), mitral and aortic valve

CONTENT REVIEW

▶ Depression and suicide are more common during adolescence than in any other age group.

PATHO PEARLS

Life Span and Disease. *The life span of individuals in most countries in the industrialized world continues to increase. This is due to many factors that include better health care, widespread availability of vaccinations, safer agricultural and manufacturing equipment, safer automobiles, the absence of major wars, and many others. With an extended life span, we are starting to commonly see diseases that were once uncommon. For example, only in the last 20 to 30 years have we started to see an increase in cases of Alzheimer's disease. But, is the incidence of Alzheimer's disease now more common or is it just that people are now living long enough for the disease to manifest itself? Although it will take structured research to determine this for sure, the latter part of the statement is surely true. Typically, approximately 10 percent of people age 65 show signs of the disease, while 50 percent of persons age 85 have symptoms of Alzheimer's. The proportion of persons with Alzheimer's begins to decrease after age 85 because of the increased mortality caused by the disease, and relatively few people over the age of 100 have the disease. Thus, the increased incidence of Alzheimer's disease may simply be due to the fact that people are living longer.*

changes, and decreased myocardial elasticity. The myocardium is less able to respond to exercise, and the SA node and other cells responsible for producing heartbeats become infiltrated with fibrous connective tissue and fat. Pacemaker cells diminish, resulting in arrhythmia. Because of prolonged contraction time, decreased response to various medications that would ordinarily stimulate the heart, and increased resistance to electrical stimulation, the heart also becomes less able to contract. Tachycardia (abnormally rapid heart action) is not well tolerated.

Functional blood volume decreases in late adulthood. Decreases also can be expected in platelet count and the number of red blood cells (RBCs), which can lead to poor iron levels.

Respiratory System

The trachea and large airways increase in diameter in late adulthood, and enlargement of the end units of the airway results in a decreased surface area of the lungs. Decreased elasticity of the lungs leads to an increase in lung volume and to a reduction in surface area. The decreased elasticity also causes the chest to expand and the diaphragm to descend. The ends of the ribs calcify to the breastbone, producing stiffening of the chest wall, which increases the workload of the respiratory muscles.

These changes lead to an increased likelihood for older adults to develop lung disease and progressive declines in lung function. Metabolic changes also may lead to decreased lung function, and because of lifelong exposure to pollutants, diffusion through alveoli is diminished. Coughing also becomes ineffective because of a weakened chest wall and bone structure. Of all the factors that influence lung function, smoking continues to produce the greatest amount of disability.

Endocrine System

During this stage of life, there is a decrease in glucose metabolism and insulin production. The thyroid shows some diminished triiodothyronine (T3) production, cortisol (from the adrenal cortex) is diminished by 25 percent, the pituitary gland is 20 percent less effective, and reproductive organs atrophy in women.

Gastrointestinal System

One way the gastrointestinal system is affected at this stage of life is by way of tooth loss. Age-related dental changes do not necessarily lead to loss of teeth. Usually tooth loss is caused by cavities or periodontal disease, both of which may be prevented by good dental hygiene. With age, the location of cavities in teeth changes and an increasing amount of root cavities and cavities around existing sites of previous dental work are seen. Tooth loss can lead to changes in diet, an increased chance of malnutrition, and serious vitamin and mineral deficiencies.

This is also true when the individual has false teeth, which do not completely restore normal chewing ability and can reduce taste sensation. In addition, alterations in swallowing are more common in older people without teeth because they tend to swallow larger pieces of food. Swallowing takes 50 to 100 percent longer, probably because of subtle changes in the swallowing mechanism. Peristalsis is decreased and the esophageal sphincter is less effective.

In general, the gastrointestinal system shows less age-associated change in function than other body systems. Stomach contractions appear to be normal, but it does take longer to empty liquids from the stomach. The amount of stomach acid secretions decreases, probably because of the loss of the cells that produce gastric acid. There is usually a small amount of atrophy to the lining of the small intestine. In the large intestine, expect to see atrophy of the lining, changes in the muscle layer, and blood vessel abnormalities. Approximately one of every three people over 60 has diverticula, or outpouchings, in the lining of the large intestine resulting from increased pressure inside the intestine. Weakness in the bowel wall also may be a contributing factor.

The number of some opiate receptors increases with aging, which may lead to significant constipation when narcotics are ingested. Changes may occur in the metabolism and in absorption of some sugars, calcium, and iron. Highly fat-soluble compounds such as vitamin A appear to be absorbed faster with age. The activity of some enzymes such as lactase—which aids in the digestion of some sugars, particularly those found in dairy products—appears to decrease. The absorption of fat also may change, and the metabolism of specific compounds, including drugs, can be significantly prolonged in elderly people.

Renal System

With aging, there is a 25 to 30 percent decrease in kidney mass. About 50 percent of nephrons are lost and abnormal glomeruli are more common. Reduced kidney function leads to a decreased clearance of some drugs and decreased elimination. The kidney's hormonal response to dehydration is reduced as is the ability to retain salt under conditions when it should be conserved. The ability of the kidneys to modify vitamin D to a more active form may also lessen.

The Senses

Taste buds diminish during this stage of life, which leads to a loss of taste sensation. Smell declines rapidly after the age of 50 and the parts of the brain involved in smell degenerate significantly so that, by age 80, the detection of smell is almost 50 percent poorer than it was at its peak. Since taste and smell work together to make enjoyment of food possible, appetite often declines. Response to painful stimuli is diminished as is kinesthetic sense, or the ability to sense movement.

Visual acuity and reaction time is diminished, and there are actual changes in the organs of hearing. The ear canal atrophies, the eardrum thickens, and there may be degenerative and even arthritic changes in the small joints connecting the bones in the middle ear. Significant changes take place in the inner ear. These changes in structure significantly affect hearing. Hearing loss for pure tones, which increases with age in men and women, is called "presbycusis." With presbycusis, higher frequencies become less audible than lower frequencies. Pitch discrimination plays an important role in speech perception so, with age, speech discrimination declines. When exposed to loud background noise or indistinct speech, older people hear less, but at the same time, they may be very sensitive to loud sounds.

Nervous System

With aging, there is a decrease of neurotransmitters and a loss of neurons in the cerebellum, which controls coordination, and the hippocampus, which is involved in some aspects of memory function. The sleep-wake cycle also is disrupted, causing older adults to have sleep problems.

Psychosocial Development

While disease may reduce physical and mental capabilities, the ability to learn and adjust continues throughout life, and is greatly influenced by interests, activity, motivation, health, and income (Figure 2-9 ●). However, there is a **terminal-drop hypothesis** that there is a decrease in cognitive functioning over a five-year period prior to death. The individual may or may not be aware of diffuse changes in mood, mental functioning, or the way his body responds.

Housing

While most older adults would rather stay in their own homes, it is not always possible because home-care services are not affordably available in all communities as a viable alternative to nursing homes. Home-care services usually provide assistance with household chores such as preparing meals, cleaning and laundry, and performing personal care tasks such as feeding and bathing. Health care services in the home are provided

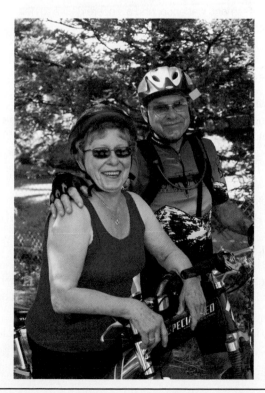

● **Figure 2-9**   The ability to learn and adjust continues throughout life.

by nurses and physical or speech therapists. In order to be eligible for these services under Medicare, the patient must be home-bound, need an intensive level of services, and be expected to benefit from such services over a reasonable amount of time. Home-care services are usually time-limited.

An alternative to home-care services is "assisted living," or living in a facility that offers a combination of home care and nursing home facilities. There is a greater sense of control, independence, and privacy because the older adult has more choices while still being in an institutional setting. Bedrooms and bathrooms can be locked by residents, but dining and recreational facilities are usually shared.

About 95 percent of older adults live in communities, from simple groupings of homes where mostly older adults live to a relatively new type of living arrangement called the "continuing-care retirement community." The appeal of these communities is that future health care needs are covered in a setting that is an attractive residential campus where cultural and recreational activities are available. Entrance fees to this type of community may be as much as $250,000, plus monthly fees which average $1,000.

Challenges

One of the major challenges for the older adult is maintaining a sense of self-worth. Senior citizens are commonly seen as "over the hill," less intelligent than younger adults, and certainly less able to care for themselves. Many older adults are forced into retirement because they are seen as less productive. In reality, although older workers may have slowed down a bit, they are often more concerned with producing quality work than younger workers. Another problem older adults face at this stage of life is a feeling of declining well-being. It is not until adults reach the age of 40 that ill health—as opposed to accidents, homicide, and suicide—becomes the major cause of death. Arteriosclerotic heart disease is the major killer after the age of 40 in all age, sex, and racial groups.

Financial Burdens

The duration of each state in the life cycle, and the ages of family members for each stage, will vary from family to family. Obviously, this will have an effect on the financial status of families. For example, a couple who completes their family while in their early adult years will have a different lifestyle when their last child leaves home than a couple with a "change-of-life" child. Late children can cause serious economic problems for retirees on fixed incomes who are trying to meet the staggering costs of education.

Retirement brings about changes for both spouses, but it seems to be particularly stressful for those wives who are not prepared emotionally or financially. Retirement usually means a decrease in income and in the standard of living, which can be very difficult to handle.

A decreasing level of interest in work is natural as one grows older, but it has a severe impact on the income of older people.

CONTENT REVIEW

▶ In late adulthood, heart rate, respiratory rate, and blood pressure depend on the individual's physical health.

Almost 22 percent of all older people live in households below the poverty level. More than 50 percent of all single women above the age of 60 live at or below the poverty level. Older women in the United States make up the single poorest group in our society.[3–6]

Dying Companions or Impending Death

Whether it is the death of a companion or one's own impending death, fear and grief seem to have a great deal in common. Grief not only follows death, but when there is advance warning, grief may well precede death. Frequently, the death or impending death of a companion leads us to fear for our own lives. Psychiatrist Elisabeth Kübler-Ross believes that regardless of whether it is one's own death or the death of a companion, everyone must go through certain emotions. While the five stages in her theory may sometimes overlap, everyone must deal with each of the stages of death before the grieving process ends. (Review Volume 1, Chapter 4 for Kübler-Ross's five stages.)

Note: Human physiologic and psychosocial development are discussed in more detail in Volume 3, *Patient Assessment;* Volume 4, *Medicine;* Volume 5, *Trauma;* and in Volume 6, *Special Patients.*

SUMMARY

The changes that take place during the span of a lifetime are innumerable. At some stages, especially birth through preschool, the changes seem to occur almost daily. The stages infant through adolescent constitute our pediatric population. By knowing the typical developmental characteristics of each age group, you will be better prepared to evaluate a sick or injured pediatric patient. This is especially important when a caregiver may not be readily available. You can compare the child's current state to an established norm and determine if there is a significant difference. Remember, however, not every person develops at the same rate and in the same way, and established norms are only guidelines that should never take the place of a thorough assessment and history obtained from someone who is intimately familiar with the patient.

Only through experience with patients at all the various stages of life—adult as well as pediatric—will you come to feel comfortable dealing with patients at each of these stages. Remember that no matter what the stage of development, a thorough assessment, patience, and a sincere desire to help will guide you to make the right emergency care decisions for each patient.

YOU MAKE THE CALL

You are dispatched to respond to a patient who is complaining of abdominal pain. When you arrive at the scene, you are met at the door by a middle-aged man who tells you the patient is his daughter. She is upstairs in her bedroom, and her mother is with her. You climb the stairs, followed closely by the father. When you enter the bedroom, you find a 16-year-old female lying on the bed. Her mother is sitting beside her, holding a damp cloth to her forehead. A younger sister is hovering around, trying to help.

The mother tells you that the patient woke about an hour ago, crying that her stomach hurt. The pain has gotten progressively worse over the last hour, and the patient has been complaining of nausea as well.

You begin your assessment of the patient, but she will not allow you to examine her abdomen. When you attempt to ask questions about what led up to this pain, the date of her last menstrual period, and whether or not she could possibly be pregnant, she refuses to answer you, shifting her eyes toward her parents and sister who are still in the room. Her mother tells her to please answer your questions, but the patient just begins to cry.

1. Do you believe that this is normal behavior for a patient of this age and in this particular situation?

2. What is a likely reason for this behavior?

3. What might you do to make this patient more cooperative?

See Suggested Responses at the back of this book.

REVIEW QUESTIONS

1. At birth, the heart rate ranges from _____ to _____ beats per minute during the first 30 minutes of life.
   a. 90, 120
   c. 100, 180
   b. 100, 120
   d. 160, 240

2. The infant's head is equal to _____ percent of total body weight.
   a. 10
   c. 20
   b. 15
   d. 25

3. The _____ _____, a blood vessel that connects the pulmonary artery and the aorta in the fetus, constricts after birth.
   a. ductus venosus
   b. foramen ovale
   c. ductus arteriosus
   d. ligamentum venosum

4. The _____ _____, which is sometimes referred to as the "startle reflex," is the characteristic reflex of newborns.
   a. Moro reflex
   b. rooting reflex
   c. sucking grasp
   d. palmar grasp

5. Parents who are _____ encourage independence but will enforce rules.
   a. dismissive
   c. authoritative
   b. permissive
   d. authoritarian

6. In this stage of moral development, children are concerned with interpersonal norms, seeking the approval of others, and developing the "good boy" or "good girl" mentality.
   a. permissive reasoning
   b. conventional reasoning
   c. preconventional reasoning
   d. postconventional reasoning

7. The theoretical, species-specific, longest duration of life, excluding premature or "unnatural" death, is:
   a. life expectancy.
   b. early adulthood.
   c. maximum life span.
   d. middle adulthood.

8. As adults reach the age of _____, ill health—as opposed to accidents, homicide, and suicide—becomes the major cause of death.
   a. 25
   c. 40
   b. 30
   d. 60

See Answers to Review Questions at the back of this book.

REFERENCES

1. American Academy of Pediatrics Section on Orthopaedics, American Academy of Pediatrics Committee on Pediatric Emergency Medicine, American Academy of Pediatrics Section on Critical Care, et al. "Management of Pediatric Trauma." *Pediatrics* 121 (2008): 849-854.

2. American College of Surgeons Committee on Trauma, American College of Emergency Physicians, National Association of EMS Physicians, Pediatric Equipment Guidelines Committee-Emergency Medical Services for Children (EMSC) Partnership for Children Stakeholder Group, and American Academy of Pediatrics. "Policy Statement—Equipment for Ambulances." *Pediatrics* 124 (2009): e166–e171.

3. Peterson, L. K., R. J. Fairbanks, A. Z. Hettinger, and M. N. Shah. "Emergency Medical Service Attitudes toward Geriatric Prehospital Care and Continuing Medical Education in Geriatrics." *J Am Geriatr Soc* 57 (2009): 530–535.

4. Shah, M. N., J. J. Bazarian, E. B. Lerner, et al. "The Epidemiology of Emergency Medical Services Use by Older Adults: An Analysis of the National Hospital Ambulatory Medical Care Survey." *Acad Emerg Med* 14 (2007): 441–447.

5. Shah, M. N., T. V. Caprio, P. Swanson, et al. "A Novel Emergency Medical Services-Based Program to Identify and Assist Older Adults in a Rural Community." *J Am Geriatr Soc* 58 (2010): 2205–2211.

6. Weiss, S. J., R. Chong, M. Ong, A. A. Ernst, and M. Balash. "Emergency Medical Services Screening of Elderly Falls in the Home." *Prehosp Emerg Care* 7 (2003): 79–84.

FURTHER READING

Craig, G. J. and W. L. Dunn. *Understanding Human Development*. 2nd ed. Upper Saddle River, NJ: Pearson, 2010.

Kall, R. V. and J. C. Cavanaugh. *Human Development: A Life-Span View*. Florence, KY: Wadsworth Publishing, 2008.

3

Emergency Pharmacology

Bryan Bledsoe, DO, FACEP, FAAEM, EMT-P

STANDARD
Pharmacology (Principles of Pharmacology; Emergency Medications)

COMPETENCY
Integrates comprehensive knowledge of pharmacology to formulate a treatment plan intended to mitigate emergencies and improve the overall health of the patient.

OBJECTIVES

Terminal Performance Objective
After reading this chapter you should be able to apply concepts of pharmacology to the assessment and management of patients.

Enabling Objectives
To accomplish the terminal performance objective, you should be able to:

1. Define key terms introduced in this chapter.
2. Explain the chemical, generic, brand, and official names of drugs.
3. Give examples of drugs from each of the four main sources of drugs.
4. Identify reliable reference materials for drug information.
5. Describe each of the components of a drug profile.
6. Explain how key drug legislation applies to the paramedic's role in administering drugs.
7. Discuss the processes of drug research and bringing a drug to market.
8. Explain the paramedic's roles and responsibilities with respect to administering medications.
9. Discuss special considerations in administering drugs to pregnant, lactating, pediatric, and geriatric patients.
10. Explain key principles of pharmacokinetics.
11. Describe each of the routes of drug administration.
12. Describe the various forms of drugs.
13. Describe considerations in drug storage.
14. Explain key principles of pharmacodynamics.
15. Describe common unintended adverse effects of drug administration.
16. Anticipate how various factors, such as age, body mass, and others, can alter drug responses.
17. Describe various types of drug interactions.
18. Describe the characteristics of common types of drugs used to affect the central nervous system.

19. Describe the characteristics of common types of drugs used to affect the autonomic nervous system.

20. Describe the characteristics of drugs used to affect the cardiovascular system.

21. Describe the characteristics of drugs used to affect the respiratory system.

22. Describe the characteristics of drugs used to affect the gastrointestinal system.

23. Describe the characteristics of drugs used to affect the endocrine system.

24. Describe the characteristics of drugs used to affect the following systems and structures:

    a. the eyes
    b. the ears
    c. the female reproductive system
    d. the male reproductive system
    e. the skin

25. Describe the characteristics of drugs used to treat the following disorders:

    a. cancer
    b. infection and inflammation
    c. poisonings and overdoses

26. Describe the characteristics of drugs used to supplement the diet.

KEY TERMS

active transport, p. 146
adjunct medication, p. 157
adrenergic, p. 172
affinity, p. 152
agonist, p. 152
agonist-antagonist, p. 153
analgesia, p. 156
analgesic, p. 156
anesthesia, p. 156
anesthetic, p. 159
antacid, p. 205
antagonist, p. 153
antiarrhythmic, p. 188
antibiotic, p. 215
anticoagulant, p. 200
antiemetic, p. 206
antihistamine, p. 203
antihyperlipidemic, p. 201
antihypertensive, p. 194
antineoplastic agents, p. 213
antiplatelet, pp. 198, 200
antitussive, p. 203
assay, p. 142
autonomic ganglia, p. 172
autonomic nervous system, p. 172
bioassay, p. 142
bioavailability, p. 149
bioequivalence, p. 142
biologic half-life, p. 155
biotransformation, p. 150
blood-brain barrier, p. 150

carrier-mediated diffusion, p. 147
cholinergic, p. 172
competitive antagonism, p. 153
diffusion, p. 147
diuretic, p. 194
dose packaging, p. 144
down-regulation, p. 152
drugs, p. 139
drug-response relationship, p. 154
duration of action, p. 154
efficacy, p. 152
enteral route, p. 151
expectorant, p. 205
extrapyramidal symptoms, p. 167
facilitated diffusion, p. 147
fibrinolytics, p. 200
filtration, p. 147
first-pass effect, p. 150
free drug availability, p. 146
glucagon, p. 210
hemostasis, p. 198
histamine, p. 203
hydrolize, p. 150
hypnosis, p. 159
immunity, p. 216
insulin, p. 210
ionize, p. 148
irreversible antagonism, p. 153
laxative, p. 206

leukotriene, p. 202
medications, p. 139
metabolism, p. 150
minimum effective concentration, p. 154
mucolytic, p. 205
neuroeffector junction, p. 172
neuroleptanesthesia, p. 159
neuroleptic, p. 167
neuron, p. 172
neurotransmitter, p. 172
noncompetitive antagonism, p. 153
onset of action, p. 154
osmosis, p. 147
oxidize, p. 150
parasympatholytic, p. 173
parasympathomimetic, p. 173
parenteral route, p. 151
partial agonist, p. 153
passive transport, p. 147
pathogen, p. 216
pharmacodynamics, p. 146
pharmacokinetics, p. 146
pharmacology, p. 139
placental barrier, p. 150
plasma-level profile, p. 154
postganglionic nerves, p. 172
preganglionic nerves, p. 172
prodrug, p. 150
prototype, p. 156
psychotherapeutic medication, p. 167

CASE STUDY

Paramedics Jo Henderson and her partner, Scott Parker, are dispatched to a rural residence just outside of town on a "chest pain" call. The response time is approximately 8 minutes. Emergency Medical Responders from the Alamo Fire Department are already on the scene. As they pull up to the well-kept brick home, a woman waves to them from the front porch. She tells them she is the patient's wife and shows them through the house to the den, where her husband is seated in an overstuffed recliner. The patient is Reverend Charles Allen, a 54-year-old Methodist minister, who is well known to the paramedics. He is conscious and alert, but in obvious distress. He is breathing at a rate of 24 breaths per minute with some difficulty. His skin is pale and diaphoretic. While Jo is getting a brief history from him, she checks his radial pulse and finds that it is strong and regular at a rate of 84 beats per minute. Scott is busy attaching ECG electrodes and a pulse oximeter. The Emergency Medical Responders have already started oxygen administration with a nonrebreather mask. They inform Jo and Scott that the patient's blood pressure is 150/90 mmHg.

Reverend Allen tells Jo he is experiencing a "heaviness" in his chest, which is making it difficult for him to breathe. He says it feels as though "an elephant is sitting on it." He rates the discomfort as an 8 out of 10 and says it began about 15 minutes ago while he was watching television. He denies any other complaints and has no relevant medical history, takes no medications, and has no allergies. Per system standing orders, Jo administers 325 milligrams of chewable aspirin to her patient while she listens to his lungs. He has clear breath sounds in all fields. Jo asks Scott to place a saline lock while she administers 0.4 milligram (1/150 grain) of nitroglycerin (NitroStat) sublingually. The patient's pain has decreased somewhat, but he is still very uncomfortable and is now complaining of nausea. Jo has him place another nitroglycerin under his tongue while she administers 4 milligrams of ondansetron (Zofran) intravenously. She asks him to hold still while she runs a 12-lead ECG, and then she moves him to the ambulance for transport to the nearest cardiac center.

Jo anticipates an approximately 75-minute transport time to Our Lady of the Sea Hospital. The local community hospital closed several years ago due to financial reasons, forcing patients to drive 60 miles to a neighboring town for health care needs. Because of this, EMS has become even more important to the small community. Jo reassesses her patient and finds that he is still having chest discomfort, but he now rates it as a 6 out of 10. She administers another 2 milligrams of morphine sulfate intravenously. She notices that the ECG shows ST elevation in leads V_2 through V_6, indicating an anterolateral injury. Jo confirms the key findings of the history in order to determine if her patient is a candidate for prehospital fibrinolytic therapy. Finding no contraindications for fibrinolytic therapy, she contacts the hospital to notify them. The medical direction physician reviews the patient's risk factors and confirms that there are no contraindications to fibrinolytic therapy. Jo faxes him a copy of the 12-lead. He agrees with the paramedics' assessment of anterolateral myocardial ischemia and authorizes her to administer recombinant tissue plasminogen activator (rtPA) via a standardized protocol. The protocol includes an initial 15-milligram bolus over 1–2 minutes followed by a timed infusion over the next 90 minutes. Following the bolus, Jo prepares and starts the infusion using a programmed

IV pump. Jo carefully documents the time the rtPA bolus was administered. In addition, they are to continue titrating the morphine sulfate with the goal of eliminating all discomfort.

Jo continues to administer morphine incrementally until Reverend Allen reports he is free of discomfort. She carefully monitors his blood pressure and pulse rate throughout transport. On arrival at the hospital, the patient is moved to the chest pain unit of the emergency department. Initial laboratory studies and a chest X-ray are obtained. The patient is placed on a 12-lead ECG monitor. The paramedics note marked improvement in the ST segment elevation seen earlier in leads V_2 through V_6. The patient remains pain-free. Shortly thereafter, he is taken to the coronary care unit and has an uneventful night.

The next morning he undergoes cardiac catheterization and coronary angiography. Unfortunately, Reverend Allen has rather severe coronary artery disease with several high-grade blockages. The cardiologists determine that he has too much disease for percutaneous coronary intervention (PCI). The patient is referred to cardiovascular surgery. The next day, he undergoes four-vessel coronary artery bypass grafting (CABG). He does well in surgery and afterward. Thanks to the efforts of the paramedics, he has no permanent myocardial injury from the heart attack.

Reverend Allen is discharged from the hospital 4 days later and begins an aggressive cardiac rehabilitation program. Six weeks later, he is able to resume his usual activities and returns to the pulpit, much to the satisfaction of his parishioners.

INTRODUCTION

The use of herbs and minerals to treat the sick and injured has been documented as long ago as 2000 B.C.E. Ancient Egyptians, Arabs, and Greeks probably passed formulations down through generations by word of mouth for centuries until they were finally recorded in pharmacopeias. By the end of the Renaissance, pharmacology was a distinct and growing discipline, separate from medicine. During the seventeenth and eighteenth centuries, tinctures of opium, coca, and digitalis were available. The related concept of vaccination with biological extracts began in 1796 with Edward Jenner's smallpox inoculations. By the nineteenth century, atropine, chloroform, codeine, ether, and morphine were in use. The discoveries of animal insulin and penicillin in the early twentieth century dramatically changed the treatment of endocrine/metabolic and infectious diseases. Now, at the start of the twenty-first century, recombinant DNA technology has produced human insulin and recombinant tissue plasminogen activator (rtPA). These drugs have markedly changed the treatment of diabetes and cardiovascular disease.

Presently in the United States, the Food and Drug Administration (FDA) is allowing many previously prescription-only drugs to become available over the counter. This is due in part to growing consumer awareness in health care and also in part to consumer marketing by the pharmaceutical industry. The industry is actively seeking drugs that appeal widely to the consumer for treatments and cures. Pharmaceutical research to limit aging or increase the life span is growing rapidly. The federal government also offers incentives to pharmaceutical companies to research drugs for rare diseases. These so-called "orphan drugs" are often expensive to investigate and have a limited sales potential, making them less profitable to develop and manufacture than others.

General principles of pharmacology are presented in this chapter, which is divided into two parts:

Part 1: Basic Pharmacology

Part 2: Drug Classifications

PART 1: Basic Pharmacology

GENERAL ASPECTS

Names

Drugs are foreign substances placed into the body. Drugs or any other agents or chemicals used to diagnose, treat, or prevent disease are called **medications**. **Pharmacology** is the study of drugs and their actions on the body. To study and converse about pharmacology, health care professionals must have a systematic method for naming drugs. The most detailed name for any drug is its chemical description, which states its chemical composition and molecular structure. Ethyl-1-methyl-4-phenylisonipecotate hydrochloride, for example, is a chemical name. A generic name is usually suggested by the manufacturer and confirmed by the United States Adopted Name Council. It becomes the Federal Drug Administration's (FDA) official name when listed in the *United States Pharmacopeia* (USP), the official standard for information about pharmaceuticals in the United States.

CONTENT REVIEW

▶ Drug Names
  • Chemical name
  • Generic name
  • Official name
  • Brand name

In the case of N-Phenyl-N-(1-(2-phenylethyl)-4-piperidinyl) propanamide, the generic name is fentanyl citrate, USP. To foster brand loyalty among its customers, the manufacturer gives the drug a brand name (sometimes called a trade name or proprietary name)—in our example, Sublimaze or Duragesic. The brand name is a proper name and should be capitalized. Most manufacturers also register the name as a trademark, so the stylized® or ™ may follow the name, as in Duragesic®. Another example is the widely prescribed sedative Valium:

Chemical Name: 7-chloro-1,3-dihydro-1-methyl-5-phenyl-2H-1, 4-benzodiazepin-2-one

Generic Name: diazepam

Official Name: diazepam, USP

Brand Name: Valium®

Sources

The four main sources of drugs are plants, animals, minerals, and the laboratory (synthetic). Plants may be the oldest source of medications; primitive people probably used them directly as "herbal" medicines. Indirectly, plant extracts such as gums and oils have long been a source of medications. Examples include the purple foxglove, a source of digitalis (a glycoside), and deadly nightshade, a source of atropine (an alkaloid). Animal extracts are another important source of drugs. For many years, the primary sources of insulin for treating diabetes mellitus were the extracts of bovine (cow) and porcine (pig) pancreas. Minerals are inorganic sources of drugs such as calcium chloride and magnesium sulfate. Synthetic drugs are created in the laboratory. They may provide alternative sources of medications for those found in nature, or they may be entirely new medications not found in nature.

Reference Materials

Obtaining information on drugs can be difficult. Using multiple sources of information about drugs is usually a good idea. Every book about drugs, including this one, has a disclaimer regarding doses and current uses, referring the reader to local medical direction for the final word. Using multiple sources and comparing the authors' statements about a drug may lead you to the best available information. The *United States Pharmacopeia (USP)* is a nongovernmental, official public standards–setting authority for prescription and over-the-counter medicines and other health care products manufactured or sold in the United States. EMS providers, however, generally like small, short guides that they can carry in a shirt pocket. These usually include important details about drugs that out-of-hospital providers administer along with a long list of commonly prescribed drugs and their classes. These EMS guides will be useful if you clearly understand the drugs used in your system and have a working knowledge of commonly prescribed drug classes.

Drug inserts, the printed fact sheets that drug manufacturers supply with most medications, contain information prescribed by the United States Food and Drug Administration. The *Physician's Desk Reference,* a compilation of these drug inserts, also includes three indices and a section containing photographs of drugs. It is among the most popular references, but it contains only factual information and must be interpreted by informed readers. The American Hospital Formulary Service annually publishes *Drug Information* as a service to the American Society of Health System Pharmacists. It contains an authoritative listing of monographs on virtually every drug used in the United States. A less bulky reference to keep in an ambulance might be one of the many drug guides for nurses. They contain information on hundreds of drugs in a format much like the EMS drug guides, but they also offer information on commonly prescribed drugs rather than only on emergency drugs. The American Medical Association also publishes a useful reference, the *AMA Drug Evaluation.* The Internet provides an enormous amount of information, but you must be especially cautious when using it as a source, because it allows anyone with a computer to be a publisher, with no requirement for accuracy. Examples of Internet-based reference sites include:

● Drugs.com

● Rxlist.com

● WebMD

● *eMedicine*

● *Micromedix*

There are several widely available pharmacology reference programs for smart phones. Among these are:

● *Epocrates*

● *Skyscape/DrDrugs*

● *MediMath*

● *Lexi-comp*

Components of a Drug Profile

A drug's profile describes its various properties. As a paramedic student, you will become familiar with drug profiles as you study specific medications. A typical drug profile will contain the following information:

● *Names.* These most frequently include the generic and trade names, although the occasional reference will include chemical names.

CULTURAL CONSIDERATIONS

Folk Remedies. *Many cultures place great trust in herbal and folk remedies. Some have been proven beneficial by modern research. It is important to ask about them when you obtain your patient's history. Some folk medications can contain potentially toxic compounds such as lead or arsenic.*

- *Classification.* This is the broad group to which the drug belongs. Knowing classifications is essential to understanding the properties of drugs.
- *Mechanism of Action.* The way in which a drug causes its effects; its pharmacodynamics.
- *Indications.* Conditions that make administration of the drug appropriate (as approved by the Food and Drug Administration).
- *Pharmacokinetics.* How the drug is absorbed, distributed, and eliminated; typically includes onset and duration of action.
- *Side Effects/Adverse Reactions.* The drug's untoward or undesired effects.
- *Routes of Administration.* How the drug is given.
- *Contraindications.* Conditions that make it inappropriate to give the drug. Unlike when the drug is simply not indicated, a contraindication means that a predictable harmful event will occur if the drug is given in this situation.
- *Dosage.* The amount of the drug that should be given.
- *How Supplied.* This typically includes the common concentrations of the available preparations; many drugs come in different concentrations.
- *Special Considerations.* How the drug may affect pediatric, geriatric, or pregnant patients.

Drug profiles may also include other components, such as its interactions with other drugs or with foods, when appropriate.

LEGAL ASPECTS

Knowing and obeying the laws and regulations governing medications and their administration will be an important part of your career. These laws and regulations come from three distinct authorities: federal law, state laws and regulations, and individual agency regulations.

Federal

Drug legislation in the United States has been aimed primarily at protecting the public from adulterated or mislabeled drugs. The *Pure Food and Drug Act of 1906,* enacted to improve the quality and labeling of drugs, named the *United States Pharmacopeia* as this country's official source for drug information. The *Harrison Narcotic Act of 1914* limited the indiscriminate use of addicting drugs by regulating the importation, manufacture, sale, and use of opium, cocaine, and their compounds or derivatives. *The Federal Food, Drug and Cosmetic Act of 1938* empowered the Food and Drug Administration (FDA) to enforce and set premarket safety standards for drugs. In 1951, the *Durham-Humphrey Amendments* to the 1938 act (also known as the prescription drug amendments) required pharmacists to have either a written or verbal prescription from a physician to dispense certain drugs. It also created the category of over-the-counter medications. The *Kefauver Harris Amendment* was an amendment to the *Federal Food, Drug and Cosmetic*

Act, added in 1962, that required pharmaceutical manufacturers to provide proof of the safety and effectiveness of their drugs before being granted approval to produce and market the products. This also stopped the process of remarking inexpensive generic drugs under new "trade names." The *Comprehensive Drug Abuse Prevention and Control Act* (also known as the Controlled Substances Act) of 1970 is the most recent major federal legislation affecting drug sales and use. It repealed and replaced the Harrison Narcotic Act.

The federal government strictly regulates controlled substances because of their high potential for abuse. Since not all drugs cause the same level of physical or psychological dependence, they do not all need to be regulated in the same way. To accommodate their differences, the *Controlled Substance Act of 1970* created five schedules of controlled substances, each with its own level of control and record keeping requirements (Table 3–1). Most emergency medical services administer only a few controlled substances, usually a narcotic analgesic such as morphine sulfate or fentanyl and a benzodiazepine anticonvulsant such as diazepam or lorazepam.

The majority of the remaining drugs provided by an EMS are prescription drugs—those whose use the FDA has designated sufficiently dangerous to require the supervision of a health care practitioner (physician, dentist, and in some states, nurse practitioner or certified physician's assistant). For emergency medical services, this means the physician medical director is in effect prescribing the drugs in advance, based on the assessments and judgments of EMS providers in the field.

Over-the-counter (OTC) medications are generally available in small doses and, when taken as recommended, present a low risk to patients. Of the few OTC drugs that EMS providers administer, acetaminophen and aspirin are probably the most commonly used. Although laws vary from state to state, they still require most EMS providers to obtain a physician's order (either written, verbal, or standing) to administer OTC drugs.

Federal drug laws require that certain substances be appropriately secured, distributed, and accounted for. Because of the complexity of this issue and the large variability of drugs used in EMS systems across the country, specific answers to these concerns are not practical here. Consult your local protocols, laws, and most importantly, medical director for guidance in this area.

LEGAL CONSIDERATIONS

Follow Orders of the Medical Director. *The administration of medications by a paramedic is allowed only by express physician order. This can be either verbal or through approved written standing orders. Always follow your medical director's orders in regard to medication administration.*

CONTENT REVIEW

▶ Drug Laws and Regulations

• Federal law
• State laws and regulations
• Individual agency regulations

State

State laws vary widely. Some states have legislated which medications are appropriate for paramedics to give, while others have left those decisions to local control. Local control varies as well. In some areas, regional EMS authorities set the local standards; in others the individual medical directors and department directors do. In all cases, however, the physician medical director can delegate to paramedics the authority to administer medications, either by written, verbal, or standing order. You must know the laws of the state where you practice.

Local

In each community, local leaders are responsible for ensuring public safety. Local EMS agencies have the responsibility to create local policies and procedures to ensure the public well-being. An excellent example of a local procedure protecting the patient (and thereby the individual EMS provider and agency) would be a requirement to use a pulse oximeter whenever a patient is sedated or paralyzed. While this requirement would not have the force of law, it would locally help to ensure that local EMS providers do not overlook hypoxia in these patients.

Standards

Because some generic drugs affect patients differently than their brand name counterparts, standardization of drugs is a necessity. Despite FDA standards, drugs sold or distributed by various manufacturers may have biological or therapeutic differences. An **assay** determines the amount and purity of a given chemical in a preparation in the laboratory (in vitro). While two generically equivalent preparations may contain the same amount of a given chemical (drug), they may have different therapeutic effects. This relative therapeutic effectiveness of chemically equivalent drugs is their **bioequivalence**. Bioequivalence is determined by a **bioassay**, which attempts to ascertain the drug's availability in a biological model (*in vivo*). Again, the *United States Pharmacopeia* (USP) is the official standard for the United States.

DRUG RESEARCH AND BRINGING A DRUG TO MARKET

The pharmaceutical industry is highly motivated to bring profitable new drugs to market. Proving the safety and reliability of these new drugs, however, requires extensive research. While better understanding of biology is shortening the time needed to bring a new drug to market, the process still takes many years. To ensure the safety of new medications, the FDA has developed a process for evaluating their safety and efficacy. This process, illustrated in Figure 3-1 ●, adds even more time to the development cycle. Initial drug testing begins with the study of both male and female mammals. After testing a drug's toxicity, researchers evaluate its pharmacokinetics—how it is absorbed, distributed, metabolized (biotransformed), and excreted—in animals. These animal studies also help determine the drug's therapeutic index (the ratio of its lethal dose to its effective dose). If the results of animal testing are satisfactory, the FDA designates the drug as an investigational new drug (IND), and researchers can then test it in humans.

Phases of Human Studies

Human studies take place in four phases.

TABLE 3–1	Schedules of Drugs According to the Controlled Substances Act of 1970	
Schedule	**Description**	**Examples**
Schedule I	High abuse potential; may lead to severe dependence; no accepted medical indications; used for research, analysis, or instruction only	Heroin, LSD, mescaline
Schedule II	High abuse potential; may lead to severe dependence; accepted medical indications	Opium, cocaine, morphine, codeine, oxycodone, methadone, secobarbital
Schedule III	Less abuse potential than Schedule I and II; may lead to moderate or low physical dependence or high psychological dependence; accepted medical indications	Limited opioid amounts or combined with noncontrolled substances: Vicodin, Tylenol with codeine
Schedule IV	Low abuse potential compared to Schedule III; limited psychological and/or physical dependence; accepted medical indications	Diazepam, lorazepam, phenobarbital
Schedule V	Lower abuse potential compared to Schedule IV; may lead to limited physical or psychological dependence; accepted medical indications	Limited amounts of opioids; often for cough or diarrhea

New Drug Development Timeline

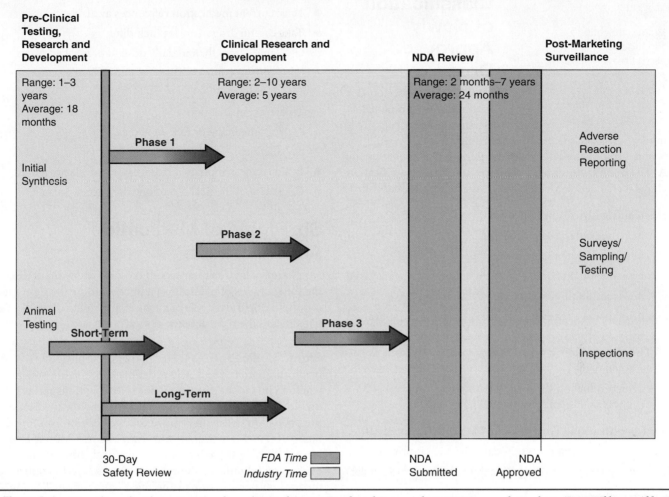

● **Figure 3-1**   New drug development timeline. (*United States Food and Drug Administration website, http://www.fda.gov/fdac/special/newdrug/testing.html*)

Phase 1   The primary purposes of phase 1 testing are to determine the drug's pharmacokinetics, toxicity, and safe dose in humans. These studies are usually carried out on limited populations of healthy human volunteers; some drugs with a high risk of untoward effects will not be tested on healthy individuals.

Phase 2   When phase 1 studies prove that the drug is safe, it is tested on a limited population of patients who have the disease it is intended to treat. The primary purposes of phase 2 studies are to find the therapeutic drug level and watch carefully for toxic and side effects.

Phase 3   The main purposes of phase 3 testing are to refine the usual therapeutic dose and to collect relevant data on side effects. Gathering the significant amounts of data needed for these goals requires a large patient population. Phase 3 studies are usually *double-blind*. That is, neither the patient nor the researcher knows whether the patient is receiving a placebo or the drug until after the study has been completed. This keeps personal biases from affecting the reporting of results. Some phase 3 studies are controlled studies, which are like placebo studies except that, instead of a placebo, the patient receives a

treatment that is known to be effective. Occasionally, a double-blind study will be ended sooner than planned if the early results are convincing.

Once phase 3 studies are completed, the manufacturer files a New Drug Application (NDA) with the Food and Drug Administration, which then evaluates the data collected in the investigation's first three phases. At this point the FDA decides whether to conditionally approve manufacturing and marketing the drug in the United States. The FDA's Abbreviated New Drug Application (ANDA) process may significantly shorten this process for generic equivalents of currently approved drugs.

Phase 4   Phase 4 testing involves postmarketing analysis during conditional approval. Once a drug is being used in the general population, the FDA requires the drug's maker to monitor its performance. Many drugs have been discontinued after marketing when previously unknown effects became apparent. One example would be the antiemetic thalidomide. Because children and pregnant women are generally excluded from the first three phases of testing, the premarket testing did not reveal that thalidomide caused birth defects in the children of pregnant women.

▶ Six Rights of Medication
Administration
• Right medication
• Right dose
• Right time
• Right route
• Right patient
• Right documentation

FDA Classification of Newly Approved Drugs

The FDA has developed a method for immediately classifying new drugs. This method of drug classification utilizes a number and a letter for each new drug in the IND phase or upon NDA review by the FDA. The manufacturer has a right to contest this classification and have it changed before the final classification is established.

Numerical Classification (Chemical)

1. A new molecular drug
2. A new salt of a marketed drug
3. A new formulation or dosage form not previously marketed
4. A new combination not previously marketed
5. A drug that is already on the market, a generic duplication
6. A product already marketed by the same company (This designation is used for new indications for a marketed drug.)
7. A drug product on the market without an approval NDA (drug was marketed prior to 1938)

Letter Classification (Treatment or Therapeutic Potential)

A. Drug offers an important therapeutic gain (P-priority)
B. Drug that is similar to drugs already on the market (S-similar)

Other Classifications

A. Drugs indicated for AIDS and HIV-related disease
B. Drugs developed to treat life-threatening or severely debilitating illness
C. An orphan drug

(*Source: US Food and Drug Administration*)

PATIENT CARE USING MEDICATIONS

Paramedics are responsible for the standard of care for patients in their charge. They are, therefore, personally responsible—legally, morally, and ethically—for the safe and effective administration of medications. The following guidelines will help you to meet that responsibility:

● Know the precautions and contraindications for all medications you administer.
● Practice proper techniques.
● Know how to observe and document drug effects.
● Maintain a current knowledge in pharmacology.
● Establish and maintain professional relationships with other health care providers.

● Understand the pharmacokinetics and pharmacodynamics.
● Have current medication references available.
● Take careful drug histories including:
  ○ Name, strength, and daily dose of prescribed drugs
  ○ Over-the-counter drugs
  ○ Vitamins
  ○ Herbal medications
  ○ Folk-medicine or folk-remedies
  ○ Allergies
● Evaluate the compliance, dosage, and adverse reactions.
● Consult with medical direction when appropriate.

Six Rights of Medication Administration

No pharmacology chapter would be complete without discussing the six rights of medication administration: the right medication, the right dose, the right time, the right route, the right patient, and the right documentation.

Right Medication When following a physician's verbal medication order, repeat the order back to him to confirm that you both intend the same thing for the patient. Inspect the label on the drug at least three times before giving the medication to the patient: first, as you remove the medication from the drug box or cabinet; second, as you draw the medication into the syringe or dole the tablet into a cup; and third, immediately before you administer the medication. Failure to confirm the medication name is one of the most common medication administration errors. If you have any question about a drug, do not administer it without confirmation. Showing the medication container to your partner and asking for confirmation is an easy way to further ensure that you are giving the right drug.

Right Dose To reduce medication errors, many drugs come in unit **dose packaging**. That is, the package contains a single dose for a single patient. Dosages of many emergency drugs, however, are based on patient weight, so a prefilled syringe may not contain the exact amount a patient needs. You will have to calculate the correct dose. One good practice for identifying potential medication errors is to consider the number of unit dose packages needed for a single dose. If your calculations tell you to open 10 vials for one dose of medication, prudence requires you to check the calculation and dose carefully. The package may contain a unit dose of the wrong medication, or you may have miscalculated.

Right Time While paramedics usually give medications in urgent and emergent situations rather than on a schedule, timing can still be very important. Giving nitroglycerin tablets too soon may precipitate hypotension; if epinephrine is not repeated on time during cardiac arrest, it may not help to lower the threshold for defibrillation. Take care to give medications punctually and to document their administration promptly.

Right Route   Often, you will have to choose from among several treatments for a particular problem. In these cases, knowing the principles of pharmacokinetics can help greatly in giving your patient the medication via the right route. For example, your knowledge that you should administer epinephrine intravenously rather than subcutaneously to the patient in anaphylactic shock because his blood is being shunted away from the skin will guide you to the proper administration route.

Right Patient   As the paramedic's role in health care expands, you will find yourself caring for more people than just "the patient in the back of the truck." You will deal with multiple patients, and the potential for giving medication to the wrong patient will be real. You will have to identify patients by name before administering medications.

Right Documentation   The drugs you administer in the field do not stop affecting your patients when they enter the hospital. As a result, you must completely document all your care, especially any drugs you have administered, so that long after you have gone on to your next call, other providers will know what drugs your patient has had.

Special Considerations

Pregnant Patients   Any time you administer drugs to a woman of childbearing years, you must consider the possibility that she is pregnant. Treating pregnant patients clearly means treating two patients. Although emphasis appropriately seems to center on the mother during care, you must understand that many drugs that affect the mother also affect the fetus. A drug's possible benefits to the mother must clearly outweigh its potential risks to the fetus. For example, some situations such as cardiac arrest justify giving the mother medications that may harm the fetus because the drug's possible harm to the fetus is clearly outweighed by the fetus's certain death if the mother dies.

Pregnancy presents two particular pharmacological problems: changes in the mother's anatomy and physiology, and the potential for drugs to harm the fetus. Because the mother is supporting the fetus entirely, her heart rate, cardiac output, and blood volume will increase. This altered maternal physiology can affect the onset and duration of action of many medications. During the first trimester of pregnancy the ingestion of some drugs (**teratogenic drugs**) may potentially deform, injure, or kill the fetus. During the last trimester, drugs administered

---

PATHO PEARLS

Medications That Cross the Placenta.   *Some medications cross the placenta and affect the fetus. Because of this, it is prudent to ask whether a female patient might be pregnant before administering a medication. In addition, some medications cross into the breast milk and can potentially affect a breast-feeding baby.*

---

to the mother may pass through the placenta to the fetus. Some of these drugs will have unwanted effects on the fetus. Others may not be metabolized and/or excreted, possibly resulting in toxic accumulations. Additionally, a breast-feeding mother's milk may pass some drugs to her infant.

Under some conditions, of course, the health and safety of mother and fetus demand the use of drugs during the pregnancy. Examples include pregnancy-induced diabetes, hypertension, and seizure disorders. To help health care providers determine when drugs are needed during pregnancy, the FDA has developed the classification system shown in Table 3–2. Always consult medical direction for any questions about drug safety in pregnancy.

Pediatric Patients   Several physiologic factors affect pharmacokinetics in newborns and young children. These patients'

TABLE 3–2 | FDA Pregnancy Categories

Category	Description
A	Adequate studies in pregnant women have not demonstrated a risk to the fetus in the first trimester or later trimesters.
B	Animal studies have not demonstrated a risk to the fetus, *but* there are no adequate studies in pregnant women. OR Adequate studies in pregnant women have not demonstrated a risk to the fetus in the first trimester and there is no risk in the last trimester, *but* animal studies have demonstrated adverse effects.
C	Animal studies have demonstrated adverse effects, *but* there are no adequate studies in pregnant women; however, benefits may be acceptable despite the potential risks. OR No adequate animal studies or adequate studies of pregnant women have been done.
D	Fetal risk has been demonstrated. In certain circumstances, benefits could outweigh the risks.
X	Fetal risk has been demonstrated. This risk outweighs any possible benefit to the mother. Avoid using in pregnant or potentially pregnant patients.

absorption of oral medications is less than an adult's due to various differences in gastric pH, gastric emptying time, and low enzyme levels. A newborn's skin is thinner than an older patient's and is therefore more permeable to topically administered drugs. This can result in unexpected toxicity. Older children still have less gastric acid than adults do, but their gastric emptying times reach an adult's around the sixth to eighth month of life. Because children up to a year old have diminished plasma protein concentrations, drugs that bind to proteins have higher **free drug availability**. That is, a greater proportion of the drug will be available in the body to cause either desired or undesired effects. Water distribution is different in the neonate as well. Neonates have a much higher proportion of extracellular fluid (nearly 80 percent) than adults (50 to 55 percent). This higher amount of water means a greater volume and, with less than expected protein binding, may require higher drug doses. The premature infant is especially susceptible to drugs penetrating the *blood-brain barrier* because his immature connective tissues form a weaker obstacle.

The newborn's metabolic rates may be much lower than an adult's, but they rise rapidly and by a few years of age may triple those of an adult. These metabolic rates then decline steadily until early adolescence, when they reach adult levels. A newborn's low metabolic rate and incompletely developed hepatic system put him at higher risk for toxic interactions. Neonates' metabolic pathways also are different from an adult's, meaning that some drugs will not have the expected effect or may have other, unexpected effects. Finally, the neonatal renal and hepatic systems' immaturity delays elimination of many drugs and their metabolites. Dosing schedules may have to be adjusted to accommodate longer half-lives until these systems mature at about 6 months to 1 year of age.

With all of these factors, a pediatric patient's drug function can differ radically from an adult's. Pediatric drug dosages must be individualized to minimize the risks of toxicity. Body surface area and weight are the two most common factors in calculating dosages. The Broselow tape gives a good approximation for children of average height/weight ratio. It bases its calculations on the child's height (length), and assumes the child's weight is at the fiftieth percentile for his height (Figure 3-2 ●). The Broselow tape primarily addresses drugs administered in the critical care setting.

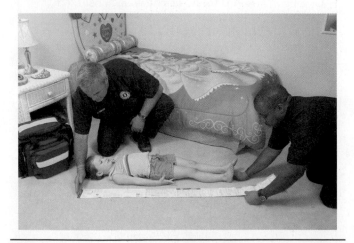

● **Figure 3-2** A Broselow tape is useful for calculating drug dosages for pediatric patients.

Geriatric Patients Significant changes in pharmacokinetics may also occur in patients older than about 60 years. They may absorb oral medications slower due to decreased gastrointestinal motility. Decreased plasma protein concentration may alter distribution of drugs in their systems, leaving drugs free that would otherwise have been protein bound. Body fat increases and muscle mass decreases with age; therefore, lipid-soluble drugs may have greater deposition, thereby lowering the amount of available drug. Absorption and distribution of intramuscular injections may change if volumes are inappropriate for the remaining muscle mass. Because the liver primarily handles biotransformation, depressed liver function in an aging patient may delay or prolong drug action. The aging process may also slow elimination by the renal system.

Older patients are also more likely to be on multiple medications or to have multiple underlying disease processes. Various medication interactions can have a severe impact on patients. For example, sildenafil (Viagra) and nitroglycerin given together may cause severe hypotension. Underlying diseases may affect therapeutics in unexpected ways. Congestive heart failure, for instance, may cause congestion of the gastrointestinal tract's vasculature, delaying the absorption of oral medications. The congestive heart failure patient may also have compromised renal function, delaying his elimination of drugs.

PHARMACOLOGY

Pharmacology is the study of drugs and their interactions with the body. Drugs do not confer any new properties on cells or tissues; they only modify or exploit existing functions. They may be given for their local action (in which case systemic absorption of the drug is discouraged) or for systemic action. Although generally given for a specific effect, drugs tend to have multiple actions at multiple sites, so they must be thought of in terms of their systemic effects rather than in terms of an isolated single effect. Pharmacology's two major divisions are pharmacokinetics and pharmacodynamics. You have already learned that **pharmacokinetics** addresses how drugs are transported into and out of the body. **Pharmacodynamics** deals with their effects once they reach the target tissues.

Pharmacokinetics

Strictly defined, pharmacokinetics is the study of the basic processes that determine the duration and intensity of a drug's effect. These four processes are absorption, distribution, biotransformation, and elimination.

Review of Physiology of Transport

Pharmacokinetics is dependent on the body's various physiologic mechanisms that move substances across the body's compartments. These mechanisms can be broken down into two broad categories based on their energy requirements and then further classified. A mechanism is referred to as **active transport** if it requires the use of energy to move a substance. This energy is achieved by the breakdown of high-energy chemical

● **Figure 3-3** Primary active transport by the Na⁺/K⁺ pump. The pump possesses three sodium-binding sites and two potassium-binding sites. ATP is used to power the pump, which transports sodium ions outside the cell and potassium ions into the cell against their electrochemical gradients. (a) Intracellular Na^+ ions bind to the pump protein. (b) The binding of three Na^+ ions triggers phosphorylation of the pump by ATP. (c) Phosphorylation induces a conformational change in the protein that allows the release of Na^+ in the extracellular fluid. (d) Extracellular K^+ ions bind to the pump protein and trigger release of the phosphate group. (e) Loss of the phosphate group allows the protein to return to its original conformation. (f) K^+ ions are released to the inside of the cell, and the Na^+ sites become again available for binding.

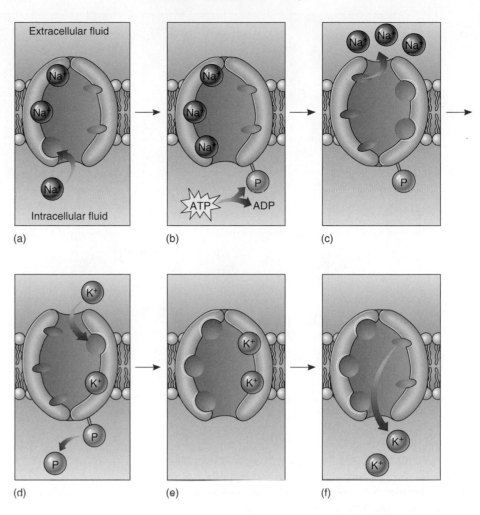

bonds found in chemicals such as ATP (adenosine triphosphate). ATP is broken down into ADP (adenosine diphosphate) liberating a considerable amount of bio-chemical energy. A common example of an active transport mechanism is the sodium-potassium (Na^+-K^+) pump. This is a protein pump that actively moves potassium ions into the cell and sodium ions out of the cell. Because this movement goes *against* the ions' concentration gradients, it must use energy (Figure 3-3 ●).

Large molecules, such as glucose and most of the amino acids, do not readily pass through the cell membrane because of their size. These molecules are moved across the cell membrane with the help of special "carrier" proteins found on the surface of the target cells. These large molecules are "carried" across the cell membrane in a special transport process called **carrier-mediated diffusion** or **facilitated diffusion**. These mechanisms typically do not require the expenditure of energy. Once the molecule to be transported binds with the carrier protein, the configuration of the cell membrane changes, allowing the large molecule to enter the target cell. Insulin, an important hormone secreted by the endocrine pancreas, can increase the rate of carrier-mediated glucose transport from 10- to 20-fold. This is the principal mechanism by which insulin controls glucose use in the body (Figure 3-4 ●).

Most drugs travel through the body by means of **passive transport**, the movement of a substance without the use of energy. This requires the presence of concentration gradients in a solution. Diffusion and osmosis are forms of passive transport. **Diffusion** involves the movement of solute in the solution, while **osmosis** involves the movement of the solvent (usually water). In diffusion, the solute's molecules or ions move *down* their

concentration gradients from an area of higher concentration to an area of lower concentration. Conversely, in osmosis the solvent's molecules move *up* the concentration gradient from an area of low solute concentration to an area of higher solute concentration. Another way of looking at this is to think of osmosis as simply the diffusion of solvent from an area of high *solvent* concentration to an area of low *solvent* concentration (Figure 3-5 ●). A final type of passive transport is **filtration**. This is simply the movement of molecules across a membrane down a *pressure* gradient, from an area of high pressure to an area of lower pressure. This pressure typically results from the hydrostatic force of blood pressure.

Absorption

When a drug is administered to a patient it must find its way to the site of action. If a drug is given orally or injected into any place except the bloodstream, its absorption into the bloodstream is the first step in this process. (Since drugs given intravenously or intraarterially enter directly into the bloodstream, no absorption needs to occur.) Several factors affect a drug's absorption. The body absorbs most drugs faster when they are given intramuscularly than when they are given subcutaneously. This is because muscles are more vascular than

Facilitated Diffusion

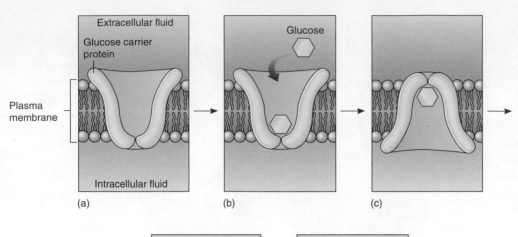

(a)　　　　　　(b)　　　　　　(c)

(d)　　　　　　(e)

● **Figure 3-4**　Transport of a glucose molecule across a cell membrane by a carrier protein. (a) A carrier protein with an empty binding site. (b) Binding of a glucose molecule to the protein's binding site, which faces the extracellular surface of the cell. (c) Conformational change in the carrier protein, such that the binding site now faces the interior of the cell. (d) Release of the glucose molecule. The binding site is once again empty. (e) Return of the carrier to its original conformation. The carrier is now ready to bind another glucose molecule.

subcutaneous tissue. Of course, anything that slows blood flow will delay absorption. Shock and hypothermia are just two examples. Conversely, processes such as fever and hyperthermia increase peripheral blood flow and speed absorption.

Drugs given orally (enterally) must first survive the digestive processes before being absorbed across the mucosa of the gastrointestinal system. If a drug is not soluble in water, it will have difficulty being absorbed. Time-released medications take advantage of this with an enteric coating that slowly releases the medication. Some drugs have an enteric coating that will not dissolve in the more acidic environment of the stomach, but will dissolve in the alkaline environment of the duodenum. This allows a drug that would irritate the stomach or be destroyed by stomach acid to be passed through the stomach into the duodenum and absorbed there. Besides being able to survive stomach acid, a drug must also be somewhat lipid (fat) soluble in order to cross the cells' lipid two-layered (bilayered) membranes. Many drugs **ionize**, or become electrically charged or polar following administration. Generally speaking, ionized drugs do not absorb across

Diffusion

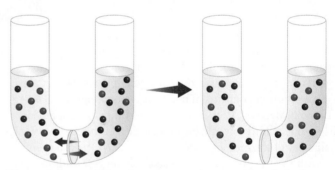

When solutes are differently concentrated on two sides of membranes, molecules cross in both directions until equilibrium is reached.

Osmosis

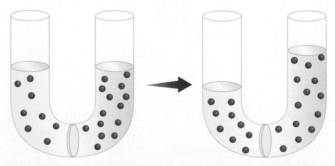

When there is more of a solute such as salt on one side of the membrane, water is drawn across the membrane to dilute the greater concentration until the concentration is equal on both sides.

● **Figure 3-5**　Diffusion is the movement of solute from an area of higher concentration to an area of lower concentration. Osmosis is the movement of water from an area of lower solute concentration to an area of higher solute concentration.

Ion Transport

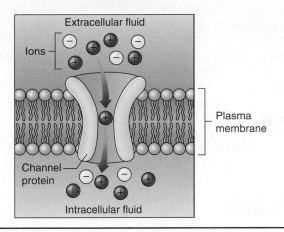

● Figure 3-6 Transport of ions across a cell membrane through a channel protein.

the membranes of cells (lipid bilayers), but fortunately, most drugs do not fully ionize. In addition, ions can be transported across the cell membrane through the use of carrier proteins (Figure 3-6 ●). In other instances, they reach an equilibrium between their ionized and nonionized forms, and the nonionized form can be absorbed. A drug's pH also affects the extent to which it ionizes. A drug that is a weak acid will ionize much more substantially in an alkaline environment than in an acidic environment; conversely, an alkaline drug will ionize more readily in an acidic environment than in an alkaline environment. For example, aspirin (an acidic drug) does not dissociate well in the stomach (an acidic environment) and is therefore readily absorbed there.

The nature of the absorbing surface and the blood flow to the administration site also affect drug absorption. The rate of absorption is directly related to the amount of surface area available for absorption. The greater the area, the faster the absorption. Much of the gastrointestinal system has multiple invaginations, or folds, that increase its surface area. Also, the greater the blood flow is to an area, the faster will be the rate of absorption. Again, the GI tract has a rich vascular system with many capillaries that perfuse its absorbing surfaces, allowing nutrients (and drugs) to diffuse into the bloodstream.

Finally, the drug's concentration affects its absorption. Because drugs diffuse in the body, the higher their concentration, the more rapidly the body will absorb them. This principle is frequently used when giving a "loading dose" of a drug and following it with a "maintenance infusion." The loading dose is typically a larger dose of the same concentration of the drug. On occasion, a more concentrated solution of the drug is used as the loading dose. Regardless, the desired effect is to rapidly raise the amount of the drug in the system to a therapeutic level. This is typically followed by a continuous infusion of the drug at a lower concentration, or slower administration rate, to keep it at the therapeutic level.

Bioavailability is the measure of the amount of a drug that is still active after it reaches its target tissue. This is the bottom line as far as absorption is concerned. The goal of administering a drug is to ensure sufficient bioavailability of the drug at the target tissue in order to produce the desired effect, after considering all the absorption factors.

Distribution

Once a drug has entered the bloodstream, it must be distributed throughout the body. Most drugs will pass easily from the bloodstream, through the interstitial spaces, into the target cells. Some drugs, however, will bind to proteins found in the blood, most commonly albumin, and remain in the body for a prolonged time. They thus have a sustained release from the bloodstream and a prolonged period of action. The therapeutic effects of a drug are primarily due to the unbound portion of the drug in the blood. A drug that is bound to plasma proteins cannot cross membranes and reach the target cells. Thus, only the unbound drug is in equilibrium with the target cells and can cross the cell membranes.

Changing the bloodstream's pH can affect the protein-binding action of a drug. Tricyclic antidepressants (TCAs), for instance, are strongly bound to plasma proteins. Making the blood more alkaline increases protein-binding of the TCA molecules. Therefore, in addition to supportive therapy, serious overdoses of TCAs are treated by administering sodium bicarbonate. Sodium bicarbonate makes the blood more alkaline (raises the pH), causing increased binding of the TCA to serum proteins. Cumulatively, this decreases the amount of free drug in the blood, thus decreasing the adverse effects. Sodium bicarbonate administration also facilitates elimination of the drug through the urine.

The presence of other serum protein-binding drugs can also affect drug-protein binding. For example, the drug warfarin (Coumadin) is highly protein bound (99 percent). Its therapeutic effects are due to the 1 percent of the drug that is unbound and circulating in the bloodstream. Aspirin molecules bind to the same binding site on the serum proteins as do warfarin molecules. Thus, when aspirin is administered to a patient on warfarin, it displaces some of the protein-bound warfarin, increasing the amount of free (unbound) warfarin in the blood. Even if it displaces only 1 percent of the total warfarin, it effectively doubles the available warfarin. This can lead to unwanted side effects such as hemorrhage.

Albumin is one of the chief proteins in the blood that is available for binding with drugs. When albumin levels are low (hypoalbuminemia), as occurs in malnutrition, drugs that are normally protein bound rise to much greater blood levels than anticipated. For example, consider a patient who has been taking warfarin without difficulty. If he develops hypoalbuminemia, his normal dose of warfarin will result in much more of the drug being available in the body, possibly leading to dangerous bleeding.

Certain organs exclude some drugs from distribution. For example, the tight junctions of the capillary endothelial cells in the central nervous system (CNS) vasculature form a

blood-brain barrier. These cells are packed together so tightly that only non-protein-bound, highly lipid-soluble drugs can cross into the CNS. The so-called **placental barrier** can likewise prevent drugs from reaching a fetus, although it is not the solid barrier that its name implies. The fetus is exposed to almost every drug that the mother takes. But because any drug must traverse the maternal blood supply and cross the capillary membranes into the placental (fetal) circulation, delivering drugs to a fetus requires them to be lipid soluble, nonionized, and non-protein-bound. This may slow some drugs or reduce their placental transfer to benign levels.

Other drugs are deposited in specific tissues. Fatty tissue, for example, can serve as a drug depot, or reservoir. Because blood flow is lower in fatty areas than in muscular areas, fatty tissue is a relatively stable depot; it can neither absorb nor release a large amount of drug in a short time. Similarly, bones and teeth can accumulate high amounts of drugs that bind to calcium, especially tetracycline antibiotics.

Biotransformation

Like other chemicals that enter the body, drugs are metabolized, or broken down into different chemicals (metabolites). The special name given to the **metabolism** of drugs is **biotransformation**. Biotransformation has one of two effects on most drugs: (1) It can transform the drug into a more or less active metabolite, or (2) it can make the drug more water soluble (or less lipid soluble) to facilitate elimination. Some drugs, such as lidocaine, are totally metabolized before elimination, others only partially, and still others not at all. The body will transform some molecules of most drugs and eliminate others without transformation. Protein-bound drugs are not available for biotransformation. Some so-called **prodrugs** (or parent drugs) are not active when administered, but biotransformation converts them into active metabolites.

Many biotransformation processes occur in the liver. The endoplasmic reticula of hepatocytes (liver cells) contain microsomal enzymes that perform much of the metabolizing. (Smaller quantities of these enzymes are also found in the kidney, lung, and GI tract.) Because the blood supply from the GI tract passes through the liver via the portal vein, all drugs absorbed in the GI tract pass through the liver before moving on through the systemic circulation. The first pass through the liver may partially or completely inactivate many drugs. This **first-pass effect** is why some drugs cannot be given orally but instead must be given intravenously to bypass the GI tract and prevent first-pass hepatic metabolism. It is also why drugs that can be given either orally or intravenously may require a much higher oral dose than IV dose. Because we can observe the extent of first-pass metabolism, we can predict how much to increase a dose of an oral medication to deliver an effective amount of the drug into the general circulation.

The liver's microsomal enzymes react with drugs in two ways: phase I, or nonsynthetic reactions; and phase II, or synthetic reactions. *Phase I reactions* most often **oxidize** the parent drug, although they may reduce it or **hydrolyze** it. These nonsynthetic reactions make the drug more water soluble to ease excretion. A number of drugs and chemicals increase the activity of, or induce, the microsomal enzyme that causes phase I reactions. This means that more enzyme is produced, and drugs will be metabolized more rapidly. Because the microsomal enzymes are nonspecific, they can be induced by one drug or chemical and then biotransform other drugs or chemicals. *Phase II reactions,* which are also called conjugation reactions, combine the prodrug or its metabolites with an endogenous (naturally occurring) chemical, usually making the drug more polar and easier to excrete.

Elimination

Whether they are unchanged or metabolized before elimination, most drugs (toxins and metabolites) are excreted in the urine. Some are excreted in the feces or in expired air.

Renal excretion occurs through two major processes: glomerular filtration and tubular secretion. Glomerular filtration is a function of glomerular filtration pressure, which in turn results from blood pressure and blood flow through the kidneys. Conditions that affect blood pressure and blood flow can affect renal elimination. Specialized transport systems in the walls of the proximal kidney tubules secrete drugs into the urine. These "pumps" are active transport systems and require energy in the form of adenosine triphosphate (ATP) to function. Some are specialized and transport only specific chemicals, while others can transport a range of similar chemicals. When drugs compete for the same pump, toxicity or other unwanted effects can result; however, combinations of some drugs can take advantage of this specialization to prolong their circulation. For example, probenecid blocks renal tubular pumps and competes for them with many antibiotics, among them penicillin, ampicillin, and oxacillin. Thus, probenecid is sometimes given with those antibiotics to increase and prolong their blood levels.

The same factors that affect absorption at any other site also affect reabsorption in the renal tubules. Of particular concern is the urine pH. Lipid soluble and nonionized molecules are readily reabsorbed. Changing the urine pH (usually by administering sodium bicarbonate to make it more alkaline) can affect the reabsorption in the renal tubules. For example, if a drug becomes ionized in a more alkaline environment, then making the urine more alkaline will interfere with reabsorption and cause more of the drug to be excreted. Some drugs and their metabolites can be eliminated in the expired air. This is the basis of the breath test that police use to determine a driver's blood alcohol level. Ethanol is released in the expired air in proportion to its concentration in the bloodstream. Although the liver degrades most ingested ethanol, exhalation releases a measurable quantity. Drugs also can be excreted in the feces. In enterohepatic circulation, if a drug (or its metabolites) is excreted into the intestines from bile, the body may reabsorb the drug and experience a sustained effect. Additionally, drugs may be excreted through sweat, saliva, and breast milk. Excretion through sweat glands is rarely a significant mechanism for elimination. Excretion through mammary glands becomes a concern when nursing mothers take medications.

Drug Routes

The route of a drug's administration clearly has an impact on the drug's absorption and distribution. The route's impact on biotransformation and elimination may not be so clear. The bloodstream will more quickly absorb and distribute water-soluble drugs if given in more vascular compartments than if given in less vascular compartments. Oral or nasogastric administration of alkaline drugs may allow the gastric acids to neutralize the drug and prevent its absorption. The liver's first-pass effect may biotransform some orally administered drugs and degrade them almost immediately.

Enteral Routes
Enteral routes deliver medications by absorption through the gastrointestinal tract, which goes from the mouth to the stomach and on through the intestines to the rectum. They may be oral, orogastric/nasogastric, sublingual, buccal, or rectal.

- *Oral (PO).* The oral route is good for self-administered drugs. Most home medications are administered by this route. The drug must be able to tolerate the acidic gastric environment and be absorbed. Few emergency drugs are administered through this route.
- *Orogastric/nasogastric tube (OG/NG).* This route is generally used for oral medications when the patient already has the tube in place for other reasons.
- *Sublingual (SL).* This is a good route for self-administration and excellent absorption from the sublingual capillary bed without the problems of gastric acidity or absorption.
- *Buccal.* Absorption through this route between the cheek and gum is similar to sublingual absorption.
- *Rectal (PR).* This route is usually reserved for unconscious or vomiting patients or patients who cannot cooperate with oral or IV administration (small children).

Parenteral Routes
Broadly defined, parenteral denotes any area outside the gastrointestinal tract; however, additional, specific criteria apply to parenteral drug administration. **Parenteral routes** typically use needles to inject medications into the circulatory system or tissues. Consequently, some forms of parenteral drug delivery afford the most rapid drug delivery and absorption.

- *Intravenous (IV).* With its rapid onset, this is the preferred route in most emergencies.[1]
- *Endotracheal (ET).* This is an alternative route for *selected* medications in an emergency.[2]
- *Intraosseous (IO).* The intraosseous route delivers drugs to the medullary space of bones. Most often used as an alternative to IV administration in pediatric emergencies, it also is used in adults.[3]

- *Umbilical.* Both the umbilical vein and umbilical artery can provide an alternative to IV administration in newborns.
- *Intramuscular (IM).* The intramuscular route allows a slower absorption than IV administration, as the drug passes into the capillaries.
- *Subcutaneous (SC, SQ, SubQ).* This route is slower than the IM route, because the subcutaneous tissue is less vascular than the muscular tissue.
- *Inhalation/Nebulized.* This route, which offers very rapid absorption, is especially useful for delivering drugs whose target tissues are in the lungs.
- *Topical.* Topical administration delivers drugs directly to the skin.
- *Transdermal.* For drugs that can be absorbed through the skin, the transdermal route allows slow, continuous release.
- *Nasal.* Useful for delivering drugs directly to the nasal mucosa, the nasal route has an expanding role in delivering systemically acting drugs.
- *Instillation.* Instillation is similar to topical administration, but places the drug directly into a wound or an eye.
- *Intradermal.* For allergy testing, intradermal administration delivers a drug or biological agent between the dermal layers.

Drug Forms

Drugs come in many forms. Solid forms, generally given orally, include:

- *Powders.* Although they are not as popular as they once were, some powdered drugs are still in use.
- *Tablets.* Powders compressed into a disklike form.
- *Suppositories.* Drugs mixed with a waxlike base that melts at body temperature, allowing absorption by rectal or vaginal tissue.
- *Capsules.* Gelatin containers filled with powders or tiny pills; the gelatin dissolves, releasing the drug into the gastrointestinal tract.

Liquid drugs are usually solutions of a solid drug dissolved in a solvent. Some can be given parenterally, while others must be given enterally.

- *Solutions.* The most common liquid preparations. Generally water based; some may be oil based.
- *Tinctures.* Prepared using an alcohol extraction process; some alcohol usually remains in the final drug preparation.

CONTENT REVIEW

▶ Types of Drug Actions

• Binding to a receptor site
• Changing the physical properties of cells
• Chemically combining with other chemicals
• Altering a normal metabolic pathway

• *Suspensions.* Preparations in which the solid does not dissolve in the solvent; if left alone, the solid portion will precipitate out.

• *Emulsions.* Suspensions with an oily substance in the solvent; even when well mixed, globules of oil separate out of the solution.

• *Spirits.* Solution of a volatile drug in alcohol.

• *Elixirs.* Alcohol and water solvent, often with flavorings added to improve the taste.

• *Syrups.* Sugar, water, and drug solutions.

Some drugs come in a gaseous form. The most common drug supplied this way is oxygen. Paramedics may also find nitrous oxide (N_2O) used as an inhaled analgesic in ambulances and emergency departments.

Drug Storage

Certain guidelines should dictate the manner in which drugs are stored; their properties may be altered by the environment in which they are stored. While some EMS units are parked in heated stations, others are kept outdoors and exposed to the elements. EMS systems must consider the storage requirements of all drugs and diluents when deciding operational issues such as vehicle design and posting policies (as occurs in system status management). This rapidly becomes a clinical issue because the actual potency of most medications is altered if they are not stored in proper conditions. Examples of variables to consider when determining the proper method of drug storage include temperature, light, moisture, and shelf life.

Pharmacodynamics

When we consider a drug's pharmacodynamics, or effects on the body, we are specifically interested in its mechanisms of action and the relationship between its concentration and its effect.

Actions of Drugs

Drugs can act in four different ways. They may bind to a receptor site, change the physical properties of cells, chemically combine with other chemicals, or alter a normal metabolic pathway. Each of these actions involves a physiochemical interaction between the drug and a functionally important molecule in the body.

Drugs That Act by Binding to a Receptor Site Most drugs operate by binding to a **receptor**. Almost all drug receptors are protein molecules on the surfaces of cells. They are part of the body's normal regulatory stimulation/inhibition function, and can be stimulated or inhibited by chemicals. Each different receptor's name generally corresponds to the drug

that stimulates it. For example, if an opiate stimulates the receptor, then the receptor is an opioid receptor. When multiple drugs stimulate the same receptor, standard practice is to use the generic name.

The force of attraction between a drug and a receptor is their **affinity**. The greater the affinity, the stronger the bond. Different drugs may bind to the same type of receptor site, but the strength of their bond may vary. The binding site's shape determines its receptivity to other chemicals, whether they are drugs or endogenous substances. These binding sites are relatively specific—a nonopiate drug generally will not affect an opiate binding site, although occasionally a drug with a similar receptor binding site will unexpectedly cross react. Receptors can also have subtypes. At least five subtypes of adrenergic receptors, for example, are important to paramedic practice.

A drug's pharmacodynamics also involves its ability to cause the expected response, or **efficacy**. Just as different drugs may have different affinities for a site, they may also have different efficacies; that is, drug A may cause a stronger response than drug B. Affinity and efficacy are not directly related. Drug A may cause a stronger response than drug B, even though drug B binds to the receptor site more strongly than drug A.

When a drug binds with its specific type of receptor, a chemical change occurs that ultimately leads to the drug's effect. In most cases, drugs will either stimulate or inhibit the cell's normal biochemical actions. In fact, a drug cannot impart a new function to a cell. Some drugs may interact with a receptor and directly result in the desired effect. Other drugs, however, may interact with a receptor and cause the release or production of a second compound. This secondary compound, or **second messenger**, includes such compounds as calcium or cyclic adenosine monophosphate (cAMP). Cyclic AMP is the most common second messenger. It has a multitude of effects inside the cell. These secondary messengers are particularly important in the endocrine system, as they principally occur in endocrine glands. Once cAMP is formed inside the cell, it activates still other enzymes, usually in a cascading action. That is, the first enzyme activates another enzyme, which activates a third enzyme, and so forth. This is important in that it amplifies the action so that even a small amount of a drug (or hormone) acting on the cell surface can initiate a powerful, cascading, activating force for the entire cell.

The number of receptors on a target cell usually does not remain constant on a daily basis, or even from minute to minute. This is because the receptor proteins are often destroyed during the course of their function. At other times, they are either reactivated or remanufactured by the protein-manufacturing mechanism of the cell. Binding of a drug (or hormone) to a target cell receptor causes the number of available receptors to decrease. This process is **down-regulation** of the receptors. It results in a decreased responsiveness of the target cell to the drug or hormone as the number of available active receptors decreases. In other cases, but less commonly, a drug (or hormone) can cause the formation of more receptors than normal. This process, **up-regulation**, increases the target tissue's sensitivity to the particular drug or hormone.

Chemicals that stimulate a receptor site generally fall into two broad categories, agonists and antagonists. **Agonists** bind to the receptor and cause it to initiate the expected response. **Antagonists** bind to a site but block agonists and prevent the receptor from initiating the expected response. Some drugs, **agonist-antagonists** (also called **partial agonists**), may do both. Nalbuphine (Nubain), for instance, stimulates some of the opioid agonists' analgesic properties but partially blocks others such as respiratory depression (Figure 3-7 ●).

Receptor-mediated drug actions work like a lock (the receptor) and key (the agonist). If you put the key in the lock and turn it, the lock will open. An antagonist is like a key that fits into the lock but will not turn and cannot open the lock. Target tissues generally have many receptors, so to take the analogy another step, imagine that to get maximal effect a single key (agonist) must move around and open many doors (trigger many biochemical responses). An agonist-antagonist would be a key that unlocks and opens a door but gets stuck in the lock. That is, the drug will cause the expected effect, but that drug will also block another drug from triggering the same receptor. This **competitive antagonism** is considered *surmountable* because a sufficiently large dose of the agonist can overcome the antagonism.

Noncompetitive antagonism can also occur. Continuing the lock, key, and door analogy, imagine the door is barred. This antagonism would be *insurmountable;* no amount of agonist could overcome it. Noncompetitive antagonism occurs because the binding of the antagonist at a different site causes a deformity of the binding site that actually prevents the agonist from fitting and binding. **Irreversible antagonism** may also occur when a competitive antagonist permanently binds with a receptor site. When this occurs, no amount of agonist will stimulate the receptor. For the effects of such an antagonist to wear off, the body must create new receptors.

Two drugs may appear to be antagonists while actually acting independently. This physiologic antagonism can occur when one drug's effects counteract another's. While neither agent chemically affects the other, their net effect is antagonistic. An example of a receptor, agonist, antagonist, and agonist-antagonist can be described using an opiate receptor. These receptors occur naturally in the brain and respond to natural endorphins. Morphine sulfate acts as an agonist. It binds to the opiate receptor and causes the expected response of pain relief. Naloxone (Narcan) acts as an antagonist. It will bind to the opiate receptor, but will not initiate the pain relief. It will prevent morphine sulfate from binding to the site and thus effectively blocks the morphine and its response. If the patient is given nalbuphine (Nubain), an agonist-antagonist, it will bind to the opiate receptor and relieve pain, but it is less efficacious than morphine. The nalbuphine blocks morphine from the receptor like an antagonist but stimulates the receptor on its own like an agonist, although to a lesser extent.

Drugs That Act by Changing Physical Properties   Some drugs change the physical properties of a part of the body. Drugs that change the osmotic balance across membranes are good examples of this type of drug action. The osmotic diuretic mannitol (Osmotrol), for instance, increases urine output by increasing the blood's osmolarity, or osmotic "pull." This increased osmolarity triggers the normal regulatory systems to decrease water reabsorption in the renal tubules, thereby reducing the total amount of water in the body.

Drugs That Act by Chemically Combining with Other Substances   Drugs that participate in chemical reactions that change the chemical nature of their substrates (the chemical or substance on which a drug acts) play a large role in paramedic practice. For example, isopropyl alcohol, which is often used to disinfect skin before percutaneous needle insertion for phlebotomy or IV cannulation, denatures the proteins on the surface of bacterial cells. This ruptures the cells, destroying the bacteria. The antacids are another example. They act by chemically neutralizing the hydrochloric acid in the stomach. Sodium bicarbonate given intravenously chemically neutralizes some of the acids in the bloodstream, effectively making the blood more alkalotic.

Drugs That Act by Altering a Normal Metabolic Pathway
Some anticancer and antiviral drugs are chemical analogs of normal metabolic substrates. In a process that has been dubbed a counterfeit incorporation mechanism, these drugs

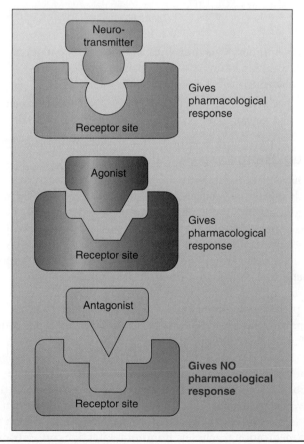

● **Figure 3-7**   Receptor site interactions. (top) Naturally occurring neurotransmitter binds to receptor site and creates a physiologic response. (middle) Administered drug (agonist) binds to the receptor site and creates a physiologic response. (bottom) A drug (antagonist) binds to the receptor site but does not cause a physiologic response and prevents agonists from binding to the receptor site.

can be incorporated into the products of metabolism of cancer cells. Since these drugs are not really the expected substrate, the anticipated product either will not form or, if formed, will be substantially or completely inactive.

Responses to Drug Administration

When a drug is administered, a response is obviously anticipated. The actual response may be the one desired, or it may be an unintended **side effect**. Most, if not all, drugs have at least some minor side effects. Because our knowledge of pharmacology and physiology has not yet arrived at the point where we can engineer the perfect drug, we must weigh the need for the desired response against the dangers of side effects. In essence, every time we give a medication, we must carefully weigh the risks against the benefits. Although undesirable, side effects are predictable. Iatrogenic responses, however, are not predicted. In general, the term *iatrogenic* refers to a disease or response induced by the actions of a care provider. Derived from the Greek *iatros* (physician) and *gennan* (to produce), it literally means *physician produced*. Negligence is not the only cause of iatrogenic responses. Some common unintended adverse responses to drugs include:

- *Allergic reaction.* Also known as hypersensitivity; this effect occurs as the drug is antigenic and activates the immune system, causing effects that are normally more profound than seen in the general population.
- *Idiosyncrasy.* A drug effect that is unique to the individual; different than seen or expected in the population in general.
- *Tolerance.* Decreased response to the same amount of drug after repeated administrations.
- *Cross tolerance.* Tolerance for a drug that develops after administration of a different drug. Morphine and other opioid agents are common examples. Tolerance for one agent implies tolerance for others as well.
- *Tachyphylaxis.* Rapidly occurring tolerance to a drug. May occur after a single dose. This typically occurs with sympathetic agonists, specifically decongestant and bronchodilation agents.
- *Cumulative effect.* Increased effectiveness when a drug is given in several doses.
- *Drug dependence.* The patient becomes accustomed to the drug's presence in his body and will suffer from withdrawal symptoms upon its absence. The dependence may be physical or psychological.
- *Drug interaction.* The effects of one drug alter the response to another drug.
- *Drug antagonism.* The effects of one drug block the response to another drug.
- *Summation.* Also known as an additive effect. Two drugs that both have the same effect are given together, analogous to $1 + 1 = 2$.
- *Synergism.* Two drugs that both have the same effect are given together and produce a response greater than the sum of their individual responses, analogous to $1 + 1 = 3$.

- *Potentiation.* One drug enhances the effect of another. A common example is promethazine (Phenergan) enhancing the effects of morphine.
- *Interference.* The direct biochemical interaction between two drugs; one drug affects the pharmacology of another drug.

Drug-Response Relationship

To have its optimal desired or therapeutic effects, a drug must reach appropriate concentrations at its site of action. The magnitude of the response therefore depends on the dosage and the drug's course through the body over time. Factors that can affect the drug's concentration may be pharmaceutical (the dosage form's disintegration and the drug's dissolution), pharmacokinetic (the drug's absorption, distribution, metabolism, and excretion), or pharmacodynamic (drug-receptor interaction). To predict how the drug will affect different people, a **drug-response relationship** thus correlates different amounts of drug to the resultant clinical response.

Most of the information needed to describe drug-response relationships comes from **plasma-level profiles**, which describe the lengths of onset, duration, and termination of action, as well as the drug's minimum effective concentration and toxic levels. The **onset of action** is the time from administration until a medication reaches its **minimum effective concentration** (the minimum level of drug necessary to cause a given effect). The length of time the amount of drug remains above this level is its **duration of action**. **Termination of action** is measured from when the drug's level drops below the minimum effective concentration until it is eliminated from the body.

The ratio of a drug's lethal dose for 50 percent of the population (LD_{50}) to its effective dose for 50 percent of the population

(ED_{50}) is its **therapeutic index** (TI) or LD_{50}/ED_{50}. The therapeutic index represents the drug's margin of safety. As the range between effective dose and lethal dose decreases, the value of TI decreases; that is, it becomes closer to one. TI values of close to one indicate a very small margin of safety. In other words, the effective dose and lethal dose of a drug whose TI value is close to one are nearly the same. This drug would be very difficult to effectively dose without causing toxicity.

The last component of the drug-response relationship, the **biologic half-life**, is the time the body takes to clear one-half of the drug. Although the rates of metabolism and excretion both affect it, a drug's half-life ($t_{1/2}$) is independent of its concentration. For example, if the concentration of a drug were 500 mcg/dL after administration and 250 mcg/dL in 10 minutes, then its half-life would be 10 minutes. After another 10 minutes, 125 mcg/dL would remain.

Factors Altering Drug Response

Different individuals may have different responses to the same drug given. Factors that alter the standard drug-response relationship include the following:

- *Age.* The liver and kidney functions of infants are not yet fully developed, so the response to drugs may be altered. Likewise, as we age, the functions of these organs begin to deteriorate. As a result, infants and the elderly are most susceptible to having an altered response to a drug.

- *Body mass.* The more body mass a person has, the more fluid is potentially available to dilute a drug. A given amount of drug will cause a higher concentration in a person with little body mass than in a much larger person. Thus, most drug dosages are stated in terms of body mass. For example, the standard dose of succinylcholine is 1–2 mg/kg. A 100-kg patient will receive 100–200 mg of succinylcholine, while a 50-kg patient would receive 50–100 mg.

- *Sex.* Most differences in drug response due to sex result from the relative body masses of men and women. The different distribution and amounts of body fat also affect the amounts of drug available at any given time.

- *Environmental milieu.* Various stimuli in a patient's environment affect his response to a given drug. This is most clearly seen with drugs affecting mood or behavior. The same dose of an antianxiety medication such as diazepam (Valium) will have different effects, depending on the patient's mood or surroundings. For example, if the patient were afraid of heights, his usual dose of diazepam would not be likely to help him remain calm while rappelling from the top of a tall building. Surrounding conditions may also affect the distribution or elimination of a drug. Heat, for example, causes vasodilation and increases perspiration, both of which may alter the rate at which the body distributes and eliminates a drug.

- *Time of administration.* If a patient takes a drug immediately after eating, its absorption will be different than if he took the same drug before breakfast in the morning.

Some drugs may cause nausea if taken on an empty stomach and must therefore be taken only after eating.

- *Pathological state.* Several disease states alter the drug-response relationship. Most notable are renal and hepatic dysfunctions, both of which may lead to excess accumulation of a drug in the body. Renal failure is likely to decrease elimination of drugs, while hepatic failure may decrease or inhibit their metabolism, prolonging their duration of action. Acid-base disturbances may alter a drug's solubility or the extent to which it ionizes, thus changing its absorption rate.

- *Genetic factors.* Genetic traits such as the lack of specific enzymes or lowered basal metabolic rate alter drug absorption or biotransformation and thus modify the patient's response.

- *Psychological factors.* A patient's mental state can also affect his response to a drug. The best-known example of this is the placebo effect. Essentially, if a patient believes that a drug will have a given effect, then he is much more likely to perceive that the effect has occurred.

Drug Interactions

Drug interactions occur whenever two or more drugs are available in the same patient. The interaction can increase, decrease, or have no effect on their combined actions. Any number of variables may cause these drug-drug interactions, including:

- One drug could alter the rate of intestinal absorption.

- The two drugs could compete for plasma protein binding, resulting in one's accumulation at the other's expense.

- One drug could alter the other's metabolism, thus increasing or decreasing either's bioavailability.

- One drug's action at a receptor site may be antagonistic or synergistic to another's.

- One drug could alter the other's rate of excretion through the kidneys.

- One drug could alter the balance of electrolytes necessary for the other drug's expected result.

In addition to drug-drug interactions, other types of interactions are possible. They include a drug's effects on the rate of absorption of food and nutrients, alteration of enzymes, and food-initiated alteration of drug excretion. Alcohol consumption and smoking may also cause interactions with drugs. Finally, some drugs are incompatible with each other. As an example, catecholamines such as epinephrine will precipitate in an alkaline solution such as sodium bicarbonate.

> **CONTENT REVIEW**
>
> ▶ Factors Affecting Drug-Response Relationship
>
> - Age
> - Body mass
> - Sex
> - Environment
> - Time of administration
> - Pathology
> - Genetics
> - Psychology

PART 2: Drug Classifications

CLASSIFYING DRUGS

The enormous amount of material that you must learn about pharmacology can easily become overwhelming. The best way to surmount this challenge is to break the information into manageable groups. Drugs can be classified in many ways. You will often find them listed by the body system they affect, by their mechanism of action, or by their indications. Drugs also can be classified by source or by chemical class. Understanding the properties of drug classes (or the model drug of a class) can increase your understanding of drugs and quicken your learning of new drugs.

Grouping medications according to their uses is a very practical way of classifying them. For example, one class of drugs is used to treat heart arrhythmias, while another treats hypertension. While the specific dosing regimens and contraindications vary among medications within any class, their general properties are consistent. If you understand those general principles, learning the specific information about individual medications becomes much easier. Thinking in terms of prototypical medications usually helps to describe each classification. A **prototype** is a drug that best demonstrates the class's common properties and illustrates its particular characteristics.

In the rest of this chapter, we will look at specific classifications of medications that as a paramedic you will commonly either administer or encounter. Even though you may not frequently administer medications from every classification, knowing how they work remains important. It will help you to understand the implications of medications your patients may be taking themselves or getting from another caregiver. An example often cited to demonstrate the importance of understanding the classes of medications, even those that you will rarely administer, is the patient who has taken an overdose of tricyclic antidepressants. Based on your knowledge of this classification, you will know to increase your index of suspicion for hypotension and abnormal cardiac rhythms.

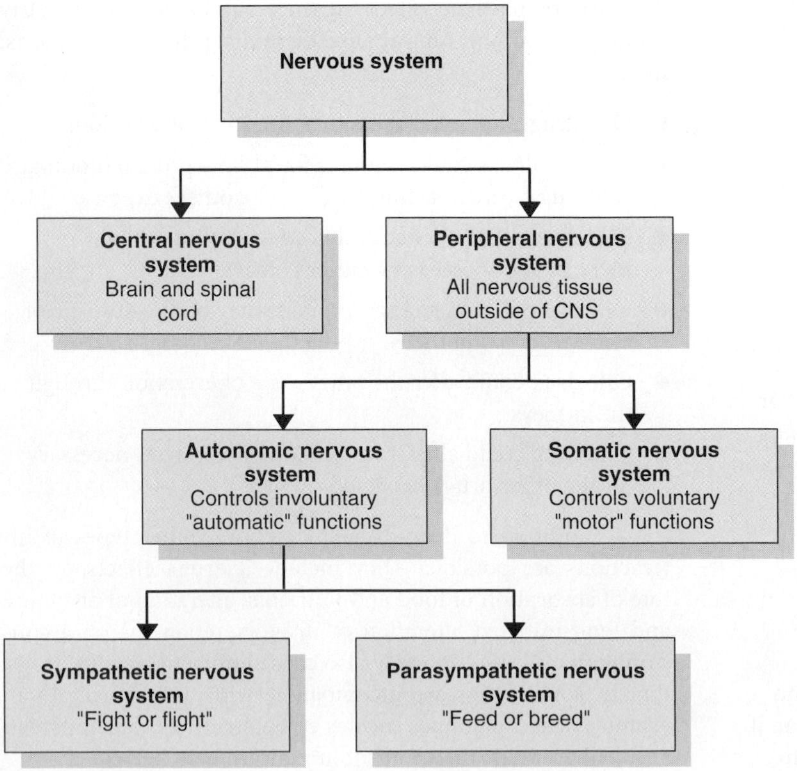

DRUGS USED TO AFFECT THE NERVOUS SYSTEM

The two major divisions of the nervous system are the central nervous system and the peripheral nervous system (Figure 3-8 ●). The *central nervous system* includes the brain and spinal cord; all nerves that originate and terminate within either the brain or the spinal cord are considered central. The *peripheral nervous system* comprises everything else. If a neuron originates within the brain and terminates outside the spinal cord, it is part of the peripheral nervous system, which in turn consists of the somatic nervous system and the autonomic nervous system. The *somatic nervous system* controls voluntary, or motor, functions. The *autonomic nervous system,* which controls involuntary, or automatic, functions, is further divided into the sympathetic and parasympathetic nervous systems. The two major groupings of medications used to affect the nervous system are those that affect the central nervous system and those that affect the autonomic nervous system.

Central Nervous System Medications

Many pathological conditions involve the central nervous system (CNS). As a result, a great number of drugs have been developed to affect the CNS, including analgesics, anesthetics, drugs to treat anxiety and insomnia, anticonvulsants, stimulants, psychotherapeutic agents (antidepressants and antimanic agents), and drugs used to treat specific nervous system disorders such as Parkinson's disease. Obviously, this is a very broad classification with many different types of agents. Having a firm grasp on the basic physiology involved will help you to understand the various drugs you encounter.

Analgesics and Antagonists

Analgesics are medications that relieve the sensation of pain. The distinction between **analgesia**, the absence of the sensation of *pain,* and **anesthesia**, the absence of *all* sensation, is important. Where an analgesic decreases the specific sensation of pain, an anesthetic prevents all sensation, often impairing consciousness in the process. A frequently used

```
                    Nervous system
                          |
          ┌───────────────┴───────────────┐
   Central nervous                  Peripheral nervous
      system                             system
  Brain and spinal              All nervous tissue
       cord                        outside of CNS
                                         |
                          ┌──────────────┴──────────────┐
                  Autonomic nervous              Somatic nervous
                      system                         system
                 Controls involuntary          Controls voluntary
                  "automatic" functions          "motor" functions
                          |
              ┌───────────┴───────────┐
      Sympathetic nervous      Parasympathetic nervous
           system                    system
        "Fight or flight"          "Feed or breed"
```

● **Figure 3-8** Functional organization of the autonomic nervous system within the overall nervous system.

class of medications, analgesics are available by prescription or over the counter. The two basic subclasses of analgesics are opioid agonists and their derivatives and nonopioid derivatives. Opioid antagonists, which we also discuss in this section, reverse the effects of opioid analgesics; **adjunct medications** enhance the effect of other analgesics.

Opioid Agonists An opioid is chemically similar to opium, which is extracted from the poppy plant and has been used for centuries for its analgesic and hallucinatory effects. Opium and all of its derivatives effectively treat pain because of their similarity to natural pain-reducing peptides called *endorphins*. Endorphins and, by extension, opioid drugs work through opiate receptors and decrease pain by decreasing the sensory neurons' ability to propagate pain impulses to the spinal cord and brain. At least five types of opiate receptors have been identified (Table 3–3).

The prototype opioid drug is morphine. Several of morphine's effects make it useful for clinical practice. At therapeutic doses, morphine causes analgesia, euphoria, sedation, and miosis (pupil constriction). It also decreases cardiac preload and afterload, which makes it useful in treating myocardial infarction and pulmonary edema. At higher doses, it may cause respiratory

TABLE 3–3 | Opiate Receptor Types

Receptor Name	Abbreviation	Effects
mu$_1$	μ$_1$	analgesia, euphoria
mu$_2$	μ$_2$	respiratory and physical depression, miosis, and reduced GI motility
delta	δ	analgesia, dysphoria, psychotomimetic effects (i.e., hallucinations), and respiratory and vasomotor stimulation
kappa	κ	analgesia, sedation, and miosis and respiratory depression and dysphoria
sigma	σ	psychotomimetic (i.e., hallucinations), dysphoria, and possibly dilation of the pupils
epsilon	ε	Effects uncertain

depression and hypotension (Figure 3-9 ●). Table 3–4 details common opioids used in EMS.[4–10]

Nonopioid Analgesics Three broad types of nonopioid medications also have analgesic properties, several of which also share antipyretic (fever-fighting) properties. These are

Opiate Receptors

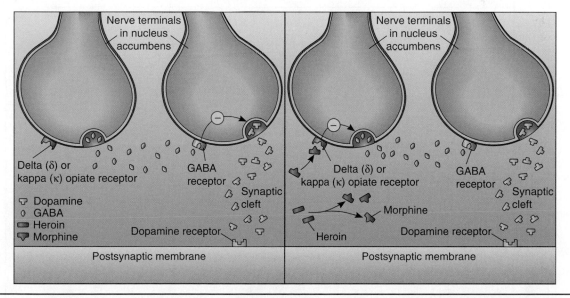

● **Figure 3-9** The effects of opiates on opiate receptors. Opiates modify the action of dopamine in selected areas of the brain, which form part of the brain's "reward pathway." After crossing the blood-brain barrier, opiates act on the various opioid receptors. This binding inhibits the release of GABA from the nerve terminal, reducing the inhibitory effect of GABA on dopaminergic neurons. The increased activation of dopaminergic neurons and the release of dopamine into the synaptic cleft results in activation of the postsynaptic membrane. Continued activation of the dopaminergic reward pathway leads to the feelings of euphoria and the "high" associated with opiate use. Morphine is a powerful agonist at the opioid mu receptor subtype, and activation of these receptors has a strong activating effect on the dopaminergic reward pathway.

TABLE 3–4 | Common Opioids

Name	Classification	Action	Indications	Contraindications	Doses	Routes	Adverse Effects	Other
Morphine *Duramorph* Ⓒ	Narcotic (opioid) Ⓒ	Analgesia and sedation through binding to opiate receptors	• Moderate–severe pain	• Hypotension • Hypersensitivity to the drug	2–10 mg	IV, IO, IM, SQ, PO	• Hypotension • Syncope • Tachycardia • Bradycardia • Apnea • Nausea • Vomiting • Respiratory depression	• Use appropriate monitors • Naloxone is an antagonist
Hydromor-phone *Dilaudid* Ⓒ	Narcotic (opioid) Ⓒ	Analgesia and sedation through binding to opiate receptors	• Moderate–severe pain	• Hypersensitivity to the drug	0.5–2.0 mg	IV, IO, IM, SQ, PO	• Nausea • Vomiting • Cramps • Respiratory depression	• Use appropriate monitors • Naloxone is an antagonist
Fentanyl *Sublimaze* Ⓒ	Narcotic (opioid) Ⓒ	Analgesia through binding to opiate receptors	• Moderate–severe pain • Anesthetic	• Hypersensitivity to the drug	50–100 mcg	IV, IO, IM, SQ, IN	• Nausea • Vomiting • Cramps • Chest wall rigidity • Respiratory depression	• Use appropriate monitors • Naloxone is an antagonist
Meperidine *Demerol* Ⓒ	Narcotic (opioid) Ⓒ	Analgesia through binding to opiate receptors	• Moderate–severe pain	• Hypersensitivity to the drug • Patients receiving monoamine oxidase inhibitors (MAOIs)	25–100 mg	IV, IO, IM, SQ, PO	• Nausea • Vomiting • Euphoria • Dysphoria • Respiratory depression	• Use appropriate monitors • Naloxone is an antagonist

salicylates such as aspirin; *nonsteroidal anti-inflammatory drugs (NSAIDs)* such as ibuprofen and ketorolac; and *para-aminophenol* derivatives such as acetaminophen. The drugs in each of these classes affect the production of prostaglandins and cyclooxygenase, important neurotransmitters involved in the pain response. Table 3–5 details common nonopioid analgesics.

Opioid Antagonists   Opioid antagonists are useful in reversing the effects of opioid drugs. Typically, this is necessary to treat respiratory depression. Naloxone (Narcan) is the prototype opioid antagonist. It competitively binds with opioid receptors but without causing the effects of opioid bonding. It is commonly used to treat overdoses of heroin and other opioid derivatives; however, it has a shorter half-life than most opioid drugs, so repeated doses may be necessary to prevent its unwanted side effects. Table 3–6 details common opiate antagonists.[11-13]

Adjunct Medications   Adjunct medications are given concurrently with other drugs to enhance their effects. While they may have only limited or no analgesic properties by themselves, combined with a true analgesic they either prolong or intensify its effect. Examples of adjunct medications are benzodiazepines (diazepam [Valium], lorazepam (Ativan), midazolam [Versed]), antihistamines (promethazine [Phenergan]), and caffeine. We will discuss many of these agents in separate sections.

Opioid Agonist-Antagonists   An opioid agonist-antagonist displays both agonistic and antagonistic properties. Pentazocine (Talwin) is the prototype for this class. Nalbuphine (Nubain) is commonly used in field care. It is an agonist because, like opioids, it decreases pain response, and it is an antagonist because it has fewer respiratory depressant and addictive side effects. Butorphanol (Stadol) is another common opioid agonist-antagonist. Although rarely used in modern EMS, they are detailed in Table 3–7.

Anesthetics

Unlike analgesics, an **anesthetic** induces a state of anesthesia, or loss of sensation to touch or pain. Anesthetics are useful during unpleasant procedures such as surgery or electrical cardioversion. At low levels of anesthesia, patients may have a decreased sensation of pain but remain conscious. **Neuroleptanesthesia**, a type of anesthesia that combines this effect with amnesia, is useful in procedures that require the patient to remain alert and responsive.

Anesthetics as a group tend to cause respiratory, central nervous system (CNS), and cardiovascular depression. Different agents affect these systems to different degrees and are typically chosen for their ability to produce the desired effect with minimal side effects. Anesthetic agents are rarely used singly; rather, several different agents are typically given together to achieve a balanced anesthetic result. For example, intubating a conscious patient requires his natural gag reflex to be inhibited. Neuromuscular blocking agents such as succinylcholine are used to induce paralysis. Because this would be a terribly frightening and potentially painful procedure, antianxiety, amnesic, and analgesic agents are also given to produce the desired anesthetic effect.

Anesthetics are given either by inhalation or injection. The gaseous anesthetics given by inhalation include halothane, enflurane, and nitrous oxide. The first clinically useful anesthetic was ether, a gas. Its discovery marked a new generation in surgical care, but it is very flammable. The modern gaseous anesthetics are much less volatile, while still decreasing consciousness and sensation as required. These drugs, by some as yet unidentified mechanism, hyperpolarize neural membranes, making depolarization more difficult. This decreases the firing rates of neural impulses and, therefore, the propagation of action potentials through the nervous system, thus reducing sensation. These effects appear to depend on the gases' solubility. The rate of onset of anesthesia further depends on several additional factors including cardiac output, inhaled concentration of gas, pulmonary minute volume, and end organ perfusion. Because these gases clear mostly through the lungs, respiratory rate and depth affect the duration of their effect. While halothane is the prototype of inhaled anesthetics, nitrous oxide is the only medication in this class with which you are likely to have much involvement.

Most anesthetics used outside the operating room are given intravenously. This gives them a considerably faster onset and shorter duration, making them much more useful in emergency care. Paramedics primarily use these agents to assist with intubation in rapid sequence intubation. They include several pharmacological classes including ultra-short-acting barbiturates (thiopental [Pentothal] and methohexital [Brevital]), benzodiazepines (diazepam [Valium] and midazolam [Versed]), and opioids (fentanyl [Sublimaze], remifentanil [Ultiva]). We discuss barbiturates' and benzodiazepines' mechanisms of action in the section on antianxiety and sedative-hypnotics.[14-15]

Anesthetics are also given locally to block sensation for procedures such as suturing and most dentistry. These agents are injected into the skin around the nerves that innervate the area of the procedure. They decrease the nerve's ability to depolarize and propagate the impulse from this area to the brain. Cocaine's first clinical use was as a topical anesthetic of the eye in 1884. The current prototype of this class is lidocaine (Xylocaine). It is frequently mixed with epinephrine. The epinephrine causes local vasoconstriction, decreasing bleeding and systemic absorption of the drug.

Antianxiety and Sedative-Hypnotic Drugs

Antianxiety and sedative-hypnotic drugs are generally used to decrease anxiety, induce amnesia, and assist sleeping and as part of a balanced approach to anesthesia. **Sedation** refers to a state of decreased anxiety and inhibitions. **Hypnosis** in this context refers to the instigation of sleep. Sleep may be categorized as either rapid-eye-movement (REM) or non-rapid-eye-movement (non-REM). REM sleep is characterized by rapid eye movements and lack of motor control. Most dreaming is thought to occur during REM sleep. Insomnia, or difficulty sleeping, typically presents with increased latency (the period of time between lying down and going to sleep) or awakening during sleep.

TABLE 3-5 | Common Nonopioid Analgesics

Name	Classification	Action	Indications	Contraindications	Doses	Routes	Adverse Effects	Other
Acetamino-phen *Tylenol*	Nonnarcotic analgesic, antipyretic (para-aminophenol derivative)	Exact mechanism uncertain but felt to inhibit cyclooxygenase	• Mild-moderate pain • Fever	• Hypersensitivity to the drug • Alcoholism • Chronic liver disease	325–650 mg	PO	• Rare	• Can be liver toxic—use minimal dose necessary
Ibuprofen *Motrin* *Advil*	NSAID	Anti-inflammatory and antipyretic through inhibition of prostaglandins	• Mild-moderate pain • Fever • Inflammation	• Hypersensitivity to the drug • Bronchospasm • Angioedema	200–800 mg	PO	• Nausea • Vomiting • GI bleeding • Allergic reactions	• Commonly causes gastric upset
Ketorolac *Toradol*	NSAID	Anti-inflammatory and antipyretic through inhibition of prostaglandins	• Mild-moderate pain • Fever • Inflammation • Renal colic	• Hypersensitivity to the drug • Bronchospasm • Angioedema	30 mg (IV and elderly) 60 mg IM	IV, IM	• Nausea • Vomiting • GI bleeding • Allergic reactions	• Can cause dizziness and headache
Aspirin	NSAID	Anti-inflammatory and antipyretic through inhibition of thromboxane A_2	• Mild-moderate pain • Fever • Platelet aggregation inhibitor	• Hypersensitivity to the drug • Bronchospasm • Angioedema • Patients receiving monoamine oxidase inhibitors (MAOIs)	350–650 mg	PO	• Nausea • Vomiting • GI bleeding • Allergic reactions	• Commonly causes gastric upset • Avoid enteric-coated aspirin in chest pain

TABLE 3-6 | Common Opioid Antagonists

Name	Classification	Action	Indications	Contraindications	Doses	Routes	Adverse Effects	Other
Naloxone *Narcan*	Opiate antagonist	Opioid antagonist without opiate agonist properties (it has no activity when given in the absence of an opiate agonist)	• Partial reversal of opiate drug effects • Opiate overdose	• Hypersensitivity to the drug	0.4–2.0 mg	IV, IO, SQ, IO, IN, nebulizer	• Fever • Chills • Nausea • Vomiting • Diarrhea • Opiate withdrawal	• Administer enough to reverse respiratory depression and avoid full narcotic withdrawal syndrome
Nalmefene *Revex*	Opiate antagonist	Opioid antagonist without opiate agonist properties (it has no activity when given in the absence of an opiate agonist)	• Partial reversal of opiate drug effects • Opiate overdose	• Hypersensitivity to the drug	0.5–1.0 mg	IV, IM, SQ, IO	• Fever • Chills • Nausea • Vomiting • Diarrhea • Opiate withdrawal	• Duration of effect much longer than naloxone

TABLE 3–7 | Opioid Agonists-Antagonists

Name	Classification	Action	Indications	Contraindications	Doses	Routes	Adverse Effects	Other
Nalbuphine *Nubain*	Opiate agonist-antagonist Ⓒᵥ	Analgesia and sedation through binding to opiate receptors. It also has some opiate receptor antagonistic properties.	• Moderate-severe pain	• Hypersensitivity to the drug • Opiate dependence • Respiratory depression	10–20 mg	IV, IO, SQ, IO	• Sedation • Dizziness • Nausea • Vomiting • Opiate withdrawal	• Use with caution in patients with liver and renal disease
Butorph-anol *Stadol*	Opiate agonist-antagonist Ⓒᵥ	Analgesia and sedation through binding to opiate receptors. It also has some opiate receptor antagonistic properties.	• Moderate to severe pain	• Hypersensitivity to the drug • Opiate dependence • Respiratory depression	1–4 mg	IV, IM, SQ, IO, IN	• Sedation • Dizziness • Nausea • Vomiting • Opiate withdrawal	• Use with caution in patients with liver and renal disease

Figure 3-10 The effects of benzodiazepines on GABA A receptors. Their binding causes a conformational change in the receptor that results in an increase in GABA A receptor activity. BDZs do not substitute for GABA, which bind at the alpha subunit, but increase the frequency of channel-opening events, which leads to an increase in chloride ion conductance and inhibition of the action potential.

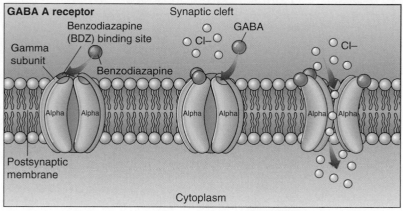

Benzodiazepine Receptors

The two main pharmacological classes within this functional class are benzodiazepines and barbiturates. Alcohol is also in this functional class. Benzodiazepines and barbiturates work in similar ways. Benzodiazepines are frequently prescribed for oral use and are relatively safe and effective for treating general anxiety and insomnia. Barbiturates, which have broader general depressant activities and a higher potential for abuse, are used much less frequently than benzodiazepines. Before the release of benzodiazepines in the 1960s, however, barbiturates were the drug of choice for treating anxiety and insomnia.

Both benzodiazepines and barbiturates hyperpolarize the membrane of central nervous system neurons, which decreases their response to stimuli. Gamma-aminobutyric acid (GABA) is the chief inhibitory neurotransmitter in the central nervous system. GABA receptors are dispersed widely throughout the CNS on proteins that make up chloride ion channels in the cell membrane. When GABA combines with these receptors, the channel "opens" and chloride, which is more prevalent outside the cell, diffuses through the channel. As chloride is an anion, or negative ion, it makes the inside of the cell more negative than the outside. This hyperpolarizes the membrane and makes it more difficult to depolarize. Depolarization therefore requires a larger stimulus to cause the cell to fire. Both benzodiazepines and barbiturates increase the GABA receptor-chloride ion channel complexes' potential for binding with

GABA, and both are dose dependent (Figure 3-10 ●). At low doses, they decrease anxiety and cause sedation (See Tables 3–8 and 3–9). As the dose increases, they induce sleep (hypnosis) and, at higher doses, anesthesia. Because benzodiazepines only increase the effectiveness of GABA, the amount of GABA present limits their effects. This actually makes benzodiazepines much safer than barbiturates, which at high doses can actually mimic GABA's effects and thus can have unlimited effects. Benzodiazepines and barbiturates are also useful in treating convulsions. Common sedatives and hypnotics are detailed in Table 3–10.

Just as opiates have an antagonist in naloxone (Narcan), benzodiazepines have an antagonist in flumazenil (Romazicon). Flumazenil competitively binds with the benzodiazepine receptors in the GABA receptor chloride ion channel complex without causing the effects of benzodiazepines. This reverses the sedation from benzodiazepines, but it can occasionally have untoward consequences, specifically if a patient depends on benzodiazepines for seizure control, is withdrawing from alcohol, or is taking tricyclic antidepressants. In these cases, the patient may develop seizures following the administration of flumazenil.

TABLE 3–8 | Levels of Sedation				
	Minimal Sedation (Anxiolysis)	**Moderate Sedation/ Analgesia (Conscious Sedation)**	**Deep Sedation/ Analgesia**	**General Anesthesia**
Responsiveness	Normal response to verbal stimulation	Purposeful response to verbal or tactile stimulation	Purposeful response after repeated or painful stimulation	Unarousable, even with painful stimulation
Airway	Unaffected	No intervention required	Intervention may be required	Intervention often required
Spontaneous Ventilations	Unaffected	Adequate	May be inadequate	Frequently inadequate
Cardiovascular Function	Unaffected	Usually maintained	Usually maintained	May be impaired

TABLE 3–9 | Ramsey Sedation Score

Score	Responsiveness
1	Patient is anxious and agitated or restless, or both.
2	Patient is cooperative, oriented, and tranquil.
3	Patient responds to commands only.
4	Patient exhibits brisk response to light glabellar (between eyebrows—just above the nose) tap or loud auditory stimulus.
5	Patient exhibits a sluggish response to light glabellar between eyebrows—just above the nose) tap or loud auditory stimulus.
6	Patient exhibits no response.

Antiseizure or Antiepileptic Drugs

Seizures are a state of hyperactivity of either a section of the brain (partial seizure) or all of the brain (generalized seizure). They may or may not be accompanied by convulsions. Therefore, although the medications in this functional class may be called anticonvulsants, they are more appropriately referred to as antiseizure or antiepileptic drugs. The goal of seizure management is to balance eliminating the seizures against the side effects of the medications used to treat them. Controlling seizures is a lifelong process for most patients and requires diligent compliance with medication dosing regimens.

Partial (or focal) seizures erupt from a specific focus and are described in terms of alterations in consciousness or behavior. These may be further divided into simple or complex partial seizures based on the specific area of the brain in which the focus is located. Complex partial seizures are also known as psychomotor seizures and are characterized by repetitive motions.

Generalized seizures involve both hemispheres of the brain and are described in terms of visible motor activity. Generalized tonic-clonic seizures involve periods of muscle rigidity (tonic stage) followed by spasmodic twitching (clonic stage) and then flaccidity and a gradual return to consciousness (postictal stage). Absence seizures are also generalized but do not have obvious convulsions. They involve brief losses of consciousness that may occur hundreds of times a day. Absence seizures are treated differently than other types of seizures. Finally, status epilepticus is a life-threatening condition characterized by uninterrupted tonic-clonic seizures lasting more than 30 minutes or by two or more tonic-clonic seizures without an intervening lucid interval. The preferred therapy for each type of seizure differs.

Seizures are treated through several general mechanisms. The most common is direct action on the sodium and calcium ion channels in the neural membranes. Phenytoin (Dilantin) and carbamazepine (Tegretol) both inhibit the influx of sodium into the cell, thus decreasing the cell's ability to depolarize and propagate seizures. Valproic acid and ethosuximide act similarly, but they interact with calcium channels in the hypothalamus, where absence seizures typically begin. These two drugs are particularly useful because they are specific to hyperactive neurons and therefore have few side effects. Other medications such as benzodiazepines and barbiturates interact with the GABA receptor-chloride ion channel complex, as explained in the section on antianxiety and sedative-hypnotic drugs.

Antiseizure medications comprise several pharmacological classes, including benzodiazepines (diazepam [Valium] and lorazepam [Ativan]), barbiturates (phenobarbital [Luminal]), hydantoins (phenytoin [Dilantin], fosphenytoin [Cerebyx]), succinimides (ethosuximide [Zarontin]), and miscellaneous medications such as valproic acid (Depakote). Table 3–11 lists the preferred medication for treating each type of seizure.

Central Nervous System Stimulants

Stimulating the central nervous system is desirable in certain circumstances such as fatigue, drowsiness, narcolepsy, obesity, and attention deficit hyperactivity disorder. Broadly, two techniques may accomplish this:

- Increasing the release or effectiveness of excitatory neurotransmitters
- Decreasing the release or effectiveness of inhibitory neurotransmitters

Within the functional class of CNS stimulants are three pharmacological classes: amphetamines, methylphenidates, and methylxanthines.

The amphetamines also include methamphetamine and dextroamphetamine. These drugs all increase the release of excitatory neurotransmitters including norepinephrine and dopamine. Norepinephrine is the primary cause of these drugs' effects, which include an increased wakefulness and awareness as well as a decreased appetite (Figure 3-11 ●). Amphetamines' most common uses, therefore, are treating drowsiness and fatigue and suppressing the appetite. Most of amphetamines' side effects result from overstimulation; they include tachycardia and other arrhythmias hypertension, convulsions, insomnia, and occasionally psychoses with hallucinations and agitation. Examples of this class include amphetamine sulfate (the prototype) and Dexedrine.

Methylphenidate, marketed as Ritalin, is the most commonly prescribed drug for attention deficit hyperactivity disorder (ADHD). While it is chemically different than the amphetamines, its pharmacological mechanism of action is similar. Also, like the amphetamines, it has a high abuse potential and is therefore listed as a Class II controlled substance. While treating hyperactivity with a stimulant may seem odd, it is quite effective. Frequently, the cause of inappropriate behavior in a child with ADHD is his inability to concentrate or focus. Ritalin's stimulant effects increase this ability, and the unwanted behavior often diminishes.

The methylxanthines include caffeine, aminophylline, and theophylline. While caffeine, the prototype drug in this class, has few clinical uses, it is frequently ingested in coffee, colas, and chocolates. Theophylline's relaxing effects on bronchial smooth muscle make it helpful in treating asthma. The methylxanthines'

TABLE 3-10 | Common Sedatives/Hypnotics

Name	Classification	Action	Indications	Contraindications	Doses	Routes	Adverse Effects	Other
Benzodiazepines								
Diazepam *Valium*	Benzodiazepine Ⓒⓥ	Binds to Type A GABA receptors causing sedation	• Anxiety • Seizures • Muscle relaxation	• History of hypersensitivity to the drug.	2–10 mg	IV, IM, IO, PO, rectal	• Hypotension • Sedation • Amnesia • Respiratory depression • Nausea • Vomiting	• Incompatible with other medications because not as water soluble. • Can cause irritation with injection. • Flumazenil is an antagonist.
Midazolam *Versed*	Benzodiazepine Ⓒⓥ	Binds to Type A GABA receptors causing sedation	• Anxiety • Sedation • Seizures	• History of hypersensitivity to the drug.	1–5 mg	IV, IM, IO,	• Hypotension • Sedation • Amnesia • Respiratory depression • Nausea • Vomiting	• Flumazenil is an antagonist.
Lorazepam *Ativan*	Benzodiazepine Ⓒⓥ	Binds to Type A GABA receptors causing sedation	• Anxiety • Sedation • Seizures	• History of hypersensitivity to the drug.	1–4 mg	IV, IM, IO, PO, rectal	• Hypotension • Sedation • Amnesia • Respiratory depression • Nausea • Vomiting	• Flumazenil is an antagonist.
Dissociative Agents								
Ketamine *Ketalar*	Dissociative anesthetic Ⓒⓘⓘⓘ	Causes dissociation between the cortical and limbic system	• Sedation • Analgesia	• History of hypersensitivity to the drug. • Hypertension	0.5–1.0 mg/kg (IV); 2–4 mg/kg (IM)	IV, IM	• Hallucinations	• All monitors should be in place. • Resuscitative equipment should be immediately available.

(Continued)

165

TABLE 3-10 | Common Sedatives/Hypnotics Continued

Miscellaneous Agents

Name	Classification	Action	Indications	Contraindications	Doses	Routes	Adverse Effects	Other
Nitrous Oxide	Sedative/ anesthetic gas	CNS depressant	• Pain • Sedation	• COPD • Pneumothorax • Bowel obstruction	Self-administered	Inhalation	• Dizziness • Hallucinations • Nausea • Vomiting • Altered mental status	• Should not be used in any patient who cannot comprehend verbal instructions or who is intoxicated with alcohol or other medications.
Propofol *Diprivan*	Nonbarbiturate, nonbenzodi-azepine sedative	Uncertain, but appears to potentiate GABA receptors	• Sedation	• History of hypersensitivity to the drug. Hypersensitivity of soy or egg products.	25–75 mcg/ kg/min	IV	• Pain on induction • Nausea • Vomiting • Respiratory depression	• All monitors should be in place. • Resuscitative equipment should be immediately available.
Etomidate *Amidate*	Nonbarbiturate, nonbenzodi-azepine sedative	Appears to modulate GABA receptors	• Sedation	• History of hypersensitivity to the drug.	0.1–0.3 mg/kg	IV	• Myoclonic jerks • Respiratory depression • Laryngospasm	• Does not have analgesic properties • Calcium-channel blockers can prolong respiratory depression • Can cause increased cortisol levels • All monitors should be in place. • Resuscitative equipment should be immediately available.

TABLE 3–11 | Antiseizure Medications

Type of Seizure	Drug of Choice
Partial Seizures	Phenytoin Carbamazepine
Grand Mal	Carbamazepine Phenytoin Phenobarbital
Absence	Valproic acid Ethosuximide

mechanism of action is unclear, but it seems to block adenosine receptors. Adenosine is an endogenous neurotransmitter which is used clinically for certain types of tachycardias. Because methylxanthines block the adenosine receptors, larger than normal doses may be needed to achieve the desired result. This class's side effects are similar to the amphetamines', but they have a much lower potential for abuse and are not controlled drugs.

Psychotherapeutic Medications

Psychotherapeutic medications treat mental dysfunction. Unlike other disease states, we do not thoroughly understand the pathophysiology of mental dysfunction; therefore, we base much of our pharmacological treatment of these conditions on our limited knowledge and on clinical correlation (scientific observation that these medications are indeed effective, even if we do not fully understand their mechanism). Medications are typically only one tactic in a balanced strategy for treating mental illness. Depending on the specific disorder, physicians will use other treatments such as psychotherapy and electroconvulsive therapy in conjunction with pharmaceutical interventions.

While we do not completely understand these diseases' specific pathologies, they seem to involve the monoamine neurotransmitters in the central nervous system. These neurotransmitters (norepinephrine, dopamine, serotonin) have been implicated in the control and regulation of emotions. Imbalances in these neurotransmitters, especially dopamine, appear to be at least involved with, if not responsible for, most mental disease. Regulating these and other excitatory and inhibitory neurotransmitters forms the basis for psychopharmaceutical therapy. Schizophrenia appears to be related to an increased release of dopamine, so

● **Figure 3-11** The mechanism of action of amphetamines. High-dose amphetamines can modify the action of dopamine and norepinephrine in the brain. At high doses, amphetamine increases the concentration of dopamine in the synaptic cleft. High-dose amphetamine has a similar effect on norepinephrine neurons; it can induce the release of norepinephrine into the synaptic cleft and inhibit the norepinephrine reuptake transporter.

treatment is aimed at blocking dopamine receptors. Depression seems to be related to inadequate amounts of these neurotransmitters, so treatment is aimed at increasing their release or duration.

The major diseases treated with psychotherapeutic medications are schizophrenia, depression, and bipolar disorder. *The Diagnostic and Statistical Manual,* fourth edition (DSM-IV), published by the American Psychiatric Association, gives schizophrenia's chief characteristics as a lack of contact with reality and disorganized thinking. Its many different manifestations include delusions, hallucinations (auditory more frequently than visual), disorganized and incoherent speech, and grossly disorganized or catatonic behavior. Schizophrenia is typically treated with antipsychotic medications, frequently in conjunction with medications from other classes such as antianxiety drugs or antidepressants. **Extrapyramidal symptoms** (EPS), a common side effect of antipsychotic medications, include muscle tremors and parkinsonism-like effects. As a result, antipsychotic medications are also known as **neuroleptic** (literally, *affecting the nerves*) drugs.

The two chief pharmaceutical classes of antipsychotics and neuroleptics are phenothiazines and butyrophenones. Both have been mainstays of psychiatry since the mid-1950s and are considered traditional antipsychotic drugs. Medications in this group block dopamine, muscarinic acetylcholine, histamine, and alpha₁ adrenergic receptors in the central nervous

CONTENT REVIEW

▶ Major Diseases Treated with Psychotherapeutic Medications

- Schizophrenia
- Depression
- Bipolar disorder

Amphetamine Actions

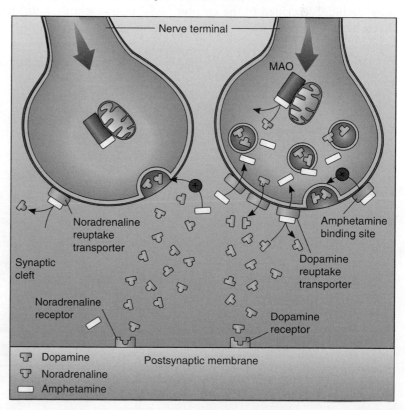

CONTENT REVIEW

▶ Major Classes of
Antipsychotic Medications

- Phenothiazines
- Butyrophenones
- Atypicals

system. These medications' therapeutic effects appear to come from blocking the dopamine receptors; their side effects are fairly well understood to originate in blocking the other receptors. The phenothiazines' and butyrophenones' mechanisms of action are the same; they differ only in potency and pharmacokinetics. The distinction between potency and strength is important. Strength refers to the drug's concentration, while potency is the amount of drug necessary to produce the desired effect. While the phenothiazines are considered low-potency and the butyrophenones are considered high-potency, they both produce the same effect. The differences in potency and pharmacokinetics determine which class of medication will be prescribed. Chlorpromazine (Thorazine) is the prototype phenothiazine; haloperidol (Haldol) is the prototype of the butyrophenones (Figure 3-12 ●).

Since the phenothiazines' and the butyrophenones' mechanisms of action are identical, their common side effects are also similar: extrapyramidal symptoms from cholinergic blockade in the basal ganglia of the cerebral hemispheres; orthostatic hypotension from blockage of alpha₁ adrenergic receptors; sedation; and sexual dysfunction. Treatment for these side effects typically involves modifying the drug dose. Diphenhydramine (Benadryl), an antihistamine with anticholinergic properties, is indicated for treating acute dystonic reactions (manifestations of EPS), which often present with tongue and neck spasm. Patients with a newly prescribed antipsychotic may experience these effects and contact EMS. Fortunately, treatment with diphenhydramine is effective and rapid. Orthostatic hypotension is treated in the usual fashion described in the chapter on hemorrhage and shock, Volume 5, Chapter 4.

Other medications used to treat psychotic conditions are considered atypical antipsychotics. While their mechanisms of action are similar to those of the traditional antipsychotics, the atypical antipsychotics block more specific receptors. This specificity allows them to function much like traditional antipsychotics but without causing the prominent extrapyramidal symptoms. These drugs include clozapine (Clozaril), risperidone (Risperdal), ziprasidone (Geodon), and olanzapine (Zyprexa). See Table 3–12.

The antidepressants are another functional class of psychotherapeutic medications. The DSM-IV characterizes major depressive episodes as causing significantly depressed mood, loss of interest in things that normally give the patient pleasure, weight loss or gain, sleeping disturbances, suicide attempts, feelings of hopelessness and helplessness, loss of energy, agitation or withdrawal, and an inability to concentrate. While the specific pathology of this disease is not yet known, it appears to be related to an insufficiency of monoamine neurotransmitters (norepinephrine and serotonin). Thus, the pharmaceutical interventions for this disease appear to increase the number of neurotransmitters released in the brain. The several ways of doing this include increasing the amount of neurotransmitter produced in the presynaptic terminal, increasing the amount of neurotransmitter released from the presynaptic terminal, and blocking the neurotransmitter's reuptake (reabsorption by the presynaptic terminal). This results in a net increase in the neurotransmitter. The antidepressants comprise three pharmacological classes: tricyclic antidepressants, selective serotonin reuptake inhibitors, and monoamine oxidase inhibitors.

Tricyclic antidepressants (TCAs) are frequently used in treating depression because they are effective, relatively safe, and have few significant side effects when taken in therapeutic dosages. TCAs act by blocking the reuptake of norepinephrine and serotonin, thus extending the duration of their action

Neuroleptic Actions

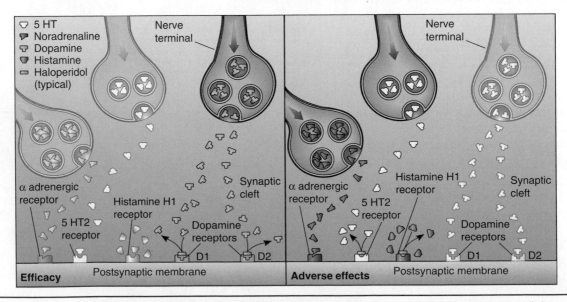

● **Figure 3-12**   The mechanism of action of haloperidol. Haloperidol is an older "typical," or "first-generation" drug. It is nonselective and binds to a broad range of receptors. It can bind to dopamine, histamine, and α₂ adrenergic receptors in the brain.

TABLE 3–12 | Antipsychotics

Name	Classification	Action	Indications	Contraindications	Doses	Routes	Adverse Effects	Other
Haloperidol *Haldol*	Butyrophenone	Blocks dopamine receptors associated with mood and behavior	• Psychosis	• Hypotension • Hypersensitivity to the drug	2–10 mg	IM, PO	• Extrapyramidal reactions • Insomnia • Restlessness • Dry mouth • Hypotension • Tachycardia	• Hypotension more common in patients taking antihypertensives
Chlorpromazine *Thorazine*	Phenothiazine	Blocks dopamine receptors associated with mood and behavior	• Psychosis • Intractable hiccoughs	• Hypotension • Hypersensitivity to the drug	25–50 mg	IM, PO	• Extrapyramidal reactions • Insomnia • Restlessness • Dry mouth • Hypotension • Tachycardia	• Hypotension more common in patients taking antihypertensives
Ziprasidone *Geodon*	Unclassified antipsychotic	Inhibits uptake of serotonin and dopamine	• Psychosis • Tourette's syndrome	• Hypersensitivity to the drug	50–100 mcg	IM, PO	• Extrapyramidal reactions • Insomnia • Restlessness • Dry mouth • Hypotension • Tachycardia	• Carbamazepine (Tegretol) can decrease ziprasidone levels

CONTENT REVIEW

▶ Major Classes of
Antidepressant Medications

• TCAs
• SSRIs
• MAOIs

(Figure 3-13 ●). Unfortunately, they also have anticholinergic properties that cause many side effects including blurred vision, dry mouth, urinary retention, and tachycardia. Another frequent side effect, orthostatic hypotension, is likely due to the alpha₁ adrenergic blockade. This is commonly seen when patients try to stand up too quickly and become dizzy. Additionally, because TCAs can lower the seizure threshold, patients with existing seizure disorders are at risk for convulsions. Unfortunately, when taken in overdose, TCAs can have very significant cardiotoxic effects that make them a favored means of attempting suicide among depressed patients. These effects include myocardial infarction and arrhythmias. Partly because of this potential for overdose, TCAs have fallen behind the newer selective serotonin reuptake inhibitors as the drug of choice for depression. Overdoses of these medications also frequently cause marked hypotension. Treatment of TCA overdoses is primarily supportive, with sodium bicarbonate given to increase the excretion of TCAs by alkalinizing the urine. The prototype tricyclic antidepressant, imipramine (Tofranil), was also the first one on the market. Other common examples include amitriptyline (Elavil), desipramine (Norpramin), and nortriptyline (Pamelor).

Selective serotonin reuptake inhibitors (SSRIs) are a recent addition to the antidepressants. The prototype, fluoxetine (Prozac), is the most widely prescribed antidepressant in the United States. These drugs' antidepressant effects are comparable to the TCAs', but because the SSRIs selectively block the reuptake of serotonin, they do not affect dopamine or norepinephrine. Nor do they block histaminic or cholinergic receptors, thus avoiding many of the TCAs' side effects (Figure 3-14 ●). The primary adverse reactions to SSRIs are sexual dysfunction, headache, and nausea. Other selective serotonin reuptake inhibitors include sertraline (Zoloft) and paroxetine (Paxil).

A third pharmacological class of psychotherapeutic medications includes the monoamine oxidase inhibitors (MAOIs). The monoamine neurotransmitters are thought to be insufficient in depression. Monoamine oxidase, an enzyme, metabolizes monoamines into inactive metabolites. MAOIs inhibit monoamine oxidase and block the monoamines' breakdown, thus increasing their availability (Figure 3-15 ●). Monoamine oxidase is also present in the liver and has a significant role in metabolizing foods that contain tyramine, a substance that increases the release of norepinephrine. The MAOIs' major side effect is hypertensive crisis brought on by the consumption of foods rich in tyramine such as cheese and red wine. By inhibiting monoamine oxidase, these drugs also decrease the body's ability to inactivate tyramine; they therefore promote the release of norepinephrine, a potent vasopressor. Because of this and

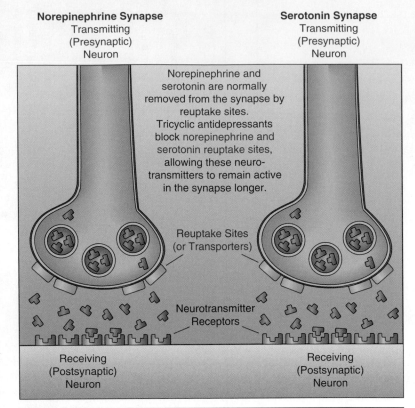

Tricyclic Antidepressants

Norepinephrine Synapse
Transmitting (Presynaptic) Neuron

Serotonin Synapse
Transmitting (Presynaptic) Neuron

Norepinephrine and serotonin are normally removed from the synapse by reuptake sites. Tricyclic antidepressants block norepinephrine and serotonin reuptake sites, allowing these neurotransmitters to remain active in the synapse longer.

Reuptake Sites (or Transporters)

Neurotransmitter Receptors

Receiving (Postsynaptic) Neuron

Receiving (Postsynaptic) Neuron

● **Figure 3-13**   The mechanism of action of tricyclic antidepressants (TCAs), blocking the reuptake of serotonin and norepinephrine.

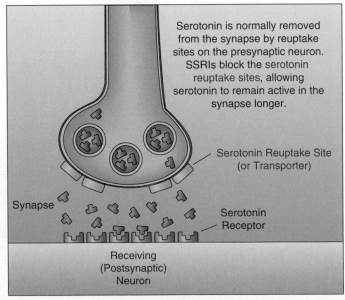

SSRI Antidepressants

Transmitting (Presynaptic) Serotonin Neuron

Serotonin is normally removed from the synapse by reuptake sites on the presynaptic neuron. SSRIs block the serotonin reuptake sites, allowing serotonin to remain active in the synapse longer.

Serotonin Reuptake Site (or Transporter)

Synapse

Serotonin Receptor

Receiving (Postsynaptic) Neuron

● **Figure 3-14**   The mechanism of action of selective serotonin reuptake inhibitors (SSRIs).

MAO Inhibitors

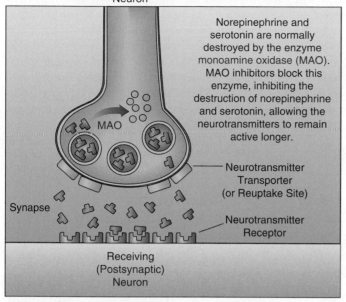

Norepinephrine or Serotonin Synapse
Transmitting (Presynaptic) Neuron

Norepinephrine and serotonin are normally destroyed by the enzyme monoamine oxidase (MAO). MAO inhibitors block this enzyme, inhibiting the destruction of norepinephrine and serotonin, allowing the neurotransmitters to remain active longer.

MAO

Synapse

Neurotransmitter Transporter (or Reuptake Site)

Neurotransmitter Receptor

Receiving (Postsynaptic) Neuron

● **Figure 3-15** The mechanism of action of monoamine oxidase inhibitors (MAOIs).

other unwanted side effects, MAOIs are not commonly used anymore; rather, they are reserved for treating depression that is refractory to TCAs and SSRIs. The prototype of this class is phenelzine (Nardil).

Patients with bipolar disorder (manic depression) exhibit cyclic swings from mania to depression with periods of normalcy in between. According to the DSM-IV, the manic phases of this disease are characterized by hyperactivity, thoughts of grandeur or inflated self-esteem, decreased need for sleep, increased goal-oriented behavior, increased productivity, flight of ideas (moving from thought to thought with little connection between them), distractibility, and increased risk taking. Lithium is the drug of choice for the management of bipolar disorder. It is frequently given in conjunction with benzodiazepines or antipsychotics. Lithium's mechanism of action is unknown, but it effectively decreases the signs of mania without causing sedation. Adverse reactions include headache, dizziness, fatigue, nausea, and vomiting. Recently, two antiseizure medications—carbamazepine (Tegretol) and valproic acid (Depakote)—have proven successful in treating bipolar disorder.

Drugs Used to Treat Parkinson's Disease

Parkinson's disease is a nervous disorder caused by the destruction of dopamine-releasing neurons in the *substantia nigra,* a part of the basal ganglia, which is a specialized area of the brain involved in controlling fine movements. Dysfunction of parts of the basal ganglia causes the extrapyramidal symptoms (EPS) often seen as a side effect of antipsychotic medications.

Parkinson's disease is characterized by dyskinesia (dysfunctional movements) such as involuntary tremors, unsteady gait,

and postural instability. Severe cases also involve bradykinesia (slow movements) and akinesia (the absence of movement). In the later stages, patients frequently present with psychological impairment including dementia, depression, and impaired memory. Parkinson's is a progressive disease that usually begins in middle age with subtle signs and progresses to a state of incapacitation. While no treatments can cure Parkinson's or even slow its progression, treating the symptoms can return some function to the patient. The goal in treating these patients is to restore their ability to function without causing unacceptable side effects. Some remarkably effective drugs are available. Unfortunately, they usually are effective for only several years. After that, signs and symptoms return and often are more severe than before treatment began.

The medications that are effective in treating Parkinson's disease are also effective in treating the extrapyramidal side effects (EPS) of antipsychotics. This is because fine motor control is based in part on a balance between inhibitory and excitatory neurotransmitters. In the basal ganglia, dopamine, an inhibitory transmitter, opposes acetylcholine, an excitatory neurotransmitter. Parkinson's disease and the medications that cause EPS both decrease the number of presynaptic terminals that release dopamine in the basal ganglia. This allows the excitatory stimulus of acetylcholine to dominate, ultimately impeding fine motor control.

Pharmacological therapy for Parkinson's disease seeks to restore the balance of dopamine and acetylcholine. This may be done either by increasing the stimulation of dopamine receptors or by decreasing the stimulation of acetylcholine receptors. Drugs can do this either through dopaminergic effects or through anticholinergic effects. Dopaminergic effects increase the release of dopamine from the neuron, directly stimulate the dopamine receptors, or decrease the breakdown of however much dopamine is being released. Anticholinergic effects prevent acetylcholine's effects either by reducing the amount of the neurotransmitter released or by directly blocking the acetylcholine receptors.

Dopamine cannot be given directly to Parkinson's disease patients because it cannot cross the blood-brain barrier and consequently would be ineffective in treating the disease while still causing many side effects. The drug of choice in treating Parkinson's disease, therefore, is levodopa, an inactive drug that readily crosses the blood-brain barrier. Levodopa is absorbed by the dopamine-releasing neuron terminals, where the enzyme decarboxylase metabolizes it into dopamine, thus increasing the amount of dopamine available for release. Levodopa is very effective and reduces symptoms in the vast majority of patients. As previously mentioned, however, symptoms will return within a period of years as the disease progresses. Levodopa's side effects include nausea, vomiting, and ironically, for unknown reasons, dyskinesias. Because it is converted to dopamine, levodopa may also have cardiovascular effects, including tachycardias and hypertension.

When given alone, levodopa is metabolized primarily outside the brain, where it is ineffective. To prevent this, Sinemet, the most popular anti-Parkinson preparation available, combines levodopa with an inactive ingredient, carbidopa. While carbidopa by itself produces no effects, it prevents levodopa's conversion into dopamine in the periphery. Because carbidopa does not cross the blood-brain barrier, however, levodopa can still be metabolized in the CNS. This decreases the incidence of cardiovascular side effects and enables lower doses of levodopa to be effective. Sinemet's side effects are essentially those of levodopa by itself. Nausea and vomiting, stimulated from within the CNS, remain problematic.

Another dopaminergic medication, amantadine (Symmetrel), promotes the release of dopamine from those dopamine-releasing neurons that remain unaffected by the disease. It has a rapid onset but generally becomes ineffective in less than a year. While it can be effective alone, it is usually given in conjunction with Sinemet or levodopa. Several other medications, such as bromocriptine, directly stimulate the dopamine receptors instead of attempting to increase the amount of dopamine released.

One additional dopaminergic approach is to decrease the breakdown of dopamine after it has been released. The enzyme responsible for breaking down monoamines such as norepinephrine, dopamine, and serotonin is monoamine oxidase. (We have previously described monoamine oxidase inhibitors in our discussion of their role in depression.) One monoamine oxidase inhibitor, selegiline (Carbex), is specific for monoamine oxidase type B. This MAO-B enzyme is involved only in the breakdown of dopamine. (MAO-A is responsible for breaking down norepinephrine and serotonin.) By selectively inhibiting the breakdown of dopamine, selegiline increases the amount available for binding with dopamine receptors, thus promoting the dopamine-acetylcholine balance. This selective blockage avoids increased norepinephrine levels that can lead to undesired tachycardia and hypertension.

As opposed to dopaminergic medications, which act on the dopamine side of the dopamine-acetylcholine balance, anticholinergic medications act on the acetylcholine side to block the acetylcholine receptors. The prototype anticholinergic, atropine, was initially used in this context with success, but it also had the typical peripheral anticholinergic side effects of blurred vision, dry mouth, and urinary hesitancy. More recently developed medications affect the CNS more than they do the peripheral nervous system. The prototype centrally acting anticholinergic medication is benztropine (Cogentin). Another example is diphenhydramine (Benadryl), which is more frequently administered for its antihistaminic properties.

Autonomic Nervous System Medications

The **autonomic nervous system** is the part of the nervous system that controls involuntary (automatic) actions. Many medications used in prehospital care directly affect the autonomic nervous system. It is essential that you have a good understanding of this aspect of the nervous system and the ways in which emergency medications affect it.

The two functional divisions of the autonomic nervous system are the sympathetic nervous system and the parasympathetic nervous system. The sympathetic nervous system allows the body to function under stress. It is often referred to as the fight-or-flight aspect of the nervous system. The parasympathetic nervous system, however, primarily controls vegetative functions such as digestion of food. It is often referred to as the feed-or-breed or the rest-and-repose aspect of the nervous system. The parasympathetic nervous system and the sympathetic nervous system work in constant opposition to control organ responses. For example, the sympathetic nervous system stimulates specific receptors in the heart that increase the heart rate. At the same time, the parasympathetic nervous system stimulates specific receptors that decrease the heart rate. The net result is the resting heart rate. When the body's physiologic needs dictate an increased heart rate, the sympathetic stimuli dominate the parasympathetic effects. Conversely, when the body needs to rest (with a decreased heart rate), the parasympathetic stimuli predominate.

Basic Anatomy and Physiology of the Autonomic Nervous System

The autonomic nervous system arises from the central nervous system. The nerves of the autonomic nervous system exit the central nervous system and subsequently enter specialized structures called **autonomic ganglia**. In the autonomic ganglia, the nerve fibers from the central nervous system interact with nerve fibers that extend from the ganglia to the various target organs. Autonomic nerve fibers that exit the central nervous system and terminate in the autonomic ganglia are called **preganglionic nerves**. Autonomic nerve fibers that exit the ganglia and terminate in the various target tissues are called **postganglionic nerves**. The ganglia of the sympathetic nervous system are located close to the spinal cord, while the ganglia of the parasympathetic nervous system are located close to the target organs (Figure 3-16 ●).

No actual physical connection exists between two nerve cells or between a nerve cell and the organ it innervates. Instead, there is a space, or **synapse**, between nerve cells. The space between a nerve cell and the target organ is a **neuroeffector junction**. Specialized chemicals called **neurotransmitters** conduct the nervous impulse between nerve cells or between a nerve cell and its target organ.

Neurotransmitters are released from presynaptic **neurons** and subsequently act on postsynaptic neurons or on the designated target organ. When released by the nerve ending, the neurotransmitter travels across the synapse and activates membrane receptors on the adjoining nerve or target tissue. The neurotransmitter is then either deactivated or taken back up into the presynaptic neuron.

The two neurotransmitters of the autonomic nervous system are acetylcholine (ACh) and norepinephrine. Acetylcholine is utilized in the preganglionic nerves of the sympathetic nervous system and in both the preganglionic and postganglionic nerves of the parasympathetic nervous system. Norepinephrine is the postganglionic neurotransmitter of the sympathetic nervous system. Synapses that use acetylcholine as the neurotransmitter are **cholinergic** synapses. Synapses that use norepinephrine as the neurotransmitter are **adrenergic** synapses.

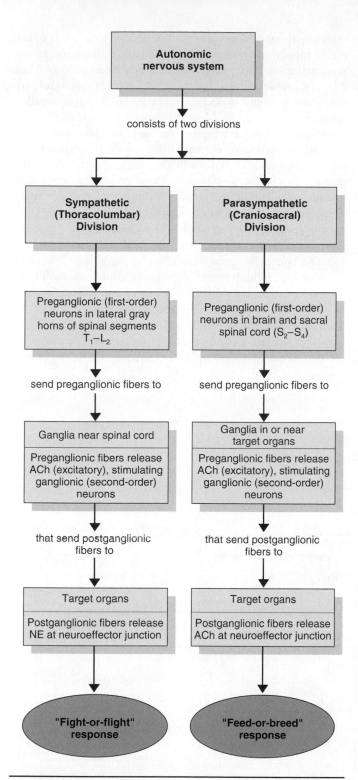

● **Figure 3-16** Components of the autonomic nervous system.

The flowchart in Figure 3-16 contains the following boxes:

Autonomic nervous system

consists of two divisions

Sympathetic (Thoracolumbar) Division | **Parasympathetic (Craniosacral) Division**

Preganglionic (first-order) neurons in lateral gray horns of spinal segments T_1–L_2 | Preganglionic (first-order) neurons in brain and sacral spinal cord (S_2–S_4)

send preganglionic fibers to | send preganglionic fibers to

Ganglia near spinal cord — Preganglionic fibers release ACh (excitatory), stimulating ganglionic (second-order) neurons | Ganglia in or near target organs — Preganglionic fibers release ACh (excitatory), stimulating ganglionic (second-order) neurons

that send postganglionic fibers to | that send postganglionic fibers to

Target organs — Postganglionic fibers release NE at neuroeffector junction | Target organs — Postganglionic fibers release ACh at neuroeffector junction

"Fight-or-flight" response | **"Feed-or-breed" response**

Drugs Used to Affect the Parasympathetic Nervous System

The parasympathetic nervous system arises from the brainstem and the sacral segments of the spinal cord. The preganglionic neurons of the parasympathetic nervous system are typically much longer than those of the sympathetic nervous system, because the ganglia are located close to the target tissues. Parasympathetic nerve fibers that leave the brainstem travel within four of the cranial nerves: the oculomotor nerve (III), the facial nerve (VII), the glossopharyngeal nerve (IX), and the vagus nerve (X). These fibers synapse in the parasympathetic ganglia with short postganglionic fibers that then continue to their target tissues. Postsynaptic fibers innervate much of the body, including the intrinsic eye muscles, the salivary glands, the heart, the lungs, and most of the organs of the abdominal cavity. The sacral segment of the parasympathetic nervous system forms distinct pelvic nerves that innervate ganglia in the kidneys, bladder, sex organs, and the terminal portions of the large intestine (Figure 3-17 ●). Stimulation of the parasympathetic nervous system results in the following conditions:

● Pupillary constriction

● Secretion by digestive glands

● Reduction in heart rate and cardiac contractile force

● Bronchoconstriction

● Increased smooth muscle activity along the digestive tract

These and other functions facilitate the processing of food, energy absorption, relaxation, and reproduction (Figure 3-18 ●).

All preganglionic and postganglionic parasympathetic nerve fibers use acetylcholine as a neurotransmitter. Acetylcholine, when released by presynaptic neurons, crosses the synaptic cleft and activates receptors on the postsynaptic neurons or on the neuroeffector junction. Acetylcholine is also the neurotransmitter for the somatic nervous system and is present in the neuromuscular junction. Acetylcholine is very short-lived. Within a fraction of a second after its release, it is deactivated by another chemical called acetylcholinesterase. Acetic acid and choline, which are produced when acetylcholine is deactivated, are taken back up by the presynaptic neuron (Figure 3-19 ●).

The parasympathetic system has two main types of ACh receptors, nicotinic and muscarinic. Knowing these receptors' locations and functions will greatly simplify learning the functions of drugs in this class (Table 3–13). Nicotinic$_N$ (neuron) receptors are found in all autonomic ganglia, where acetylcholine serves as the presynaptic neurotransmitter of both the parasympathetic and sympathetic nervous systems. Nicotinic$_M$ (muscle) receptors are found at the neuromuscular junction and initiate muscular contraction as part of the somatic nervous system. Muscarinic receptors are found in many organs throughout the body and are primarily responsible for promoting the parasympathetic response. Table 3–14 summarizes the locations and actions of the muscarinic receptors.

Because both nicotinic and muscarinic receptors are specialized for acetylcholine, they are termed cholinergic receptors. Medications that stimulate them are known as cholinergics (**parasympathomimetics**), and those that block them are known as anticholinergics or cholinergic blockers (**parasympatholytics**).

► Sludge Effects of Cholinergic Medications

- *Salivation*
- *Lacrimation*
- *Urination*
- *Defecation*
- *Gastric motility*
- *Emesis*

Cholinergics Cholinergic drugs act either directly or indirectly. Direct-acting cholinergics (also called cholinergic esters) simulate the effects of ACh by directly binding with the cholinergic receptors. Drugs in this class generally produce the same effects as cholinergic stimulation, mostly focused on the muscarinic receptors. Their adverse effects are related primarily to decreased heart rate: decreased peripheral vascular resistance resulting in hypotension and excessive salivation, urination, defecation, and sweating. Vomiting and abdominal cramps may also occur. The acronym SLUDGE (*s*alivation, *l*acrimation, *u*rination, *d*efecation, *g*astric motility, *e*mesis) is helpful for remembering these effects.

The prototype direct-acting cholinergic is bethanechol (Urecholine). Its pharmacokinetics make it a good clinical substitute for acetylcholine. It is not broken down by cholinesterase, the enzyme responsible for destroying acetylcholine, and therefore it has a longer duration of action. Most of its effects are on muscarinic receptors in the urinary bladder and gastrointestinal tract. It may be given orally or subcutaneously. Thus, it is used primarily to increase micturition (urination) and peristalsis. Adverse effects are rare but related to its parasympathomimetic effects. Another direct-acting cholinergic medication, pilocarpine, is used as a topical treatment for glaucoma.

Indirect-acting cholinergic drugs affect acetylcholinesterase. By inhibiting its actions in degrading acetylcholine, they prolong the cholinergic response. These drugs affect both muscarinic and nicotinic receptors and therefore have little specificity. Their uses are limited primarily to treating myasthenia gravis, some types of poisoning, and glaucoma as well as for reversing nondepolarizing neuromuscular blockade.

The two basic types of indirect-acting cholinergic drugs are reversible inhibitors and irreversible inhibitors. Both types bind with cholinesterase (ChE), acting as a substitute for ACh. In doing so, they prevent ChE from destroying ACh. The difference between the reversible and irreversible inhibitors is how long they remain bound with cholinesterase. The reversible inhibitors remain bound with cholinesterase much longer than

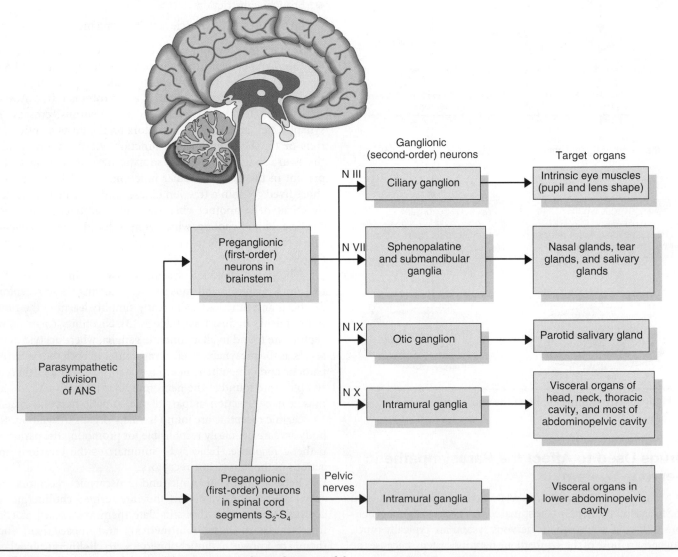

● **Figure 3-17** Organization of the parasympathetic division of the autonomic nervous system.

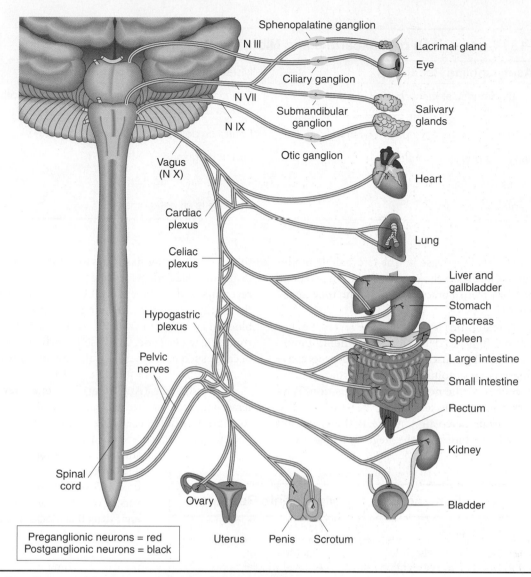

● **Figure 3-18**   Distribution of the parasympathetic postganglionic fibers.

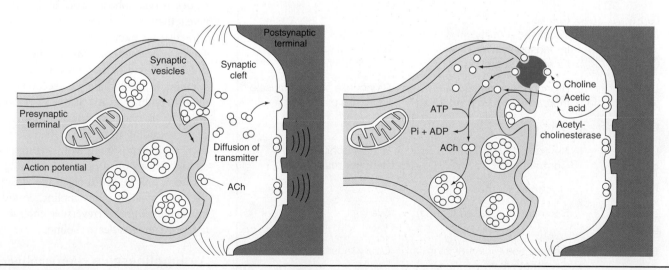

● **Figure 3-19**   Physiology of a cholinergic synapse. Acetylcholine is released from the presynaptic nerve and stimulates receptors on the postsynaptic nerve. Subsequently, acetylcholinesterase breaks down the acetylcholine and the presynaptic nerve fiber takes up the products.

TABLE 3–13 | Comparison of Muscarinic and Nicotinic Receptors

Nicotinic Acetylcholine Receptors	Muscarinic Acetylcholine Receptors
Found at the neuromuscular junction of skeletal (only) muscles.	Found at the neuromuscular junction of smooth and cardiac muscle.
Found on postganglionic parasympathetic nerves.	Found on postganglionic sympathetic nerves.
Found on many neurons in the brain.	Found on glands.
Nicotine is an agonist.	Muscarine is an agonist.
Curare is an antagonist.	Atropine is an antagonist.

acetylcholine but eventually release it. The irreversible inhibitors, too, will eventually release cholinesterase, but they remain bound for so long that, from a practical standpoint, they can be considered irreversible.

Neostigmine (Prostigmin) is the prototype reversible cholinesterase inhibitor. It is used to treat myasthenia gravis, an illness characterized by muscle weakness and progressive fatigue. This illness is an autoimmune disease that destroys the nicotinic$_M$ receptors at the neuromuscular junction. With fewer of these receptors, muscles cannot be stimulated as well and weakness occurs. Neostigmine treats the symptoms of myasthenia gravis by blocking the degradation of ACh, thereby prolonging its effects and increasing motor strength. Its primary side effects are due to the stimulation of muscarinic receptors and include the SLUDGE responses. Fortunately, these responses may be treated effectively with a cholinergic blocker. Neostigmine can also reverse a nondepolarizing neuromuscular blockade. This use is fairly uncommon, however, because such blockades typically are administered only intentionally as part of anesthesia or before intubation.

Physostigmine (Antilirium) is another reversible cholinesterase inhibitor. Its mechanism is similar to neostigmine's, with their primary difference being in their pharmacokinetics. While neostigmine is poorly absorbed across the cell membrane, physostigmine crosses rapidly and therefore has a shorter onset and may be given in lower doses. Physostigmine's chief use is for reversing overdoses of atropine, an anticholinergic drug that blocks muscarinic receptors.

Irreversible cholinesterase inhibitors have only one clinical function, the treatment of glaucoma, and only one drug, echothiophate (Phospholine Iodide), has been approved for that purpose. Cholinesterase inhibitors, however, are very useful as insecticides (organophosphates), and, unfortunately, their mechanism of action is also very attractive for makers of chemical weapons. They are the chief component in nerve gases such as VX and sarin. They cause extensive stimulation of cholinergic receptors, ultimately resulting in the SLUDGE response. Toxic levels may also affect nicotinic$_M$ receptors, leading to paralysis. Treatment for such toxic exposures involves drugs such as high doses of atropine or pralidoxime (Protopam, 2-PAM) to block the effects of the accumulating acetylcholine. Pralidoxime can encourage irreversible cholinesterase inhibitors to release cholinesterase.

TABLE 3–14 | Location and Effect of Muscarinic Receptors

Organ	Functions	Location
Heart	Decreased heart rate Decreased conduction rate	Sinoatrial node Atrioventricular node
Arterioles	Dilation Dilation Dilation	Coronary Skin and mucosa Cerebral
GI tract	Relaxed Increased motility Increased salivation Increased secretion	Sphincters Salivary glands Exocrine glands
Lungs	Bronchoconstriction Increased mucus production	Bronchiole smooth muscle Bronchial glands
Gallbladder	Contraction	
Urinary bladder	Relaxation Contraction	Urinary sphincter Detrusor muscle
Liver	Glycogen synthesis	
Lacrimal glands	Secretion (increased tearing)	Eye
Eye	Contraction for near vision Constriction	Ciliary muscle Pupil
Penis	Erection	

Anticholinergics Anticholinergic agents oppose the parasympathetic (cholinergic) nervous system. Just as there are multiple types of cholinergic receptors, there are multiple classes of cholinergic receptor antagonists. We will discuss agents that selectively block muscarinic and nicotinic receptors as well as nonselective blockers (ganglionic blockers). A special subclass of nicotinic receptor antagonists are the neuromuscular blocking drugs.

Muscarinic Cholinergic Antagonists Cholinergic antagonists block the effects of acetylcholine almost exclusively at the muscarinic receptors. They are often called anticholinergics or parasympatholytics. They work by competitively binding with muscarinic receptors without stimulating them. As a result, these receptors cannot bind with acetylcholine.

The prototype anticholinergic drug is atropine, which is widely used to block muscarinic receptors and is commonly administered in the field. Found in the plant *Atropa belladonna,* atropine is one of several drugs classified as belladonna alkaloids (scopolamine is also in this classification). Readily absorbed through both enteral and parenteral routes, it has therapeutic effects at dose dependent levels at most sites with muscarinic receptors. At low doses, atropine decreases secretion from salivary and bronchial glands as well as from the sympathetically innervated sweat glands. At moderate doses, it increases heart rate and causes mydriasis (dilated pupils) and blurry vision. At higher doses, it decreases gastric motility and stomach acid secretion. Atropine is also useful in reversing overdoses of muscarinic agonists (cholinergics or cholinesterase inhibitors). Its side effects, which are predictable, include dry mouth, blurred vision and photophobia, urinary retention, increased intraocular pressure, tachycardia, constipation, and anhidrosis (decreased sweating), which may cause hyperthermia. A helpful mnemonic for remembering the effects of atropine overdose is "hot as hell, blind as a bat, dry as a bone, red as a beet, mad as a hatter."

Scopolamine is another belladonna anticholinergic. Its actions are similar to atropine's, but unlike atropine, scopolamine causes sedation and antiemesis. Thus, its primary purpose is to prevent motion sickness. It is available as a transdermal patch.

Several synthetic medications mimic the effects of the belladonna alkaloids while minimizing their side effects. Ipratropium bromide (Atrovent), an inhaled anticholinergic, is effective in treating asthma because it relaxes the bronchial smooth muscle and causes bronchodilation. It is frequently administered along with an inhaled beta-adrenergic agonist. Because it is inhaled and has little systemic effect, ipratropium bromide avoids many of atropine's side effects (Table 3–15).

Other anticholinergic drugs include dicyclomine (Bentyl) and benztropine (Cogentin).

Nicotinic Cholinergic Antagonists Nicotinic cholinergic antagonists block acetylcholine only at nicotinic sites. They include ganglionic blocking agents that block the nicotinic$_N$ receptors in the autonomic ganglia and neuromuscular blocking agents that block nicotinic$_M$ receptors at the neuromuscular junction.

Ganglionic Blocking Agents Ganglionic blockade is produced by competitive antagonism with acetylcholine at the nicotinic$_N$ receptors in the autonomic ganglia. This can, in effect, turn off the entire autonomic nervous system. The two drugs in this class are trimethaphan (Arfonad) and mecamylamine (Inversine). Both are used to treat hypertension. The adverse effects of ganglionic blockade include signs associated with antimuscarinic drugs like atropine—dry mouth, blurred vision, urinary retention, and tachycardia. Other adverse effects arising from the vasodilation and decreased preload caused by sympathetic blockage include profound hypotension, with orthostatic hypotension even more evident. Trimethaphan is administered primarily for hypertensive crisis when other treatments are ineffective. These agents are almost never used anymore because they are not selective and many superior agents are available.

Neuromuscular Blocking Agents Neuromuscular blockade produces a state of paralysis without affecting consciousness. Imagine how terrifying it would be to be fully conscious and aware but completely paralyzed, unable to move or breathe. Neuromuscular blockade is caused by competitive antagonism of nicotinic$_M$ receptors at the neuromuscular junction. This is useful during surgery as part of anesthesia and during electroconvulsive therapy for depression. These agents are most often used in the field to facilitate intubation.

Neuromuscular blocking agents are either depolarizing or nondepolarizing, depending on their mechanism of action. Most are nondepolarizing; only one depolarizing drug, succinylcholine (Anectine), is commonly used in the clinical setting. Tubocurarine, while not frequently used clinically, is the oldest neuromuscular blocker and the prototype nondepolarizing agent. It produces neuromuscular blockade by binding with the nicotinic$_M$ receptor sites without causing muscle depolarization. Succinylcholine acts in the same manner, but like acetylcholine, it does cause muscle depolarization when it binds with the nicotinic$_M$ receptor. It is useful as a neuromuscular blocker because, in contrast to ACh, which rapidly separates from the receptor, it remains bound, preventing the muscle's repolarization. Several nondepolarizing agents are available; the specific agent chosen depends on its rate of onset and duration of action. Succinylcholine has the shortest onset and duration of action because it has a naturally occurring enzyme, pseudocholinesterase, which degrades it.[16–17] See Table 3–16.

Ganglionic Stimulating Agents Nicotinic$_N$ receptors reside at the ganglia of both the parasympathetic and sympathetic nervous systems. The alkaloid nicotine stimulates these receptors. Nicotine is found in tobacco and, although it has no therapeutic uses, is of interest for two reasons. Historically, nicotine, along with muscarine, led to a much better understanding of the autonomic nervous system's specific receptors. Also, it is one of the most abused drugs in the world.

Nicotine may cause a variety of responses, most of which are dose related. At low doses, like those from smoking, nicotine causes excitation at the autonomic ganglia. This affects both the parasympathetic and sympathetic nervous systems. The parasympathetic response causes increased salivation, peristalsis, and secretion of gastric acid. The sympathetic response causes the release of norepinephrine and epinephrine. These lead to

CONTENT REVIEW

▶ Types of Parasympathetic Acetylcholine Receptors

- Muscarinic
- Nicotinic
  - Nicotinic$_N$ (neuron)
  - Nicotinic$_M$ (muscle)

TABLE 3–15 | Parasympatholytic Medications

Name	Classification	Action	Indications	Contraindications	Doses	Routes	Adverse Effects	Other
Atropine	Muscarinic anticholinergic (Parasympatholytic)	Selectively blocks muscarinic receptors inhibiting parasympathetic stimulation	• Bradycardia • Antidote for organophosphate poisoning • Premedication for RSI	• Hypersensitivity to the drug	0.5–2.0 mg	IV, IO	• Blurred vision • Dry mouth • Dilated pupils • Confusion	• Organophosphate poisonings may require a significantly higher dose
Ipratropium *Atrovent*	Muscarinic anticholinergic (parasympatholytic)	Selectively blocks muscarinic receptors inhibiting parasympathetic stimulation	• Bronchospasm associated with obstructive lung disease (asthma, COPD)	• Hypersensitivity to the drug	500 mcg	Inhaled	• Blurred vision • Dry mouth • Dilated pupils • Cough • Confusion	• Typically administered with a beta agonist (although not as frequently)

TABLE 3–16 | Neuromuscular Blocking Agents

Name	Classification	Action	Indications	Contraindications	Doses	Routes	Adverse Effects	Other
Succinyl-choline *Anectine*	Depolarizing neuromuscular blocker	Binds to acetylcholine receptors at the neuromuscular junction causing depolarization and subsequent paralysis	• Rapid sequence intubation (RSI)	• Hyperkalemia • Neuromuscular disease • Crush injury • Burns • Increased intracranial pressure • Severe trauma	1–2 mg/kg	IV, IO,	• Hyperkalemia • Bradycardia • Prolonged paralysis • Malignant hyperthermia • Increased intracranial pressure • Muscle fasciculations • Trismus	• These agents should only be used by person skilled in their use, competent at complicated airway management, and with all necessary resuscitative equipment available.
Vecuronium *Norcuron*	Nondepolarizing neuromuscular blocker	Binds to acetylcholine receptors at the neuromuscular junction causing paralysis	• Rapid sequence intubation (RSI)	• Hypersensitivity to the drug	0.1–0.15 mg/kg	IV, IO,	• Skeletal muscle weakness • Malignant hyperthermia • Apnea	• These agents should only be used by person skilled in their use, competent at complicated airway management, and with all necessary resuscitative equipment available.
Rocuronium *Zemuron*	Nondepolarizing neuromuscular blocker	Binds to acetylcholine receptors at the neuromuscular junction causing paralysis	• Rapid sequence intubation (RSI)	• Hypersensitivity to the drug	1 mg/kg	IV, IO	• Hypertension • Hypotension • Skeletal muscle weakness • Malignant hyperthermia • Apnea	• These agents should only be used by person skilled in their use, competent at complicated airway management, and with all necessary resuscitative equipment available.

CONTENT REVIEW

▶ Effects of Atropine Overdose

- Hot as hell
- Blind as a bat
- Dry as a bone
- Red as a beet
- Mad as a hatter

increases in heart rate, myocardial contractility, vasoconstriction, and blood pressure, all of which increase the heart's workload. Sympathetic stimulation also increases awareness and suppresses fatigue and appetite.

Nicotine administration devices such as gum and transdermal patches are available for use in smoking cessation. Their actions are similar to the actions of nicotine inhaled in smoke.

Drugs Used to Affect the Sympathetic Nervous System

The sympathetic nervous system arises from the thoracic and lumbar regions of the spinal cord. Preganglionic nerves leave the spinal cord through the spinal nerves and end in the sympathetic ganglia. There are two types of sympathetic ganglia: sympathetic chain ganglia and collateral ganglia (Figure 3-20 ●). In addition, special preganglionic sympathetic nerve fibers innervate the adrenal medulla. Postganglionic nerves that exit the sympathetic chain ganglia extend to several peripheral target tissues of the sympathetic nervous system. When stimulated, these fibers have several effects. They include:

- Stimulation of secretion by sweat glands
- Constriction of blood vessels in the skin
- Increase in blood flow to skeletal muscles
- Increase in the heart rate and force of cardiac contractions
- Bronchodilation
- Stimulation of energy production

The collateral ganglia are located in the abdominal cavity. Nerves leaving the collateral ganglia innervate many of the organs of the

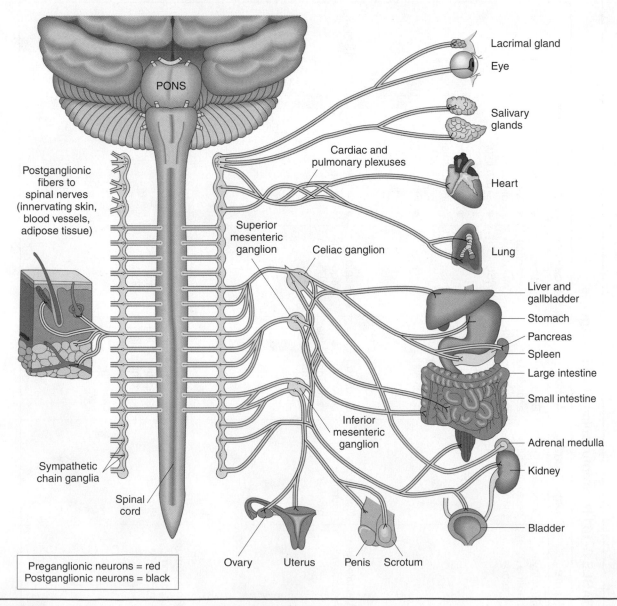

● **Figure 3-20** Distribution of sympathetic postganglionic fibers.

abdomen. Stimulation of these fibers causes several conditions. They include:

- Reduction of blood flow to abdominal organs
- Decreased digestive activity
- Relaxation of smooth muscle in the wall of the urinary bladder
- Release of glucose stores from the liver

Sympathetic nervous system stimulation also results in direct stimulation of the adrenal medulla, the inner portion of the adrenal gland (Figure 3-21 ●). The adrenal medulla in turn releases the hormones norepinephrine (noradrenalin) and epinephrine (adrenalin) into the circulatory system. Approximately 80 percent of the hormones released by the adrenal medulla are epinephrine, while norepinephrine constitutes the remaining 20 percent. Once released, these hormones are carried throughout the body where they cause their intended effects by acting on hormone receptors. The release of norepinephrine and epinephrine by the adrenal medulla stimulates tissues that are not innervated by sympathetic nerves. In addition, it prolongs the effects of direct sympathetic stimulation. All of these effects serve to prepare the body to deal with stressful and potentially dangerous situations.

Adrenergic Receptors Sympathetic stimulation ultimately results in the release of the hormone norepinephrine from postganglionic nerves. The norepinephrine subsequently crosses the synaptic cleft and interacts with adrenergic receptors on the postsynaptic nerves. Shortly thereafter, the norepinephrine is either taken up by the presynaptic neuron for reuse or broken down by enzymes present within the synapse (Figure 3-22 ●). Sympathetic stimulation also results in the release of the hormones epinephrine and norepinephrine from the adrenal medulla. In addition, both epinephrine and norepinephrine interact with specialized adrenergic receptors on the membranes of the target organs. These receptors are located throughout the body. Once stimulated by the appropriate hormone, they cause a response in the organ or organs they control.

The two known types of sympathetic receptors are the adrenergic receptors and the dopaminergic receptors. The adrenergic receptors are generally divided into four types. These five receptors are designated alpha 1 (α_1), alpha 2 (α_2), beta 1 (β_1), beta 2 (β_2), and beta 3 (β_3). The alpha$_1$ receptors cause peripheral vasoconstriction, mild bronchoconstriction, and stimulation of metabolism. The alpha$_2$ receptors are found on the presynaptic surfaces of sympathetic neuroeffector junctions. Stimulation of alpha$_2$ receptors is inhibitory. These receptors serve to prevent

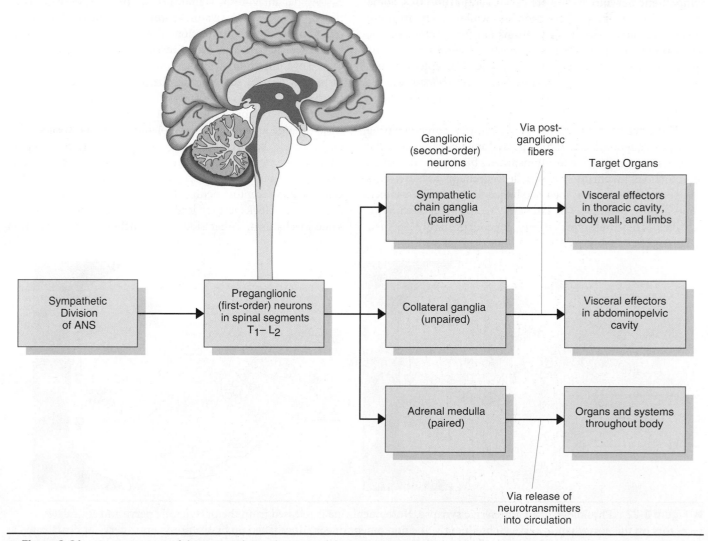

● **Figure 3-21**   Organization of the sympathetic division of the autonomic nervous system.

CONTENT REVIEW

▶ Types of Sympathetic
Receptors

- Adrenergic
  - alpha₁ (α₁)
  - alpha₂ (α₂)
  - beta₁ (β₁)
  - beta₃ (β₃)
- Dopaminergic

overrelease of norepinephrine in the synapse. When the level of norepinephrine in the synapse gets high enough, the alpha₂ receptors are stimulated, and norepinephrine release is inhibited. Stimulation of beta₁ receptors causes increases in heart rate, cardiac contractile force, and cardiac automaticity and conduction. Stimulation of beta₂ receptors causes vasodilation and bronchodilation. Stimulation of beta₃ receptors promotes the breakdown of lipids for energy production. It has been long thought that dopaminergic receptors cause some degree of dilation of the renal, coronary, and cerebral arteries. However, recent studies have questioned whether such an effect exists. Several studies have demonstrated that low-dose dopamine infusions actually worsen renal function instead of improving it. Other studies have not been able to demonstrate improved bowel perfusion with dopamine administration.

Medications that stimulate the sympathetic nervous system are **sympathomimetics**. Medications that inhibit the sympathetic nervous system are called **sympatholytics**. Some medications are pure alpha agonists, while others are pure alpha antagonists. Some medications are pure beta agonists, while others are pure beta antagonists. Medications such as epinephrine stimulate both alpha and beta receptors. Other medications, such as the bronchodilators, are termed beta selective, since they act more on beta₂ receptors than on beta₁ receptors.

The sympathetic nervous system releases norepinephrine from postganglionic end terminals and epinephrine from the adrenal medulla. These neurotransmitters bind with adrenergic receptors. (Epinephrine is also called adrenalin because of its release from the adrenal medulla; hence the term *adren*-ergic.) There are two main types of adrenergic receptors, each with two subtypes. These receptors' effects depend primarily on their

locations. Table 3–17 describes the chief locations and primary actions of each receptor.

The primary clinical purpose for medications that stimulate alpha₁ receptors is peripheral vasoconstriction. Constriction of the arterioles increases afterload, while constriction of venules increases preload (decreasing venous capacitance or "pooling"). Both of these effects increase systolic and diastolic blood pressure and represent the chief therapeutic indication for alpha₁ agonists. Stimulation of alpha₁ receptors locally may be useful in combination with local anesthetics. The main reason to add the alpha₁ agonist in this context is to cause local vasoconstriction so that the systemic absorption of the anesthetic will decrease, and its duration will increase. Alpha₁ agonists are also useful topically to decrease nasal congestion caused by dilation and engorgement of nasal blood vessels. The primary adverse responses to alpha₁ agonist agents are hypertension and local tissue necrosis. If a medication with significant alpha₁ properties infiltrates the surrounding tissue or distal body parts such as fingers, toes, earlobes, or nose, inadequate local blood flow due to profound vasoconstriction will likely kill the tissue. Also, alpha₁ stimulation may cause reflex bradycardia due to the feedback mechanism that regulates blood pressure. As baroreceptors detect a rise in blood pressure, heart rate decreases to compensate.

Alpha₁ antagonism is indicated almost exclusively for controlling hypertension. By preventing the peripheral vasoconstriction of alpha₁ stimulation, these agents decrease blood pressure. They are also useful in treating local tissue necrosis caused by infiltration of alpha₁ agonists. Injecting alpha₁ antagonists into the area surrounding the infiltration prevents tissue death from excessive vasoconstriction. The effects of pheochromocytoma, a tumor of the adrenal medulla that causes the release of large amounts of catecholamine, may be treated with an alpha₁ blocker. The most common adverse effects of alpha₁ antagonism are orthostatic hypotension and reflex tachycardia. Just as alpha₁ stimulation may increase blood pressure and cause a baroreceptor-mediated bradycardia, the hypotension from alpha₁ blockage may lead to reflex tachycardia from the same mechanism. Other side effects include nasal congestion

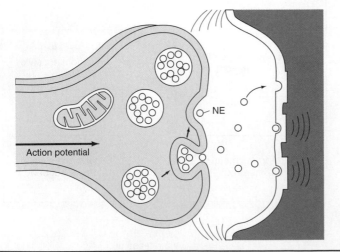
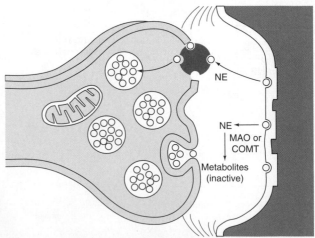

● **Figure 3-22**   Physiology of an adrenergic synapse. Norepinephrine is released from the presynaptic nerve and stimulates receptors on the postsynaptic nerve. Subsequently, the norepinephrine is either taken up by the presynaptic nerve or deactivated by enzymes in the synapse.

TABLE 3–17 | Location of Adrenergic Receptors and Effects of Stimulation

Receptor	Response to Stimulation	Location
Alpha₁ (α_1)	Constriction	Arterioles
	Constriction	Veins
	Mydriasis	Eye
	Ejaculation	Penis
Alpha₂ (α_2)	Presynaptic terminals inhibition*	
Beta₁ (β_1)	Increased heart rate	Heart
	Increased conductivity	
	Increased automaticity	
	Increased contractility	
	Renin release	Kidney
Beta₂ (β_2)	Bronchodilation	Lungs
	Dilation	Arterioles
	Inhibition of contractions	Uterus
	Tremors	Skeletal muscle
Beta₃ (β_3)	Lipolysis	Adipose tissue
Dopaminergic	Vasodilation (increased blood flow)	Kidney

*Stimulation of α_2 adrenergic receptors inhibits the continued release of norepinephrine from the presynaptic terminal. It is a feedback mechanism that limits the adrenergic response at that synapse. These receptors have no other identified peripheral effects.

and inhibition of ejaculation. These agents may also increase blood volume. This is ironic, since their primary indication is hypertension. As another feedback mechanism detects hypotension, the kidneys begin to reabsorb sodium and water to increase blood volume. This is typically addressed by use of a diuretic concomitant with the alpha₁ antagonist.

Beta₁ stimulation increases heart rate, contractility, and conduction. Its primary indications are cardiac arrest and hypotension resulting from inadequate pumping. During cardiac arrest, beta₁ activation may stimulate contractions or increase the force of any existing contractions. Even if the heart is only fibrillating, these agents may increase the effectiveness of electrical defibrillation. In cardiogenic shock, when the heart is not pumping with enough force to overcome the afterload created by peripheral vascular resistance, beta₁ agonists can adequately increase the contractions' force. The chief adverse effects of beta₁ agonists include tachycardia, arrhythmias, and chest pain from increasing workload.

Beta₁ antagonists are among the most frequently prescribed medications in the United States. Their most common use is to control blood pressure. By blocking the effects of beta₁ stimulation, they decrease heart rate (chronotropy) and contractility (inotropy). These agents are also effective in treating supraventricular tachycardias because they decrease the rate of impulse generation at the SA node (negative chronotropic effects) while also slowing conductivity through the AV node (negative dromotropic effects). Blocking beta₁ stimulation also helps treat angina pectoris and reduces the recurrence of myocardial infarction. Its

main adverse effects are symptomatic bradycardia, hypotension, and AV block.

Beta₂ agonists are used to treat asthma and other conditions with excessive narrowing of the bronchioles. By stimulating beta₂ receptors in the lungs, these agents relax the bronchial smooth muscle and cause bronchodilation. Beta₂ agonists can also cause uterine smooth muscle relaxation, which may help to suppress preterm labor. Their primary adverse effects are muscle tremors and "bleed over" effects on unintended beta₁ stimulation such as tachycardias.

While beta₂ blockade serves no clinically useful purpose, nonselective beta-blockers have side effects of beta₂ blockade. Chief among these is bronchoconstriction and inhibition of glycogenolysis, the release of stored glycogen by the liver and skeletal muscles. Beta₂ stimulation causes glycogenesis. Antagonizing the beta₂ receptors can inhibit this release. While this is not typically a problem for most people, it can be very problematic for diabetics. It not only makes hypoglycemia more likely but also masks one of its common early warning signs, tachycardia.

Adrenergic Agonists Drugs that stimulate the effects of adrenergic receptors work either directly, indirectly, or through a combination of the two. The direct-acting agents bind with the receptor and cause the same response as the normal neurotransmitter. In fact, most of the drugs in this category are either synthetically produced versions of the naturally occurring neurotransmitter or derivatives of those synthetically produced versions. The indirect-acting agents stimulate the release of epinephrine from the adrenal medulla and of norepinephrine from the presynaptic terminals. In turn, the epinephrine and norepinephrine stimulate the adrenergic receptors. The mixed actions of direct-indirect-acting medications combine these mechanisms.

The most frequently used adrenergic agents are chemically and functionally similar to the endogenous neurotransmitters. These drugs, which are called catecholamines, include norepinephrine, epinephrine, and dopamine.[18-19] Synthetic catecholamines are also available. They include dobutamine and isoproterenol. Noncatecholamine adrenergic agents, including ephedrine, phenylephrine, and terbutaline, also affect the adrenergic receptors and have useful clinical applications.

PATHO PEARLS

Adrenergic Agonists: Effects of Repeated Doses. *Many adrenergic agonists (Table 3–18), particularly decongestants and respiratory drugs, can result in tachyphylaxis. That is, repeated doses of the same drug have decreasing effects. In these cases, it may be prudent to change to a similar drug in the same family. The effects of a different drug can often be significantly better.*

TABLE 3-18 | Adrenergic Agonists

Name	Classification	Action	Indications	Contraindications	Doses	Routes	Adverse Effects	Other
Vasopressors								
Epinephrine	Sympathetic agonist	α- and β-adrenergic agonist (β effects more pronounced although dose-related)	• Cardiac arrest • Symptomatic bradycardia • Normovolemic hypotension • Allergies/anaphylaxis • Severe bronchospasm	• Few in the emergency setting	0.3–1.0 mg	IV, IO, IM, SQ, ET, Inhaled	• Palpitations • Anxiety • Tremulousness • Headache • Dizziness • Hypertension • Can worsen cardiac ischemia	• Two preparations are commonly available: • *1:1,000 (1 mg/mL)* • *1:10,000 (1 mg/10 mL)*
Norepinephrine *Levophed*	Sympathetic agonist	α- and β-adrenergic agonist (α effects more pronounced)	• Normovolemic hypotension • Septic shock • Cardiogenic shock	• Should not be used in hypovolemia until volume replacement has occurred	0.1–0.5 mcg/kg/min (titrate to effect)	IV	• Palpitations • Anxiety • Tremulousness • Headache • Dizziness • Hypertension • Can worsen cardiac ischemia • Reflex bradycardia	• Extravasation can cause localized tissue damage • Best administered through a central line
Dopamine *Intropin*	Sympathetic agonist	α- and β-adrenergic agonist	• Normovolemic hypotension • Symptomatic bradycardia • Septic shock • Cardiogenic shock	• Should not be used in hypovolemia until volume replacement has occurred	2–20 mcg/kg/min (titrated to effect)	IV	• Palpitations • Anxiety • Tremulousness • Headache • Dizziness • Hypertension • Can worsen cardiac ischemia • Reflex bradycardia	• Extravasation can cause localized tissue damage • Best administered through a central line • Proposed renal benefit has been disproven
Dobutamine *Dobutrex*	Synthetic sympathetic agonist	α- and β-adrenergic agonist (inotropic properties more pronounced than chronotropic properties)	• Congestive heart failure	• Should not be used in hypovolemia until volume replacement has occurred	2–20 mcg/kg/min (titrate to effect)	IV	• Palpitations • Anxiety • Tremulousness • Headache • Dizziness • Hypertension • Can worsen cardiac ischemia • Reflex bradycardia	• Extravasation can cause localized tissue damage • Best administered through a central line • Other agents preferred in cardiogenic shock

Drug	Class	Mechanism	Indications	Contraindications	Dose	Route	Side Effects	Notes
Phenylephrine *Neo-Synephrine*	Sympathetic agonist	Almost a pure α- agonist causing vasoconstriction	• Normovolemic hypotension • Septic shock • Spinal shock	• Avoid in cardiogenic shock	100–180 mcg/min (0.5–2.0 mcg/kg/min and titrate to effect)	IV	• Palpitations • Anxiety • Tremulousness • Headache • Dizziness • Can worsen cardiac ischemia • Reflex bradycardia	• Can be applied topically to nasal mucosa to shrink tissues prior to nasal procedures
Bronchodilators								
Albuterol *Ventolin, Proventil*	β-agonist	β-agonist with preference for β₂ adrenergic receptors	• Bronchospasm • Allergies/anaphylaxis • Hyperkalemia	• Known hypersensitivity to the medication	2.5 mg (SVN); 90 mcg (MDI)	Inhalation	• Palpitations • Anxiety • Tremulousness • Headache • Dizziness • Tachycardia	• The patient's heart rate and SpO₂ should be monitored during treatment.
Levalbuterol *Xopenex*	β-agonist	β-agonist with preference for β₂ adrenergic receptors. It is a racemic isomer of albuterol.	• Bronchospasm • Allergies/anaphylaxis • Hyperkalemia	• Known hypersensitivity to the medication	0.63 mcg (SVN)	Inhalation	• Palpitations • Anxiety • Tremulousness • Headache • Dizziness • Tachycardia	• The patient's heart rate and SpO₂ should be monitored during treatment.
Metaproterenol *Alupent*	β-agonist	β-agonist with preference for β₂ adrenergic receptors	• Bronchospasm • Allergies/anaphylaxis • Hyperkalemia	• Known hypersensitivity to the medication	0.2–0.3 mL of solution containing 15 mg/mL (SVN); 0.65 mg (MDI)	Inhalation	• Palpitations • Anxiety • Tremulousness • Headache • Dizziness • Tachycardia	• The patient's heart rate and SpO₂ should be monitored during treatment.
Terbutaline *Brethine*	β-agonist	Relatively nonselective β-agonist	• Bronchospasm • Allergies/anaphylaxis • Hyperkalemia • Preterm labor	• Known hypersensitivity to the medication	0.25 mg	Inhalation SQ	• Palpitations • Anxiety • Tremulousness • Headache • Dizziness • Tachycardia	• The patient's heart rate and SpO₂ should be monitored during treatment.
Racemic Epinephrine *S₂*	Sympathetic agonist	Relatively nonselective β-agonist. It is a mix of both racemic isomers of epinephrine	• Croup	• Known hypersensitivity to the medication	0.25–0.75 mL of a 2.5% solution	Inhalation	• Palpitations • Anxiety • Tremulousness • Headache • Dizziness • Tachycardia	• The patient's heart rate and SpO₂ should be monitored during treatment.

CONTENT REVIEW

► Common Catecholamines

- Natural
  - Epinephrine
  - Norepinephrine
  - Dopamine
- Synthetic
  - Isoproterenol
  - Dobutamine

Almost all the drugs in this section act on more than one type of receptor. Their specificity varies and is important in determining their uses. Table 3–19 lists their actions on various receptors.[20-21]

Adrenergic Antagonists
Unlike most adrenergic agonists, the majority of available adrenergic antagonists are remarkably selective in which receptor they affect. This selectivity, however, occurs only at therapeutic doses. At higher doses, most agents lose their selectivity and begin affecting other receptors as well.

The two basic subcategories of alpha adrenergic antagonists are "noncompetitive, long-acting" and "competitive, short-acting." They differ chiefly in the stability of their bond with the receptor. The prototype noncompetitive, long-acting alpha antagonist is phenoxybenzamine (Dibenzyline). The prototype competitive, short-acting antagonist is prazosin (Minipress). Prazosin also is the prototype for all alpha adrenergic antagonists. Phentolamine (Regitine) is an important nonselective alpha antagonist because of its effects in reversing tissue necrosis caused by catecholamine infiltration.

Beta adrenergic antagonists are more commonly referred to as beta-blockers. Propranolol (Inderal) is the prototype beta-blocker. It is a nonselective antagonist, which means that it blocks both beta$_1$ and beta$_2$ receptors. It is used to treat tachycardia, hypertension, and angina, all results of beta$_1$ blockade. Because it is nonselective, it also has the side effects of beta$_2$ blockade—bronchoconstriction and inhibited glycogenolysis. Propranolol was the first clinically employed beta-blocker, but its use has declined since the development of more selective beta$_1$ antagonists. The prototype of these cardioselective beta-blockers is metoprolol (Lopressor). At normal doses, metoprolol is selective for only beta$_1$ receptors; therefore, it does not cause propranolol's problematic side effects for asthmatics and diabetics. Atenolol (Tenormin) is another commonly used cardioselective beta-blocker.

Skeletal Muscle Relaxants Skeletal muscle relaxants are used to treat muscle spasm from injury and muscle spasticity from CNS injuries or diseases such as multiple sclerosis. Treatment can involve centrally acting agents or direct-acting agents.

The centrally acting muscle relaxants' mechanism is not clear, but it appears to be associated with general sedation. The prototype centrally acting skeletal muscle relaxant is baclofen (Lioresal), which is indicated in the treatment of spasticity. While baclofen is effective in the treatment of muscle spasticity, it is generally ineffective in muscle spasm. Several drugs are effective in treating muscle spasm, including cyclobenzaprine (Flexeril) and carisoprodol (Soma).

The prototype of the direct-acting muscle relaxants is dantrolene (Dantrium). Unlike the centrally acting agents, dantrolene's mechanism is well understood. It decreases the release of calcium from the sarcoplasmic reticulum in response to action potentials propagated from the neuromuscular junction. This calcium is required for the cross-bridge binding of the actin and myosin filaments in the muscle fibers responsible for contraction. Dantrolene is indicated for treating the spasticity associated with multiple sclerosis and cerebral palsy. It is also indicated for treating malignant hyperthermia, which is seen, on rare occasion, with some anesthetics and succinylcholine. This hyperthermia results from muscular contractions. Since dantrolene decreases these contractions, the heat that they generate also decreases. Dantrolene is not effective in treating muscle spasm.

DRUGS USED TO AFFECT THE CARDIOVASCULAR SYSTEM

Cardiovascular drugs have traditionally comprised one of the largest parts of the paramedic's pharmacological "toolbox." While this is changing with the expansion of paramedic practice, cardiovascular care (and agents used in that care) remains an important and integral part of a paramedic's knowledge base.

Cardiovascular Physiology Review

To understand cardiovascular pharmacology, you must first understand how electrical conduction and mechanical contraction work together to produce an organized and effective pumping action. We will briefly review the anatomy and physiology of the heart and then discuss the generation of electrical impulses and

TABLE 3–19 | Adrenergic Receptor Specificity

Medication	Receptor				
	Alpha$_1$	Alpha$_2$	Beta$_1$	Beta$_2$	Dopaminergic
Phenylephrine	✓				
Norepinephrine	✓	✓	✓		
Ephedrine	✓	✓	✓	✓	
Epinephrine	✓	✓	✓	✓	
Dobutamine			✓		
Dopamine*			✓		✓
Isoproterenol			✓	✓	
Terbutaline				✓	

*More recent research has questioned the dopaminergic effects of dopamine.

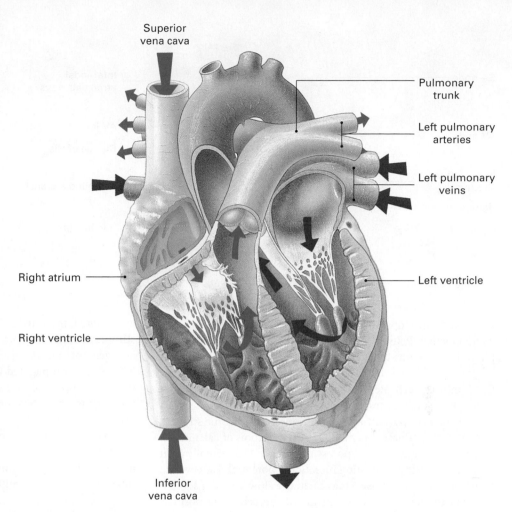

● **Figure 3-23** Blood flow through the heart.

the creation of arrhythmias. Then we will discuss how each classification acts on arrhythmias.

The heart is essentially a two-sided pump. The right side is a low-pressure pump responsible for pulmonary circulation, and the left side is a high-pressure pump responsible for systemic circulation. The human heart has four chambers: two atria and two ventricles. The atria receive blood from the pulmonary and systemic circulation and pass it on to the ventricles, where most of the pumping pressure originates (Figure 3-23 ●). Because the left side of the heart has to generate substantially higher pressures than the right, the left ventricle's muscular wall is much larger than those of the other chambers. The atria accept blood and allow it to pour passively into the ventricles. Just before the ventricles contract, the atria contract to "top off" the volume of blood in the ventricles. After this atrial "kick" fills the ventricles, they contract, forcing blood out of the heart. The myocardial muscle contraction depends on three factors: (1) electrical stimulation from the conduction system, (2) adequate amounts of ATP (energy), and (3) adequate amounts of the calcium ion. ATP and calcium are both needed for the thin and thick filaments to combine and shorten the muscle. To pump blood effectively, the entire heart must contract in a precise sequence. Both atria contract at the same time from the top down (toward the AV valves). A slight delay allows the ventricles to fill completely with blood, and then both ventricles contract simultaneously from the bottom up (toward the semilunar valves). This entire cycle must repeat itself continually.

Impulse Generation and Conduction

The key to the precise cardiac cycle is the electrical conduction system (Figure 3-24 ●). This system is composed of specialized cardiac tissue that generates electrical impulses and conducts them rapidly throughout the heart to ensure the chambers contract in proper sequence. The sinoatrial (SA) node is the heart's dominant pacemaker. It spontaneously generates electrical impulses (action potentials) that are propagated through intraatrial pathways to the atrioventricular (AV) node, where conduction is delayed momentarily. This delay gives the ventricles time to fill completely. The impulse then travels from the AV node throughout the ventricles via the bundle of His and the Purkinje network.

All myocardial tissue, both contractile and conductive, has the ability to self-generate electrical impulses (automaticity) and to propagate those impulses to surrounding tissue. It does this through the movement of ions across the cell membrane. At rest (when not stimulated), the cell membrane is polarized with a slight electrical charge. This charge is present because there are more positive ions outside the cell than inside, resulting in a slight negative charge on the inside. The primary ions involved are sodium (Na^+) on the outside of the cell and potassium (K^+) on the inside. Calcium (Ca^{++}), which is responsible for muscle contraction, is present in storage vesicles surrounding the cell. These vesicles are called the sarcoplasmic reticulum. The cell membrane is said to depolarize when this charge is eliminated or reversed. When an impulse is generated and conducted to the muscle cells, the process of depolarization and repolarization begins. Figure 3-25 ● depicts the sequence of ion movements in the depolarization and repolarization of both slow and fast potentials. Fast potentials occur in cardiac muscle tissue as well as in the ventricular conduction system; slow potentials occur in the pacemaker cells of the SA and AV nodes.

Cyclic activity in the fast potentials has five phases. Phase 0, which represents depolarization, results from a rapid influx of Na^+ ions into the cell. This makes the inside of the cell more positive than the outside and is normally caused by the arrival of an impulse generated elsewhere in the heart, such as the SA

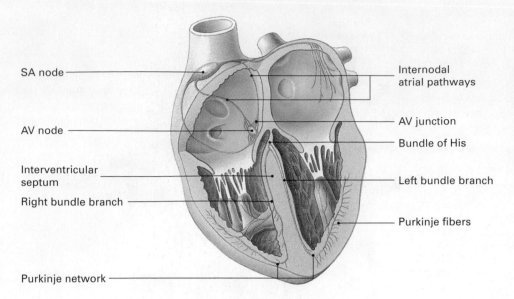

SA node

AV node

Interventricular septum

Right bundle branch

Purkinje network

Internodal atrial pathways

AV junction

Bundle of His

Left bundle branch

Purkinje fibers

node. Sodium stops entering the cell once the inside has become positive. Phases 1 through 3 represent repolarization. In phase 1, K^+ begins to leave the cell, slowly returning the cell to its normal negative charge. Phase 2 interrupts with an influx of Ca^{++} into the cell. Remember, the muscles are using calcium inside the cell for contraction. This plateau phase delays repolarization and is important for medications that affect the strength of contraction. Phase 3 is marked by a cessation of calcium influx and the rapid efflux of potassium. Phase 4 is normally a flat stage representing the resting membrane potential. However, in pathological states, phase 4 may include a slow influx of sodium that will gradually make the inside of the cell more positive. When the interior of the cell reaches a point called its threshold potential, the cell will depolarize without waiting for an impulse. Many antiarrhythmics have their mechanism of action during this phase 4 depolarization.

The slow potentials, while similar to the fast ones, have several important distinctions. First, they are located in the dominant pacemakers of the heart. Second, they depolarize differently. Notice in Figure 3-25 how phase 4 normally exhibits a gradually increasing slope toward threshold potential. While sodium causes depolarization (phase 0) of the fast potentials, a gradual influx of calcium causes it in the slow potentials. The slow potentials normally undergo a gradual, phase 4 depolarization. While we do not know the exact mechanism, this gradual depolarization clearly is responsible for the spontaneous generation of impulses in the SA and AV nodes. While the AV node also has these slow potentials, the SA node's rate of depolarization is faster, making it the heart's dominant pacemaker.

Arrhythmia Generation

Arrhythmias are generated at various places in the heart through either abnormal impulse formation (automaticity) or abnormal conductivity. The most prevalent types of arrhythmias are tachycardia (too fast) and bradycardia (too slow). An imbalance between the sympathetic and parasympathetic nervous systems most often causes these arrhythmias. Typically, excessive parasympathetic stimulation through muscarinic receptors causes bradycardias, which are treated with anticholinergic

medications. Tachycardias, however, have a variety of causes and are treated with the antiarrhythmics we discuss in this section.

As mentioned earlier, fast-potential means of depolarization dominate most of the heart, including the muscle cells and the ventricular conduction system. This process normally does not include a phase 4 depolarization; rather, depolarization most often happens in response to an impulse generated in the SA node and propagated to the cell. In pathological conditions such as ischemia, myocardial infarction, and excessive sympathetic stimulation, these tissues will develop phase 4 depolarization and generate an impulse abnormally. This abnormal impulse will then be propagated throughout the heart. These are considered ectopic foci, meaning the focus for the electrical impulse generation originated someplace other than where it normally should.

Another cause of both abnormal beats and abnormal rhythms is abnormal conduction. Figure 3-26 ● shows how an irregularity in the conduction system can generate arrhythmias. The inverted Y in that diagram represents the Purkinje network attaching to a single muscle fiber (represented by the horizontal bar under the Y). Impulses normally travel down both legs of the Y and begin depolarizing the muscle tissue. The muscle tissue depolarizes in both directions and meets in the middle of the Y, where it ends because the tissue is now refractory in both directions. In pathological conditions, a section of one of the Purkinje fibers has what amounts to a one-way valve that allows impulses to travel in only one direction. The impulse travels down the good leg and depolarizes the muscle fiber, which then propagates the impulse in both directions, unhindered by a refractory period in the opposing direction. Then the impulse will travel up the other leg of the Y, through the one-way valve. If the tissue of the other leg is no longer in the absolute refractory phase, the impulse will continue back down the first leg. This can create either an early beat or, if circumstances are just right, a very rapid reentrant rhythm (a so-called "circus rhythm").

Classes of Cardiovascular Drugs

The drugs used to treat cardiovascular disease generally fall into the two broad functional classifications of antiarrhythmics, also called antiarrhythmics, and antihypertensives.

Antiarrhythmics

Antiarrhythmic drugs are used to treat and prevent abnormal cardiac rhythms. Table 3–20 describes the pharmacological classes of antiarrhythmics. While these medications are

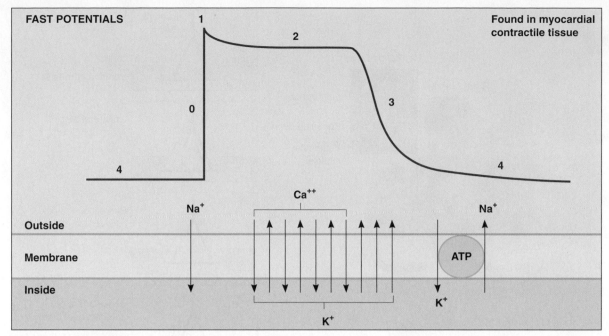

Action potential of cardiac contractile (muscle) tissue depends upon activation of fast sodium channels (opening the gates) via stimulus from pacing cells.

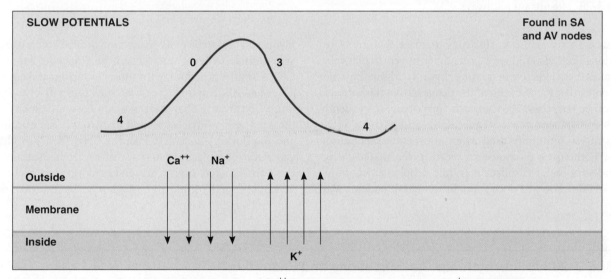

Action potential of cardiac pacing cells slows influx of Ca^{++} (leaking) and, to a lesser extent, Na^+ is responsible for automaticity or spontaneous depolarization. Class IV antiarrhythmics inhibit these calcium channels and decrease heart rate.

● **Figure 3-25** Ion movements in the depolarization and repolarization of slow and fast potentials.

useful in treating arrhythmias, they can also cause them or deterioration in existing rhythms when used inappropriately (Table 3–21).

Sodium Channel Blockers (Class I) All the medications in this general class affect the sodium influx in phases 0 and 4 of fast potentials. This slows the propagation of impulses down the specialized conduction system of the atria and ventricles, although it does not affect the SA or AV node.

Class IA drugs include quinidine (Quinidex), procainamide (Pronestyl), and disopyramide (Norpace). In addition to slowing conduction, these drugs also decrease the repolarization rate. This widens the QRS complex and prolongs the QT interval. While quinidine is usually considered the prototype for this class, we will use procainamide here because it is administered more frequently in emergency medicine. Procainamide is indicated in the treatment of atrial fibrillation with rapid ventricular response and ventricular arrhythmias. Quinidine has a similar mechanism of action, but it also has anticholinergic properties that may induce unintended tachycardias.

Class IB drugs include lidocaine (Xylocaine), phenytoin (Dilantin), tocainide (Tonocard), and mexiletine (Mexitil).

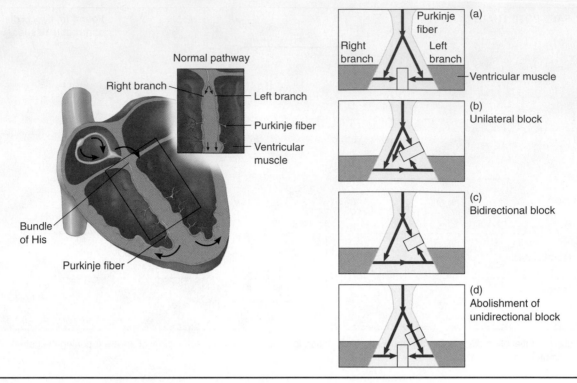

● **Figure 3-26** Reentrant pathways.

Unlike Class IA drugs, Class IB drugs increase the rate of repolarization. They also reduce automaticity in ventricular cells, which makes them effective in treating rhythms originating from ectopic ventricular foci. Several of the drugs in this class are also used for other purposes. Lidocaine, the prototype, is frequently used with epinephrine as a local anesthetic, and phenytoin (Dilantin) is most commonly used as an antiseizure medication. Lidocaine is the drug of choice for treating ventricular tachycardia and ventricular fibrillation. While prophylactic administration of lidocaine was once thought to benefit patients with myocardial infarction, its use is now limited to life-threatening arrhythmias. When given in overdose, lidocaine has significant CNS side effects including tinnitus, confusion, and convulsions.

Class IC drugs include flecainide (Tambocor) and propafenone (Rythmol). They decrease conduction velocity through the atria and ventricles as well as through the bundle of His and the Purkinje network. Like the Class IA drugs, they delay ventricular repolarization. Both of these medications, which are administered orally, are given to prevent recurrence of ventricular arrhythmias, but both also have prodysrhythmic

TABLE 3–20 | Antiarrhythmic Classifications and Examples

General Action	Class	Prototype	ECG Effects
Sodium Channel Blockers	IA	Quinidine, procainamide*, disopyramide	Widened QRS, prolonged QT
	IB	Lidocaine*, phenytoin, tocainide, mexiletine	Widened QRS, prolonged QT
	IC	Flecainide*, propafenone	Prolonged PR, widened QRS
	I (Miscellaneous)	Moricizine*	Prolonged PR, widened QRS
Beta-Blockers	II	Propranolol*, acebutolol, esmolol	Prolonged PR, bradycardias
Potassium Channel Blockers	III	Bretylium*, amiodarone	Prolonged QT
Calcium Channel Blockers	IV	Verapamil*, diltiazem	Prolonged PR, bradycardias
Miscellaneous		Adenosine, digoxin	Prolonged PR, bradycardias

*Prototype.

TABLE 3–21 | Antiarrhythmics

Name	Classification	Action	Indications	Contraindications	Doses	Routes	Adverse Effects	Other
Amiodarone *Cordarone*	Class III antiarrhythmic	Prolongs action potential and duration in cardiac tissues through sodium, potassium, and calcium channels; blocks α- and β-adrenergic receptors.	• Ventricular tachycardia • Ventricular fibrillation • Narrow-complex tachycardias	• Breast feeding • Bradycardia • High-grade heart block • Hypersensitivity to the drug	150–300 mg	IV	• Hypotension • Bradycardia • Prolonged PR, QRS, and QT.	• Constant ECG monitoring • Now first-line agent in ventricular fibrillation and tachycardia
Lidocaine *Xylocaine*	Class IB antiarrhythmic; local anesthetic	Amide-type local anesthetic; slows depolarization and automaticity	• Ventricular tachycardia and fibrillation refractory to amiodarone • Local anesthetic	• Should not be administered to patients receiving IV calcium channel blockers	1.0–1.5 mg/kg	IV	• Drowsiness • Slurred speech • Confusion • Seizures • Hypotension	• Use with caution when administered with other antiarrhythmics
Procainamide *Pronestyl*	Class IA antiarrhythmic; local anesthetic	Ester-type local anesthetic; reduces automaticity and AV conduction	• Ventricular tachycardia with pulse • Pre-excited atrial fibrillation	• Should not be administered to patients receiving IV calcium channel blockers	20–50 mg/min	IV	• Drowsiness • Slurred speech • Confusion • Seizures • Hypotension	• Carefully monitor ECG (QRS duration) during administration
Phenytoin *Dilantin*	Class IB antiarrhythmic; anticonvulsant	Depresses automaticity and AV conduction; reduces voltage and spread of electrical discharges in motor cortex	• Life-threatening arrhythmias from digitalis toxicity • Seizures	• Bradycardia • High-grade heart block • Hypersensitivity to the drug	15–18 mg/kg	IV	• Drowsiness • Dizziness • Headache • Hypotension • Arrhythmias • Nausea • Vomiting	• Fosphenytoin is preferred for seizure management
Adenosine *Adenocard*	Nucleoside	Slows AV conduction; short half-life	• Supraventricular tachyarrhythmias	• Atrial fibrillation • *Torsades des pointes* • Atrial fibrillation	6 mg	IV	• Facial flushing • Headache • Chest pain • Nausea	• Should be given by rapid IV push followed by saline bolus • Arrhythmias common following administration

(Continued)

TABLE 3–21 | Antiarrhythmics Continued

Name	Classification	Action	Indications	Contraindications	Doses	Routes	Adverse Effects	Other
Esmolol *Brevibloc*	Class II antiarrhythmic; beta-blocker	Slows heart rate through selective blockade of β_1 receptors; short half-life	• Tachycardia	• Asthma • Heart block • Bradycardia • Cardiogenic shock	50–100 mcg/ kg/min	IV	• Bradycardia • Hypotension • Congestive heart failure • Lethargy	• Hypotension is common but dose-related • Should not be administered to patients receiving IV calcium channel blockers
Labetalol *Trandate, Normodyne*	Class II antiarrhythmic; beta-blocker	Lowers blood pressure through nonselective blockade of β receptors (and limited blockade of α_2 receptors)	• Hypertensive emergency	• Asthma • Heart block • Bradycardia • Cardiogenic shock	10–20 mg	IV, PO	• Bradycardia • Hypotension • Congestive heart failure • Lethargy	• Should not be administered to patients receiving IV calcium channel blockers
Diltiazem *Cardizem*	Class IV antiarrhythmic; calcium channel blocker	Lowers blood pressure by relaxing vascular smooth muscle; slows AV conduction	• Rapid ventricular rate associated with atrial fibrillation • Stable narrow-complex tachyarrhythmias	• Hypotension • Congestive heart failure • Cardiogenic shock • Wide-complex ventricular tachycardia	15–20 mg	IV	• Nausea • Vomiting • Dizziness • Headache • Hypotension	• Can be given as IV bolus or IV infusion • Calcium chloride can reverse some of the untoward effects
Magnesium Sulfate	Mineral/ electrolyte	Physiologic calcium-channel blocker; bronchodilator	• *Torsades des pointes* • Asthma • Hypertensive disorders of pregnancy	• High-degree heart blocks • Shock • Dialysis • Hypocalcemia	1–2 g	IV	• Flushing • Sweating • Bradycardia • Respiratory depression • Hypothermia	• Can cause cardiac conduction problems in conjunction with digitalis

properties; that is, they are likely to cause arrhythmias as well as treat them. They also depress myocardial contractility and are therefore reserved for potentially lethal ventricular arrhythmias that do not respond to any other conventional therapy.

Moricizine (Ethmozine) is similar to the other Class I drugs but has additional properties that exclude it from the other subclasses. Like the other drugs in this class, it blocks sodium influx during fast potential depolarization, thereby decreasing conduction velocity, but it can also depress myocardial contractility. Like the Class IC drugs, it is reserved for the treatment of ventricular arrhythmias refractory to other conventional therapy.

Beta-Blockers (Class II)

The drugs in this class, propranolol (Inderal), acebutolol (Sectral), and esmolol (Brevibloc), are all beta adrenergic antagonists. Propranolol is nonselective, while acebutolol and esmolol are both selective for the $beta_1$ receptors in the heart. (The mechanism of action at the $beta_1$ receptor is described in the section on adrenergic antagonists.) Of the many beta-blockers, these are the only ones approved for the treatment of arrhythmias. They are indicated in the treatment of tachycardias resulting from excessive sympathetic stimulation. The $beta_1$ receptor in the heart is attached to the calcium channels. Blocking the $beta_1$ receptors thus blocks the calcium channel and prevents the gradual influx of calcium in phase 0 of the slow potential. As a result, the effects of beta-blocker therapy on arrhythmias are almost identical to those of calcium channel blockers. Propranolol is the prototype Class II drug. Because it is nonselective, it also blocks the effect of $beta_2$ receptors, which leads to many of its side effects. Other side effects are consistent with those discussed in the section on drugs that affect the sympathetic nervous system.

Potassium Channel Blockers (Class III)

Potassium channel–blocking drugs are also known as antiadrenergic medications because of their complex actions on sympathetic terminals. They include bretylium (Bretylol) and amiodarone (Cordarone); bretylium is the prototype. Their mechanism of action is on the potassium channels in the fast potentials. By blocking the efflux of potassium, bretylium prolongs repolarization and the effective refractory period. It is indicated in the treatment of ventricular fibrillation and refractory ventricular tachycardia. It causes an initial release of norepinephrine at the sympathetic end terminals, followed by an inhibition of that neurotransmitter's release. This delayed repolarization prolongs the QT interval; consequently, bretylium's primary and frequent side effect is hypotension.[22]

Calcium Channel Blockers (Class IV)

Calcium channel blockers' effect on the heart is almost identical to that of beta-blockers. They decrease SA and AV node automaticity, but most of their usefulness arises from decreasing conductivity through the AV node. They effectively slow the ventricular conduction of atrial fibrillation and flutter, and they can terminate supraventricular tachycardias originating from a reentrant circuit. Verapamil (Calan) and diltiazem (Cardizem) are the only two calcium channel blockers that affect the heart. Verapamil is the prototype. Their chief side effect is hypotension and bradycardia. The section on antihypertensives discusses calcium channel blockers in more detail.

Miscellaneous Antiarrhythmics

Adenosine (Adenocard) and digoxin (Lanoxin) are both effective antiarrhythmics. Magnesium is the drug of choice in *torsades de pointes*, a type of polymorphic ventricular tachycardia. We will briefly discuss each.

Adenosine does not fit any of the previous categories. It is an endogenous nucleoside with a very short half-life (about 10 seconds). It acts on both potassium and calcium channels, increasing potassium efflux and inhibiting calcium influx. This results in a hyperpolarization that effectively slows the conduction of slow potentials such as those found in the SA and AV nodes. It has little effect on the fast potentials in the ventricles and is not particularly effective on ventricular tachycardias or atrial fibrillation or flutter. Because of its short half-life, its side effects are short lived, but they can be alarming. They include facial flushing, shortness of breath, chest pain, and marked bradycardias. Adenosine must be given as a rapid IV push, as the drug is rapidly metabolized. Doses should be increased in patients taking adenosine blockers such as aminophylline or caffeine. They should be decreased in patients taking adenosine uptake inhibitors like dipyridamole (Persantine) and carbamazepine (Tegretol).

Digoxin (Lanoxin) is a paradoxical drug. Its many effects on the heart make it both an effective antiarrhythmic and a potent prodysrhythmic (generator of arrhythmias). While we do not clearly understand its specific actions on the heart's electrical activity, we do understand its effects. Digoxin decreases the intrinsic firing rate in the SA node, whereas it decreases conduction velocity in the AV node. Both of these effects are due to its increasing the strength of the parasympathetic effects on the heart. In the Purkinje fibers and ventricular myocardial cells, it decreases the effective refractory period and increases automaticity, both of which may explain its ability to increase ventricular arrhythmias. To compound this, by depressing SA node activity, digoxin makes ectopic ventricular beats more likely to assume the pacing activity of the heart. Its side effects include bradycardias, AV blocks, PVCs, ventricular tachycardia, ventricular fibrillation, and atrial fibrillation. Actually, there are few arrhythmias that digoxin does not produce. In addition, digoxin has a very narrow therapeutic index, meaning that it is difficult to find a patient's effective dose without producing side effects. Digoxin also increases cardiac contractility. It is indicated for atrial fibrillation with rapid ventricular conduction and chronic treatment of congestive heart failure.

CONTENT REVIEW

▶ Pharmacological Classes
of Antihypertensives

- Diuretics
- Beta-blockers and
  antiadrenergic drugs
- ACE inhibitors
- Calcium channel blockers
- Direct vasodilators

Magnesium is the drug of choice in *torsades de pointes,* a polymorphic ventricular tachycardia, and in other ventricular arrhythmias refractory to other therapy. Its mechanism of action is not known, but it may act on the sodium or potassium channels or on $Na^+K^+ATPase$.

Antihypertensives

Hypertension affects more than 50 million people in the United States alone and is a major contributor to coronary artery disease, stroke, and blindness. Fortunately, available drugs can effectively manage blood pressure with limited side effects in the vast majority of patients. Multiple studies have shown conclusively that controlling blood pressure decreases both morbidity and mortality.

Blood pressure is the force of blood against the arteries' walls as the heart contracts and relaxes. It is equal to cardiac output times the peripheral vascular resistance:

Blood pressure = Cardiac output × Peripheral vascular resistance

Cardiac output is equal to the heart rate times the stroke volume:

Cardiac output = Heart rate × Stroke volume

Antihypertensive agents can manipulate each of these factors. The primary determinant of peripheral vascular resistance is the diameter of peripheral arterioles, which are affected by $alpha_1$ receptors. Heart rate is affected by both muscarinic receptors of the parasympathetic nervous system and $beta_1$ receptors of the sympathetic nervous system; however, hypertension control typically manipulates only $beta_1$ receptors. Stroke volume is affected by contractility and volume. Recall that Starling's law says that preload and stroke volume are proportionate; that is, as preload increases, stroke volume increases (up to a point), and as preload decreases, stroke volume decreases. Drugs that affect blood volume control hypertension by manipulating preload.

Several pharmacological classes of medications are used to control blood pressure. The major approaches to dealing with hypertension are diuretics, beta-blockers and other antiadrenergic drugs, angiotensin converting enzyme (ACE) inhibitors, calcium channel blockers, and direct vasodilators. Of these, diuretics and beta-blockers are the most frequently prescribed, and they are effective in many patients. The remaining agents are used when diuretics or beta-blockers are contraindicated or when those approaches are not effective, although ACE inhibitors are gaining increasing popularity. Often, physicians must prescribe multiple drugs to manage hypertension effectively. In these cases, they will pick one drug from two or more classes that complement each other. For example, a physician might prescribe a diuretic with a beta-blocker.[23]

Diuretics **Diuretics** reduce circulating blood volume by increasing the amount of urine. This reduces preload to the heart, which in turn reduces cardiac output. The main categories of diuretics include loop diuretics (high-ceiling diuretics), thiazides, and potassium-sparing diuretics. They all affect the reabsorption of sodium and chloride and create an osmotic gradient that decreases the reabsorption of water. These classes differ according to which area of the nephron they affect. In general, the earlier in the nephron the drug works, the more sodium and water will be affected. Almost all electrolytes and other small particles in the blood are filtered through the glomerulus. Most sodium and water (approximately 65 percent) is reabsorbed in the proximal convoluted tubule. Another 20 percent is reabsorbed in the thick portion of the ascending loop of Henle, while only about 1 to 5 percent is recaptured in the distal convoluted tubule and collecting duct. Therefore, a drug that decreases sodium reabsorption in the proximal convoluted tubule will cause the kidneys to excrete more water than will a drug that works on the distal convoluted tubule.

Loop diuretics profoundly affect circulating blood volume. In fact, they decrease blood volume so well that they are typically considered excessive for treating moderate hypertension. They are, however, one of the primary tools in treating left ventricular heart failure (congestive heart failure). Their use for hypertension is typically because other diuretics have failed. Furosemide (Lasix) is the prototype of this class. Furosemide blocks sodium reabsorption in the thick portion of the ascending loop of Henle (hence, the name *loop diuretic*). In doing so, it decreases the pull of water from the tubule and into the capillary bed, thus decreasing fluid volume. Furosemide's main side effects are hyponatremia, hypovolemia, hypokalemia, and dehydration. Because the decrease in volume is most noticeable as decreased preload, orthostatic hypotension is a problem. Reflex tachycardia may also occur as the baroreceptors detect a decreased blood pressure and attempt to compensate by increasing heart rate. This happens in individuals with hypertension because the homeostatic "thermostat" has been set too high. In other words, the body believes that what is actually hypertension is normal and tries to maintain a higher blood pressure than is healthy. This reflex tachycardia is frequently treated with concurrent administration of a loop diuretic with a $beta_1$ blocker. Hypokalemia is frequently treated by increasing dietary potassium intake (bananas are rich in potassium) or by prescribing potassium supplements. An unexplained side effect of loop diuretics is ototoxicity (tinnitus and deafness). Administering loop diuretics slowly can decrease ototoxicity.

Thiazides have a mechanism similar to loop diuretics. The main difference is that the thiazides' mechanism affects the early part of the distal convoluted tubules and therefore cannot block as much sodium from reabsorption. Thiazides are often the drugs of choice in hypertension treatment because they can decrease fluid volume sufficiently to prevent hypertension but not so much that they promote hypotension. The prototype thiazide is hydrochlorothiazide (HydroDIURIL). This class has essentially the same side effects as loop diuretics. One important distinction is that thiazides depend on the glomerular filtration rate, while loop diuretics do not. Thus, loop diuretics may be preferred for patients with renal disease.

Potassium-sparing diuretics have a slightly different mechanism than other diuretics. Although they still affect sodium absorption, they do so by inhibiting either the effects of aldosterone on the distal tubules (as does spironolactone) or the specific sodium-potassium exchange mechanism (as does triamterene). Acting so late in the nephritic loop, these agents are not very potent diuretics. In fact, they are rarely used alone but instead are typically administered in conjunction with either a loop diuretic or a thiazide diuretic. They are useful as adjuncts to other diuretics because they not only decrease sodium reabsorption (although in small volumes) but also increase potassium reabsorption. This helps to limit the other diuretics' hypokalemic effects. Spironolactone (Aldactone) is the prototype potassium-sparing diuretic.

While not used in the treatment of hypertension, osmotic diuretics are important because they alter the reabsorption of water in the proximal convoluted tubule. To do this, they use an osmotically large sugar molecule that is freely filtered through the glomerulus and pulls water after it. Mannitol (Osmitrol), the prototype osmotic diuretic, is used to treat increased intracranial and intraocular pressure.

Adrenergic Inhibiting Agents Inhibiting the effects of adrenergic stimulation can also control hypertension. Several broad mechanisms accomplish this: beta adrenergic antagonism, centrally acting alpha adrenergic antagonism, adrenergic neuron blockade, alpha$_1$ blockade, and alpha/beta blockade.

Beta Adrenergic Antagonists From Table 3–17 in our earlier discussion of beta$_1$ blockers, you will recall that most beta$_1$ receptors are in the heart but some also exist in the juxtaglomerular cells of the kidney. Selective beta$_1$ blockade is useful in treating hypertension for several reasons. It decreases contractility, thereby directly decreasing cardiac output. It also reduces reflex tachycardia by inhibiting sympathetically induced compensatory increases in heart rate. Finally, it represses renin release from the kidneys, which in turn inhibits the vasoconstriction activated by the renin-angiotensin-aldosterone system. The prototype selective beta$_1$ blocker is metoprolol (Lopressor); the prototype nonselective beta-blocker is propranolol (Inderal). The section on beta$_1$ blockers discussed these agents' side effects.

Centrally Acting Adrenergic Inhibitors Centrally acting adrenergic inhibitors reduce hypertension by inhibiting CNS stimulation of adrenergic receptors. In effect, they are CNS alpha$_2$ agonists. Recall that alpha$_2$ receptors are located on the presynaptic end terminals in the sympathetic nervous system. When stimulated, they inhibit the release of norepinephrine to counterbalance sympathetic stimulation. By increasing the stimulation of alpha$_2$ receptors in the section of the CNS responsible for cardiovascular regulation, centrally acting adrenergic inhibitors decrease the sympathetic stimulation of both alpha$_1$ and beta$_2$ receptors. The net effect is to decrease heart rate and contractility by decreasing release of norepinephrine at beta$_1$ receptors and to promote vasodilation by decreasing norepinephrine release at alpha$_1$ receptors at vascular smooth muscle. The prototype drug in this category is clonidine (Catapres). While it does have some side effects, notably drowsiness and dry mouth, clonidine is a relatively safe and frequently prescribed antihypertensive agent. Methyldopa (Aldomet) is another centrally acting antihypertensive with a mechanism similar to clonidine.

Peripheral Adrenergic Neuron Blocking Agents Like the centrally acting adrenergic inhibitors, peripheral adrenergic neuron blocking agents work indirectly to decrease stimulation of adrenergic receptors. They do this by decreasing the amount of norepinephrine released from sympathetic presynaptic terminals. These agents are no longer commonly used.

The prototype of this class is reserpine (Serpalan). Reserpine has two actions that decrease the amount of norepinephrine released. First, it decreases the synthesis of norepinephrine. Second, it exposes norepinephrine in the terminal vesicles to monoamine oxidase, an enzyme that destroys it. This decreases stimulation of alpha$_1$ receptors, resulting in peripheral vasodilation, and of beta$_1$ receptors, resulting in decreased heart rate and contractility. The decreased peripheral vascular resistance and cardiac output in turn lower blood pressure.

Reserpine also decreases synthesis of several CNS neurotransmitters (serotonin and other catecholamines). This causes reserpine's primary adverse effect, depression. Reserpine, therefore, is not frequently used as an antihypertensive. Additional side effects include gastrointestinal cramps and increased stomach acid production. Other drugs with similar actions include guanethidine (Ismeline) and guanadrel (Hylorel).

Alpha$_1$ Antagonists This chapter's section on drugs affecting the sympathetic nervous system discusses the alpha$_1$ receptor antagonists in detail. Only their specific action will be repeated here. The prototype selective alpha$_1$ antagonist is prazosin (Minipress). It decreases blood pressure by competitively blocking the alpha$_1$ receptors, thereby inhibiting the sympathetically mediated increases in peripheral vascular resistance. By causing the arterioles to dilate, prazosine directly decreases afterload. By causing the venules to dilate, it promotes venous pooling, which decreases preload. The decreased afterload and preload help to lower blood pressure. Terazosin (Hytrin) is another drug with similar properties.

Combined Alpha/Beta Antagonists Labetalol (Normodyne) and carvedilol (Coreg) competitively bind with both alpha$_1$ and beta$_1$ receptors, increasing their antihypertensive actions. Hypertension is treated by decreasing alpha$_1$-mediated vasoconstriction, which, again, decreases both preload and afterload. Beta$_1$ blockade decreases heart rate, contractility, and renin release from kidneys. By blocking the release of renin, which promotes vasoconstriction, these agents decrease peripheral vascular resistance even further. Labetalol is commonly used to treat hypertensive crisis and is rapidly replacing the use of sublingual nifedipine (Procardia) for this purpose.

Angiotensin Converting Enzyme (ACE) Inhibitors Agents in this class interrupt the renin-angiotensin-aldosterone system (RAAS) by preventing the conversion of angiotensin I to angiotensin II. Angiotensin II is one of the most potent vasoconstrictors yet discovered. By decreasing the amount of circulating angiotensin II, peripheral vascular resistance can be decreased, which leads to a decrease in blood pressure.

The juxtaglomerular apparatus in the kidneys releases renin in response to decreases in blood volume, sodium concentration, and blood pressure. Renin acts as an enzyme to convert the inactive protein angiotensinogen into angiotensin I. Neither angiotensinogen nor angiotensin I has much pharmaceutical effect, but angiotensin-converting enzyme (ACE) almost immediately converts angiotensin I in the blood into angiotensin II. (ACE is found in the lumen of almost all vessels and is found in the lungs in very high concentrations.) Angiotensin II causes both systemic and local vasoconstriction, with more pronounced effects on arterioles than on venules. It also lessens water loss by decreasing renal filtration secondary to renal vasoconstriction. Finally, angiotensin II also increases the release of aldosterone, a corticosteroid produced in the adrenal cortex. Aldosterone in turn increases sodium and water reabsorption in the distal convoluted tubule of the nephrons (Figure 3-27 ●).

Angiotensin converting enzyme inhibitors are very effective in treating hypertension and have also seen success in managing heart failure and renal failure. ACE inhibitors block the conversion of angiotensin I to angiotensin II, thereby providing a host of beneficial effects for patients with hypertension. These include a rapid decrease in arteriolar constriction, which lowers peripheral vascular resistance and afterload. While it does cause some dilation of the venules, this effect is limited. Because of the limited decrease in preload, orthostatic hypotension, common in other antihypertensives, is not a significant concern with ACE inhibitors. These agents also appear to be effective in preventing some of the untoward structural changes in the heart and blood vessels that angiotensin II causes over time.

The prototype ACE inhibitor is captopril (Capoten). Captopril acts like all ACE inhibitors to prevent hypertension. Its main advantage is the absence of side effects common to other antihypertensives. It does not interfere with beta receptors, so it does not decrease the ability to exercise or respond to hemorrhage. It does not cause potassium loss like many diuretics, and it does not cause depression or drowsiness. Because it has no effect on sexual desire or performance, it is much more attractive to many patients who might not comply with other medications. Other common ACE inhibitors include enalapril (Vasotec) and lisinopril (Zestril). These medications are all taken orally. For intravenous use in hypertensive crisis, enalaprilat (Vasotec I.V.) is available.

The most dangerous side effect of ACE inhibitors is pronounced hypotension after the first dose. This can be minimized by reducing initial doses, and it does not reoccur. The main adverse effects of continual use are a persistent cough and angioedema.

Angiotensin II Receptor Antagonists   This recently developed classification of antihypertensive drugs also acts on the renin-angiotensin-aldosterone system. Angiotensin II receptor antagonists achieve the same effects as the ACE inhibitors

Renin-Angiotensin-Aldosterone System

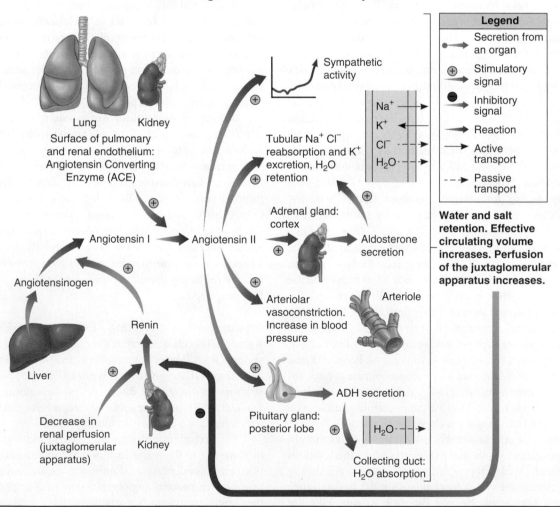

● **Figure 3-27**   The renin-angiotensin-aldosterone system.

without the side effects of cough or angioedema. The prototype of this new class is losartan (Cozaar).

Calcium Channel Blocking Agents We have already discussed two calcium channel blockers, verapamil and diltiazem, in the section on antiarrhythmics. Another structural subclass of calcium channel blockers is the dihydropyridines. The prototype dihydropyridine is nifedipine (Procardia, Adalat). Nifedipine, as well as the other members of the dihydropyridines, differs from verapamil and diltiazem in that it does not affect the calcium channels of the heart at therapeutic doses. Rather, it acts only on the vascular smooth muscle of the arterioles. These agents act by blocking the calcium channels in the arterioles. Calcium, which is required for muscle contraction, is released from the sarcoplasmic reticulum upon activation by an action potential. When it enters the muscle cell through calcium channels, muscle contraction ensues. Blocking the calcium channels prevents the arterioles' smooth muscle from contracting and therefore dilates these vessels. When this occurs, peripheral vascular resistance decreases, and blood pressure falls as a result of lower afterload. Because nifedipine has little effect on veins, it does not cause a corresponding drop in preload and consequently avoids orthostatic hypotension. While nifedipine does not affect the cardiac electrical conduction system, it is effective in dilating the coronary arteries and arterioles and thereby helps to increase coronary perfusion. The primary indications for nifedipine are angina pectoris and chronic treatment of hypertension. Its primary side effects include reflex tachycardia (responding to baroreceptor response to decreased blood pressure), facial flushing, dizziness, headache, and peripheral edema. It has been used commonly for the emergent reduction of blood pressure in the field; however, labetalol is replacing it.

Direct Vasodilators We have already discussed several drugs that cause vasodilation. Two specific classes of vasodilators are those that dilate arterioles and those that dilate both arterioles and veins. All of these drugs are used to decrease blood pressure.

Selective dilation of arterioles causes a decrease in peripheral vascular resistance or afterload. This is the resistance that the heart must overcome in order to eject blood. Decreasing peripheral vascular resistance lowers blood pressure, increases cardiac output, and reduces cardiac workload. However, dilating the veins increases capacitance and decreases preload, the amount of blood in the heart prior to contraction. Starling's law tells us that as preload increases, so do stroke volume and cardiac output (up to a point). By decreasing preload, venodilators decrease both blood pressure and cardiac output.

Hydralazine (Apresoline) is the prototype for the selective arteriole dilators. It is effective in decreasing peripheral vascular resistance and afterload and thus lowering blood pressure. Its primary side effects are reflex tachycardia and increased blood volume. Both occur as a compensatory mechanism to lowered blood pressure, and both have the effect of increasing cardiac workload. As a result, hydralazine is almost always prescribed in conjunction with a beta-blocker and a diuretic. It is frequently used in the treatment of pregnancy-induced hypertension.

Minoxidil (Loniten) is another selective arteriole dilator with properties similar to those of hydralazine. One side effect deserves comment. It produces hypertrichosis (excessive hair growth) in about 80 percent of those taking it. While this is particularly irritating when it occurs all over a patient's body, it can become a therapeutic effect when the drug is applied as a topical ointment. Minoxidil is marketed in this form as Rogaine for promoting hair growth in men.

Unlike hydralazine, sodium nitroprusside (Nipride) acts on both arterioles and veins. It is the fastest acting antihypertensive available and is the drug of choice in hypertensive emergencies. It is very potent and is given via controlled IV infusion. Its effects are almost immediate and end within minutes of drug cessation; therefore, blood pressure must be carefully and continuously monitored during infusion, preferably in the ICU. Sodium nitroprusside has several significant side effects. Obviously, hypotension can be a problem when this medication is not carefully administered. Because cyanide and thiocyanate are by-products of nitroprusside metabolism, other adverse effects include cyanide poisoning and thiocyanate toxicity.

Ganglionic Blocking Agents Ganglionic blocking agents are nicotinic$_N$ antagonists. The prototype is trimethaphan (Arfonad). Since nicotinic$_N$ receptors exist at the ganglia of both the sympathetic and the parasympathetic nervous systems, competitive antagonism of these receptors turns off the entire autonomic nervous system, which is obviously not a very selective approach. When this happens, the effects on each organ system are determined by the predominant autonomic tone (the division of the ANS that normally has the greater influence on that organ). Because the arteries and veins have predominant sympathetic control, they dilate in response to trimethaphan administration. This reduces both preload and afterload, and blood pressure drops. Trimethaphan also directly affects vascular smooth muscle, causing dilation and the release of histamine, which is also a vasodilator. Mecamylamine (Inversine) is the other ganglionic blocking drug available in the United States, although it is not commonly used anymore.

Cardiac Glycosides The cardiac glycosides occur naturally in the foxglove plant. The two drugs in the class, digoxin (Lanoxin) and digitoxin (Crystodigin), are chemically related. These drugs are also known as digitalis glycosides. Digoxin is the prototype. One of the ten most frequently prescribed medications in the country, it is indicated for heart failure and some types of arrhythmias. Digoxin's mechanism of action is complex. It blocks the effects of Na$^+$K$^+$ATPase, an enzyme responsible for returning ion flow to normal levels after muscle depolarization. By interfering with this sodium-potassium pump, digoxin increases the intracellular levels of sodium. Because sodium is also involved in a reciprocal exchange with calcium, a buildup of intracellular sodium leads to a similar buildup of intracellular calcium. These elevated levels of intracellular calcium increase the strength of muscle contraction and are the basis for digoxin's primary indication. Digoxin reduces the symptoms of congestive heart failure by increasing myocardial contractility and cardiac output. This diminishes the dilation of the heart's chambers frequently seen in left heart failure because it enables the heart to effectively pump blood out of its ventricles, thus decreasing the engorgement typical of this condition. Increasing cardiac output decreases the sympathetic discharge mediated by baroreceptor reflexes, resulting in reduced afterload. Furthermore, digoxin indirectly lessens preload by increasing renal blood flow, which results in higher glomerular filtration and decreased blood volume. Digoxin also has antiarrhythmic effects, which we discuss more thoroughly in the section on antiarrhythmic medications.

While digoxin effectively treats the symptoms of heart failure, it also is potentially dangerous. Its therapeutic index is very small, and the individual variability is large. This leads to toxicity in some individuals even though they have normal digoxin levels. Digoxin's chief adverse effects are arrhythmias. In fact, digoxin frequently induces some of the same arrhythmias it is used to treat. Other side effects include fatigue, anorexia, nausea and vomiting, and blurred vision with a yellowish haze and halos around dark objects.

Other Vasodilators and Antianginals The drugs discussed in this section have vasodilatory properties that are useful in reducing blood pressure, but they are most commonly used to treat angina. The three basic types of angina pectoris (chest pain) are stable (exertional) angina; unstable angina; and variant, or Prinzmetal's, angina. Stable and unstable angina have the same pathophysiology and differ only by causation: Stable angina occurs after exercise as a result of increased myocardial oxygen demand; unstable angina occurs without exertion. Both result from an imbalance between myocardial supply and demand. A buildup of plaque (atherosclerosis) along the walls of coronary arteries decreases these vessels' diameter and, as a result, the amount of blood flow to the heart. The same imbalance causes Prinzmetal's angina but it results from vasospasm instead of plaque buildup. The medications discussed in this section all either increase oxygen supply or decrease oxygen demand.

In addition to their previously discussed use as antihypertensives and antiarrhythmics, calcium channel blockers have a role in the treatment of angina. The three calcium channel blockers most frequently used for this purpose are verapamil (Calan, Isoptin), diltiazem (Cardizem), and nifedipine (Procardia). Recall that calcium is an integral part of both depolarization and muscle contraction. The effects of blocking its entry into the cells are twofold. All of these agents directly affect vascular smooth muscle, leading to dilation of the arterioles and, to a lesser degree, of the venules. This arterial dilation decreases peripheral vascular resistance and, as a result, afterload, which in turn directly decreases the workload of the heart and myocardial oxygen demand. Verapamil and diltiazem also reduce SA and AV node conductivity, which can decrease reflex tachycardia and arrhythmias. Nifedipine has relatively few effects on the heart and, thus, has limited antiarrhythmic properties. The calcium channel blockers are effective in all forms of angina. A primary side effect of these agents is hypotension.

Organic nitrates are potent vasodilators used to treat all forms of angina. First used clinically in 1879, nitroglycerin (Nitrostat) is the oldest of these drugs and is the category's prototype. Other agents include isosorbide (Isordil, Sorbitrate) and amyl nitrite. Nitroglycerin acts on vascular smooth muscle via a complex series of events to decrease intracellular calcium, thus causing vasodilation. Nitroglycerin primarily dilates veins rather than arterioles. This decreases preload and thus decreases myocardial workload, which is its primary antianginal effect. In Prinzmetal's angina, nitroglycerin reverses coronary artery spasm and increases oxygen supply.

Nitroglycerin is very lipid soluble, which allows it to cross membranes easily. Because of this, it is readily absorbed and can be administered via sublingual, buccal, and transdermal routes. The primary concern with nitroglycerin is orthostatic hypotension, a side effect more common in the presence of right ventricular failure. Other common side effects include headache and reflex tachycardia. Headache is frequently used as an indicator of the effectiveness of nitroglycerin, which rapidly loses its potency when exposed to light. While orthostatic hypotension is a serious concern with the administration of nitroglycerin, this condition typically responds well to fluid infusions.[24] Table 3–22 details common nitrates.

Hemostatic Agents

Hemostasis is the stoppage of bleeding. It is a series of events in response to a tear in a blood vessel. Damage to the vessel's intima (innermost layer) exposes the underlying collagen and triggers a release of two naturally occurring substances, adenosine diphosphate (ADP) and thromboxane A_2 (TXA_2). Both ADP and TXA_2 stimulate the aggregation of platelets and vasoconstriction. The vasoconstriction decreases the flow of blood past the tear, thus allowing the newly "sticky" platelets to form a plug that temporarily occludes the bleeding.

While this plug effectively halts bleeding for the short term, it must be reinforced to continue the stoppage until the tear can be permanently repaired. Stabilizing the plug requires a complex cascade of events involving the activation of naturally occurring factors and ending with the conversion of prothrombin into thrombin. The thrombin then converts fibrinogen into fibrin, a strandlike substance that attaches to the vessel's surface and contracts in a mesh web over the platelet plug to form a blood clot. Several of the factors involved need vitamin K to carry out their functions. A vitamin K deficiency inhibits clotting and makes uncontrolled bleeding more likely. Conversely, limiting the clotting cascade to the immediate area of the vessel injury is important for obvious reasons. The protein antithrombin III is key in this process. Antithrombin III binds with several of the factors needed for clotting, thus inhibiting their ability to coagulate.

Once the vessel has been permanently repaired, the fibrin mesh must be broken down. This process, called fibrinolysis, involves another cascading system that ends with the activation of plasminogen into plasmin, which in turn breaks up the clot. Tissue plasminogen activator, a substance in the tissue, activates this last conversion.

Thrombi (blood clots that obstruct vessels or heart cavities) are the primary pathology in several clinical conditions, including myocardial infarction, stroke, and pulmonary embolism. Drugs can effectively treat the causes of these conditions by decreasing platelet aggregation (**antiplatelet** drugs), by interfering with the clotting cascade (anticoagulants), or by directly breaking up the thrombus (fibrinolytics).

TABLE 3-22 | Nitrates

Name	Classification	Action	Indications	Contraindications	Doses	Routes	Adverse Effects	Other
Nitroglycerin *Nitrostat*	Nitrate	Relaxes vascular smooth muscle causing vasodilation, decreased cardiac work, and improved coronary blood flow.	• Chest pain • Congestive heart failure	• Hypotension • Increased intracranial pressure	0.4 mg	SL (tablet or spray)	• Headache • Dizziness • Weakness • Tachycardia • Hypotension	• Tablets will lose effectiveness after exposure to air • Monitor BP closely
Nitroglycerin Paste	Nitrate	Relaxes vascular smooth muscle causing vasodilation, decreased cardiac work, and improved coronary blood flow.	• Chest pain • Congestive heart failure	• Hypotension • Increased intracranial pressure	0.5– 1.0 inch	Transdermal	• Headache • Dizziness • Weakness • Tachycardia • Hypotension	• Do not get paste on your finger as this may cause a headache • Monitor BP closely

CONTENT REVIEW

▶ Drugs Used to Treat
Thrombi

• Antiplatelets
• Anticoagulants
• Fibrinolytics

Platelet Aggregation Inhibitors Platelet aggregation inhibitors (**antiplatelets**) decrease the formation of platelet plugs. The prototype antiplatelet drug is aspirin. Aspirin inhibits cyclooxygenase, an enzyme needed for the synthesis of thromboxane A_2 (TXA_2). Remember that TXA_2 causes platelets to aggregate and promotes local vasoconstriction. By inhibiting TXA_2, aspirin decreases the formation of platelet plugs and potential thrombi. Aspirin, as well as other antiplatelet and anticoagulant drugs, has no effect on existing thrombi; it only curbs the formation of new thrombi. Aspirin is indicated in the acute treatment of developing myocardial infarction. It is also useful in preventing the reoccurrence of MI and of ischemic stroke following transient ischemic attacks (TIAs).

One of aspirin's primary side effects is bleeding. Aspirin also may lead to an increase in gastric ulcers, which are a frequent source of gastrointestinal hemorrhage. By both stimulating the development of a potential source of bleeding as well as blocking an important mechanism for stopping that bleeding, aspirin can cause dangerous blood loss. Other antiplatelet drugs include dipyridamole (Persantine). A major class of drugs in this family includes the adenosine diphosphate (ADP) and glycoprotein IIB/IIIA inhibitors such as ticlopidine (Ticlid), abciximab (ReoPro), clopidogrel (Plavix), eptifibatide (Integrilin), tirofiban (Aggrastat), and ticlopidine (Ticlid).[25]

Anticoagulants **Anticoagulants** interrupt the clotting cascade. The two main types of anticoagulants are parenteral and oral. The prototype parenteral anticoagulant is heparin, a substance derived from the lungs of cattle or the intestines of pigs. Its primary mechanism of action is to enhance antithrombin III's ability to inhibit the clotting cascade. Because heparin is very polar, it is very poorly absorbed and must be given parenterally. Heparin injections and infusions are indicated in treating and preventing deep vein thrombosis, pulmonary embolism, and some forms of stroke. Heparin also is used frequently in conjunction with fibrinolytics to treat myocardial infarction. Finally, it is used to keep rubber-capped IV catheters (Hep-Locks) free from clots. As you would expect, bleeding is heparin's primary side effect. Other untoward effects include thrombocytopenia (decreased platelet counts) and allergic reactions. Heparin is measured in units rather than milligrams. A unit is that amount of heparin necessary to keep 1 mL of sheep plasma from clotting for 1 hour. Using this measurement is necessary because heparin's potency varies greatly when measured in milligrams.

Low-molecular-weight heparin (enoxaparin [Lovenox]) has become increasingly popular in emergency medicine. Normal heparin has a molecular weight of 5,000 to 30,000 Da, whereas low-molecular-weight heparin has a molecular weight of 1,000 to 10,000 Da. Because of this, low-molecular-weight heparin has greater bioavailability, is easier to dose, and has fewer effects on platelet function.

Protamine sulfate is available as a heparin antagonist. Protamine can reverse the effects of heparin in the presence of dangerous and unintended bleeding by binding with heparin. This prevents heparin from binding with antithrombin III and enhancing its anticlotting abilities.

The prototype oral anticoagulant is warfarin (Coumadin). Warfarin's history serves as a useful reminder of its primary side effect. Warfarin was first developed as a rat poison that killed through uncontrolled bleeding. After noticing that a patient who attempted suicide by ingesting warfarin did not, in fact, die, its clinical use was investigated. Needless to say, this drug's primary side effect is bleeding.

Warfarin prevents coagulation by antagonizing the effects of vitamin K, which is needed for the synthesis of multiple factors involved in the clotting cascade. It is prescribed for chronic use to prevent thrombi in high-risk patients such as those who have hip replacements or artificial heart valves or those who are in atrial fibrillation. Because warfarin easily crosses the placental barrier and has dangerous *teratogenic* (capable of causing malformations) properties, it is contraindicated in pregnant patients. It also interacts adversely with many other medications. Like heparin, warfarin may lead to bleeding. In cases of overdose, you may give vitamin K as an antidote.

Fibrinolytics **Fibrinolytics** (also called *thrombolytics*) act directly on thrombi to break them up. The several available fibrinolytics share a similar mechanism of action. Through a chemical conversion, these drugs activate enzymes that dissolve thrombi or clots. The prototype drug of this class is streptokinase (Streptase). Other fibrinolytics include alteplase (rtPA), tenecteplase (TNKase), and anistreplase (Eminase). These medications all dissolve clots effectively; they differ primarily in their administration and risk of bleeding side effects.

Streptokinase, which is derived from the streptococci bacterium, is the oldest available fibrinolytic. Its mechanism of action is to promote plasminogen's conversion to plasmin. Since plasmin dissolves the fibrin mesh of clots, it can directly treat the cause of most myocardial infarctions and some strokes, as opposed to antiplatelet agents and anticoagulants, which can only prevent potential future thrombi. Streptokinase also breaks down fibrinogen, the precursor to fibrin. While this action does not serve a clinical purpose (the problematic clot has already been formed), it does play an important role in streptokinase's chief side effect, bleeding. Other side effects include allergic reaction, hypotension, and fever.

Alteplase (Activase) is produced by recombinant DNA technology that is identical to the naturally occurring tissue plasminogen activator (hence its common name, rtPA). The window of opportunity for fibrinolytic therapy is limited. Because of this, some EMS systems administer fibrinolytics in the prehospital setting.[26]

Antihyperlipidemic Agents

Elevated levels of low-density lipoproteins (LDLs) have been clearly indicated as a causative factor in coronary artery disease. Lipoproteins are essentially transport mechanisms for lipids (triglycerides and cholesterol). Because lipids are insoluble in plasma, the body coats them in a plasma-soluble shell in order to transport them to their target destinations. Lipoproteins are categorized as very low-density (VLDL), low-density (LDL), intermediate-density (IDL), and high-density (HDL). Low-density lipoproteins contain most of the cholesterol in the blood and are required for transporting cholesterol from the liver to the peripheral tissues. Conversely, high-density lipoproteins (HDLs) carry cholesterol from the peripheral tissues to the liver, where it is broken down.

HDLs have been described as good cholesterol because they lower blood cholesterol levels and decrease the risk of coronary artery disease (CAD). LDLs are known as bad cholesterol because they increase blood cholesterol levels and the risk of CAD. As blood cholesterol levels increase, fatty plaque is deposited under the arteries' endothelial tissues. Atherosclerosis then develops, and coronary arteries decrease in diameter. Coronary vasoconstriction in turn reduces blood flow to the heart and, in times of increased myocardial oxygen demand, may lead to angina. Also, newly deposited plaque is often unstable. Typically, the plaque is under the endothelial tissues, which cap the plaque deposits. As the deposits age, the cap usually becomes fairly stable. In some cases, however, the cap breaks open and exposes the plaque to the blood. When this happens, platelet aggregation and coagulation begin. If the developing clot breaks free of the vessel, it becomes a thrombus and may completely occlude a coronary artery, leading to myocardial infarction.

The goal in lowering LDL levels is to prevent atherosclerosis and subsequent CAD. While raising HDL levels would help accomplish this, no pharmaceutical means of doing so currently exists. By far, the best way to lower LDL levels remains dietary modification. If this is not sufficient, several classifications of **antihyperlipidemic** medications may be used. The most common are drugs that inhibit hydroxymethylglutaryl coenzyme A (HMG CoA) reductase. The liver must have HMG CoA to synthesize cholesterol. By inhibiting this enzyme, HMG CoA agents lower LDL levels; however, they also increase the number of LDL receptors in the liver, causing a further uptake of LDL.

Five HMG CoA reductase inhibitors are available. Because the names of all five end in *statin,* these agents are also known as statins. They include lovastatin (Mevacor) and simvastatin (Zocor). Lovastatin is the HMG CoA reductase inhibitors' prototype. Overall, these drugs are well tolerated. Their chief side effects are headache, rash, and flushing. In rare cases, they may cause hepatotoxicity and lead to liver failure.

Bile acid–binding resins can also reduce LDL levels. Inert substances that have no direct biological activity, these agents pass straight through the GI system without being absorbed and are excreted in feces. They are useful, however, in that they indirectly increase the number of LDL receptors in the liver by binding with bile acids, thus decreasing their availability. Because the liver needs cholesterol to synthesize bile acids, it must have more cholesterol to compensate for the decrease in bile acids. The body therefore increases the LDL receptors on the liver. As more LDLs remain in the liver, their levels in the blood drop. Since the body does not absorb bile acid–binding agents, they have no systemic effects. Their chief untoward effect is constipation. Cholestyramine (Questran) is the prototype.

DRUGS USED TO AFFECT THE RESPIRATORY SYSTEM

Drugs that affect the respiratory system are useful for several purposes. The most obvious is the treatment of asthma, but this class also includes cough suppressants, nasal decongestants, and antihistamines.

Antiasthmatic Medications

Asthma is a common disease that decreases pulmonary function and may limit daily activities. It typically presents with shortness of breath, wheezing, and coughing. Its basic pathophysiology has two components, bronchoconstriction and inflammation. Typically, a response to some sort of allergen sets both of these processes in motion. Common culprits include pet dander, mold, and dust. In patients with existing asthma, cold air, tobacco smoke, or other pollutants may bring on acute episodes of shortness of breath.

The response to asthma typically begins with an allergen's binding to an antibody on mast cells. This causes the mast cell membrane to rupture and release its contents, including histamine, leukotrienes, and prostaglandins. These cause immediate bronchoconstriction followed by a slower inflammatory response that can lead to mucus plugs and a further decrease in airway size. The inflammation may in turn cause a hyperreactivity to stimuli, and allergens that might not normally produce dyspnea may lead to an acute attack.

Drug treatment of asthma aims to relieve bronchospasm and decrease inflammation. Specific approaches are categorized as beta$_2$ selective sympathomimetics, nonselective sympathomimetics, methylxanthines, anticholinergics, glucocorticoids, and leukotriene antagonists. Cromolyn (Intal), a frequently used anti-inflammatory agent, does not fit neatly into any of those categories. Table 3–23 summarizes these agents.

Beta$_2$ Specific Agents Drugs that are selective for beta$_2$ receptors are the mainstay in treating asthma-induced shortness of breath. Albuterol (Proventil, Ventolin) is the prototype of this class. In general, these agents relax bronchial smooth muscle, which results in bronchodilation and relief from bronchospasm. Agents from this class are first-line therapy for acute shortness of breath and may also be used daily for prophylaxis. Most are administered via metered dose inhaler or nebulizer. Albuterol and terbutaline may both be taken orally, and terbutaline may be given by injection. These medications' beta$_2$ specificity is not absolute; some patients may experience beta$_1$ effects such as tachycardia or arrhythmias. Patients may also experience tremors resulting from the stimulation of beta$_2$ receptors in smooth muscles. Overall, these agents are very safe.

Nonselective Sympathomimetics Medications that stimulate both beta$_1$ and beta$_2$ receptors, as well as alpha receptors, are rarely used to treat asthma because they have the undesired effects of increased peripheral vascular resistance and increased risks for tachycardias and other arrhythmias.

TABLE 3–23	Drugs Used in the Treatment of Asthma	
Mechanism of Action	**Medication**
Bronchodilators	
Nonspecific agonists	Epinephrine Ephedrine
Beta$_2$ specific agonists	
Inhaled (short acting)	Albuterol (Ventolin, Proventil) Metaproterenol (Alupent) Terbutaline (Brethine) Bitolterol (Tornalate)
Inhaled (long-acting)	Salmeterol (Serevent)
Methylxanthines	Theophylline (Theo-Dur, Slo-Bid) Aminophylline
Anticholinergics	Atropine Ipratropium (Atrovent)
Anti-inflammatory agents	
Glucocorticoids	
Inhaled	Beclomethasone (Beclovent) Flucticasone (Flovent) Triamcinolone (Azmacort)
Oral	Prednisone (Deltasone)
Injected	Methylprednisolone (Solu-Medrol) Dexamethasone (Decadron)
Leukotriene Antagonists	Zafirlukast (Accolate) Zileuton (Zyflo)
Mast-Cell Membrane Stabilizer	Cromolyn (Intal)

Nonselective drugs include epinephrine, ephedrine, and isoproterenol. Epinephrine is the only nonselective sympathomimetic in common use today, due to the availability of selective agents. It may be given subcutaneously for patients who have severe bronchospasm that does not respond to other treatments.

Methylxanthines The methylxanthines are CNS stimulants that have additional bronchodilatory properties. While they were once first-line therapy for asthma, now they are used only when other drugs such as beta$_2$ specific agents are ineffective. We do not know the methylxanthines' specific action, but they may block adenosine receptors. The prototype methylxanthine, theophylline, is taken orally. Aminophylline, an IV medication, is rapidly metabolized into theophylline and, therefore, has identical effects. These agents' chief side effects are nausea, vomiting, insomnia, restlessness, and arrhythmias. Aminophylline

is still used occasionally in the emergency treatment of acute asthma attacks.

Anticholinergics Ipratropium (Atrovent) is an atropine derivative given by nebulizer. Because stimulating the muscarinic receptors in the lungs results in constriction of bronchial smooth muscle, ipratropium, a muscarinic antagonist, causes bronchodilation. Ipratropium is inhaled and, therefore, has no systemic effects. Ipratropium and beta$_2$ agonists like albuterol act along different pathways, so their concurrent administration has an additive effect. Ipratropium's most common side effect is dry mouth. It results from the local effects of the drug that remains in the oropharynx after administration.

Glucocorticoids Glucocorticoids have anti-inflammatory properties. They lower the production and release of inflammatory substances such as histamine, prostaglandins, and leukotrienes, and they reduce mucus and edema secondary to decreasing vascular permeability. These drugs may be inhaled or taken orally, or they may be given intravenously in emergencies. The prototype inhaled glucocorticoid is beclomethasone; the prototype oral glucocorticoid is prednisone. Primarily preventive, they are taken on a regular schedule as opposed to the as-needed administration of the beta$_2$ agonists. An injectable glucocorticoid (methylprednisolone) is available for use secondary to beta$_2$ agonists in emergencies. When inhaled, glucocorticoids cause few side effects. Those are due mostly to direct exposure on the oropharynx, and gargling after taking the drug can decrease them. Likewise, side effects from the intravenous administrations of methylprednisolone in emergencies are not likely. Given orally or intravenously over long periods, however, glucocorticoids may have profound side effects, including adrenal suppression and hyperglycemia.

Another anti-inflammatory agent used to prevent asthma attacks is cromolyn (Intal), an inhaled powder. While it is not a glucocorticoid, its actions are similar. While the inhaled glucocorticoids are relatively safe, cromolyn is even safer. In fact, it is the safest of all antiasthma agents. Its only side effects are coughing or wheezing due to local irritation caused by the powder. Cromolyn is often used for preventing asthma in adults and children. It is also a useful prophylaxis before activities known to cause shortness of breath such as exercise or mowing grass.

Leukotriene Antagonists Leukotrienes are mediators released from mast cells upon contact with allergens. They contribute powerfully to both inflammation and bronchoconstriction. Consequently, agents that block their effects are useful in treating asthma. Leukotriene antagonists can either block the synthesis of leukotrienes or block their receptors. Zileuton (Zyflo) is the prototype of those that block the synthesis of leukotrienes. Zafirlukast (Accolate) is the prototype of those that block their receptors.

Drugs Used for Rhinitis and Cough

Rhinitis (inflammation of the nasal lining) comprises a group of symptoms including nasal congestion, itching, redness, sneezing, and rhinorrhea (runny nose). Either allergic reactions or viral infections such as the common cold may cause it. Drugs that treat the symptoms of rhinitis and cold are commonly found in over-the-counter remedies. In addition, nasal decongestants, antihistamines, and cough suppressants are available in prescription medications. Although manufacturers of cold medications often combine several drugs in one product intended to treat multiple symptoms, we will discuss each class separately.

Nasal Decongestants   Nasal congestion is caused by dilated and engorged nasal capillaries. Drugs that constrict these capillaries are effective nasal decongestants. The main pharmacological classification in this functional category is alpha$_1$ agonists. Alpha$_1$ agonists may be given either topically or orally. The chief examples of these agents, phenylephrine, pseudoephedrine, and phenylpropanolamine, can be administered either as a mist or in drops. Topical administration reduces systemic effects but has the undesired local effect of rebound congestion, a form of tolerance. Rebound congestion occurs after long-term use (greater than 7 consecutive days). As the drug wears off, congestion becomes progressively worse. This effect ends when the patient stops taking the drug; however, the longer the patient has been using the drug, the more unpleasant stopping becomes. While pseudoephedrine is an over-the-counter (OTC) medication, it is often placed behind the pharmacy counter because pseudoephedrine is one of the ingredients used in the clandestine manufacturing of methamphetamine.

Antihistamines   **Antihistamines** arrest the effects of histamine by blocking its receptors. **Histamine** is an endogenous substance that affects a wide variety of organ systems. It is noted for its role in allergic reaction. In the vasculature, histamine binds with H$_1$ receptors to cause vasodilation and increased capillary permeability. In the lungs, H$_1$ receptors cause bronchoconstriction. In the gut, H$_2$ receptors cause an increase in gastric acid release. Histamine also acts as a neurotransmitter in the central nervous system. Histamine is synthesized and stored in two types of granulocytes: tissue-bound mast cells and plasma-bound basophils. Both types are full of secretory granules, which are vesicles containing inflammatory mediators such as histamine, leukotrienes, and prostaglandins, among others. When these cells are exposed to allergens, they develop antibodies on their surfaces. On subsequent exposures, the antibodies bind with their specific allergen. The secretory granules then migrate toward the cell's exterior and fuse with the cell membrane. This causes them to release their contents. While some available medications stabilize this membrane to prevent the release of these substances, the traditional antihistamines work by antagonizing the histamine receptors.

Commonly thought of as a nuisance, histamines are useful in our immune systems. Only when our immune systems overreact do allergies such as hay fever or cedar fever send us running for the antihistamines. The typical symptoms of allergic reaction include most of those associated with rhinitis. Severe allergic reactions (anaphylaxis) may cause hypotension. While histamines play a major role in mild and moderate allergic reactions, their part in anaphylaxis is minimal; therefore,

antihistamines are at best only a secondary drug for treating anaphylaxis. (Epinephrine is the drug of choice.)

Just as there are H$_1$ and H$_2$ histamine receptors, there are H$_1$ and H$_2$ histamine receptor antagonists. When most people refer to antihistamines, they are thinking of H$_1$ receptor antagonists. These agents were in popular use long before the discovery of the H$_2$ receptors. (We discuss H$_2$ receptor antagonists in the section on drugs used to treat peptic ulcer disease.) The chief side effect of antihistamines is sedation, which the early antihistamines all caused to some degree. Now a second generation of antihistamines that do not cause sedation is available.

The first-generation antihistamines comprise several chemical subclasses. Examples include alkylamines (chlorpheniramine [Chlor-Trimeton]), ethanolamines (diphenhydramine [Benadryl], clemastine [Tavist]), and phenothiazines (promethazine [Phenergan]). While the different classes of agents have the same actions, they differ in the degree of sedation they cause and in their ability to block other, nonhistamine receptors. Several antihistamines also have significant anticholinergic properties. In fact, some are used specifically for their anticholinergic effects, notably promethazine and dimenhydrinate (Dramamine), which are used to reduce motion sickness. Other than the sedation that first-generation antihistamines cause, these agents' primary side effects are constipation and the effects of muscarinic blockade, such as dry mouth. Because they can thicken bronchial secretions, antihistamines should not be used in patients with asthma.

The second-generation antihistamines include loratadine (Claritin), cetirizine (Zyrtec), and fexofenadine (Allegra). These agents' actions are similar to the first generation's, with the notable exception that they do not cross the blood-brain barrier and therefore do not cause sedation. In addition, their H$_1$ receptor antagonism is more pronounced, and their anticholinergic actions are greatly diminished. See Table 3–24 for common antihistamines.

Cough Suppressants   Coughing is a complex reflex that depends on functions in the CNS, the PNS, and the respiratory muscles. It is a defense mechanism that aids the removal of foreign particles such as smoke and dust. A productive cough is one in which these particles are actually being coughed up. In general, treating a productive cough is not appropriate, as it is performing a useful function. An unproductive cough, however, usually results from an irritated oropharynx and can be troublesome. The three classifications of cough suppressants include one that is supported by evidence and two that are not. **Antitussive** medications suppress the stimulus to cough in the central nervous system. This functional class includes two specific pharmacological types, opioids and nonopioids. The two most common opioid antitussives are codeine and hydrocodone. Both inhibit the stimulus for coughing in the brain but also produce varying degrees of euphoria. The doses required for cough suppression are not high enough to cause euphoria, but these drugs still have the potential for abuse. The nonopioid antitussives, in contrast, do not have the potential for abuse. Dextromethorphan is the leading drug in this class. While it is almost never given alone, it is the most common antitussive used in over-the-counter combination products for treating cold and flu symptoms. Diphenhydramine (Benadryl)

TABLE 3-24 | Antihistamines

Name	Classification	Action	Indications	Contraindications	Doses	Routes	Adverse Effects	Other
Diphenhydramine *Benadryl*	Antihistamine	Nonselectively blocks H_1 and H_2 histamine receptors	• Allergies • Extrapyramidal reactions • Parkinson's disease • Sedation • Anaphylaxis	• Hypersensitivity to the drug • Glaucoma • Pregnancy	25–50 mg	IV, IM, IO, PO	• Drowsiness • Dizziness • Sedation • Dry mouth	• If given IM, give deep in muscle
Cimetidine *Tagamet*	Antihistamine	Selectively blocks H_2 histamine receptors	• Duodenal/peptic ulcer • Anaphylaxis	• Hypersensitivity to the drug	300 mg	IV, IM, IPO	• Diarrhea • Drowsiness • Dizziness	• Can be used as an adjunct for severe allergic reactions and anaphylaxis

is also used as a nonopioid antitussive, although its mechanism of action is not clear. Finally, the locally acting anesthetic benzonatate (Tessalon) depresses the cough stimulus by directly reducing oropharyngeal irritation. **Expectorants** are intended to increase the productivity of cough, and **mucolytics** make mucus more watery and, therefore, easier to cough up; however, little data support the effectiveness of either of these approaches to cough suppression.

DRUGS USED TO AFFECT THE GASTROINTESTINAL SYSTEM

The main purposes of drug therapy in the gastrointestinal system are to treat peptic ulcers, constipation, diarrhea, and emesis, and to aid digestion.

Drugs Used to Treat Peptic Ulcer Disease

Peptic ulcer disease (PUD) is characterized by an imbalance between factors in the gastrointestinal system that increase acidity and those that protect against acidity. PUD may manifest as indigestion, heartburn, or, more seriously, as perforated ulcers. If the imbalance becomes too severe, parts of the lining of the GI system may be eaten away, exposing the tissue and vasculature underneath to the highly acidic environment of the stomach or duodenum. The GI system's structure fits its function. Many mucus-lined folds surround the GI lumen. The cells of these folds secrete acids needed to help break down foods; they secrete protective mucus that prevents the acid from injuring the underlying tissue; and finally, they secrete bicarbonates, which buffer the effects of acids on the GI system's absorbing surfaces. To absorb the digested nutrients and supply the mucus-producing cells of the lumen wall with oxygen, the entire GI system is very vascular. If the protective lining covering these vessels is removed, hemorrhage may occur.

Several pathological factors oppose the GI system's defenses. Contrary to popular belief, the most common cause of peptic ulcer disease is not stress or alcohol, but the *Helicobacter pylori* bacterium. *H. pylori* infests the space between the endothelial cells and the mucus lining of the stomach and duodenum. It can remain there for decades, protected against the acid environment by the mucus layer. While we are still uncertain how this bacteria promotes ulcers, it apparently decreases the body's ability to produce the protective mucus lining. *H. pylori* by itself, however, does not cause ulcers. Many people remain infected for years and years without signs of PUD. Evidently, predisposing and contributing factors combine with *H. pylori* to cause ulceration. Some of these factors include smoking and long-term use of nonsteroidal anti-inflammatory drugs (NSAIDs) such as aspirin and acetaminophen.

The approaches to treating PUD include antibiotics and drugs that block or decrease the secretion of gastric acid. Most often they are used in conjunction with each other. First, and most effective, are antibiotics. When the *H. pylori* infection is eliminated, the signs of PUD resolve, and recurrence is low. Typically, three antibiotics will be utilized to ensure elimination of the bacteria and prevent resistance. Common medications for this purpose include bismuth (Pepto-Bismol), metronidazole (Flagyl), amoxicillin (Amoxil), and tetracycline (Achromycin V).

Drugs that block or decrease the secretion of gastric acid include H_2 receptor antagonists (H_2RAs), proton pump inhibitors, and anticholinergic agents. Mucosal protectants and antacids are also used.

H_2 receptors occur throughout the gut on the membranes of the parietal cells lining the GI lumen. When stimulated with histamine, they increase the action of H^+K^+ATPase, an enzyme that exchanges potassium for hydrogen, leading to increased gastric acid secretion. Acetylcholine and prostaglandin receptors appear along with H_2 receptors. Stimulating the ACh receptors (muscarinic receptors) increases gastric acid secretion; stimulating the prostaglandin receptors inhibits it.

H_2 Receptor Antagonists H_2RA agents block the H_2 receptors in the gut. This inhibits gastric acid secretion and helps return the balance between protective and aggressive factors. Four approved H_2RAs are in use: cimetidine (Tagamet), ranitidine (Zantac), famotidine (Pepcid), and nizatidine (Axid Pulvules). Cimetidine is the oldest of these and serves as the prototype. These agents' primary therapeutic use is for ulcers, gastroesophageal reflux, heartburn or acid indigestion, and preventing aspiration pneumonia during anesthesia. Most of these agents have few significant side effects, with the exception of cimetidine, which may lead to decreased libido, impotence, and CNS effects in some patients. While these agents could technically be called antihistamines, that name by tradition is reserved for the H_1 antagonists. The H_2RAs have no effect on the H_1 receptors and are of no value in allergic reaction.

Proton Pump Inhibitors Proton pump inhibitors act directly on the K^+/H^+ATPase enzyme that secretes gastric acid. Omeprazole (Prilosec) and lansoprazole (Prevacid) are examples. Omeprazole is the prototype. These agents irreversibly block this enzyme, which means that the body must produce new enzyme in order to begin secreting acid again. This gives proton pump inhibitors a long duration of effect. Side effects are minor and rare, occurring in less than 1 percent of patients. They include diarrhea and headache.

Antacids **Antacids** are alkalotic compounds used to increase the gastric environment's pH. Most available products are either aluminum, magnesium, calcium, or sodium compounds. They are used in conjunction with other approaches to PUD and are available over the counter for relief of acid indigestion and heartburn.

Anticholinergics While it might seem that all muscarinic blocking agents would be effective in decreasing gastric acid secretion, most atropine-like drugs produce too many

CONTENT REVIEW

► Categories of Laxatives

- Bulk-forming
- Stimulant
- Osmotic
- Surfactant

unwanted effects and, therefore, are not used. The one exception is pirenzepine (Gastrozepine), because of its ability to selectively block the ACh receptors in the gut.

Drugs Used to Treat Constipation

Laxatives decrease the firmness of stool and increase the water content. While an uninformed public frequently uses these agents unnecessarily, they are effective in some situations, specifically with patients for whom excessive strain is inappropriate. These patients include those with recent episiotomy, hemorrhoids, colostomies, or cardiovascular disease (for whom excessive straining may decrease heart rate).

Laxatives are traditionally grouped into four categories based on their mechanism of action: bulk-forming, surfactant, stimulant, and osmotic. The bulk-forming agents such as methylcellulose (Citrucel) and psyllium (Metamucil) produce a response almost identical to normal dietary fiber intake. Fiber is undigestible and unabsorbable; therefore, it remains in the lumen of the GI system and is passed more or less intact in stool. Most water absorption takes place in the colon. Fiber (or bulk-forming laxatives) in the colon absorbs water, leading to a softer, more bulky stool. Fiber can also provide nutrients for bacteria living in the colon. These bacteria feed and provide even more bulk. The enlarged stool stimulates stretch receptors in the colonic wall, which increases peristalsis. Softening the stool also lessens strain on defecation.

The **surfactant** laxatives include docusate sodium (Colace). They decrease surface tension, which increases water absorption into the feces. They also increase water secretion and limit its reabsorption by the intestinal wall.

Stimulant laxatives increase motility. Like the surfactant laxatives, they also increase water secretion and decrease its absorption. The prototype stimulant laxative is phenolphthalein (Ex-Lax, Correctol). Bisacodyl (Bisacolax) is another example.

The osmotic laxatives are poorly absorbed salts that increase the feces' osmotic pull, thereby increasing their water content. Magnesium hydroxide, the active ingredient in Milk of Magnesia, is the prototype of this class.

Drugs Used to Treat Diarrhea

Diarrhea is the abnormally frequent passage of soft, liquid stool. It is a symptom of an underlying disease, usually a bacterial infection. It may be caused by an increased gastric motility (the stool does not stay in the colon long enough to have much water absorbed), increased water secretion, or decreased water absorption. While it is a nuisance, diarrhea is often a helpful process because it increases the expulsion of the offending agent. It is usually self-correcting and does not need to be treated. When treatment is necessary, either specific or nonspecific agents may be used. A specific agent directly treats the cause, usually a bacteria. As you would expect, antibiotics are a common specific antidiarrheal medication.

Drugs Used to Treat Emesis

Emesis is a complex process that involves different parts of the brain as well as receptors and muscles in the stomach and inner ear. The two involved parts of the brain are the vomiting center in the medulla and the chemoreceptor trigger zone (CTZ). The vomiting center stimulates vomiting directly, while the CTZ does so indirectly.

The vomiting center is stimulated by H_1 and ACh receptors in the pathway between itself and the inner ear, by sensory input from the eyes and nose (unpleasant or disturbing sights and smells), and by other parts of the brain in response to anxiety or fear. The CTZ stimulates the vomiting center in response to stimuli from serotonin receptors in the stomach and bloodborne substances such as opioids and ipecac.

Stimulating emesis is rarely desired, but it can be useful in treating certain types of overdoses or poisonings. Ipecac is the drug of choice when stimulating emesis is indicated. It stimulates the CTZ which, in turn, stimulates the vomiting center.

Antiemetics Unlike causing emesis, preventing emesis is frequently desirable. **Antiemetics** are indicated in conjunction with chemotherapy, which may cause violent nausea and vomiting. Antiemetics are also indicated in the prophylactic treatment of motion sickness.

Multiple transmitters are involved in the vomiting reflex. They include serotonin, dopamine, acetylcholine, and histamine. Drugs that interfere with any of these transmitters can decrease or prevent nausea and vomiting. This functional class includes several pharmacological subclasses: serotonin antagonists, dopamine antagonists, anticholinergics, and cannabinoids.

Serotonin Antagonists The prototype serotonin antagonist is ondansetron (Zofran). It blocks the serotonin receptors in the CTZ, the stomach, and the small intestine. It is very effective in the treatment of nausea and vomiting associated with chemotherapy, and unlike the dopamine antagonists, it does not cause extrapyramidal effects like dystonia and ataxia. Its most common side effects are headache and diarrhea.

Dopamine Antagonists Both phenothiazines and butyrophenones effectively block dopamine receptors in the CTZ. (This chapter's section on psychotherapeutic medications discusses both of these medications at length.) The phenothiazines include prochlorperazine (Compazine) and promethazine (Phenergan), while the butyrophenones include haloperidol (Haldol) and droperidol (Inapsine). Agents from both classes cause side effects of extrapyramidal effects and sedation. Another dopamine antagonist, metoclopramide (Reglan), is neither a phenothiazine nor a butyrophenone. It is unique in that it blocks both serotonin and dopamine receptors in the CTZ. Table 3–25 details common antiemetics.

Cannabinoids The cannabinoids are derivatives of tetrahydrocannabinol (THC) and are effective antiemetics used to treat chemotherapy-induced nausea and vomiting. The two available agents are dronabinol (Marinol) and nabilone (Cesamet). Because both agents are essentially the same as THC (the active

TABLE 3-25 | Antiemetics

Name	Classification	Action	Indications	Contraindications	Doses	Routes	Adverse Effects	Other
Prochlorperazine *Compazine*	Phenothiazine	Suppresses the CTZ; has antihistaminic effects	• Nausea • Vomiting • Anxiety • Psychosis	• Hypersensitivity to the drug or the phenothiazine class • Small children • Pregnancy	5–10 mg	IV, IM, IO, PO	• Drowsiness • Dizziness • Sedation • Dry mouth • Extrapyramidal symptoms	• Can potentiate CNS depressants (e.g., alcohol)
Promethazine *Phenergan*	Phenothiazine	Suppresses the CTZ; has antihistaminic effects	• Nausea • Vomiting	• Hypersensitivity to the drug	12.5–25 mg	IV, IM, PO	• Drowsiness • Dizziness • Sedation • Dry mouth • Extrapyramidal symptoms	• Can potentiate CNS depressants (e.g., alcohol) • Extravasation can cause local tissue injury • Rarely used
Ondansetron *Zofran*	Serotonin antagonist	Selectively blocks 5-HT$_3$ serotonin receptors including those in the CTZ and vagus nerve terminals	• Nausea • Vomiting	• Hypersensitivity to the drug	4–8 mg	IV, IM, PO	• Dizziness • Lightheaded	• Commonly used in emergency medicine because of good safety profile

ingredient in marijuana), their side effects include euphoria similar to that of marijuana. While those effects may be desirable for some, they may be intensely unpleasant for others.

Drugs Used to Aid Digestion

Several drugs are available to aid the digestion of carbohydrates and fats. These agents are similar to endogenous digestive enzymes released into the duodenum in response to vagal stimulation. Occasionally, supplemental enzymes are necessary for patients whose vagal stimulus has been surgically severed or whose duodenum has been bypassed. Two of these drugs are pancreatin (Entozyme) and pancrelipase (Viokase). Their chief side effects are nausea, vomiting, and abdominal cramping.

DRUGS USED TO AFFECT THE EYES

Ophthalmic drugs are used to treat conditions involving the eyes, primarily glaucoma and trauma. In addition, some ophthalmic agents are used in diagnosing and examining the eyes.

Glaucoma is a degenerative disease that affects the optic nerve. Its causative factors are not clear; however, correlations are known between it and several risk factors including intraocular pressure, race (its rate is three times higher among African Americans than among whites), and age. The medications used to treat glaucoma are all aimed at reducing intraocular pressure (IOP). Beta-blockers and cholinergics are the most common. Beta-blockade decreases IOP by an unknown mechanism. Timolol (Timoptic) and betaxolol (Betoptic) are examples of this class. Pilocarpine (Isopto Carpine) is the prototype cholinergic drug for treating glaucoma. It stimulates muscarinic receptors in the eye to cause miosis (pupil constriction) and ciliary muscle contraction, which indirectly lowers IOP. Drugs from these classes are given topically. Beta-blockers have few side effects, while pilocarpine causes blurred vision and local irritation.

Some diagnostic procedures call for causing mydriasis (pupil dilation) and cycloplegia (paralysis of the ciliary muscles used to focus vision). The two pharmacological approaches to doing this involve anticholinergics or adrenergic agonists. In this functional class, atropine solutions (such as Atropisol) and scopolamine solutions (such as Isopto Hyoscine) are typical anticholinergics; phenylephrine solution (AK-Dilate) is the class's principal adrenergic agonist. This chapter's sections on anticholinergics and adrenergic agonists discuss these pharmacological classes in more detail.

Tetracaine (Pontocaine) is a local anesthetic of the ester class. (It is related to cocaine, another ester, but not to lidocaine, an amide.) It is used to decrease pain and sensation in the eye from trauma or during ophthalmic procedures.

DRUGS USED TO AFFECT THE EARS

Most drugs used to treat conditions involving the ear are aimed at eliminating underlying bacterial or fungal infections or at breaking up impacted earwax. Chloramphenicol (Chloromycetin Otic) and gentamicin sulfate otic solution (Garamycin) are common antibiotics; carbamide peroxide (Auro Ear Drops) and carbamide peroxide and glycerin (Ear Wax Removal System) are both used to treat earwax. Finally, several drugs are available to treat swimmer's ear, an inflammation/irritation of the external ear. They include isopropyl alcohol (Auro-Dri Ear Drops) and boric acid and isopropyl alcohol (Aurocaine 2).

Some drugs that are used for other purposes have ototoxic (harmful to the organs or nerves that produce hearing or balance) properties if taken in overdose or administered too quickly. The most common ototoxic symptom is tinnitus, or ringing in the ears. Drugs with ototoxic properties include aspirin and other NSAIDs, some antibiotics (including erythromycin and vancomycin), and the diuretic furosemide (Lasix).

DRUGS USED TO AFFECT THE ENDOCRINE SYSTEM

The endocrine system and nervous system together are chiefly responsible for the regulatory activities that maintain homeostasis. The nervous system, with its direct connections between nerves and organs, may be thought of as a "wired" system, while the endocrine system, which releases hormones directly into the bloodstream, may be thought of as "wireless." The endocrine system comprises the following glands: pituitary (anterior and posterior lobes), pineal, thyroid, parathyroid, thymus, adrenal, pancreas, ovaries, and testes. (Table 3–26 lists the specific hormones that each gland releases.) Of these, the pituitary is commonly referred to as the master gland because of its role in controlling the other endocrine glands. (The hypothalamus in turn controls many of the pituitary's functions.) Once in the bloodstream, the hormones from these glands circulate widely throughout the body. To be effective, however, they must bind with very specific receptors. This discussion will focus on the pharmacological actions of drugs that affect the various endocrine glands.

Drugs Affecting the Pituitary Gland

The pituitary gland is made up of a posterior lobe and an anterior lobe. It sits in the *sella turcica*, a depression of the sphenoid bone, and is physically connected to the hypothalamus. The posterior pituitary hormones are actually synthesized in the hypothalamus and then migrate into the posterior pituitary, where they are released upon hypothalamic stimulation. In contrast, the hormones of the anterior pituitary are actually synthesized in that lobe. The hypothalamus secretes releasing hormones into a portal system that carries them into the anterior pituitary, where they stimulate the release of the anterior pituitary hormones. There are six main anterior pituitary hormones.

Anterior Pituitary Drugs The only conditions treated with anterior pituitary-like drugs are those associated with abnormal growth, specifically dwarfism, acromegaly, and gigantism. Dwarfism is caused by a deficiency of growth hormone, and therapy is aimed at hormone replacement. Somatrem

TABLE 3–26 | Summary of Hormone Actions

Gland	Hormone	Action
Posterior pituitary	Oxytocin	Uterine contraction, milk ejection
	Vasopressin (ADH)	Retains salt and water, increases ECF volume
Anterior pituitary	Thyroid-stimulating hormone (TSH)	Increases metabolic rate
	Growth hormone (GH)	Increases use of stored fats, decreases glucose use
	Adrenocorticotropic hormone (ACTH)	Stimulates adrenal cortex to release hormones
	Follicle-stimulating hormone (FSH)	Males: sperm production
		Females: stimulates growth and development of ovarian follicles
	Luteinizing hormone (LH)	Males: responsible for secretion of testosterone by testes
		Females: ovulation, secretion of estrogen and progesterone
	Prolactin (PRL)	Enhances breast development and milk production
Thyroid	Thyroid hormone	Increases metabolic rate
Parathyroid	Parathyroid hormone	Increases calcium in ECF
Pancreas	Insulin	Decreases blood glucose
	Glucagon	Increases blood glucose
Adrenal	Glucocorticoids	Increase blood glucose, prevent inflammation

(Protropin) and somatropin (Humatrope) are both essentially the same as the endogenous growth hormone, acting indirectly to increase skeletal growth as well as cell numbers by stimulating another hormone, insulinlike growth factor 1 (IGF-1), to cause its effects. These drugs' primary side effects are pain and redness at the injection site. Some cases of inadvertent gigantism have been reported, but this can be avoided with careful observation.

Acromegaly and gigantism are caused by excesses of growth hormone, usually resulting from a tumor. While the treatment of choice is surgical removal of the tumor, octreotide (Sandostatin) is available for pharmacological intervention. Octreotide is a synthetic drug with actions similar to somatostatin, the endogenous growth hormone inhibiting hormone. Its main action inhibits the release of growth hormone. Octreotide's many side effects include bradycardia, diarrhea, and stomach distress.

Posterior Pituitary Drugs The two posterior pituitary hormones are oxytocin and antidiuretic hormone. Oxytocin is discussed in the section on drugs affecting labor and delivery. Antidiuretic hormone (ADH) increases water reabsorption in the renal collecting tubules, thus promoting the retention of water and a more concentrated urine. Physiologically, ADH is a key component in regulating blood volume, blood pressure, and electrolyte balance. Clinically, ADH analogues are used to treat diabetes insipidus and nocturnal enuresis (bed-wetting). Diabetes insipidus, unlike diabetes mellitus, is caused by inadequate amounts of centrally acting ADH. This causes a profound polyuria and polydipsia. At higher doses, ADH can cause vasoconstriction and increased blood pressure; hence its other name, vasopressin. Vasopressin (Pitressin), desmopressin

(Stimate), and lypressin (Diapid) are all available to reverse this ADH deficiency. Desmopressin is also available for administration via intranasal spray for nocturnal enuresis.[27]

Drugs Affecting the Parathyroid and Thyroid Glands

The parathyroid glands are primarily responsible for regulating calcium levels. Hypoparathyroidism leads to decreased levels of calcium and vitamin D. Treatment, therefore, is through calcium and vitamin D supplements. Hyperparathyroidism leads to high levels of calcium. Because it usually results from tumors, the treatment of choice is surgical removal of all or part of the parathyroid glands.

The thyroid gland produces thyroid hormones, which play a vital role in regulating growth, maturation, and metabolism. Hypothyroidism can occur in children or adults. When it develops in children, it is known as cretinism and manifests itself as dwarfism and mental retardation with characteristic features. Because most growth and maturation in adults is complete, adult onset of hypothyroidism appears as decreased metabolic rate, weight gain, fatigue, and bradycardia. In some cases, myxedema (facial puffiness) may be present. Treatment is aimed at thyroid hormone replacement. The prototype drug, levothyroxine (Synthroid), is also the most commonly used. A synthetic analogue of T_4 (thyroxine), one of the thyroid hormones, levothyroxine generally has no significant side effects when taken in therapeutic doses. Overdose may lead to thyrotoxicosis or thyroid storm. Thyrotoxicosis is a condition in which hyperthyroidism causes an increase in thyroid hormones. Thyroid storm is a severe form of thyrotoxicosis where the manifestations of the disease increase to life-threatening proportions. Thyroid storm is characterized by tachycardic arrhythmias, angina, hypertension, and hyperthermia.

Goiters are enlargements of the thyroid gland. They are typically caused by insufficient dietary iodine. In developed countries, goiter is much rarer than in undeveloped countries and is most commonly caused by Hashimoto's disease, a chronic autoimmune disease. Treatment of goiters is aimed at supplementing the inadequate iodine.

Hyperthyroidism is caused by excessive release of thyroid hormones, typically as a result of tumors. The most common cause of hyperthyroidism in the United States is Graves' disease. It presents with tachycardia, hypertension, hyperthermia, nervousness, insomnia, increased metabolic rate, and weight loss. In severe cases, exophthalmos (protrusion of the eyeballs) may occur. Treatment is typically surgical removal of all or part of the thyroid gland. Radioactive iodine (^{131}I) may also be given for radiation therapy. Propylthiouracil (PTU) may be given alone or as adjunct therapy to surgery or radiation in treating hyperthyroidism.

Drugs Affecting the Adrenal Cortex

The adrenal cortex synthesizes and secretes three classes of hormones: glucocorticoids, mineralocorticoids, and androgens. The glucocorticoids and mineralocorticoids are referred to collectively as corticosteroids, adrenocorticoids, or corticoids. As their name implies, glucocorticoids increase the production of glucose by enhancing carbohydrate metabolism, promoting gluconeogenesis, and reducing peripheral glucose utilization. The most important glucocorticoid is cortisol. The mineralocorticoids regulate salt and water balance. The primary mineralocorticoid is aldosterone. The androgens are important hormones in regulating sexual maturation and development.

Two diseases typify the disorders associated with the adrenal cortex: Cushing's disease and Addison's disease. Cushing's disease is characterized by hypersecretion of adrenocorticotropic hormone, an anterior pituitary tropic hormone that increases the synthesis of corticoids, leading to excessive glucocorticoid secretion. Common signs and symptoms include hyperglycemia, obesity, hypertension, and electrolyte imbalances. Addison's disease is characterized by hyposecretion of corticoids as a result of damage to the adrenal gland. Common signs and symptoms include hypoglycemia, emaciation, hypotension, hyperkalemia, and hyponatremia.

Treatment of Cushing's disease is typically surgical. Symptomatic pharmacological intervention with an antihypertensive (potassium-sparing diuretics such as spironolactone [Aldactone] or ACE inhibitors such as captopril [Capoten]) may be necessary. Drugs that may inhibit the synthesis of corticosteroids (antiadrenals) may also be used as an adjunct to surgery or radiation. In high doses, the antifungal agent ketoconazole (Nizoral) is an effective temporary antiadrenal drug. At such doses, however, it may cause liver dysfunction.

Treatment of Addison's disease is aimed at replacement therapy. Cortisone (Cortistan) and hydrocortisone (Solu-Cortef) are the drugs of choice. Occasionally, a specific mineralocorticoid is necessary. Fludrocortisone (Florinef Acetate) is the only mineralocorticoid available.[28]

Drugs Affecting the Pancreas

Diabetes mellitus is the most important disease involving the pancreas. Diabetes mellitus (as opposed to diabetes insipidus, which involves inadequate ADH secretion) involves inappropriate carbohydrate metabolism. Traditionally, the term *diabetes* used alone refers to diabetes mellitus, of which the two main types are, logically, type I and type II. Type I diabetes is also known as insulin-dependent diabetes mellitus, or IDDM. It results from an inadequate release of insulin from the beta cells of the pancreatic islets. Patients with type I diabetes rely on insulin replacement therapy to survive. Because type I diabetes typically manifests itself at an early age (usually before 30 years) it is also commonly called juvenile onset diabetes. Most diabetics have type II diabetes, which is also referred to as non-insulin-dependent diabetes mellitus (NIDDM) or adult onset diabetes. It results from a decreased responsiveness to insulin and a lack of synchronization between insulin release and blood glucose levels. Type II diabetes typically begins later in life (after 40 years) and almost always occurs in patients with obesity. Because they have functioning beta cells that release insulin, type II diabetics usually do not depend on insulin replacement. Gestational diabetes, a third type, occurs transitionally during pregnancy. Gestational diabetes is a form of stress-induced diabetes in which the mother cannot effectively manage her blood glucose levels during pregnancy without medical intervention. Gestational diabetes resolves itself within hours to days after delivery.

The two main substances involved with regulating blood glucose are insulin and glucagon. Both are secreted from the pancreas and both are used to manage diabetes. Secreted from the beta cells of the pancreatic islets of Langerhans in response to increased blood glucose levels, **insulin** increases cellular transport of glucose, potassium, and amino acids. It also converts glucose into glycogen for storage in the liver and in skeletal muscle. Finally, insulin promotes cell growth and division.

Glucagon, too, is secreted from the pancreatic islets, but by alpha cells rather than by the insulin-producing beta cells. Glucagon's actions are the direct opposite of insulin's; it increases both glycogenolysis (glycogen breakdown into glucose) and gluconeogenesis (the synthesis of glucose from glycerol and amino acids). So, while insulin decreases blood glucose levels, glucagon increases them.

Patients with either type I or type II diabetes may experience both hyperglycemia and hypoglycemia. While hyperglycemia more often results from the disease, hypoglycemia is a common side effect of treatment. The main intervention for patients with type I diabetes is insulin-replacement therapy. Several insulin preparations are available. The most effective therapy for patients with type II diabetes is usually weight loss through diet modification and exercise. When this is not effective, oral hypoglycemic agents and, occasionally, insulin are used. Finally, glucagon and diazoxide (both can be considered hyperglycemic agents) are occasionally used for treating emergency hypoglycemia.

Insulin Preparations Insulin comes from one of three sources. Initially, it came from either beef or pork intestines.

TABLE 3–27 | Insulin Preparations

Classification	Trade Name	Source	Onset (Hrs)	Peak (Hrs)	Duration (Hrs)
Rapid-Acting			0.25+	<0.75–2.5	3.5–5.0
Lispro Insulin	Humalog	Human			
Aspart Insulin	NovoRapid	Human			
Short-Acting or Regular	Humulin R Novolin R Iletin II R	Human Human Pork	0.5–10	2.0–5.0	5.0–8.0
Intermediate-Acting or NPH	Humulin N Novolin N Iletin II NPH	Human Human Pork	1–2	4–12	14–18
Premixed	Humulin 70/30 Humulin 50/50 Novolin 70/30 Novolin 50/50	Human Human Human Human	0.5–1.0	2–12	14–18
Intermediate-Acting	Humulin L Iletin II Lente	Human Pork	2–4	7–15	12–24
Long-Acting	Humulin U Ultralente	Human	3–4	8–24	24–28
Insulin Glargine	Lantus	Human	>1.5	No peak	>20

Now, recombinant DNA technology has made human insulin available (that is, insulin synthesized with a human RNA template, not harvested directly from humans). Insulin preparations differ primarily in their onset and duration of action and in their incidence of allergic reaction. Insulin preparations may be short acting, intermediate acting, or long acting, depending on their onset and duration of action. (Table 3–27 lists insulin preparations.)

Insulin is also classified as natural (regular) or modified. As their name suggests, the natural insulins are used as they occur in nature. The other insulin preparations have been modified to increase their duration of action and thus decrease the frequency of their administration. All insulin preparations are given subcutaneously, with the exception of regular insulin, which may also be given intravenously. Insulin is not available as an oral medication because the digestive enzymes would rapidly render it inactive; therefore, type I patients must take multiple injections every day of their lives. This may discourage compliance in some patients.

The modified insulin preparations include NPH (neutral protamine Hagedorn) insulin, which is regular insulin attached to a large protein designed to delay absorption, and the Lente series, which is attached to zinc. Two preparations of Lente insulin are available by themselves, Lente and Ultralente. A third, Semilente insulin, is available only in a combination product with other insulins.

Insulin preparations are used for lifelong replacement therapy in type I diabetes and for emergency treatment of hyperglycemia and hyperkalemia in nondiabetics. (Recall that insulin also increases potassium uptake by cells and is therefore useful in lowering potassium levels.) These preparations' primary side effect is unintended hypoglycemia. Because beta$_2$ adrenergic blockers can hide the effects of hypoglycemia, patients may not recognize this condition's signs until they cannot care for themselves. Also, beta-blockers decrease the release of glucagon, so these patients' hypoglycemia may be even worse. Insulin preparations derived from beef or pork, as well as the Lentes, may lead to allergic reactions. The natural human insulin preparations do not have this effect.

Oral Hypoglycemic Agents Oral hypoglycemic agents are used to stimulate insulin secretion from the pancreas in patients with type II diabetes. These agents are ineffective in people with type I diabetes since those patients cannot secrete insulin. This functional class comprises four pharmacological classes: sulfonylureas, biguanides, alpha-glucosidase inhibitors, and thiazolidinediones. The sulfonylureas were the first class of oral hypoglycemics available and as such are also known as first-generation or second-generation oral hypoglycemics, depending on when they were released. Drugs in this class include tolbutamide (Orinase), chlorpropamide (Diabinese), glipizide (Glucotrol), and glyburide (Micronase). They work by increasing insulin secretion from the pancreas and may also increase tissue response to insulin. Their major side effect is hypoglycemia.

The only agent in the biguanide class is metformin (Glucophage). It decreases glucose synthesis and increases glucose uptake. It does not stimulate the release of insulin from the pancreas and therefore does not cause hypoglycemia. Its primary side effects are nausea, vomiting, and decreased appetite.

Alpha-glucosidase inhibitors include acarbose (Precose) and miglitol (Glyset). They work by delaying carbohydrate metabolism, which moderates the increase in blood glucose that occurs after meals. These agents' primary side effects are flatulence, cramps, diarrhea, and abdominal distention resulting from colonic bacteria feeding on the increased number of carbohydrates remaining in fecal matter.

Thiazolidinediones are a new class of oral hypoglycemic agents unrelated to the others. The only drug in this class is troglitazone (Rezulin). It works by promoting tissue response to insulin and thus making the available insulin more effective. Troglitazone has no major side effects.

Hyperglycemic Agents

Two hyperglycemic agents, glucagon and diazoxide (Proglycem), act to increase blood glucose levels. Glucagon is indicated for the emergency treatment of patients with hypoglycemia. It will frequently be given intramuscularly to hypoglycemic patients in whom an IV line is unobtainable. Occasional side effects are nausea and vomiting and, rarely, allergic reactions. Diazoxide (Proglycem) inhibits insulin release and is typically used only for patients with hyperinsulin secretion resulting from pancreatic tumors; it is more commonly used for hypertension. It is not indicated for treating diabetes-induced hypoglycemia.

$D_{50}W$ (50 percent dextrose in water) is a sugar solution given intravenously for acute hypoglycemia. Its primary side effect is local tissue necrosis if infiltration occurs.

Drugs Affecting the Female Reproductive System

The main groups of drugs affecting the female reproductive system are estrogens, progestins, oral contraceptives, drugs affecting uterine contraction, and those used to treat infertility.

Estrogens and Progestins

Estrogens are produced in females by the ovaries and the ovarian follicles, and in pregnancy, the placenta. Outside of pregnancy, the ovaries are the principal source of estrogens. The principal ovarian estrogen is estradiol, of which there are many commercial preparations. The principal indication for estrogen is replacement therapy in postmenopausal women. After menopause, estrogen levels drop significantly and have been indicated as the cause of menopausal symptoms such as hot flashes and vaginal dryness and as an increased risk factor for osteoporosis. Hormone replacement therapy (HRT) with estrogen has been shown to alleviate menopausal symptoms and reverse the increased risk for osteoporosis; however, it is not without its own risks. Recent studies have shown increased chances of breast cancer and stroke associated with hormone replacement therapy. Side effects include nausea, fluid retention, and breast tenderness. The nausea usually diminishes after

several months of therapy. Estrogen is also administered in cases of delayed puberty in girls as a result of hypogonadism.

The progestins' principal noncontraceptive use is to counteract the untoward effects of estrogen on the endometrium in hormone replacement therapy for postmenopausal women. They are also used to treat amenorrhea, endometriosis, and dysfunctional uterine bleeding.

Oral Contraceptives

Oral contraception is an effective means of preventing pregnancy. All oral contraceptives' primary mechanism of action is the prevention of ovulation, which makes the endometrium less favorable for implantation and promotes the development of a thick mucus plug that blocks access to sperm through the cervix. These contraceptives are either a combination of estrogen and progestin or, in the case of "minipills," progestin only. They may also be classified based on their administration cycle as monophasic, biphasic, or triphasic. These classes differ in how they alter the dose of estrogen or progestin throughout the menstrual cycle. Many different preparations are available, although they all work in similar fashion. In general, these drugs are well tolerated and have few side effects. The oral contraceptives' chief side effects are unintended pregnancy (in less than 3 percent of users), thromboembolism (this risk is much lower with the newer low-estrogen dose preparations), hypertension, and abnormal uterine bleeding. They are in wide use and are one of the most widely prescribed drug classes. They are the second most popular means of birth control after surgical sterilization (male and female combined).

Uterine Stimulants and Relaxants

Drugs that increase uterine contraction (uterine stimulants) are oxytocics (oxytocin means rapid birth). Drugs that relax the uterus or inhibit uterine contraction are tocolytics.

The primary indications for administration of an oxytocic are to induce labor and to treat severe postpartum hemorrhage. Oxytocin is available commercially as Pitocin and Syntocinon. The uterus becomes increasingly sensitive to oxytocin throughout gestation, progressing from relatively insensitive before pregnancy to very sensitive around the time of labor. Oxytocin's chief side effect, water retention, is rarely significant and only so if large volumes of fluid have been administered without careful ongoing assessment. Ergonovine (Ergotrate), a derivative of a rye fungus, is a powerful uterine stimulant. It increases both the force and duration of contraction. Because of this increased duration, ergonovine is only used in the treatment of postpartum hemorrhage.

The tocolytics relax uterine smooth muscle by stimulating the $beta_2$ receptors in the uterus. The two $beta_2$ agonists commonly used for this purpose are terbutaline (Brethine) and ritodrine (Yutopar). Terbutaline's primary use is to treat asthma, but it is commonly used to delay labor even though the FDA does not currently approve it for that purpose. Both agents decrease both the force and frequency of contraction. Their chief side effects are the same as those of the other $beta_2$ agonists used to treat asthma: tremors and tachycardia. Occasionally, hyperglycemia may result from glycogenolysis in the liver.

Infertility Agents

A number of conditions may cause infertility, which is the inability to become pregnant, and medications can treat only some of them. Most infertility drugs are developed for women and promote maturation of ovarian follicles. Clomiphene (Clomid), urofollitropin (Metrodin), and menotropins (Pergonal) are all within this class, although they each act by a different mechanism. These agents' side effects include ovarian enlargement or cysts, abdominal pain, and menstrual irregularities.

Drugs Affecting the Male Reproductive System

Drugs that affect the male reproductive system include those that treat testosterone deficiency and benign prostatic hyperplasia. Testosterone replacement therapy may be indicated in testosterone deficiency caused by cryptorchidism (failure of one or both of the testes to descend during puberty), orchitis (testicular inflammation), or orchidectomy (testicular removal). It is also used in delayed puberty. Preparations include testosterone enanthate, methyltestosterone (Metandren), and fluoxymesterone (Halotestin).

Benign prostatic hyperplasia is an enlarged prostate. This is a common but problematic age-related disease. By the age of 70, close to 75 percent of men will have symptoms severe enough to seek therapy. These symptoms may include urinary hesitancy and retention. Treatment has traditionally been surgery, but several drugs are available, including finasteride (Proscar), which interferes with the production of an enzyme involved with prostate growth. Side effects may include rash, breast tenderness, headache, impotence, and decreased libido.

Drugs Affecting Sexual Behavior

For centuries, cultures have searched for drugs that would increase libido and sexual potency. Ironically, the reverse has most commonly been found. The largest category of drugs affecting sexual behavior do so as a side effect of their intended purpose. Many drug classifications decrease libido in both sexes and inhibit erection and ejaculation. Examples include antihypertensives (beta-blockers, centrally acting alpha antagonists, and diuretics) and antianxiety/antipsychotic medications (benzodiazepines, phenothiazines, MAO inhibitors, and tricyclic antidepressants).

Many drugs are purported to increase libido. The most notable of these is cantharis (Spanish fly). Despite common belief, no evidence indicates that cantharis actually increases sexual appetite. Indeed, it can produce some very dangerous side effects. Hallucinogens such as LSD and marijuana, as well as alcohol, are also commonly believed to heighten sexuality. Any such effect from these agents is likely an indirect result of decreased inhibitions or anxiety. These drugs all have very different effects, depending on each individual's unique physiology, expectations before use, and surrounding circumstances. They have no proven direct physiologic effect on sexual gratification.

Levodopa (L-dopa), an anti-Parkinson's drug, has demonstrated increased libido and improved erectile ability as a side effect of treatment. Whether this results directly from increased autonomic stimulation or indirectly from improved self-esteem achieved in therapy, any improvement seems to be only temporary. Several drugs have been developed that aid in erectile dysfunction. Erectile dysfunction becomes more frequent with age or with certain diseases such as diabetes or cardiovascular disease. Drugs that aid in erectile dysfunction increase blood supply to the penis. These include sildenafil (Viagra), vardenafil (Levitra), and tadalafil (Cialis). These drugs act by relaxing vascular smooth muscle, which increases blood flow to the corpus cavernosum, the spongelike tissue on the sides of the penis responsible for erection. These drugs are unique in that they have no effect in the absence of sexual stimulation. Other drugs used to treat impotence have caused prolonged and painful erections (priapism). The chief side effect of sildenafil is seen when it is used in combination with nitrates. The combined effect of relaxing vascular smooth muscle may lead to a dangerously decreased preload, which may lower blood pressure and lead to myocardial infarction. Prehospital personnel should be aware of this important interaction.

If you are called on to treat a patient with chest pain who has taken sildenafil, vardenafil, or tadalafil recently, do not give him nitroglycerin or any other nitrate. Table 3–28 details hormones and related agents.

DRUGS USED TO TREAT CANCER

Drugs used to treat cancer are called **antineoplastic agents**. A detailed discussion of the many different antineoplastic agents is beyond the scope of this text; however, this section will briefly overview their main classes and prototype drugs.

Cancer involves the modification of cellular DNA leading to an abnormal growth of tissues. Of the many known types of cancer, only a few are successfully treated with chemotherapy. In fact, most cancers are best treated by surgical removal of the tumor. Unfortunately, many of the more lethal cancers do not involve a compact growth; rather, they affect the formed elements of the blood, especially leukocytes. Treating these widely dispersed cancers with surgery is not possible, as there is nothing for the surgeon to remove.

Chemotherapy is not nearly as safe or devoid of side effects as antibiotic therapy; however, scientists have yet to identify any unique characteristics of cancer cells that would allow them to develop drugs specific to those cells. Because cancer is the abnormal growth of normal cells, drugs that kill cancerous cells therefore also kill noncancerous cells. Chemotherapy is thus largely a balancing act aimed at maximizing the kill rate of cancer cells while minimizing the death of normal tissue. The one characteristic that most cancer cells share is rapid cell division and replication. Consequently, most antineoplastic agents have their greatest effect on cancer cells during mitosis and on young, small cancers that are undergoing rapid growth.

The agents used to kill cancer cells are grouped according to their mechanism of action. Antimetabolite drugs mimic some of the enzymes and proteins needed for DNA replication but do not have the same effects; therefore, they prevent cells from reproducing. Their prototype is fluorouracil (Adrucil). Alkylating agents that interfere with DNA splitting include cyclophosphamide (Cytoxan) and mechlorethamine (Mustargen).

TABLE 3–28 | Hormones and Related Agents

Name	Classification	Action	Indications	Contraindications	Doses	Routes	Adverse Effects	Other
Vasopressin *Pitressin*	Hormone (analog of antidiuretic hormone)	Non-adrenergic vasoconstrictor; promotes fluid retention in the kidney	• Cardiac arrest • Normovolemic hypotension	• Few in the emergency setting	40 units	IV	• Blanching of the skin • Abdominal cramping • Nausea • Hypertension	• Benefits in cardiac arrest are questionable
Oxytocin *Pitocin*	Hormone (oxytocin)	Oxytocic; causes uterine contractions and lactations	• Postpartum vaginal bleeding • Induction/ augmentation of labor	• Anything other than post-partum bleeding (in the prehospital setting)	10–20 units in 500 mL IV; 3–10 units (IM)	IV, IM	• Anaphylaxis • Arrhythmias	• Ensure placenta (and possible additional baby) has delivered before administering
Glucagon	Hormone (glucagon)	Elevates blood glucose levels through conversion of glycogen to glucose and other factors	• Hypoglycemia • Beta-blocker overdose	• Hypersensitivity to the drug	0.25– 0.5 u (IV); 1.0 mg IM	IV, IM, IO	• Few in the emergency setting	• Less effective in patients with decreased glycogen stores (e.g., alcoholics)
Insulin *Humulin, NovoLog, Novolin*	Hormone (insulin)	Causes glucose uptake by the cells thus lowering blood glucose levels	• Diabetes • Hyper-glycemia • Diabetic ketoacidosis	• Hypoglycemia • Normoglycemia	Varies	IV, SQ	• Few in the emergency setting	• Dosages of the various insulin types vary significantly
Dextrose, 50%	Carbohydrate	Substrate for carbohydrate metabolism	• Hypoglycemia	• None in the emergency setting	12.5– 25.0 g	IV, PO	• Local venous irritation common • Tissue injury	• Less concentrated solutions (e.g., 10%) equally effective with fewer side-effects
Methylpred-nisolone	Hormone (analog of corticosteroid)	Anti-inflammatory; suppresses immune response	• Asthma • COPD • Anaphylaxis	• Hypersensitivity to the drug	125– 250 mg	IV, IO	• GI bleeding • Increases blood glucose levels	• Effects are delayed and not typically seen in the prehospital setting

Mitotic inhibitors also interfere with cell division; they include vinblastine (Velban) and vincristine (Oncovin).

Chemotherapy's primary side effects include nausea, vomiting, and other gastrointestinal disturbances, as well as hair loss and weakness. Almost all antineoplastic agents cause severe side effects and are given in conjunction with antiemetics.

DRUGS USED TO TREAT INFECTIOUS DISEASES AND INFLAMMATION

Infectious diseases are typically caused by bacteria, viruses, or funguses and may be treated with antimicrobial drugs developed to fight those particular invaders. We will discuss each broad class.

Antibiotics An **antibiotic** agent may either kill the offending bacteria (bactericidal agents) or so decrease the bacteria's growth that the patient's immune system can effectively fight the infection (bacteriostatic agents). In general, all of these agents share one of several mechanisms. Drugs in the penicillin and cephalosporin classes, as well as vancomycin (Vancocin), are bactericidal and act by inhibiting cell wall synthesis. Unlike animal cells, bacteria have hypertonic cell cytoplasm and depend on the rigid and relatively impermeable cell wall to maintain integrity. When cell wall synthesis is inhibited, osmotic pressure pulls water into the cell, and the cell ruptures, killing the bacteria. The macrolide, aminoglycoside, and tetracycline antibiotics inhibit protein synthesis, preventing the bacterial cell from replicating and thus spreading infection. These agents are usually bacteriostatic but can be bactericidal at high doses. Typical side effects from antibiotics include gastrointestinal dysfunction, which commonly results from a decrease in the natural gastrointestinal bacteria that inhabit the colon.

Antifungal and Antiviral Agents Fungi are parasitic microorganisms that cannot synthesize their own food. Fungal infections (mycoses) may be treated with several drugs. The azole antifungals inhibit fungal growth. Their prototype is ketoconazole (Nizoral). Drugs used to treat viruses work by a variety of mechanisms and include acyclovir (Zovirax) and zidovudine (Retrovir), which is commonly known as AZT. Protease inhibitors are one of the more promising classes of drugs for treating viruses such as HIV. Indinavir (Crixivan) is the prototype of this class.

Other Antimicrobial and Antiparasitic Agents While most diseases treated with the medications discussed in this section are uncommon in developed countries, they are leading causes of death in third-world countries. They include malaria, tuberculosis, leprosy, amebiasis, and helminthiasis. Tuberculosis is increasingly appearing in the United States in patients with compromised immune systems.

Malaria is a parasitic infection common in the tropics. It is transmitted by certain types of mosquitoes or, less commonly, by blood transfusion. Drugs used to treat malaria are called schizonticides. They include chloroquine (Aralen), mefloquine (Lariam), and quinine. Treatment is aimed at either preventing

infestation (prophylactic treatment for individuals traveling to high-risk areas) or killing the parasites in infected patients.

Tuberculosis is caused by bacteria that are transmitted through airborne droplets from the coughing and sneezing of infected patients. The bacteria can grow only in well-oxygenated areas. Because of the route of infection and the need for oxygen, most patients with tuberculosis have infections in the lungs. Once in the lungs, the bacteria are typically "walled off," or enclosed in tubercles, and become dormant and noninfective. If the patient's immune system is compromised, the bacteria may become active again and begin to cause symptoms. Drugs commonly used to treat tuberculosis include isoniazid (Nydrazid, INH) and rifampin (Rifadin).

Amebiasis is a parasitic infection of the intestines common in tropical areas. Transmission most frequently occurs via the oral-fecal route from eating poorly cooked food contaminated by cooks who inadequately wash their hands. Drugs used to treat amebiasis include paromomycin (Humatin) and metronidazole (Flagyl).

Helminthiasis is caused by parasitic worms (helminths) including flatworms and roundworms. These worms usually invade the host's intestinal tract and attach themselves to the lumen wall with hooks or suckers. They cause symptoms by depriving the host of nutrients (especially in children); by obstructing the intestinal lumen, which leads to bowel obstruction; and by producing toxins. Treatment is aimed at either killing the organism outright or destroying its ability to latch onto the intestinal wall so it passes with the patient's feces. These drugs include mebendazole (Vermox) and niclosamide (Niclocide).

Leprosy, also known as Hansen's disease, is caused by bacteria. It leads to characteristic lesions, footdrop (plantar flexion), and plantar ulceration. Drugs used to treat it include dapsone (DDS, Avlosulfon) and clofazimine (Lamprene).

Nonsteroidal Anti-Inflammatory Drugs NSAIDs (nonsteroidal anti-inflammatory drugs) are commonly used as analgesics and antipyretics (fever reducers). Many are available over the counter, including acetaminophen and ibuprofen. As a group, these agents interfere with the production of prostaglandins, thereby interrupting the inflammatory process. NSAIDs are indicated for the relief of pain, fever, and inflammation associated with common headache, arthritis, dysmenorrhea, and orthopedic injuries. They are also commonly prescribed to relieve pain following trauma and surgery. Other NSAIDs include ketorolac (Toradol), piroxicam (Feldene), and naproxen (Naprosyn).

Uricosuric Drugs Uricosuric drugs are used to treat and prevent acute episodes of gout. Gout is an inflammatory disease caused by an altered metabolism of uric acid and marked by hyperuricemia (high levels of uric acid in the blood). It may present with acute episodes characterized by pain and swelling of joints. Left untreated, gout may lead to crystal deposits in various parts of the body that can cause kidney stones, nephritis, and atherosclerosis. Drugs used to treat gout include colchicine and allopurinol (Zyloprim).

Serums, Vaccines, and Other Immunizing Agents The human body has a complex series of systems that help prevent disease. The most important of these are the anatomic barriers such as the skin and mucous membranes that block the entrance of **pathogens** (disease-causing organisms including viruses and bacteria). If pathogens get past these protective barriers, our immune system comes into play. This system consists of the spleen, lymph nodes, thymus, leukocytes, and proteins called antibodies in plasma. The ability to respond to pathogens is called **immunity**.

Immunity may be acquired passively or actively. It is passively acquired when antibodies pass directly into a person, either through artificial routes such as injection or through natural routes such as the placenta or breast milk. Immunity may also be actively acquired in response to the presence of a pathogen.

Actively acquired immunity occurs when T lymphocytes (a type of leukocyte that becomes specialized in the thymus gland) comes in contact with a new pathogen. The body produces an infinite variety of T cell configurations. When the pathogen comes into contact with a T cell that is specific to it, that T cell begins to rapidly reproduce. Some of these cells become involved in the immune response to the pathogen, while others act as "memory" cells. The cells involved in the immune response either directly attack the pathogen (cell-mediated immunity) or activate the complement system, a complex cascade of events that leads to the immune response. The memory cells remain in the body in higher numbers so that the next time this specific pathogen enters the body, a much faster response is possible. At the same time, B cells (lymphocytes that differentiate or become more specialized in the body, as opposed to the thymus) that are specific for the invading pathogen begin to produce antibodies for that antigen. This process is called humoral immunity or antibody immunity. When an antibody contacts its specific antigen, it forms a complex that triggers the complement system, leading to the immune response.

Serums and vaccines may augment the immune system. A **serum** is a solution containing whole antibodies for a specific pathogen. The antibodies give the recipient temporary, passive immunity. A **vaccine** contains a modified pathogen that does not actually cause disease but still stimulates the development of antibodies specific to it. These pathogens may be either dead or attenuated (having a decreased disease-causing ability).

The best age for vaccination against disease is within the first 2 years of life, as the immune system is fairly immature. Tables 3–29 and 3–30 summarize the recommended schedule for immunization.

Immune Suppressing and Enhancing Agents Available drugs can either suppress the immune system (immunosuppressants) or enhance it (immunomodulators). Suppressing the immune system is indicated to prevent the rejection of transplanted organs and grafted skin. Azathioprine (Imuran) is a commonly used immunosuppressant that acts by decreasing cell-mediated reactions and suppressing antibody production.

Immunomodulating agents enhance the natural immune reaction in immunosuppressed patients such as those with HIV. Zidovudine (Retrovir), commonly known as AZT, and several protease inhibitors such as ritonavir (Norvir) and saquinavir (Invirase) are examples of these agents.

DRUGS USED TO AFFECT THE SKIN

Dermatologic drugs are used to treat skin irritations. They are common over-the-counter medications. The many different general preparations include baths, soaps, solutions, cleansers, emollients (Lubriderm, Vaseline), skin protectants (Benzoin), wet dressings or soaks (Domeboro Powder), and rubs and liniments (Ben-Gay, Icy Hot). Prophylactic agents such as sunscreens are also available to help prevent skin disease and irritation.

DRUGS USED TO SUPPLEMENT THE DIET

Many disease processes affect the production, distribution, and utilization of essential dietary nutrients. Additionally, the body's intricate balance of fluid (including specific amounts of electrolytes) is a vital component of maintaining homeostasis. Dietary supplements can help to maintain needed levels of these essential nutrients and fluids.

Vitamins and Minerals

Vitamins are organic compounds necessary for many different physiologic processes including metabolism, growth, development, and tissue repair. The body absorbs most vitamins through the gastrointestinal tract following dietary ingestion. Vitamins must be obtained from the diet, as the body cannot manufacture them. In developed countries, healthy adults usually receive adequate amounts of vitamins and do not need supplements. Vitamin supplements may, however, be indicated for special populations including pregnant and nursing women, patients with absorption disorders, the chronically ill, surgery patients, alcoholics, and the malnourished. Additionally, people on a strict vegetarian diet may need supplemental vitamins. Vitamins are either fat-soluble or water soluble. The liver stores the fat-soluble vitamins (A, D, E, and K), so the patient will become deficient only after long periods of inadequate vitamin intake. Vitamin D is unique in that the skin produces it with exposure to sunlight. The water-soluble vitamins (C and those in the B complex) must be routinely ingested, as the body does not store them. After short periods of deprivation, patients may begin to experience vitamin deficiency. The B complex vitamins are grouped only because they occur together in foods; otherwise, they share no significant characteristics. The individual B vitamins are named for the order in which they were discovered (B_1, B_2, B_3, and so forth). These vitamins also have specific names. For example, B_1 is also known as thiamine, a vitamin that plays a key role in carbohydrate metabolism. It was once commonly administered in the prehospital setting for presumed Wernicke's encephalopathy (a disease commonly seen in chronic alcoholics that results from a deficiency in thiamine).[29] However, it has been determined that delaying administration to the hospital setting saves money and is just as effective. Table 3–31 details selected vitamins. Iron is an essential mineral necessary for oxygen transport and several metabolic processes. Iron supplements are the most common mineral supplement. They are indicated for iron deficiency.

TABLE 3–29 | Recommended Childhood (0–6 Years) Immunization Schedule United States, 2011

Recommended Immunization Schedule for Persons Aged 0 Through 6 Years—United States • 2011

For those who fall behind or start late, see the catch-up schedule

Vaccine ▼ Age ▶	Birth	1 month	2 months	4 months	6 months	12 months	15 months	18 months	19–23 months	2–3 years	4–6 years
Hepatitis B[1]	HepB	HepB				HepB					
Rotavirus[2]			RV	RV	RV[2]						
Diphtheria, Tetanus, Pertussis[3]			DTaP	DTaP	DTaP	see footnote[3]	DTaP				DTaP
Haemophilus influenzae type b[4]			Hib	Hib	Hib[4]	Hib					
Pneumococcal[5]			PCV	PCV	PCV	PCV				PPSV	
Inactivated Poliovirus[6]			IPV	IPV		IPV					IPV
Influenza[7]						Influenza (Yearly)					
Measles, Mumps, Rubella[8]						MMR		see footnote[8]			MMR
Varicella[9]						Varicella		see footnote[9]			Varicella
Hepatitis A[10]						HepA (2 doses)				HepA Series	
Meningococcal[11]										MCV4	

Range of recommended ages for all children

Range of recommended ages for certain high-risk groups

This schedule includes recommendations in effect as of December 21, 2010. Any dose not administered at the recommended age should be administered at a subsequent visit, when indicated and feasible. The use of a combination vaccine generally is preferred over separate injections of its equivalent component vaccines. Considerations should include provider assessment, patient preference, and the potential for adverse events. Providers should consult the relevant Advisory Committee on Immunization Practices statement for detailed recommendations: **http://www.cdc.gov/vaccines/pubs/acip-list.htm**. Clinically significant adverse events that follow immunization should be reported to the Vaccine Adverse Event Reporting System (VAERS) at **http://www.vaers.hhs.gov** or by telephone, **800-822-7967**. Use of trade names and commercial sources is for identification only and does not imply endorsement by the U.S. Department of Health and Human Services.

1. **Hepatitis B vaccine (HepB).** (Minimum age: birth)
   At birth:
   • Administer monovalent HepB to all newborns before hospital discharge.
   • If mother is hepatitis B surface antigen (HBsAg)-positive, administer HepB and 0.5 mL of hepatitis B immune globulin (HBIG) within 12 hours of birth.
   • If mother's HBsAg status is unknown, administer HepB within 12 hours of birth. Determine mother's HBsAg status as soon as possible and, if HBsAg-positive, administer HBIG (no later than age 1 week).
   Doses following the birth dose:
   • The second dose should be administered at age 1 or 2 months. Monovalent HepB should be used for doses administered before age 6 weeks.
   • Infants born to HBsAg-positive mothers should be tested for HBsAg and antibody to HBsAg 1 to 2 months after completion of at least 3 doses of the HepB series, at age 9 through 18 months (generally at the next well-child visit).
   • Administration of 4 doses of HepB to infants is permissible when a combination vaccine containing HepB is administered after the birth dose.
   • Infants who did not receive a birth dose should receive 3 doses of HepB on a schedule of 0, 1, and 6 months.
   • The final (3rd or 4th) dose in the HepB series should be administered no earlier than age 24 weeks.
2. **Rotavirus vaccine (RV).** (Minimum age: 6 weeks)
   • Administer the first dose at age 6 through 14 weeks (maximum age: 14 weeks 6 days). Vaccination should not be initiated for infants aged 15 weeks 0 days or older.
   • The maximum age for the final dose in the series is 8 months 0 days
   • If Rotarix is administered at ages 2 and 4 months, a dose at 6 months is not indicated.
3. **Diphtheria and tetanus toxoids and acellular pertussis vaccine (DTaP).** (Minimum age: 6 weeks)
   • The fourth dose may be administered as early as age 12 months, provided at least 6 months have elapsed since the third dose.
4. *Haemophilus influenzae* **type b conjugate vaccine (Hib).** (Minimum age: 6 weeks)
   • If PRP-OMP (PedvaxHIB or Comvax [HepB-Hib]) is administered at ages 2 and 4 months, a dose at age 6 months is not indicated.
   • Hiberix should not be used for doses at ages 2, 4, or 6 months for the primary series but can be used as the final dose in children aged 12 months through 4 years.
5. **Pneumococcal vaccine.** (Minimum age: 6 weeks for pneumococcal conjugate vaccine [PCV]; 2 years for pneumococcal polysaccharide vaccine [PPSV])
   • PCV is recommended for all children aged younger than 5 years. Administer 1 dose of PCV to all healthy children aged 24 through 59 months who are not completely vaccinated for their age.
   • A PCV series begun with 7-valent PCV (PCV7) should be completed with 13-valent PCV (PCV13).
   • A single supplemental dose of PCV13 is recommended for all children aged 14 through 59 months who have received an age-appropriate series of PCV7.
   • A single supplemental dose of PCV13 is recommended for all children aged 60 through 71 months with underlying medical conditions who have received an age-appropriate series of PCV7.

• The supplemental dose of PCV13 should be administered at least 8 weeks after the previous dose of PCV7. See *MMWR* 2010:59(No. RR-11).
• Administer PPSV at least 8 weeks after last dose of PCV to children aged 2 years or older with certain underlying medical conditions, including a cochlear implant.
6. **Inactivated poliovirus vaccine (IPV).** (Minimum age: 6 weeks)
   • If 4 or more doses are administered prior to age 4 years an additional dose should be administered at age 4 through 6 years.
   • The final dose in the series should be administered on or after the fourth birthday and at least 6 months following the previous dose.
7. **Influenza vaccine (seasonal).** (Minimum age: 6 months for trivalent inactivated influenza vaccine [TIV]; 2 years for live, attenuated influenza vaccine [LAIV])
   • For healthy children aged 2 years and older (i.e., those who do not have underlying medical conditions that predispose them to influenza complications), either LAIV or TIV may be used, except LAIV should not be given to children aged 2 through 4 years who have had wheezing in the past 12 months.
   • Administer 2 doses (separated by at least 4 weeks) to children aged 6 months through 8 years who are receiving seasonal influenza vaccine for the first time or who were vaccinated for the first time during the previous influenza season but only received 1 dose.
   • Children aged 6 months through 8 years who received no doses of monovalent 2009 H1N1 vaccine should receive 2 doses of 2010–2011 seasonal influenza vaccine. See *MMWR* 2010;59(No. RR-8):33–34.
8. **Measles, mumps, and rubella vaccine (MMR).** (Minimum age: 12 months)
   • The second dose may be administered before age 4 years, provided at least 4 weeks have elapsed since the first dose.
9. **Varicella vaccine.** (Minimum age: 12 months)
   • The second dose may be administered before age 4 years, provided at least 3 months have elapsed since the first dose.
   • For children aged 12 months through 12 years the recommended minimum interval between doses is 3 months. However, if the second dose was administered at least 4 weeks after the first dose, it can be accepted as valid.
10. **Hepatitis A vaccine (HepA).** (Minimum age: 12 months)
    • Administer 2 doses at least 6 months apart.
    • HepA is recommended for children aged older than 23 months who live in areas where vaccination programs target older children, who are at increased risk for infection, or for whom immunity against hepatitis A is desired.
11. **Meningococcal conjugate vaccine, quadrivalent (MCV4).** (Minimum age: 2 years)
    • Administer 2 doses of MCV4 at least 8 weeks apart to children aged 2 through 10 years with persistent complement component deficiency and anatomic or functional asplenia, and 1 dose every 5 years thereafter.
    • Persons with human immunodeficiency virus (HIV) infection who are vaccinated with MCV4 should receive 2 doses at least 8 weeks apart.
    • Administer 1 dose of MCV4 to children aged 2 through 10 years who travel to countries with highly endemic or epidemic disease and during outbreaks caused by a vaccine serogroup.
    • Administer MCV4 to children at continued risk for meningococcal disease who were previously vaccinated with MCV4 or meningococcal polysaccharide vaccine after 3 years if the first dose was administered at age 2 through 6 years.

The Recommended Immunization Schedules for Persons Aged 0 Through 18 Years are approved by the Advisory Committee on Immunization Practices (**http://www.cdc.gov/vaccines/recs/acip**), the American Academy of Pediatrics (**http://www.aap.org**), and the American Academy of Family Physicians (**http://www.aafp.org**).
Department of Health and Human Services • Centers for Disease Control and Prevention

TABLE 3–30 | Recommended Childhood (7–18 Years) Immunization Schedule United States, 2011

Recommended Immunization Schedule for Persons Aged 7 Through 18 Years—United States • 2011
For those who fall behind or start late, see the schedule below and the catch-up schedule

Vaccine ▼ Age ►	7–10 years	11–12 years	13–18 years	
Tetanus, Diphtheria, Pertussis[1]		Tdap	Tdap	Range of recommended ages for all children
Human Papillomavirus[2]	see footnote [2]	HPV (3 doses)(females)	HPV Series	
Meningococcal[3]	MCV4	MCV4	MCV4	
Influenza[4]		Influenza (Yearly)		Range of recommended ages for catch-up immunization
Pneumococcal[5]		Pneumococcal		
Hepatitis A[6]		HepA Series		
Hepatitis B[7]		Hep B Series		
Inactivated Poliovirus[8]		IPV Series		Range of recommended ages for certain high-risk groups
Measles, Mumps, Rubella[9]		MMR Series		
Varicella[10]		Varicella Series		

This schedule includes recommendations in effect as of December 21, 2010. Any dose not administered at the recommended age should be administered at a subsequent visit, when indicated and feasible. The use of a combination vaccine generally is preferred over separate injections of its equivalent component vaccines. Considerations should include provider assessment, patient preference, and the potential for adverse events. Providers should consult the relevant Advisory Committee on Immunization Practices statement for detailed recommendations: **http://www.cdc.gov/vaccines/pubs/acip-list.htm**. Clinically significant adverse events that follow immunization should be reported to the Vaccine Adverse Event Reporting System (VAERS) at **http://www.vaers.hhs.gov** or by telephone, **800-822-7967**.

1. **Tetanus and diphtheria toxoids and acellular pertussis vaccine (Tdap).**
   (Minimum age: 10 years for Boostrix and 11 years for Adacel)
   - Persons aged 11 through 18 years who have not received Tdap should receive a dose followed by Td booster doses every 10 years thereafter.
   - Persons aged 7 through 10 years who are not fully immunized against pertussis (including those never vaccinated or with unknown pertussis vaccination status) should receive a single dose of Tdap. Refer to the catch-up schedule if additional doses of tetanus and diphtheria toxoid–containing vaccine are needed.
   - Tdap can be administered regardless of the interval since the last tetanus and diphtheria toxoid–containing vaccine.
2. **Human papillomavirus vaccine (HPV).** (Minimum age: 9 years)
   - Quadrivalent HPV vaccine (HPV4) or bivalent HPV vaccine (HPV2) is recommended for the prevention of cervical precancers and cancers in females.
   - HPV is recommended for prevention of cervical precancers, cancers, and genital warts in females.
   - HPV4 may be administered in a 3-dose series to males aged 9 through 18 years to reduce their likelihood of genital warts.
   - Administer the second dose 1 to 2 months after the first dose and the third dose 6 months after the first dose (at least 24 weeks after the first dose).
3. **Meningococcal conjugate vaccine, quadrivalent (MCV4).** (Minimum age: 2 years)
   - Administer MCV4 at age 11 through 12 years with a booster dose at age 16 years.
   - Administer 1 dose at age 13 through 18 years if not previously vaccinated.
   - Persons who received their first dose at age 13 through 15 years should receive a booster dose at age 16 through 18 years.
   - Administer 1 dose to previously unvaccinated college freshmen living in a dormitory.
   - Administer 2 doses at least 8 weeks apart to children aged 2 through 10 years with persistent complement component deficiency and anatomic or functional asplenia, and 1 dose every 5 years thereafter.
   - Persons with HIV infection who are vaccinated with MCV4 should receive 2 doses at least 8 weeks apart.
   - Administer 1 dose of MCV4 to children aged 2 through 10 years who travel to countries with highly endemic or epidemic disease and during outbreaks caused by a vaccine serogroup.
   - Administer MCV4 to children at continued risk for meningococcal disease who were previously vaccinated with MCV4 or meningococcal polysaccharide vaccine after 3 years (if first dose administered at age 2 through 6 years) or after 5 years (if first dose administered at age 7 years or older).
4. **Influenza vaccine (seasonal).**
   - For healthy nonpregnant persons aged 7 through 18 years (i.e., those who do not have underlying medical conditions that predispose them to influenza complications), either LAIV or TIV may be used.
   - Administer 2 doses (separated by at least 4 weeks) to children aged 6 months through 8 years who are receiving seasonal influenza vaccine for the first

time or who were vaccinated for the first time during the previous influenza season but only received 1 dose.
   - Children 6 months through 8 years of age who received no doses of monovalent 2009 H1N1 vaccine should receive 2 doses of 2010-2011 seasonal influenza vaccine. See *MMWR* 2010;59(No. RR-8):33–34.
5. **Pneumococcal vaccines.**
   - A single dose of 13-valent pneumococcal conjugate vaccine (PCV13) may be administered to children aged 6 through 18 years who have functional or anatomic asplenia, HIV infection or other immunocompromising condition, cochlear implant or CSF leak. See *MMWR* 2010;59(No. RR-11).
   - The dose of PCV13 should be administered at least 8 weeks after the previous dose of PCV7.
   - Administer pneumococcal polysaccharide vaccine at least 8 weeks after the last dose of PCV to children aged 2 years or older with certain underlying medical conditions, including a cochlear implant. A single revaccination should be administered after 5 years to children with functional or anatomic asplenia or an immunocompromising condition.
6. **Hepatitis A vaccine (HepA).**
   - Administer 2 doses at least 6 months apart.
   - HepA is recommended for children aged older than 23 months who live in areas where vaccination programs target older children, or who are at increased risk for infection, or for whom immunity against hepatitis A is desired.
7. **Hepatitis B vaccine (HepB).**
   - Administer the 3-dose series to those not previously vaccinated. For those with incomplete vaccination, follow the catch-up schedule.
   - A 2-dose series (separated by at least 4 months) of adult formulation Recombivax HB is licensed for children aged 11 through 15 years.
8. **Inactivated poliovirus vaccine (IPV).**
   - The final dose in the series should be administered on or after the fourth birthday and at least 6 months following the previous dose.
   - If both OPV and IPV were administered as part of a series, a total of 4 doses should be administered, regardless of the child's current age.
9. **Measles, mumps, and rubella vaccine (MMR).**
   - The minimum interval between the 2 doses of MMR is 4 weeks.
10. **Varicella vaccine.**
   - For persons aged 7 through 18 years without evidence of immunity (see *MMWR* 2007;56[No. RR-4]), administer 2 doses if not previously vaccinated or the second dose if only 1 dose has been administered.
   - For persons aged 7 through 12 years, the recommended minimum interval between doses is 3 months. However, if the second dose was administered at least 4 weeks after the first dose, it can be accepted as valid.
   - For persons aged 13 years and older, the minimum interval between doses is 4 weeks.

The Recommended Immunization Schedules for Persons Aged 0 Through 18 Years are approved by the Advisory Committee on Immunization Practices (**http://www.cdc.gov/vaccines/recs/acip**), the American Academy of Pediatrics (**http://www.aap.org**), and the American Academy of Family Physicians (**http://www.aafp.org**). Department of Health and Human Services • Centers for Disease Control and Prevention

TABLE 3–31 | Vitamin Sources and Deficiencies

Vitamin	Problems Resulting from Deficiency	Source
Fat Soluble		
A	Night blindness, skin lesions	Butter, yellow fruit, green leafy vegetables, milk
D	Bone and muscle pain, weakness, softening of bones	Fish, fortified milk, exposure to sunlight
E	Hyporeflexia, ataxia, anemia	Nuts, green leafy vegetables, wheat
K	Increased bleeding	Liver, green leafy vegetables
Water Soluble		
B_1 (thiamine)	Peripheral neuritis, depression, anorexia, poor memory	Whole grain, beef, pork, peas, beans, nuts
B_2 (riboflavin)	Sore throat, stomatitis, painful or swollen tongue, anemia	Milk, eggs, cheese, green leafy vegetables
B_3 (niacin)	Skin eruptions, diarrhea, enteritis, headache, dizziness, insomnia	Meat, eggs, milk
B_6 (pyridoxine)	Skin lesions, seizures, peripheral neuritis	Liver, meats, eggs, vegetables
B_9 (folic acid)	Megaloblastic anemia	Liver, fresh green vegetables, yeast
B_{12} (cyanocobalamin)	Irreversible nervous system damage, pernicious anemia	Fish, egg yolk, milk
C	Scurvy	Citrus fruits, tomatoes, strawberries

Fluids and Electrolytes

Water comprises approximately 60 percent of a person's total body weight. The specific composition and amounts of this fluid are vital to a patient's well-being. The specific amounts of electrolytes such as calcium, potassium, sodium, and chlorine are similarly important. This book's chapter on pathophysiology reviews the physiology of fluids and electrolytes and discusses acid-base balance. The indications and contraindications for administering fluids and electrolytes, as well as these medications' interactions, are covered in the chapter on medication administration in this book and in the chapter on hemorrhage and shock, Volume 5, Chapter 4.

DRUGS USED TO TREAT POISONING AND OVERDOSES

The treatment for poisoning and overdose depends greatly on the substance involved. In general, therapy aims at eliminating the substance by emptying the gastric contents, by increasing gastric motility in order to decrease the time available for absorption, by alkalinizing the urine with sodium bicarbonate (for tricyclic antidepressant and salicylate overdose), or by filtering the substance from the blood with dialysis. Activated charcoal may be used as a gastric absorbent.[30]

Actual antidotes are few; however, some medications are effective in treating certain overdoses or poisonings. General mechanisms for antidote action include receptor site antagonism, blocking enzyme actions involved with metabolism of the substance, and chelation (binding the substance with a stable compound such as iron so that it becomes inactive). Specific antidotes include acetylcysteine (Mucomyst) for acetaminophen overdose and deferoxamine for iron chelation. Organophosphates are a common ingredient in insecticides and herbicides as well as chemical weapons. They are aggressive acetylcholinesterase (AChE) inhibitors that prevent the breakdown of acetylcholine, leading to overstimulation of the parasympathetic nervous system as well as neuromuscular junctions. Signs and symptoms of this overstimulation may be remembered by the acronym SLUDGE (salivation, lacrimation, urination, defecation, gastric motility, and emesis). Other signs include bradycardia, hypotension, bronchospasm, muscle fasciculations, miosis (pupil constriction), and respiratory arrest. The antidotes for organophosphate poisoning are atropine and pralidoxamine (2-PAM, Protopam). Atropine antagonizes ACh, while pralidoxamine breaks the organophosphate-acetylcholinesterase bond, freeing AChE to break down the excess ACh. Hydroxocobalamin is now available as an antidote for cyanide poisoning. Hydroxocobalamin is a precursor to cyanocobalamin (vitamin B_{12}). When administered, it chelates the cyanide molecule from cytochrome oxidase, thus restoring normal energy production. It has largely replaced the old cyanide antidote kit.[31] See Table 3–32 for common antidotes.

TABLE 3-32 | Common Antidotes

Name	Classification	Action	Indications	Contraindications	Doses	Routes	Adverse Effects	Other
Naloxone *Narcan*	Opiate antagonist	Opioid antagonist without opiate agonist properties (it has no activity when given in the absence of an opiate agonist)	• Partial reversal of opiate drug effects • Opiate overdose	• Hypersensitivity to the drug	0.4– 2.0 mg	IV, IO, SQ, IO, IN, nebulizer	• Fever • Chills • Nausea • Vomiting • Diarrhea • Opiate withdrawal	• Administer enough to reverse respiratory depression and avoid full narcotic withdrawal syndrome
Flumazenil *Romazicon*	Benzodiazepine antagonist	Competitively blocks benzodiazepines at the GABA/benzodiazepine receptor complex	• Benzodiazepine overdose	• Hypersensitivity to the drug	0.2 mg	IV	• Fatigue • Headache • Nervousness • Dizziness	• Administer with caution in patients dependent on benzodiazepines as life-threatening withdrawal (including seizures) can occur
Hydroxoco-balamin *Cyanokit*	Cyanide antidote	Chelates cyanide from cytochrome oxidase forming cyanocobalamin (vitamin B_{12})	• Cyanide or suspected cyanide poisoning	• None in the emergency setting	5–10 g	IV	• Chromaturia • Red skin • Rash • Hypertension • Nausea • Headache	• Be prepared to continue full resuscitative measures following administration

Drug		Mechanism	Indication	Contraindications	Dose	Route	Adverse effects	Notes
Amyl nitrite	Cyanide antidote	Vasodilator; oxidizes hemoglobin to methemoglobin which reacts with cyanide ion to form cyanomethemoglobin, that is enzymatically degraded	• Cyanide poisoning	• None in the emergency setting	1–2 inhalants	Inhaled	• Headache • Weakness • Dizziness • Flushing • Tachycardia • Orthostatic hypotension	• Headache and hypotension common • Can worsen hypoxia in the setting of carbon monoxide poisoning
Sodium nitrite	Cyanide antidote	Vasodilator; oxidizes hemoglobin to methemoglobin which reacts with cyanide ion to form cyanomethemoglobin, that is enzymatically degraded	• Cyanide poisoning	• Should not be administered to asymptomatic patients	150–300 mg	IV	• Headache • Weakness • Dizziness • Flushing • Tachycardia • Orthostatic hypotension	• Headache and hypotension common • Can worsen hypoxia in the setting of carbon monoxide poisoning
Sodium thiosulfate	Cyanide antidote	Converts cyanide to thiocyanate which is removed by the kidneys	• Cyanide poisoning	• None in the emergency setting	12.5 g	IV	• Nausea • Vomiting • Joint pain • Psychosis	• Should be administered as part of the standard (Pasadena) cyanide kit
Pralidoxime *2-PAM, Protpam*	Organophosphate antidote	Reactivates cholinesterase; deactivates certain organophosphates	• Organophosphate poisoning	• Poisonings other than organophosphates	1–2 g over 30 minutes	IV	• Excitement • Manic behavior • Laryngospasm • Tachycardia	• Always protect rescue personnel from the poison • 2-PAM administration should always follow atropinization

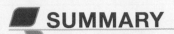

SUMMARY

Pharmacology is a cornerstone of paramedic practice. Paramedics must have a solid understanding of its foundations (legal issues, terminology, drug forms, and routes), pharmacokinetics, and pharmacodynamics if they are to practice their profession safely. Additionally, paramedics must understand not only the medications they personally administer, but also the medications that their patients are taking on an ongoing basis. You are personally, ethically, and legally responsible for every medication you administer. If medical direction orders you to give a medication or a dosage that is potentially dangerous, it is your responsibility to question and even refuse to administer a harmful medication or dosage.

While you are not likely to remember everything in this chapter after your first reading, with diligent study and practice you can master this information. This chapter has barely broken the surface of pharmacology. To continue your education, you should take the time to understand the mechanisms and interactions of the medications your patients are taking. If you do not already know them (you will not in the majority of cases as you begin your career), look them up. Many very useful drug references are available today. Most are small and can be easily carried with you on a smart phone, on your unit, or in your station.

Pharmacology is a dynamic field with new discoveries being made every day. Emergency treatments are constantly changing, based on the latest results of pharmacological studies. If you take your responsibilities as a paramedic seriously and practice lifelong learning, remaining current on the latest changes in this field, you can be confident in your ability to give your patients the care they deserve.

YOU MAKE THE CALL

You and your partner are caring for a 62-year-old male with acute pulmonary edema and cardiogenic shock. He is responsive only to painful stimuli, has ashen skin, and is very diaphoretic. He is in obvious respiratory distress with a rate of 36 per minute. You note bilateral crackles in all fields. His blood pressure is 82/50, and his heart rate is 108. The ECG shows atrial fibrillation. You immediately have your partner begin assisting the patient's ventilations with a bag-valve mask and 100 percent high-flow, high-concentration oxygen. You establish a saline lock and begin to administer a dopamine infusion through one of them at 6 mcg/kg/min and move the patient to your unit for transport to the hospital.

The dopamine appears to be helping, as your patient's blood pressure rises to 110/60; however, your partner is having an increasingly difficult time bagging the patient, whose oxygen saturation has not risen above 86 percent. You decide to perform a facilitated intubation and administer the following medications: 0.5 mg of atropine, 1.0 mg/kg of lidocaine, and 5.0 mg of midazolam (Versed). Your partner applies cricoid pressure, and you then administer 1.5 mg/kg of succinylcholine. After placing a size 8.0 ET tube, you confirm placement and secure the tube. Now that the patient is being successfully ventilated, you turn your attention back to the pulmonary edema. As you are delivering your patient to the ED staff, you note that his color and breath sounds have improved remarkably and the pulse oximeter now reads 96 percent.

1. What is dopamine and what is its mechanism of action?

2. What was the purpose of the dopamine infusion?

3. What is atropine's mechanism of action?

4. What is the purpose of giving lidocaine to this patient?

5. Why was midazolam administered before succinylcholine?

6. What are succinylcholine's classification and mechanism of action?

See Suggested Responses at the back of this book.

REVIEW QUESTIONS

1. The study of drugs and their interactions with the body is called:
a. physiology.
c. pharmacology.
b. toxicology.
d. pharmacopeia.

2. A drug or other substance that blocks the actions of the sympathetic nervous system is called:
a. adrenergic.
c. sympathomimetic.
b. sympatholytic.
d. anticholinergic.

3. _____ is the preferred antihypertensive for the management of pregnancy-induced hypertension.
   a. Coreg
   b. Apresoline
   c. Captopril
   d. Nifedipine

4. Because they can thicken bronchial secretions, you should not use _____ in patients with asthma.
   a. mucolytics
   b. antitussives
   c. antihistamines
   d. antiarrrhythmics

5. The following describes a Schedule _____ drug: High abuse potential; may lead to severe dependence; accepted medical indications.
   a. I   c. III
   b. II   d. IV

6. An example of an anticholinergic drug used in the treatment of asthma is:
   a. atropine.
   b. ephedrine.
   c. proventil.
   d. beclovent.

7. The drug name found in the *United States Pharmacopeia* (USP) is its:
   a. official name.   c. generic name.
   b. chemical name.   d. trade name.

8. The drug name that is derived from its chemical composition is referred to as its:
   a. official name.
   b. chemical name.
   c. generic name.
   d. trade name.

9. The proprietary name of a drug, such as Valium, is the same as the:
   a. official name.
   b. chemical name.
   c. generic name.
   d. trade name.

10. Drug legislation was instituted in 1906 by the:
    a. Narcotics Act.
    b. Cosmetics Act.
    c. Pure Food and Drug Act.
    d. Pharmacology Act.

11. _____ drug sources may provide alternative sources of medications to those found in nature, or they may be entirely new medications not found in nature.
    a. Plant
    b. Animal
    c. Synthetic
    d. Mineral

12. The six rights of medication administration include the right:
    a. dose.
    b. time.
    c. route.
    d. all of the above.

13. Which of the following routes is the least appropriate for medication administration in the prehospital setting?
    a. oral
    b. sublingual
    c. subcutaneous
    d. intravenous

14. Drugs manufactured in gelatin containers are called:
    a. pills.
    b. tablets.
    c. capsules.
    d. extracts.

15. A drug's pharmacodynamics involves its ability to cause the expected response, or:
    a. affinity.
    b. efficacy.
    c. side effect.
    d. contraindication.

16. A type of anesthesia that combines decreased sensation of pain with amnesia, while the patient remains conscious, is a(n):
    a. opioid.
    b. nonopioid.
    c. anesthetic.
    d. neuroleptanesthesia.

17. _____ agents oppose the parasympathetic nervous system.
    a. Cholinergic
    b. Adrenergic
    c. Antiadrenergic
    d. Anticholinergic

18. In antiarrhythmic classifications, Class IA drugs include all of the following except:
    a. quinidine.
    b. lidocaine.
    c. procainamide.
    d. disopyramide.

19. One of aspirin's primary side effects is:
    a. stasis.   c. headache.
    b. bleeding.   d. seizures.

20. _____ are mediators released from mast cells upon contact with allergens.
    a. Histamines
    b. Leukotrienes
    c. Glucocorticoids
    d. Methylxanthines

See Answers to Review Questions at the back of this book.

REFERENCES

1. Olasveengen, T. M., K. Sunde, C. Brunborg, J. Thowsen, P. A. Steen, and L. Wik. "Intravenous Drug Administration during Out-of-Hospital Cardiac Arrest: A Randomized Trial." *JAMA* 302 (2009): 2222–2229.

2. Niemann, J. T., S. J. Stratton, B. Cruz, and R. J. Lewis. "Endotracheal Drug Administration during Out-of-Hospital Resuscitation: Where Are the Survivors?" *Resuscitation* 53 (2002): 153–157.

3. Fowler, R., J. V. Gallagher, S. M. Isaacs, E. Ossman, P. Pepe, and M. Wayne. "The Role of Intraosseous Vascular Access in the Out-of-Hospital Environment (Resource Document to NAEMSP Position Statement)." *Prehosp Emerg Care* 11 (2007): 63–66.

4. Thomas, S. H., O. Rago, T. Harrison, P. D. Biddinger, and S. K. Wedel. "Fentanyl Trauma Analgesia Use in Air Medical Scene Transports." *J Emerg Med* 29 (2005): 179–187.

5. Galinski, M., F. Dolveck, S. W. Borron et al. "A Randomized, Double-Blind Study Comparing Morphine with Fentanyl in Prehospital Analgesia." *American Journal of Emergency Medicine* 23 (2005): 114–119.

6. Green, R., B. Bulloch, A. Kabani, B. J. Hancock, and M. Tenenbein. "Early Analgesia for Children with Acute Abdominal Pain." *Pediatrics* 116 (2005): 978–983.

7. Kanowitz, A., T. M. Dunn, E. M. Kanowitz, W. W. Dunn, and K. Vanbuskirk. "Safety and Effectiveness of Fentanyl Administration for Prehospital Pain Management." *Prehosp Emerg Care* 10 (2006): 1–7.

8. Meine, T. J., M. T. Roe, A. Y. Chen et al. "Association of Intravenous Morphine Use and Outcomes in Acute Coronary Syndromes: Results from the CRUSADE Quality Improvement Initiative." *Am Heart J* 149 (2005): 1043–1049.

9. Rickard, C., P. O'Meara, M. McGrail, D. Garner, A. McLean, and P. Le Lievre. "A Randomized Controlled Trial of Intranasal Fentanyl vs. Intravenous Morphine for Analgesia in the Prehospital Setting." *Am J Emerg Med* 25 (2007): 911–917.

10. Pace, S. and T. F. Burke. "Intravenous Morphine for Early Pain Relief in Patients with Acute Abdominal Pain." *Acad Emerg Med* 3 (1996): 1086–1092.

11. Barton, E. D., C. B. Colwell, T. Wolfe et al. "Efficacy of Intranasal Naloxone as a Needleless Alternative for Treatment of Opioid Overdose in the Prehospital Setting." *J Emerg Med* 29 (2005): 265–271.

12. Kelly, A. M., D. Kerr, P. Dietze, I. Patrick, T. Walker, and Z. Koutsogiannis. "Randomised Trial of Intranasal versus Intramuscular Naloxone in Prehospital Treatment for Suspected Opioid Overdose." *Med J Aust* 182 (2005): 24–27.

13. Robertson, T. M., G. W. Hendey, G. Stroh, and M. Shalit. "Intranasal Naloxone Is a Viable Alternative to Intravenous Naloxone for Prehospital Narcotic Overdose." *Prehosp Emerg Care* 13 (2009): 512–515.

14. Holsti, M., B. L. Sill, S. D. Firth, F. M. Filloux, S. M. Joyce, and R. A. Furnival. "Prehospital Intranasal Midazolam for the Treatment of Pediatric Seizures." *Pediatr Emerg Care* 23 (2007): 148–153.

15. Kress, J. P. and Hall J. B. "Sedation in the Mechanically Ventilated Patient." *Crit Care Med* 34 (2006): 2541–2546.

16. Bulger, E. M., M. K. Copass, D. R. Sabath, R. V. Maier, and G. J. Jurkovich. "The Use of Neuromuscular Blocking Agents to Facilitate Prehospital Intubation Does Not Impair Outcome after Traumatic Brain Injury." *J Trauma* 58 (2005): 718–723; discussion 723–724.

17. Wyer, P. C., P. Perera, Z. Jin et al. "Vasopressin or Epinephrine for Out-of-Hospital Cardiac Arrest." *Ann Emerg Med* 48 (2006): 86–97.

18. Ong, M. E., E. H. Tan, F. S. Ng et al. "Survival Outcomes with the Introduction of Intravenous Epinephrine in the Management of Out-of-Hospital Cardiac Arrest." *Ann Emerg Med* 50 (2007): 635–642.

19. De Backer, D., P. Biston, J. Devriendt et al. "Comparison of Dopamine and Norepinephrine in the Treatment of Shock." *N Engl J Med* 362 (2010): 779–789.

20. Delbridge, T., R. Domeier, and C. B. Key. "Prehospital Asthma Management." *Prehosp Emerg Care* 7 (2003): 42–47.

21. Christianson, G., A. Woolf, and K. R. Olson. "β-Blocker Ingestion: An Evidence-Based Consensus Guideline for Out-of-Hospital Management." *Clinical Toxicology* 43 (2005): 131–146.

22. Marill, K. A., I. S. deSouza, D. K. Nishijima, T. O. Stair, G. S. Setnik, and J. N. Ruskin. "Amiodarone Is Poorly Effective for the Acute Termination of Ventricular Tachycardia." *Ann Emerg Med* 47 (2006): 217–224.

23. Kessler, C. S. and Y. Joudeh. "Evaluation and Treatment of Severe Asymptomatic Hypertension." *Am Fam Physician* 81 (2010): 470–476.

24. Tang, W. H. "Pharmacological Therapy for Acute Heart Failure." *Cardiol Clin* 25 (2007): 539–551; vi.

25. Anderson, J. L., C. D. Adams, E. M. Antman et al. "ACC/AHA 2007 Guidelines for the Management of Patients with Unstable Angina/Non ST-Elevation Myocardial Infarction: A Report of the American College of Cardiology/American Heart Association Task Force on Practice Guidelines (Writing Committee to Revise the 2002 Guidelines for the Management of Patients with Unstable Angina/Non ST-Elevation Myocardial Infarction): Developed in Collaboration with the American College of Emergency Physicians, the Society for Cardiovascular Angiography and Interventions, and the Society of Thoracic Surgeons: Endorsed by the American Association of Cardiovascular and Pulmonary Rehabilitation and the Society for Academic Emergency Medicine." *Circulation* 116 (2007): e148–e304.

26. Pedley, D. K., K. Bissett, E. M. Connolly et al. "Prospective Observational Cohort Study of Time Saved by Prehospital Thrombolysis for ST Elevation Myocardial Infarction Delivered by Paramedics." *BMJ* 327 (2003): 22–26.

27. Gueugniaud, P. Y., J. S. David, E. Chanzy et al. "Vasopressin and Epinephrine vs. Epinephrine Alone in Cardiopulmonary Resuscitation." *N Engl J Med* 359 (2008): 21–30.

28. Knapp, B. and C. Wood. "The Prehospital Administration of Intravenous Methylprednisolone Lowers Hospital Admission Rates for Moderate to Severe Asthma." *Prehosp Emerg Care* 7 (2003): 423–426.

29. Donnino, M. W., J. Vega, J. Miller, and M. Walsh. "Myths and Misconceptions of Wernicke's Encephalopathy: What Every Emergency Physician Should Know." *Ann Emerg Med* 50 (2007): 715–721.

30. Manoguerra, A. S. and D. J. Cobaugh. "Guidelines for the Management of Poisoning Consensus Panel. Guideline on the Use of Ipecac Syrup in the Out-of-Hospital Management of Ingested Poisons." *Clin Toxicol (Phila)* 43 (2005): 1–10.

31. Borron, S. W., F. J. Baud, P. Barriot, M. Imbert, and C. Bismuth. "Prospective Study of Hydroxocobalamin for Acute Cyanide Poisoning in Smoke Inhalation." *Ann Emerg Med* 49 (2007): 794–801, 801.e1–e2.

 FURTHER READING

Bledsoe, Bryan E. and Dwayne E. Clayden. *Prehospital Emergency Pharmacology.* 7th ed. Upper Saddle River, NJ: Pearson/Prentice Hall, 2012.

Katzung, Bertram G. *Basic and Clinical Pharmacology.* 11th ed. Philadelphia: McGraw-Hill Medical, 2009.

Shannon, Margaret T., Billie Ann Wilson, and Carolyn L. Stang. *Prentice Hall's Health Professionals Drug Guide 2009–2010.* Upper Saddle River, NJ: Pearson/Prentice Hall, 2010.

4

Intravenous Access and Medication Administration

Bryan Bledsoe, DO, FACEP, FAAEM, EMT-P

STANDARD
Pharmacology (Medication Administration)

COMPETENCY
Integrates comprehensive knowledge of pharmacology to formulate a treatment plan intended to mitigate emergencies and improve the overall health of the patient.

OBJECTIVES

Terminal Performance Objective
After reading this chapter you should be able to apply concepts of pharmacology to the assessment and management of patients.

Enabling Objectives
To accomplish the terminal performance objective, you should be able to:

1. Define key terms introduced in this chapter.

2. Apply the six rights of medication administration when administering patient medications.

3. Identify the boundaries of your scope of practice pertaining to medication administration.

4. Recognize situations involving medication administration in which you should communicate directly with a medical direction physician.

5. Select the appropriate standard precautions for all medication administration situations.

6. Demonstrate principles of medical asepsis in the administration of medications.

7. Accurately and completely document the pertinent details of administering medication to a patient.

8. Describe the procedures, precautions, risks, equipment, advantages, and disadvantages of each of the routes of percutaneous, pulmonary, enteral, and parenteral medication administration.

9. Demonstrate the safe administration of medications allowed in your scope of practice under the supervision of a lab instructor or clinical preceptor, including medications administered by percutaneous, pulmonary, enteral, and parenteral routes.

10. Prepare medications for administration from a variety of types of packaging, including vials, non-constituted vials, ampules, prefilled syringes, and packaging for intravenous solutions.

11. Describe the indications, contraindications, procedure, equipment, and risks associated with peripheral intravenous access.

12. Describe devices used for central venous access.

13. Describe the characteristics of various intravenous fluids, including colloids, crystalloids, and oxygen-carrying solutions.

14. Given a variety of scenarios, select an appropriate intravenous fluid, infusion set, catheter, and infusion rate.

15. Assemble an intravenous infusion line.

16. Establish a peripheral intravenous line under the supervision of a lab instructor or clinical preceptor.

17. Troubleshoot an intravenous infusion.

18. Recognize complications of intravenous infusion.

19. Change an intravenous solution bag or bottle.

20. Establish a heparin or saline lock under the supervision of a lab instructor or clinical preceptor.

21. If permitted in your scope of practice, access an implanted venous access device under the supervision of a lab instructor or clinical preceptor.

22. Demonstrate venous blood sampling under the supervision of a lab instructor or clinical preceptor.

23. Discontinue a peripheral intravenous infusion.

24. Establish an intraosseous infusion in adult and pediatric patients under the supervision of a lab instructor or clinical preceptor.

25. Troubleshoot an intraosseous infusion.

26. Recognize complications of an intraosseous infusion.

27. Identify indications and contraindications for intraosseous infusion.

28. Given a variety of scenarios involving medication orders and patient factors, precisely calculate intravenous infusion rates and drug dosages.

KEY TERMS

administration tubing, p. 257
air embolism, p. 268
ampule, p. 244
anticoagulant, p. 268
antiseptic, p. 232
asepsis, p. 231
aural medication, p. 236
blood tube, p. 275
blood tubing, p. 259
bolus, p. 242
buccal, p. 234
burette chamber, p. 259
cannula, pp. 257, 260
cannulation, p. 254
catheter inserted through the needle, p. 261
central venous access, p. 255
circulatory overload, p. 268
colloidal solution, p. 256
concentration, p. 286
crystalloid, p. 256
desired dose, p. 286
disinfectant, p. 232
dosage on hand, p. 286
drip chamber, p. 258
drip rate, p. 258
drop former, p. 258
drops, p. 258
drugs, p. 229
embolus, p. 268

enema, p. 242
enteral route, p. 238
extension tubing, p. 258
extravasation, p. 266
extravascular, p. 274
gauge, p. 243
hemoconcentration, p. 277
hemolysis, p. 277
heparin lock, p. 272
hepatic alteration, p. 240
hollow-needle catheter, p. 261
Huber needle, p. 273
hypertonic, p. 256
hypodermic needle, p. 243
hypotonic, p. 256
induced therapeutic hypothermia (ITH), p. 257
infusion, p. 247
infusion controller, p. 274
infusion pump, p. 274
infusion rate, p. 289
inhalation, p. 236
injection, p. 236
intracatheter, p. 261
intradermal, p. 249
intramuscular, p. 251
intraosseous, p. 277
intravenous (IV) access, p. 254

intravenous fluid, p. 256
isotonic, p. 256
IV catheter, p. 260
local, p. 231
Luer sampling needle, p. 276
macrodrip tubing, p. 258
measured volume administration set, p. 259
medically clean, p. 231
medicated solution, p. 247
medication injection port, p. 258
medications, p. 229
metered dose inhaler, p. 237
microdrip tubing, p. 258
Mix-o-Vial, p. 246
nasal medication, p. 235
nebulizer, p. 236
necrosis, p. 268
needle adapter, p. 258
nonconstituted medication vial, p. 246
ocular medication, p. 235
over-the-needle catheter, p. 260
parenteral route, p. 242
peripheral venous access, p. 255
peripherally inserted central catheter (PICC), p. 255

CASE STUDY

It is early in February, and clouds heavy with snow loom not far in the distance. Paramedic Susan Adams watches the sky and hopes she will get off work on time, before the storm hits. Suddenly the tones drop, alerting her and her partner, Advanced EMT Todd Michaels, of a 28-year-old female patient with shortness of breath. After acknowledging the call and confirming the location with their GPS device, Susan and Todd get under way. In preparation, Susan dons gloves and eye protection. Additionally, she reviews the likely causes of shortness of breath in a 28-year-old patient.

As Susan and Todd pull up to the residence, they observe a well-kept house. A woman frantically waves them inside, shouting that her daughter cannot breathe. Quickly, they grab the airway kit, cardiac monitor, and medication bag, then cautiously enter the residence.

Once inside, Susan and Todd begin to size up the scene. Immediately to their left, they find the female patient seated on a chair in the tripod position. Quick observation reveals her to be in considerable respiratory distress and exhibiting cyanosis around the lips and in the extremities. Even without a stethoscope, Susan detects expiratory wheezing.

Promptly, Susan introduces herself and Todd to the patient and asks what is wrong. As the patient can barely talk, Susan cannot obtain a specific chief complaint. Recognizing a life-threatening situation, she gains consent for treatment and turns her attention to the primary assessment.

The patient is responsive but exhibits lethargy and fatigue from the increased work of breathing and hypoxia. Inspection of her oral cavity reveals no foreign bodies or other obstructions. Susan deems the patient able to maintain her airway and forgoes a nasopharyngeal airway adjunct.

The patient presents tachypneic at 36 breaths per minute. Tidal and minute volumes are shallow. Todd obtains a pulse oximetry reading of 86 percent on room air. Exhaled carbon dioxide ($EtCO_2$) is 55 mmHg. A quick 2-point auscultation reveals expiratory wheezing in the upper lobes of both the right and left lungs. As the patient will not tolerate the assistance of ventilations with a bag-valve mask, Susan applies a nonrebreather face mask with 15 liters per minute of supplemental oxygen.

Without missing a beat, Susan proceeds to evaluate the circulatory system. The patient's radial pulse is weak and rapid, with accompanying cool, diaphoretic skin. Again Susan notes cyanosis.

Realizing the situation is critical, Susan turns to the patient's mother while Todd applies the cardiac monitor and obtains vital signs. When Susan asks about a history of asthma, the mother confirms it and adds that this particular episode has been occurring over the past day and a half. Her daughter's metered-dose inhaler of albuterol has not provided any relief, as it has in the past. Aside from the asthma, the patient has no other medical history. She has no allergies and has not eaten or drunk anything today.

Confident that she is dealing with an asthmatic patient, Susan performs a detailed secondary assessment. She accordingly notes bilateral distention of the jugular veins and retractions at the suprasternal notch and intercostal spaces, along with nasal flaring and pursed lips. Quickly she auscultates breath sounds from the posterior thorax in a 6-point pattern. She observes bilateral expiratory wheezing in the apices of the lungs with no net air movement in the bases.

Todd informs Susan of the patient's vital signs: pulse, 116 beats per minute; respirations, 56 per minute; and blood pressure, 152/94 mmHg. With the primary assessment and history obtained, Susan begins emergency interventions. The cardiac monitor displays sinus tachycardia with no ectopy.

As Todd obtains a venous blood sample and establishes an IV line, Susan assembles a nebulizer and adds a solution of 2.5 mg of albuterol and 500 mcg of ipratropium (diluted in 3 mL of normal saline) to the chamber. She gives the nebulizer complete with medication to the patient for self-administration. Susan proceeds to administer 125 mg of methyl-prednisolone (Solu-Medrol) intravenously. Todd prepares the cot and loads the patient for transport. The patient is exhibiting minimal improvement with the nebulizer treatment. Susan places a continuous-positive airway pressure (CPAP) mask and begins CPAP with 100 percent oxygen. The patient quickly starts to pink up. The albuterol is placed in an in-line delivery system so that the patient receives the medication through the CPAP device.

En route to the hospital, Susan performs reassessment by evaluating the components of the primary assessment and the effects of all interventions. The patient now is more alert and breathes easier. Her pulse oximetry reads 92 percent, and her expiratory wheezing has subsided significantly. Her $EtCO_2$ has dropped to 50 mmHg. Susan now notes air movement in the bases of the lungs. Additionally, the cyanosis and diaphoresis have almost subsided, and vital signs have returned to normal limits. Because the pulse oximeter reading is still low and some residual wheezing persists, Susan gives another nebulized treatment of 2.5 mg of albuterol (without ipratropium). She alerts the receiving hospital.

Once at the hospital, Susan and Todd turn over care to the emergency department staff. Later they find out that the woman was admitted for overnight observation with the diagnosis of acute exacerbation of asthma. She is doing fine and is expected to be released in the morning.

INTRODUCTION

Drugs are foreign substances placed into the human body. **Medications** are drugs used for medical purposes. They serve a variety of purposes, such as controlling specific diseases like hypertension or helping the body cure diseases like cancer and infection.

Medication administration will be an important part of the medical care you provide as a paramedic. You may have to use medications to correct or prevent many life-threatening situations. You may also use them to stabilize or comfort a patient in distress. In addition to your knowledge of particular medications and their properties from the previous chapter on pharmacology, you must also be thoroughly skilled in medication administration. Specific medications require specific routes and administration techniques. Their effectiveness depends directly on their correct route of delivery. Incorrect or sloppy medication administration can have tremendous legal implications for the paramedic. More important, it equates to poor care that can harm or even kill the patient.

This chapter discusses the routes and techniques you will use to correctly deliver your patient's medications. It is divided into three parts:

Part 1: Principles and Routes of Medication Administration

Part 2: Intravenous Access, Blood Sampling, and Intraosseous Infusion

Part 3: Medical Mathematics

PART 1: Principles and Routes of Medication Administration

GENERAL PRINCIPLES

As a paramedic, you are responsible for ensuring that all emergency medications are in place and ready for immediate use. Therefore, you must know your local medication distribution

CONTENT REVIEW

▶ Six Rights of Drug Administration

• Right person
• Right drug
• Right dose
• Right time
• Right route
• Right documentation

system. You will have to know where to obtain and replace each medication as it expires or is used, as another patient may require it at any time. You also will have to thoroughly document the administration and restocking of narcotics, as many local, state, and federal agencies mandate such record keeping.

Always be certain that you correctly give all medications in the right dose. Medication errors may prove disastrous in terms of patient care and legal responsibility. Your knowledge of medication indications, contraindications, side effects, dosages, and routes of administration is crucial to effective patient care. (See Volume 2, Chapter 3.)

You can attain effective pharmacological therapy and eliminate medication errors by following the six rights of medication administration:

Right person. Ensure that the patient receiving the medication is the right person. Generally, you will provide one-on-one attention. In a clinical setting, however, keeping track of multiple patients proves more challenging.

Right medication. Ensure that you administer the proper medication. Many medications are contained in similar appearing packages. To avoid inadvertently delivering the incorrect medication, read the label! Administering the incorrect medication can have disastrous consequences.

Right dose. Be certain that you administer the exact dosage of any medication. The correct dose may be standardized or require calculation. Never underdose or overdose a patient.

Right time. Timing their administration is important for many medications. Typically, in the emergent setting, you will quickly administer the necessary emergency medications. During transfers and critical care transports, you may have to administer other medications at preestablished intervals.

Right route. Specific medications require specific delivery routes. You must not only be familiar with the properties of individual medications but also with their different routes of administration.

Right documentation. Documenting medication administration is of paramount importance. You must record all appropriate information about every medication you administer. Pertinent information includes, but is not limited to, medication name(s), dose, route of delivery, person administering, time administered, and patient response to the medication—both good and bad.

In the field, you will be responsible for the safe and appropriate delivery of medications. If you ever doubt the use or dosage of a medication, contact medical direction immediately. You must repeat back, or echo, all medication orders issued by on-line medical direction. For example, if medical direction ordered you to administer 25 mg of diphenhydramine (Benadryl), you would echo, "Medic 101 copies the medication order for 25 mg of diphenhydramine to be administered slow IV push." By echoing, you confirm your reception and understanding of the order. If medical direction has issued an inappropriate medication or dosage, echoing may bring it to light and elicit an immediate correction. If you still find the order questionable after echoing, diplomatically request clarification or ask about the intent.

Pharmacological therapy permits you to function as an extension of the physician. No room exists for medication errors, as once a medication is given it is difficult, if not impossible, to retrieve. In addition, withholding a needed medication can have catastrophic consequences. Concentration and knowledge are the keys to this component of paramedical care.

Medical Direction

Paramedics do not practice autonomously. You will operate under the license of a medical director who is responsible for all of your actions. This responsibility extends to the administration of medications.

The medical director (or the EMS system) determines which medications you will use and the routes by which you will deliver them. Some states have a "state medication list" whereby the medications a service carries are dictated by law or a legislative or regulatory agency. While some medications can be administered via off-line medical direction (written standing orders), you may need specific authorization for others after consulting on-line or direct medical direction. You must strictly abide by all of your medical director's guidelines.

Knowing all medication administration protocols is essential, especially which medications to administer under standing orders and which to deliver only after getting authorization from medical direction. You can ill afford to waste valuable time looking up procedures and directives for the critical patient who requires immediate medication therapy. Furthermore, because inappropriate medication delivery can have serious consequences, you may face severe legal ramifications even if your patient suffers no harm.[1, 2]

Standard Precautions

Establishing routes for medication delivery presents the constant potential for exposure to blood and other body fluids. Formerly called *body substance isolation (BSI),* the strategy is now called **Standard Precautions**. In 1996 (and updated in 2007), the Centers for Disease Control and Prevention (CDC) established a single set of guidelines called Standard Precautions. These guidelines are measures to decrease your risk of exposure. The purpose of Standard Precautions is to ensure that you take the same precautions for every patient. (Table 4–1).

During most patient care, you will wear gloves and eye protection (Figure 4-1 ●). A mask is often required for procedures and patient care conditions where there is an increased likelihood

TABLE 4–1 | Summary of Standard Precautions

Component	Recommendations
Hand hygiene	After touching blood, body fluids, secretions, excretions, and contaminated items; immediately after removing gloves; between patient contacts.
Personal protective equipment (PPE)	*Gloves* For touching blood, body fluids, secretions, excretions, contaminated items; for touching mucous membranes and nonintact skin.
	Gown During procedures and patient-care activities when contact of clothing/exposed skin with blood/body fluids, secretions, and excretions is anticipated.
	Mask, eye protection (goggles), face shield* During procedures and patient-care activities likely to generate splashes or sprays of blood, body fluids, or secretions, especially suctioning or endotracheal intubation
Soiled patient-care equipment	Handle in a manner that prevents transfer of microorganisms to others and to the environment; wear gloves if visibly contaminated; perform hand hygiene.
Environmental control	Develop procedures for routine care, cleaning, and disinfection of environmental surfaces, especially frequently touched surfaces in patient-care areas.
Textiles and laundry	Handle in a manner that prevents transfer of microorganisms to others and to the environment.
Needles and other sharps	Do not recap, bend, break, or hand-manipulate used needles; if recapping is required, use a one-handed scoop technique only; use safety features when available; place used sharps in puncture-resistant container.
Patient resuscitation	Use mouthpiece, resuscitation bag, other ventilation devices to prevent contact with mouth and oral secretions.
Patient placement	Prioritize for single-patient room if patient is at increased risk of transmission, is likely to contaminate the environment, does not maintain appropriate hygiene, or is at increased risk of acquiring infection or developing adverse outcome following infection.
Respiratory hygiene/cough etiquette	Instruct symptomatic persons to cover mouth/nose when sneezing/coughing; use tissues and dispose in no-touch receptacle; observe hand hygiene after soiling of hands with respiratory secretions; wear surgical mask if tolerated or maintain spatial separation, >3 feet if possible.

During aerosol-generating procedures on patients with suspected or proven infections transmitted by respiratory aerosols (e.g., SARS), wear a fit-tested N95 or higher respirator in addition to gloves, gown, and face/eye protection.

that splashes or sprays of blood, body fluids, or secretions may occur. This is especially important during suctioning, endotracheal intubation, and other airway procedures. Remarkably, the simplest standard precaution is often the most neglected: hand washing. Washing your hands before and after patient contact is one of the most effective ways to decrease your exposure to infectious material. Volume 1, Chapter 4 on workforce safety and wellness includes a thorough discussion of Standard Precautions.

Medical Asepsis

Medical **asepsis** (*a-*, without; *sepsis,* infection) describes a medical environment free of pathogens. Many paramedical procedures, especially those related to medication administration, place the patient at increased risk for infection. The external environment is full of microorganisms, many of them pathogenic. Techniques such as intravenous access or endotracheal intubation can allow pathogens to enter the patient's body, where they may cause **local** or **systemic** complications. Medical asepsis practices, including the use of sterilization, disinfectants, and antiseptics, guard against this hazard.

Sterilization

A truly aseptic environment is a sterile one. A **sterile** environment is free of all forms of life. Generally, environments are sterilized with extensive heat or chemicals. A sterile environment is difficult to attain in the prehospital setting. Consequently, you must practice medically clean techniques to minimize your patient's risk of infection. **Medically clean** techniques involve the careful

CONTENT REVIEW

► Needle Handling
Precautions

• Minimize tasks in a moving
  ambulance.
• Properly dispose of all
  sharps.
• Recap needles only as
  a last resort.

handling of sterile equipment to prevent contamination. For example, much of the equipment used for medication administration is packaged sterilely. Once you open the package, you must use a medically clean technique to keep the equipment clean and uncontaminated until you use it. If you drop a piece of equipment on a dirty surface, you should discard it and obtain a new piece. Other medically clean techniques, including hand washing, glove changing, and discarding equipment that is in opened packages, help to prevent equipment and patient contamination. Remember, too, that many patients have lowered immunity levels or carry infectious diseases. Thus, keeping the ambulance and equipment clean is another essential medically clean procedure.

Disinfectants and Antiseptics

When administering medications, you must use disinfectants and antiseptics to ensure local cleanliness. Do not confuse disinfectants and antiseptics; the distinction between them is important. **Disinfectants** are toxic to living tissue. You will therefore use them only on nonliving surfaces or objects such as the inside of an ambulance or laryngoscope blades after use. Never use disinfectants on living tissue. **Antiseptics** are not toxic to living tissue. They destroy or inhibit pathogenic microorganisms that already exist on living surfaces and are generally used to cleanse the local area before a needle puncture. Common antiseptics include alcohol and iodine preparations, used either alone or together. Frequently, antiseptics are diluted disinfectants.

Disposal of Contaminated Equipment and Sharps

Blood and body fluid can harbor infectious material that endangers the health care provider, family, bystanders, or the patient himself. Many times, the patient is infected with pathogenic organisms long before signs and symptoms appear. Therefore, you must treat all blood and body fluids as potentially infectious.

Medication administration commonly involves needles in direct contact with the patient's blood and body fluid. Once used, a needle presents a significant risk. Inadvertent needlesticks, the most common accident in health care, can transmit diseases between the patient and paramedic. Properly handling needles and other sharps before and after patient use can prevent many of these accidental needlesticks. To minimize or eliminate the risk of an accidental needlestick, take these precautions:

• *Minimize the tasks you perform in a moving ambulance.* Use needles as sparingly as possible in the back of a moving ambulance. When appropriate, perform all interventions involving needles on scene. If en route, it may occasionally be necessary to have the driver pull the ambulance to the side of the road and stop briefly. Most paramedics become quite proficient at completing these procedures in a moving ambulance.

• *Immediately dispose of used sharps in a sharps container.* A **sharps container** is a rigid, puncture-resistant container clearly marked as biohazardous. You can deposit whole needles and prefilled syringes in it, thus eliminating the need for bending or cutting. Some sharps containers have adapters that permit the easy removal of needles from blood draw equipment and syringes. You should also dispose of items such as used ampules in the sharps container. Avoid dropping sharps onto the floor for later disposal. In the heat of the moment, you may forget the sharp or mentally misplace it.

• *Recap needles only as a last resort.* If you absolutely must recap a needle, never use two hands to do so. Instead, use the "one-handed scoop" method. First, place the cap on the bench top and hold the syringe in one hand. Keep the other hand by your side. Next, slip the needle into the cap. Finally, lift it up and snap it on securely using only one hand and dispose of it properly (Figure 4-2 ●).

By law, every medical organization must have a biological hazard exposure plan. Be familiar with yours. If you are exposed to blood or other body substances, follow the plan and immediately notify the appropriate resources. Remember that prevention is the best medicine.[3]

Medication Administration and Documentation

When administering medications, proper and thorough documentation is extremely important. You must record all information concerning the patient and the medication including:

• Indication for medication administration

• Dosage and route delivered

• Patient response to the medication—both positive and negative

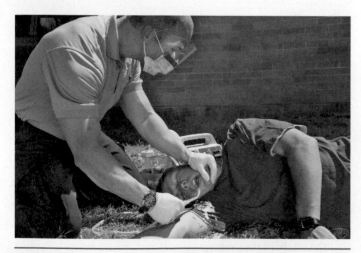

● **Figure 4-1** Standard Precautions should be followed on each possible patient encounter.

You must also document the patient's condition and vital signs before medication administration as well as after. In addition to communicating all information to those to whom you transfer care, you must record it on a copy of the patient care report.

In emergent and nonemergent situations alike, you will administer a variety of medications through a variety of delivery routes. The routes of medication administration fall into four basic categories: percutaneous, pulmonary, enteral, and parenteral. Technically, medications delivered through the rectum and pulmonary system are **topical medications**; however, accepted practice classifies these routes separately. Which route you use will depend on the medication you are administering and your patient's status.

PERCUTANEOUS MEDICATION ADMINISTRATION

Percutaneous medications are those that are applied to and absorbed through the skin or the mucous membranes. They are easy to administer, and they bypass the digestive tract, making their absorption more predictable.

Transdermal Administration

Medications given by the **transdermal** (*trans-*, across; *dermal*, skin) route promote slow, steady absorption. Nitroglycerin, hormones, and analgesics are commonly administered transdermally. Transdermal delivery can also produce localized effects, as with anti-inflammatories and other bacteriostatic and softening agents. Applying medication locally avoids passing larger quantities of the medication through the entire body, where it is not needed. Transdermal medications include lotions, ointments, creams, foams, wet dressings, adhesive-backed applications, and suppositories.

To administer a transdermal medication, use the following technique:

1. Use Standard Precautions and avoid contaminating the medication and inadvertently getting it on your skin.
2. Clean and dry your patient's skin at the administration site.

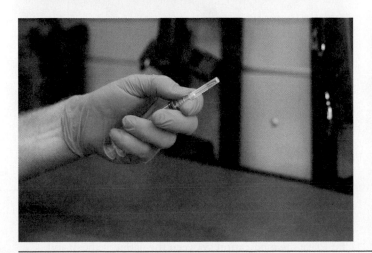
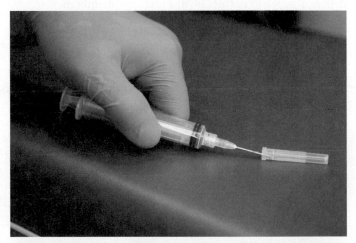
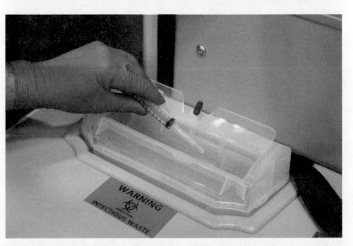

● **Figure 4-2** The "one-hand scoop" is the safest way to recap a needle when it must be recapped.

3. Apply medication to the site as specified by the manufacturer. Avoid overdosing or underdosing when using lotion, ointment, cream, or foam.

4. Leave the medication in place for the required time. Monitor the patient for desirable or adverse effects.

You may need to place a dressing over the medication to protect the site and quantity of medication. Carefully follow all recommendations. Administration may vary subtly, depending on the form of medication and the specific manufacturer's instructions.

Several factors can affect how quickly the skin absorbs transdermal medications. Thin skin, overdose, or penetrating solvents can increase the absorption rate. Conversely, thick skin, scar tissue, or peripheral vascular disease can decrease the rate. If these factors are present, consider alternative sites or dosage adjustments.

Mucous Membranes

The mucous membranes absorb medications at a moderate to rapid rate. Similar to transdermal administration, medication delivery through the mucous membranes avoids the digestive tract and complications associated with that route. You can deliver medications through the mucous membranes at several sites (sublingual, buccal, ocular, nasal, and aural). However, specific medications are made for specific sites and generally are not interchangeable.

Sublingual

Sublingual medications are absorbed through the mucous membranes beneath the tongue (*sub-*, below; *lingual,* tongue). The sublingual region is extremely vascular and permits rapid absorption with systemic delivery. These medications are generally dissolvable tablets or sprays. One commonly administered sublingual medication is nitroglycerin.

To administer a medication via the sublingual route, follow these steps (Figure 4-3 ●):

1. Use Standard Precautions.

2. Confirm the indication, medication, dose, sublingual route, and expiration date.

3. Have your patient lift his tongue toward the top and back of his oral cavity.

4. Place the pill or direct spray between the underside of the tongue and the floor of the oral cavity. Have your patient relax his tongue and mouth. If administering a tablet, instruct the patient to let the tablet dissolve and not to swallow it.

5. Monitor the patient for desirable or adverse effects.

Buccal

The **buccal** region lies in the oral cavity between the cheek and gums. Buccal medications are generally tablets. Hormonal and enzyme preparations are typically given buccally.

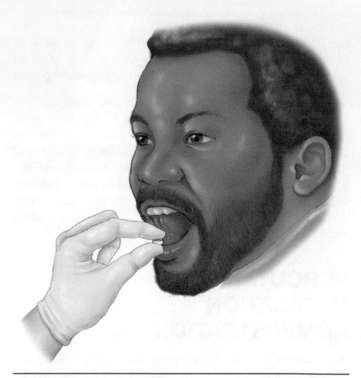

● **Figure 4-3**   Sublingual medication administration. Place the pill or direct spray between the underside of the tongue and the floor of the oral cavity.

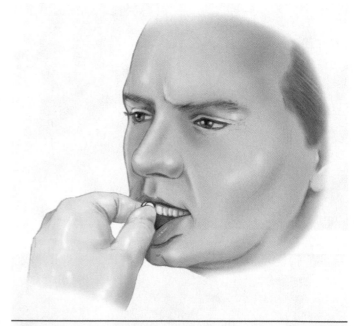

● **Figure 4-4**   Buccal medication administration. Place the medication between the patient's cheek and gum.

To administer a medication buccally, follow these steps (Figure 4-4 ●):

1. Use Standard Precautions.

2. Confirm the indication, medication, dose, buccal route, and expiration date.

3. Place the medication between the patient's cheek and gum. Instruct the patient to allow the pill or other

preparation to dissolve. Ensure that the patient does not swallow the medication.

4. Monitor the patient for desirable or adverse effects.

Ocular

Ocular medications are topical medications that are administered through the mucous membranes of the eye. These are typically local medications for alleviating eye pain, treating infection, decreasing intraocular pressure, or lubricating the eyelid. Medications delivered by way of the eye are labeled for ophthalmic use and packaged as drops or ointments.

If medication is to be administered only to one eye, be sure to medicate the correct eye. The following abbreviations were formerly used to designate right, left, or both eyes:

o.d.   right eye (*oculus dexter*)

o.s.   left eye (*oculus sinister*)

o.u.   both right and left eyes (*oculus uterque*)

However, to avoid confusion, it is preferred to simply write "left eye", "right eye" or "both eyes."

To administer a medication via eye drops, use the following technique (Figure 4-5 ●):

1. Use Standard Precautions.
2. Have your patient lie supine or lay his head back and look toward the ceiling.
3. Pull the lower eyelid downward to expose the conjunctival sac. Never touch the eye.
4. Use a medicine dropper to place the prescribed dosage on the conjunctival sac. Never administer medications directly on the eye unless specifically instructed.
5. Instruct the patient to hold his eye(s) shut for 1 to 2 minutes.

Ocular medications may also be packaged as ointments. To apply an ointment, follow the same procedure as above, but carefully squeeze the ointment onto the conjunctival sac. If you administer too much medication, carefully blot away the excess drops or ointment with sterile gauze. The ointment will melt as it warms to body temperature and will spread smoothly across the surface of the eye.

Nasal

The mucous membranes of the nose are another port for topical medication delivery. Given through the nares (nostrils), these **nasal medications** are usually drops or sprays intended for local effect. A commercial device called the mucosal atomization device (MAD) is commonly used. Often, these medications are aerosolized to provide better distribution to the nasal mucosa. The intranasal route can be used for analgesia (particularly in children), sedation, epistaxis, and to reduce nasal congestion from nasotracheal intubation.[4-7]

To administer a medication via the nose, use the following technique (Figure 4-6 ●):

1. Use Standard Precautions including face mask.
2. Have the patient blow his nose and tilt his head backwards.
3. Use a medicine dropper or squeezable nebulizer to administer the medication into the appropriate nare(s) according to the manufacturer's instructions (Figure 4-7 ●).

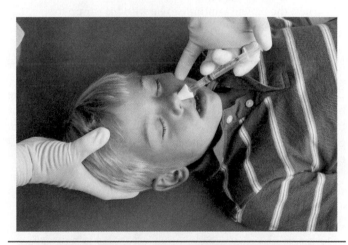

● **Figure 4-6**   Nasal medication administration.

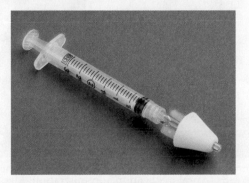

● **Figure 4-7**   Mucosal atomization device (MAD) for intranasal administration of emergency medications.

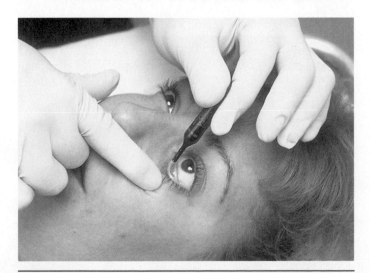

● **Figure 4-5**   Eyedrop administration. Use a medicine dropper to place the prescribed dosage on the conjunctival sac.

4. Hold the nare(s) shut and/or tilt the head forward to distribute the medication.

5. Monitor the patient for desirable and undesirable effects.

Aural

Some medications are delivered to the mucous membranes of the ear and ear canal through drops or medicated gauze. These **aural medications** primarily treat local infections and ear pain. Use the following technique to administer medicated drops (Figure 4-8 ●):

1. Use Standard Precautions.

2. Confirm the indication, medication, dose, and expiration date.

3. Determine the correct ear for administration.

4. Have the patient lie in the lateral recumbent position with the affected ear upward.

5. Manually open the ear canal: for adult patients, pull the ear up and back; for pediatric patients, pull it down and back.

6. Administer the appropriate dose of medication with a medicine dropper.

7. Have the patient continue to lie with his ear up for 10 minutes.

8. Monitor the patient for desirable and undesirable effects.

Using medicated gauze or cotton is generally reserved for the hospital setting. If your local protocols permit you to administer these medications, follow the procedure previously outlined, gently inserting the gauze into the ear instead of instilling medicated drops. Avoid tightly packing the ear canal.

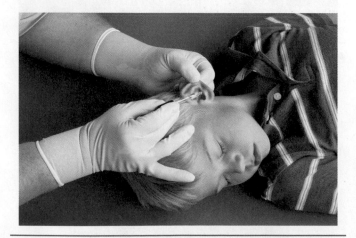

● **Figure 4-8** Aural medication administration. Manually open the ear canal and administer the appropriate dose.

PULMONARY MEDICATION ADMINISTRATION

Special medications can be administered into the pulmonary system via **inhalation** or **injection**. Generally in the form of gases, powders, fine mists, or liquids, these medications include those that promote bronchodilation for respiratory emergencies. Other inhaled medications are mucolytics, antibiotics, and topical steroids. Inhalation can also be used for humidification and pulmonary decongestion.

Nebulizer

Typically, medications administered by inhalation are delivered with the aid of a small volume nebulizer (SVN) or handheld nebulizer (HHN). A **nebulizer** uses pressurized oxygen or air to disperse a liquid into a fine aerosol spray or mist. Inhalation carries the aerosol into the lungs. Figure 4-9 ● illustrates a typical nebulizer. The specific design depends on the manufacturer, but they all work on the same principle and typically have the same parts:

● Mouthpiece
● Medication reservoir
● Oxygen port
● Relief valve
● Oxygen tubing
● Oxygen source

To administer a medication with a nebulizer, follow these steps:

1. Use Standard Precautions including a mask.

2. Put the medication in the medication reservoir. If the medication is not diluted, combine it with 3 to 5 cc sterile saline solution. This will allow adequate aerosolization. Screw the reservoir in place.

3. Assemble the nebulizer.

4. Attach oxygen tubing to the oxygen port and oxygen source.

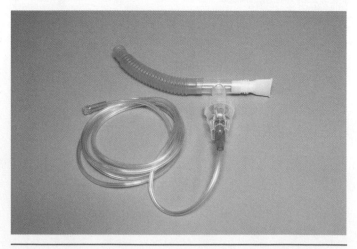

● **Figure 4-9** Typical small-volume nebulizer (SVN) setup.

5. Set the oxygen source regulator for 5 to 8 liters per minute.

   Note: Never set the oxygen pressure outside of this range. Less than 5 liters per minute will not create enough pressure to aerosolize the medication. More than 8 liters per minute will create too much pressure and destroy the oxygen tubing or nebulizer at its weakest point. Furthermore, because of pressure restrictions, do not attach the nebulizer to an oxygen humidifier.

6. Place the nebulizer in the patient's mouth. Instruct him to exhale and then seal his lips around the mouthpiece. Now have him hold the nebulizer and slowly inhale as deeply as possible. On maximum inhalation, instruct the patient to hold in the medication for 1 to 2 seconds before exhaling. This permits maximum deposition and absorption. Continue this process until the medication is completely gone. Typically, this takes 3 to 5 minutes.

Nebulizers also come preattached to an oxygen face mask in both pediatric and adult sizes (Figure 4-10 ●). Use nebulization face masks for pediatric or adult patients who cannot hold the nebulizer. Nebulizers can also be used with continuous-positive

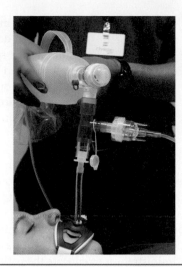

● **Figure 4-12** In-line administration of nebulized medication in an intubated patient.

airway pressure (CPAP) devices when indicated (Figure 4-11 ●).[8] They can also be used in patients who are intubated and receiving mechanical ventilation (Figure 4-12 ●)

For a nebulizer to be effective, the patient must have an adequate tidal volume and respiratory rate. If the tidal volume is shallow or respiratory rate low, the medication will not move from the nebulizer into the lungs. For patients with a poor tidal and/or respiratory rate who cannot pull the medication into their lungs, you can connect the nebulizer to a bag-valve mask, CPAP devices, and/or an endotracheal tube.

Metered Dose Inhaler

Inhaled medications may also be delivered through a **metered dose inhaler** (MDI). These small, handheld devices produce a medicated spray for inhalation. Patients with conditions such as asthma or COPD use metered dose inhalers to deliver a specific, or metered, dose of medication. A metered dose inhaler consists of two parts, a medication canister and a plastic shell and mouthpiece (Figure 4-13 ●). Some metered dose inhalers come equipped with a spacer. The spacer is a cylindrical canister between the inhaler and the mouthpiece. Prior to self-administration, the patient will

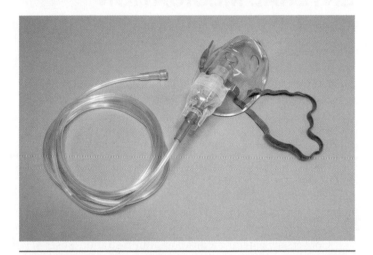

● **Figure 4-10** SVN medication administration through mask.

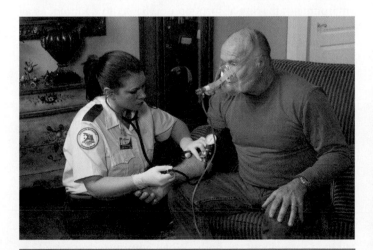

● **Figure 4-11** Nebulized medications can be administered through most CPAP masks.

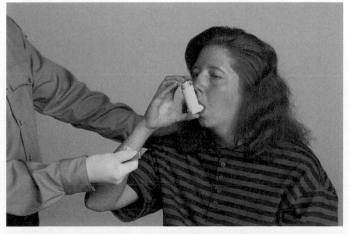

● **Figure 4-13** Metered dose inhaler.

CONTENT REVIEW

► Endotracheal Medications

 • Lidocaine
 • Vasopressin
 • Epinephrine
 • Atropine
 • Naloxone

depress the inhaler, sending a measured dose of medication into the spacer. The patient will then breathe in and out of the spacer through the mouthpiece, thus inhaling the medication into the lungs. The spacer system is particularly useful for patients who have a hard time operating and inhaling directly from the metered dose inhaler, which is common in the elderly and in young children. The spacer, when used in conjunction with a metered dose inhaler, is very effective.

Metered dose inhalers are usually self-administered. However, if your patient is incapacitated, you may have to physically assist with the administration or educate the patient or his caregivers in its use. To assist a patient in the use of a metered dose inhaler, follow this technique:

1. Insert the medication canister into the plastic shell.

2. Remove the cap from the mouthpiece. Make sure the cap is clean.

3. Gently shake the MDI for 2 to 5 seconds.

4. Instruct the patient to maximally exhale.

5. Place the mouthpiece in the patient's mouth and have him form a seal with his lips.

6. As the patient inhales, press the canister's top downward to release the medication.

7. Have the patient hold his breath for several seconds.

8. Remove the inhaler from the patient's mouth and instruct him to breathe slowly.

9. If a second dose is necessary, wait according to the manufacturer's instructions. Then repeat.

In an acute respiratory emergency involving a patient with a metered dose inhaler, always use a nebulizer instead of the MDI. While the metered dose inhaler delivers a small amount of medication, the nebulizer delivers larger quantities of medication mixed with water and oxygen.

Nebulizers and metered dose inhalers offer several advantages. In respiratory emergencies, less medication is needed because it reaches its exact site of action. The lower dosage is less likely to promote side effects, and if the patient has an adverse reaction, implementing or discontinuing medication delivery is easy. Furthermore, because the patient can hold the nebulizer, he will benefit from feeling more in control of his overall therapy. Most importantly, if your patient is hypoxic you can administer inhaled medications with supplemental oxygen.

The nebulizer and metered dose inhaler also have disadvantages. Moving the aerosolized medication into the lungs depends on adequate ventilation. For the patient with a poor tidal and minute volume, nebulized medications are ineffective, as the medication cannot reach its site of action. In these cases, you should use the nebulizer in conjunction with a bag-valve mask and/or endotracheal tube. In addition, the patient must exhibit an adequate level of consciousness and manual dexterity to hold the nebulizer and follow instructions correctly.

Endotracheal Tube

Although infrequently used, you can administer certain medications such as lidocaine (Xylocaine), vasopressin, epinephrine, atropine, and naloxone (Narcan) through an endotracheal tube if an intravenous line or intraosseous line is unavailable. Delivering liquid medications into the lungs theoretically permits rapid absorption through the pulmonary capillaries. However, recent research has shown the administration of medications via an endotracheal tube is not as effective as once thought.

When using an endotracheal tube, you must increase conventional IV dosages from two to two-and-one-half times. You also should dilute the medication in normal saline to create 10 mL of solution and then quickly inject it down the endotracheal tube. Several ventilations must follow to aerosolize the medication and enhance its absorption. Ideally, you can pass a commercially manufactured catheter through the endotracheal tube and inject the medication through it.[9]

ENTERAL MEDICATION ADMINISTRATION

Enteral route is the delivery of medication to be absorbed through the gastrointestinal tract. The gastrointestinal tract, or alimentary canal, travels from the mouth to the stomach and on through the intestines to the rectum (Figure 4-14 ●). You can administer enteral medications orally, through a gastric tube, or rectally.

Several advantages make the gastrointestinal tract the most common route for medication delivery. Aside from sheer convenience, it is the least expensive route, and its use requires little equipment and minimal training. In some instances, after you have delivered a medication you may be able to retrieve it by inducing vomiting, by removing it from the rectum, or simply by having the patient spit it out.

Conversely, enteral medication administration poses several disadvantages. Physical activity, emotions, or food can significantly alter the gastrointestinal tract's chemical and physical environment, making absorption unreliable. In addition, as all blood from the stomach and small intestine must pass through the hepatic circulatory system (portal circulation), the liver's condition can reduce the medication's effectiveness. A dysfunctional liver can significantly alter medication distribution and, in extreme cases, metabolize therapeutic medications into inert or harmful substances. Furthermore, a patient resistant to or *noncompliant* in taking medications makes administration via the enteral route very difficult.

Oral Administration

Oral medication administration denotes any medication taken by mouth (oral) and swallowed into the gastrointestinal (GI) tract. From the GI tract, the medication is absorbed and distributed throughout the body. When administering a medication by the oral route, you must be sure that the patient has an adequate level of consciousness to support his airway. Administering an oral medication to a patient who cannot support his airway may result in an airway occlusion or aspiration into the lungs. If aspiration into the lungs occurs, aspiration pneumonia and its deadly consequences may occur.

Medications for oral delivery come in a variety of forms, either solid or liquid.

- **Capsules.** Capsules contain liquid, dry, or beaded medication in a soluble casing. For maximum effectiveness, the patient must swallow them whole.
- **Tablets.** Tablets comprise medicated powder compressed into a small, solid disk. Typically, tablets may be scored to permit breaking in half or quarters when lesser dosages are required.
- **Enteric coated/time-release capsules and tablets.** These forms of medication release the medication gradually as layers of the capsule or tablet slowly erode. Time-release capsules or tablets must be swallowed whole.
- **Elixirs.** Elixirs are liquid medications combined with alcohol or placed in a sweetened fluid.
- **Emulsions.** Emulsions are medications combined with a fat or oil emulsifier.
- **Lozenges.** Lozenges are solid forms of medication that slowly dissolve in the mouth, thus permitting gradual swallowing.
- **Suspensions.** A suspension is a liquid that contains small particles of solid medication.
- **Syrups.** A syrup is a concentrated solution of sugar in water or another liquid to which a medication is added.

Equipment for Oral Administration

Administering oral medications is simple and easy. The basic equipment that you may need depends on the medication and the patient's status:

- **Soufflé cup.** A soufflé cup is a paper or plastic cup. Placing a solid medication in a soufflé cup makes it easy to see and minimizes contact with the provider's hands.
- **Medicine cup.** A medicine cup is a plastic or glass cup with volumetric measurements on the side. It facilitates giving specific amounts of liquid medication. When you pour medication into the cup, the liquid does not form a flat surface but clings to the sides at a higher level, forming a *meniscus*. To compensate for the meniscus, measure the medication toward the center, at its lowest level.
- **Medicine dropper.** A medicine dropper has markings for measuring liquid volumes. You will use it for special medications and to administer medications to children or patients who cannot tolerate other forms of oral medication.
- **Teaspoon.** You will use these accurately sized measuring spoons to administer liquid medications. A teaspoon normally holds

5 milliliters of fluid; however, the volume of household teaspoons varies significantly. To ensure accurate medication administration, use a measured teaspoon or syringe.

- **Oral syringe.** Oral syringes are calibrated plastic syringes without a hypodermic needle. They are considered the most accurate oral means of administering liquid-based medications. When administering a medication with the oral syringe, place the end of the syringe in the patient's mouth and deliver only as much medication as the patient can safely swallow. Several administrations may be necessary to deliver a complete dose.
- **Nipple.** For the neonate or infant, liquid medication can be delivered with a plastic nipple.

General Principles of Oral Administration

To administer medications orally, use the following technique:

1. Use Standard Precautions.
2. Note whether to administer the medication with food or on an empty stomach.

CONTENT REVIEW

► Enteral Routes
- Oral
- Gastric tube
- Rectal

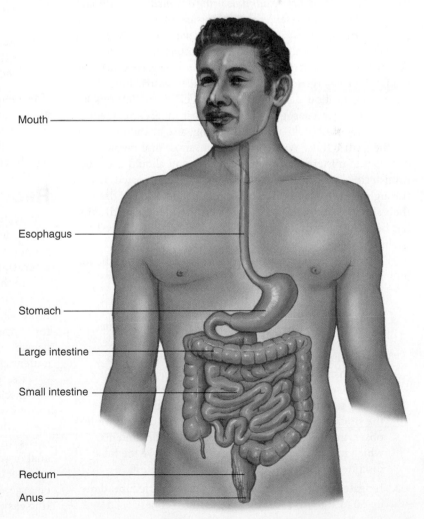

- **Figure 4-14** Gastrointestinal tract.

Mouth

Esophagus

Stomach

Large intestine

Small intestine

Rectum

Anus

3. Gather any necessary equipment such as a soufflé cup or teaspoon; mix liquids or suspensions, or otherwise prepare medications as needed.

4. Have your patient sit upright (when not contraindicated).

5. Place the medication into your patient's mouth. Allow self-administration when possible; assist when needed.

6. Follow administration with 4 to 8 ounces of water or other liquid. Swallowing a liquid pushes the medication into the stomach.

7. Ensure that the patient has swallowed the medication and it is not hidden in his mouth. For some pediatric and psychiatric patients, you may have to visually confirm that the patient has swallowed the medication by inspecting the oral cavity.

Gastric Tube Administration

For patients who have difficulty swallowing or whose nutritional status is poor, you may place a gastric tube to support or completely supplement nutritional requirements. Gastric tubes are also used in instances of medication overdose, trauma, and upper gastrointestinal bleeding. They may be surgically inserted directly into the stomach through the abdomen or indirectly through the nose (nasogastric tube) or mouth (orogastric tube). Placing a gastric tube through the abdominal wall is reserved for the hospital setting. *Before administering any medication through a gastric tube or other enteral tube, ensure that it is indeed an enteral tube and not a similar-looking device such as a chronic ambulatory peritoneal dialysis (CAPD) catheter.* In some EMS systems, paramedics insert orogastric or nasogastric tubes in the field for emergencies. A properly placed gastric tube allows enteral medication delivery. Few emergency medications are administered via a nasogastric or orogastric tube. Other medications, many used in the nonacute setting, also are administered via the gastric tube. With modification, most oral medications can be administered this way. However, you should avoid administering time-release capsules and enteric-coated tablets through a gastric tube, as crushing them for delivery destroys their slow-release mechanism. Also, ensure that the medication has been sufficiently crushed so as not to become trapped and occlude the gastric tube.

To administer a medication via a gastric tube, use the following technique (Procedure 4-1):

1. Use Standard Precautions.

2. Confirm proper tube placement. Disconnect the tube from the drainage or suction unit or clamping device. Clamp the tube from the drainage or suction unit to avoid gastric contents' spilling from either device. Attach a cone-tipped syringe to the proximal end of the gastric tube. Gently inject air while auscultating over the stomach. Following this, withdraw the plunger while observing for the presence of gastric fluid or contents, which indicates appropriate placement. Leave the tube disconnected from the drainage or suction unit.

3. Irrigate the gastric tube. To irrigate the gastric tube, draw up 50 to 100 mL of normal saline into a cone-tipped

syringe. Insert the syringe into the open end of the gastric tube. With the syringe tip pointed at the floor, gently inject the saline into the tube. If the saline encounters resistance, look for problems such as tube kinking. Also, have the patient lie on his left side and reattempt injection. If the saline still meets resistance, reattach the tube to the drainage or suction unit and contact medical direction for further directives.

4. Prepare the medication(s) for delivery. Crush tablets or empty capsules into 30 cc of warm water. Ensure that all particles are small so that they will not occlude the tube. You may administer liquid medications without further preparation.

5. Draw the medication into a 30 to 50 mL cone-tipped syringe and place the tip into the open gastric tube. Gently administer the medication into the gastric tube. Forceful application may create considerable distention and patient discomfort.

6. Draw 50 to 100 mL of warm normal saline into a cone-tipped syringe and attach it to the open end of the gastric tube. Gently inject the saline. This facilitates the medication's passage into the stomach and rinses the tube, ensuring that the patient receives the entire dose. Repeated administrations may be necessary.

7. Clamp off the distal tube. Use a commercially manufactured device or hemostat to clamp shut the distal portion of the gastric tube for approximately 30 minutes after you administer the medication. Do not reattach to the drainage or suction unit. This will prevent the medication's inadvertent removal from the stomach.

If you must refill the syringe in order to administer the full dosage of medication, do not allow the syringe to empty completely before you detach it from the gastric tube. This prevents drawing air into the syringe and then introducing it into the stomach, which causes discomfort.

Rectal Administration

The rectum's extreme vascularity promotes rapid medication absorption. Additionally, because medications given rectally do not pass through the liver, they are not subject to **hepatic alteration**; thus, their absorption is more predictable.

In the emergency setting, you may give certain medications rectally if you cannot establish an intravenous line or use the oral route. These include diazepam (Valium) or lorazepam (Ativan) for protracted seizures or aspirin for cardiac or neurologic emergencies. In the nonacute setting, you may administer sedatives, antiemetics, or other specially prepared medications rectally.

Rectal administration may prove advantageous with the unconscious or pediatric patient, or when administering medications with an objectionable taste or odor. Unfortunately, medication absorption may be erratic if gross fecal matter exists. In addition, some medications may cause considerable anal or rectal irritation.

Rectal medications come in a variety of forms. In the emergency setting, they are typically liquid, thus permitting easy administration and rapid absorption. To administer

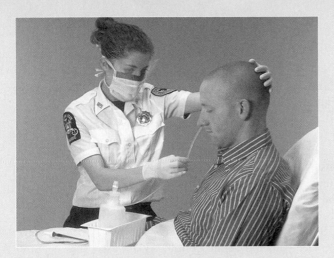

4-1a ● Confirm proper tube placement.

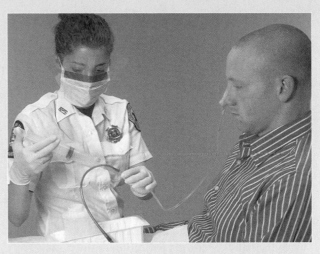

4-1b ● Withdraw the plunger while observing for the presence of gastric fluid or contents.

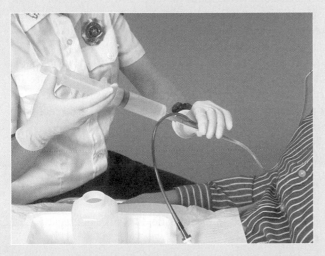

4-1c ● Instill medication into the gastric tube.

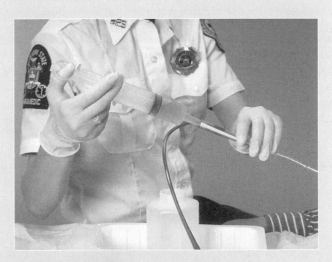

4-1d ● Gently inject the saline.

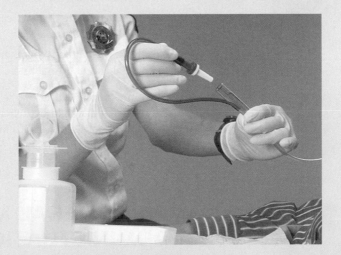

4-1e ● Clamp off the distal tube.

CONTENT REVIEW

▶ Parenteral Routes

• Intradermal injection
• Subcutaneous injection
• Intramuscular injection
• Intravenous access
• Intraosseous infusion

a rectal medication in the emergent setting follow this technique:

1. Use Standard Precautions.

2. Confirm the indication for administration and dose, and draw the correct quantity of medication into a syringe.

3. Place the hub of a 14-gauge Teflon catheter (removed from the IV catheter) on the end of a needleless syringe (Figure 4-15 ●).

4. Insert the Teflon catheter into the patient's rectum and inject the medication. Try to keep the medication in the lower part of the rectum. Administration higher in the rectum may result in the medication's being absorbed by veins that deliver the medication to the portal circulation.

5. Withdraw the catheter and hold the patient's buttocks together, thus permitting retention and absorption.

An alternative technique utilizes a small endotracheal tube instead of the Teflon IV catheter. Remove the 15/22-mm BVM adapter and connect a syringe to the proximal end of the tube (Figure 4-15). Lubricate the tube and insert it into the rectum. Inject the medication, remove the tube, and hold the buttocks together. A small endotracheal tube attached to a syringe can be used as well (Figure 4-16 ●).

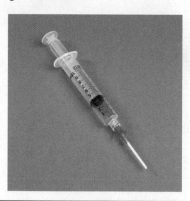

● **Figure 4-15** Catheter placement on needleless syringe.

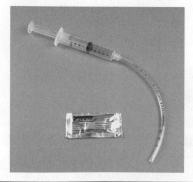

● **Figure 4-16** Syringe attached to endotracheal tube for rectal administration.

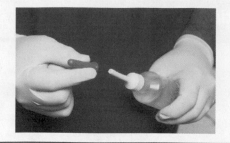

● **Figure 4-17** Prepackaged enema container.

In the nonemergent setting, suppositories or enemas are common methods for rectal administration. Because your responsibilities as a paramedic may include nonemergent clinical settings, you should master these techniques. Additionally, the rectal route may prove beneficial for a pediatric patient who resists oral administration or for whom IV access proves impractical.

Suppositories are medications packaged in a soft, pliable form. Generally refrigerated until they are used, they begin to melt at body temperature in the rectum. Some are lubricated to ease insertion. Suppositories can be lubricated by running a small amount of lukewarm tap water over the suppository prior to insertion. To administer a suppository, manually insert it into the rectum. Hold the buttocks shut for 5 to 10 minutes to allow for retention and absorption.

An **enema** is typically a liquid **bolus** of medication that is injected into the rectum. Medications given via this route are typically referred to as small volume enemas. They are typically prepackaged in a squeezable container with a rectal tip (Figure 4-17 ●).

To administer a medicated small volume enema, use the following technique:

1. Use Standard Precautions and confirm the need for administration via a small volume enema.

2. Place the patient on his left side. Flex his right leg to expose the anus.

3. Insert the prelubricated rectal tip into the anus and advance 3 to 4 inches.

4. Gently squeeze the medicated solution of the bottle into the rectum and colon.

5. Hold the buttocks together to enhance absorption into the rectal and intestinal tissue.

Only those medications with specific guidelines for rectal administration should be delivered through this route. Do not administer rectal medications in the presence of diarrhea, rectal bleeding, hemorrhoids, or any other situation involving severe anal irritation.

PARENTERAL MEDICATION ADMINISTRATION

Parenteral route denotes the administration of medication outside the gastrointestinal tract. Broadly, this encompasses pulmonary and some topical forms of medication delivery;

Accidental Needlesticks. *Administering medications in an emergency setting increases the chances of accidental needlestick injuries for all involved. It is paramount that paramedics anticipate potential dangers and avoid them. For example, a natural reaction to pain (such as occurs with a medication injection) is to withdraw. This sudden movement can cause an accidental needlestick injury. Similarly, the combative or agitated patient poses a significant risk. Always make sure that medication administration is safe. If it is not, defer administration until additional resources or personnel are available. Your safety and the safety of your partner come first.*

however, additional, specific criteria apply to parenteral administration. Typically, the parenteral route involves the use of needles as medications are injected into the circulatory system or tissues. Consequently, some forms of parenteral medication delivery afford the most rapid medication delivery and absorption.

Syringes and Needles

Frequently, giving medications via the parenteral route requires a syringe and hypodermic needle.

Syringe

A **syringe** is a plastic tube with which liquid medications can be drawn up, stored, and injected. Syringes range in size from 1 to 100 cc and greater. Remember that while medication dosages are generally given by weight (g/mg/mcg), syringes represent volume. Therefore, you must be prepared to mathematically convert these measurements.

A syringe's two major components are a barrel and a plunger (Figure 4-18 ●). The tube-like barrel, or body, functions as a reservoir for medication. Markings on its side calibrate its overall volume. Smaller syringes are calibrated in 0.10-mL intervals, larger syringes in 1.0-mL intervals.

The plunger is a device that fits into the barrel. At one end it has a handle for pulling or pushing. At the opposite end, a rubber stopper fits snugly into the barrel. Pulling on the plunger draws material into the barrel; pushing on it expels material

from the barrel. The rubber end forms a tight seal from which the fluid medication cannot escape.

The junction of the fluid and rubber stopper measures the total volume of liquid in the syringe. The barrel's maximum volume should correspond closely to the volume of medication needed. For example, to administer 2 mL of medication, a 3-mL syringe would prove most appropriate.

An adapter at the syringe's distal end is compatible with the hub of an IV catheter or, as many cases will require, a hypodermic needle.

Hypodermic Needle

The **hypodermic needle** is a hollow metal tube used with the syringe to administer medications. It is sharp enough to easily puncture tissues, blood vessels, or IV medication ports.

The hypodermic needle's primary components include a hilt and shaft. The hilt is a threaded plastic tube that screws securely onto the syringe's distal adapter. The shaft is a thin metal tube through which medications can flow from the syringe into the delivery site. A bevel at the shaft's distal end accounts for its sharpness (Figure 4-19 ●).

Hypodermic needles come in a variety of gauges and lengths. A needle's **gauge** describes its diameter. Generally, hypodermic needle gauges range from 18 to 27. The gauge and actual diameter are inversely related: the higher the gauge, the smaller the diameter. Thus, a 25-gauge needle's diameter is smaller than an 18-gauge needle's. Conversely, a 20-gauge needle's diameter is larger than a 22-gauge needle's. Hypodermic needle lengths generally range from 3/8 to 1½ inches. The package label lists the size of the syringe and the gauge and length of the hypodermic needle.

Because syringes and hypodermic needles frequently involve invasive procedures, they are packaged sterile. Never use either a syringe or a hypodermic needle from a package that has been opened or tampered with. Used hypodermic needles are sharp and present a biohazard. Dispose of them immediately after you complete any task involving their use. Many modern needles are designed for safe needle disposal without recapping the needle (Figure 4-20 ●). These decrease the possibility of accidental needlestick injuries and are preferred in the emergency setting.

Medication Packaging

All medications delivered by the parenteral route are liquids. They are packaged in a variety of containers with which you must be familiar, as obtaining medication from each type

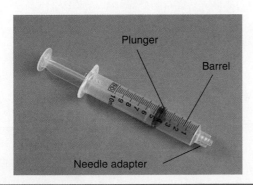

● **Figure 4-18**   Syringe.

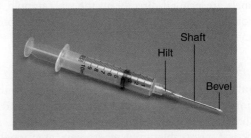

● **Figure 4-19**   Hypodermic needle.

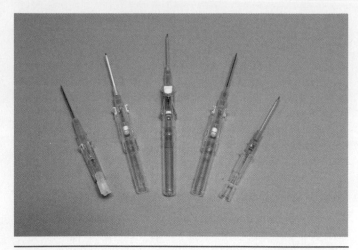

● **Figure 4-20** Safety needles help to minimize the possibility of needlestick injuries.

requires a different procedure. The kinds of parenteral medication containers include:

- Glass ampules
- Single and multidose vials
- Nonconstituted medication vials
- Nebulizer vials
- Prefilled syringes
- Intravenous medication fluids

You must also be thoroughly familiar with the information included on the labels of all medication containers:

- *Name of medication.* The label lists both the generic and trade name of the medication. Always ensure that you have selected the right medication.
- *Expiration date.* All medications have an expiration date after which they cannot be used. Never use an expired medication.
- *Total dose and concentration.* The total dose of medication is the total weight (g/mg/mcg) of medication in the container. The concentration represents the weight of the medication per volume of fluid. For example, if 10 mg of a medication were packaged in 10 mL of fluid, the total dose would be 10 mg, and the concentration would be 10 mg/10 mL or 1 mg/mL. Beware, identical medications can be packaged in different dosages and concentrations.

These labels are printed directly on the vial, ampule, prefilled syringe, or IV medication bag. Always use them to confirm the correct medication.

Glass Ampules

An **ampule**, or amp, is a breakable glass vessel containing liquid medication. It has a cone-shaped top, thin neck, and circular tubular base for storing the medication (Figure 4-21 ●). The thin neck is a vulnerable point where you intentionally break the ampule to retrieve its contents. Ampules usually range in

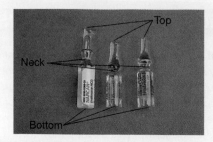

● **Figure 4-21** Ampules.

volume from 1 to 5 mL. The least-expensive form of medication packaging, they contain single doses of medication. It is essential to use a filter needle when drawing medication up from a glass ampule. This will help to filter any small glass shards that may be present.

To obtain medication from a glass ampule you will need a syringe and needle. Use the following technique (Procedure 4-2):

1. Confirm medication indications and patient allergies.
2. Confirm the ampule label (medication name, dose, and expiration).
3. Hold the ampule upright and tap its top to dislodge any trapped solution.
4. Place gauze around the thin neck and snap it off with your thumb.
5. Place the tip of the hypodermic needle inside the ampule and withdraw the medication into the syringe.
6. Reconfirm the indication, medication, dose, and route of administration.
7. Administer the medication appropriately via the indicated route.
8. Properly dispose of the needle, syringe, and broken glass ampule.

Single and Multidose Vials

Vials are plastic or glass containers with a self-sealing rubber top (Figure 4-22 ●). Vials may contain single or multiple doses of medication; the self-sealing rubber top prevents leakage from punctures and permits multiple accesses with a syringe and hypodermic needle. The medication inside the vial is packaged in a vacuum.

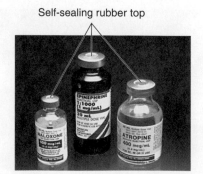

Figure 4-22 Vials.

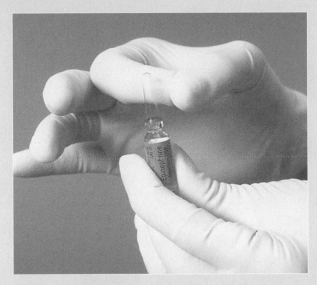

4-2a ● Hold the ampule upright and tap its top to dislodge any trapped solution.

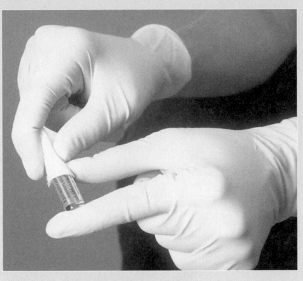

4-2b ● Place gauze around the thin neck . . .

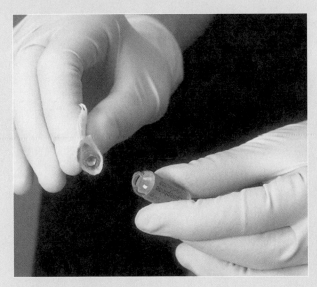

4-2c ● . . . and snap it off with your thumb.

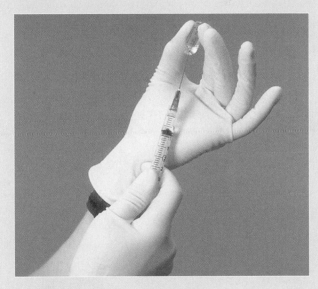

4-2d ● Draw up the medication.

To obtain medication from a vial, follow these steps (Procedure 4-3):

1. Confirm medication indications and patient allergies.
2. Confirm the vial label (name, dose, and expiration).
3. Determine the volume of medication to be administered.
4. Prepare the syringe and hypodermic needle. Because the vial is vacuum packed, you will have to replace the volume of medication removed with air in order to maintain equilibrium in the vial. Withdraw the plunger to draw a volume of air into the syringe equal to the volume of medication to be administered. This technique permits easy medication retrieval from the vial.
5. Cleanse the vial's rubber top with an antiseptic alcohol preparation.
6. Insert the hypodermic needle into the rubber top and inject the air from the syringe into the vial. Then withdraw the appropriate volume of medication.
7. Reconfirm the indication, medication, dose, and route of administration.
8. Administer appropriately via the indicated route.
9. Properly dispose of the needle, syringe, and vial.

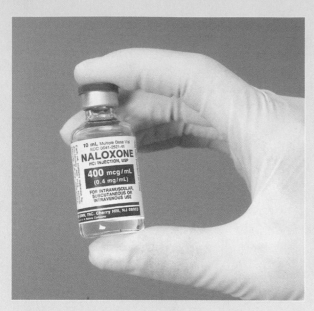

4-3a ● Confirm the vial label.

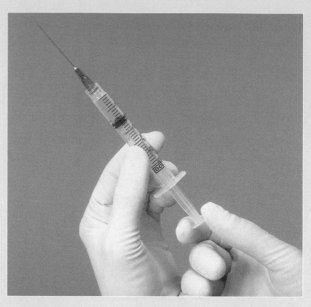

4-3b ● Prepare the syringe and hypodermic needle.

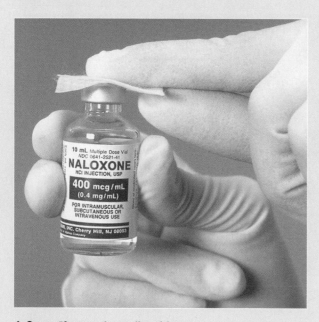

4-3c ● Cleanse the vial's rubber top.

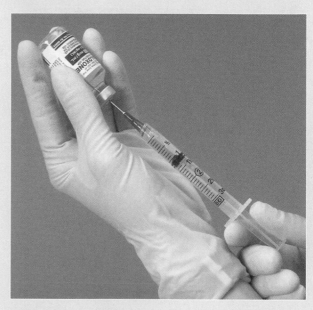

4-3d ● Insert the hypodermic needle into the rubber top and inject the air from the syringe into the vial.

Nonconstituted Medication Vial

The **nonconstituted medication vial** extends the viability and storage time of medications that have a short shelf life or are unstable in liquid form. The nonconstituted medication vial actually consists of two vials, one containing a powdered medication and one containing a liquid mixing solution (Figure 4-23 ●). To prepare the medication you must mix it, or reconstitute it, by withdrawing the liquid solution from its vial and placing it in the powdered medication's vial. In a **Mix-o-Vial** system, the two vials are joined and you must squeeze them together to break the seal and mix.

To prepare a medication from a nonconstituted medication vial, use the following technique (Procedure 4-4):

1. Confirm medication indications and patient allergies.

2. Confirm the vial's label (name, dose, expiration date).

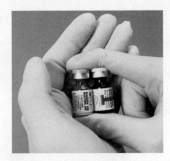

● **Figure 4-23** The nonconstituted drug vial actually consists of two vials, one containing a powdered medication and one containing a liquid mixing solution.

3. Remove all solution from the vial containing the mixing solution, using the same procedure as you would to withdraw medication from a single or multidose vial.

4. With an alcohol preparation, cleanse the top of the vial containing the powdered medication and inject the mixing solution.

5. Gently agitate or shake the vial to ensure complete mixture.

6. Determine the volume of newly constituted medication to be administered.

7. Prepare the syringe and hypodermic needle. Because the vial is vacuum packed, you will have to replace the volume of medication removed with air in order to retain equilibrium in the vial. By withdrawing the plunger, place into the syringe a volume of air equal to the volume of medication that will be removed. This technique permits easy medication retrieval from the vial.

8. Cleanse the medication vial's rubber top with an antiseptic alcohol preparation.

9. Insert the hypodermic needle into the rubber top and withdraw the appropriate volume of medication.

10. Reconfirm the indication, medication, dose, and route of administration.

11. Administer appropriately via the indicated route.

12. Monitor the patient for the desired effects.

13. Properly dispose of the needle and syringe.

Prefilled or Preloaded Syringes

Prefilled or **preloaded syringes** are packaged in tamper-proof containers with the medication already in the syringe. Because the syringe is prefilled, you do not need to draw the medication from another source. Generally, prefilled syringes contain standard dosages, thus decreasing the chance of dosage error.

The prefilled syringe consists of two parts, a syringe and a glass tube prefilled with liquid medication. The plastic syringe is similar to those described earlier; however, it does not have a plunger. Rather, you screw the prefilled glass tube into the syringe barrel and secure it (Figure 4-24 ●). Pushing the glass container into the syringe barrel expels the medication through the attached hypodermic needle.

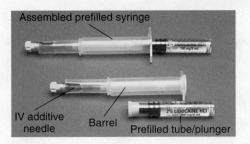

● **Figure 4-24** Prefilled syringes.

Follow these steps to administer a medication from a prefilled syringe:

1. Confirm medication indications and patient allergies.

2. Confirm the prefilled syringe label (name, dose, and expiration date).

3. Assemble the prefilled syringe. Remove the pop-off caps and screw together.

4. Reconfirm the indication, medication, dose, and route of administration.

5. Administer appropriately via the indicated route.

6. Properly dispose of the needle and syringe.

Intravenous Medication Solutions

Medicated solutions are another form of parenteral medication. They are packaged in an IV bag and administered as an IV **infusion**. IV medication solutions may be premixed, or you may have to mix them. The section on intravenous medication infusions later in this chapter discusses their actual preparation and administration.

Parenteral Routes

Parenterally administered medications can be absorbed locally or systemically. In addition, depending on the route of administration, their absorption rate may be slow, sustained, or rapid. Parenteral delivery bypasses the digestive tract, thus making the medication's absorption, action, and onset more predictable. Because parenteral routes use hypodermic needles that contact body fluids, the risk of disease transmission is ever present.

Parenteral medication delivery employs the following routes:

● Intradermal injection

● Subcutaneous injection

● Intramuscular injection

● Intravenous access

● Intraosseous infusion

Specific medications require specific routes of parenteral delivery; therefore, you must be competent with every route. In this section we will discuss the specialized equipment, medications, and routes for intradermal, subcutaneous, and intramuscular injections. Because of their complexity, we will discuss

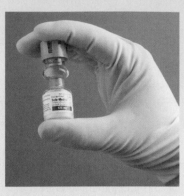

4-4a ● Inspect the medication. Check the label and the expiration date.

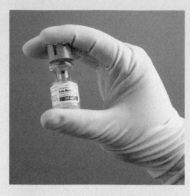

4-4b ● Compress the plunger to mix the solution and the solvent.

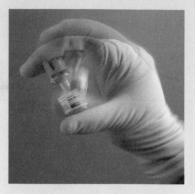

4-4c ● Shake the vial to adequately mix the solution.

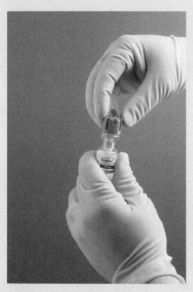

4-4d ● Remove the protective covering to expose the diaphragm.

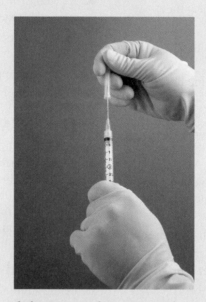

4-4e ● Uncap the syringe and prepare to withdraw the medication.

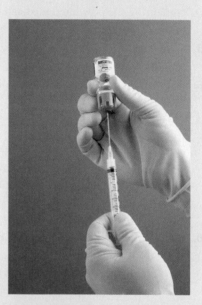

4-4f ● Insert the needle through the diaphragm.

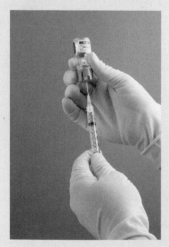

4-4g ● Withdraw the medication from the vial.

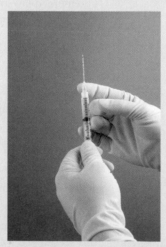

4-4h ● Expel any air from the syringe.

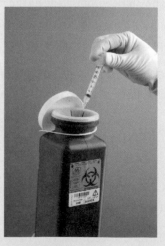

4-4i ● Administer the medication and properly dispose of the needle.

intravenous access and intraosseous infusions separately in the following sections.

Whether you are administering a parenteral injection or an IV bolus or infusion, you should explain the entire procedure to the patient to help alleviate his anxiety. Finally, remember that hypoperfusion (hypovolemia or peripheral vascular disease, for instance) may significantly reduce parenteral absorption.

Intradermal Injection

Using a syringe and hypodermic needle, **intradermal** injections deposit medication into the dermal layer of the skin (*intra-*, within; *derma*, skin). The amount of medication placed in the dermal layer is quite small, typically less than 1 mL (Figure 4-25 ●).

Capillaries in the dermis afford a very slow rate of absorption, with little or no systemic distribution. Rather, the bulk of medication remains localized in the area of administration. Intradermal delivery proves useful for allergy testing and tuberculin skin testing (PPD or Mantoux) and for administering local anesthetics during suturing, wound debridement, and IV establishment.

The forearm and upper back are preferred sites for intradermal injections. They have little hair and are highly visible. Additionally, you should look for sites free of superficial blood vessels, which increase the chance for systemic absorption.

To administer an intradermal injection, you will need the following equipment:

- Personal protective equipment
- Antiseptic preparations
- Packaged medication
- Tuberculin syringe (1 cc)
- 25- to 27-gauge needle, 3/8 to 1 inch long
- Sterile gauze and adhesive bandage

To administer an intradermal injection, follow these steps (Procedure 4-5):

1. Assemble and prepare the needed equipment.
2. Use Standard Precautions and confirm the medication, indication, dosage, and need for intradermal injection.

3. Draw up medication as appropriate.
4. Prepare the site with antiseptic solution. The intended site must be cleansed of pathogens, therein decreasing the likelihood of infection. Generally, you will use alcohol or similar antiseptics. To appropriately cleanse the site, start at the site itself and work outward with an expanding circular motion. This motion will push pathogens away from the intended site of puncture.
5. Pull the patient's skin taut with your nondominant hand.
6. Insert the needle, bevel up, just under the skin, at a 10° to 15° angle.
7. Slowly inject the medication; look for a small bump or wheal to form as medication is deposited and collects in the intradermal tissue.
8. Remove the needle and dispose of it in the sharps container.
9. Place the adhesive bandage over the site; use the gauze for hemorrhage control if needed.

Do not rub or massage the injection site. This promotes systemic absorption and nullifies the advantage of localized effect.

Subcutaneous Injection

Subcutaneous injections place medication into the subcutaneous tissue (*sub-*, below; *cutaneous*, skin). The subcutaneous layer consists of loose connective tissue between the skin and muscle (Figure 4-26 ●). The subcutaneous tissue has few blood vessels and thus promotes slow, sustained absorption, which prolongs a medication's effect on the body. Like intradermal injections, no more than 1.0 mL of medication is administered subcutaneously. Administering more than 1.0 mL of medication can cause irritation and, possibly, an abscess.

Administer subcutaneous injections where you can easily pinch the skin on the upper arms, thighs, or occasionally, the abdomen (Figure 4-27 ●). Easily pinched skin contains more subcutaneous tissue and readily separates from the muscle. All sites should be free of superficial blood vessels, nerves, and tendons. Additionally, avoid areas with tattoos or bruising.

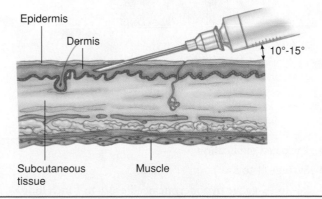

● **Figure 4-25**   Intradermal injection.

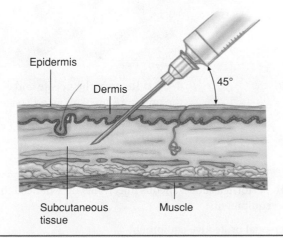

● **Figure 4-26**   Subcutaneous injection.

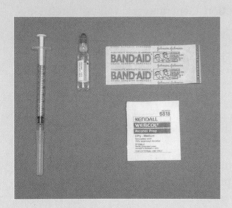

4-5a ● Assemble and prepare the needed equipment.

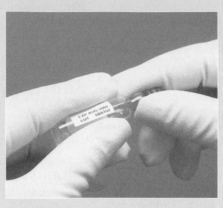

4-5b ● Check the medication.

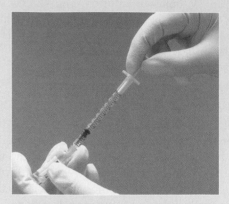

4-5c ● Draw up the medication.

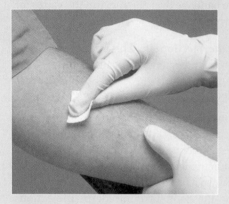

4-5d ● Prepare the administration site.

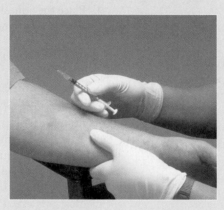

4-5e ● Pull the patient's skin taut.

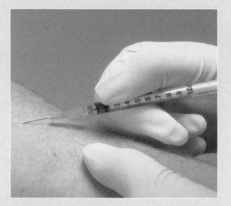

4-5f ● Insert the needle, bevel up, at a 10° to 15° angle.

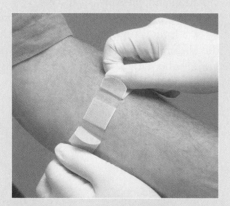

4-5g ● Remove the needle and cover the puncture site with an adhesive bandage.

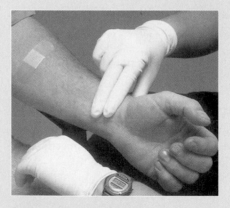

4-5h ● Monitor the patient.

To perform a subcutaneous injection, you will need the following equipment:

● Personal protective equipment
● Antiseptic preparations

● Packaged medication
● Syringe (1 to 3 cc)
● 24- to 26-gauge hypodermic needle, 3/8 to 1 inch long
● Sterile gauze and adhesive bandage

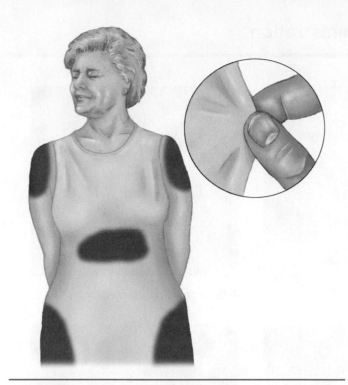

● **Figure 4-27** Subcutaneous injection sites (injection sites shown in red).

To administer a subcutaneous injection, use the following technique (Procedure 4-6):

1. Assemble and prepare equipment.
2. Use Standard Precautions and confirm the medication, indication, dosage, and need for subcutaneous injection.
3. Draw up the medication as appropriate.
4. Prepare the site with antiseptic solution.
5. Gently pinch a 1-inch fold of skin.
6. Insert the needle just into the skin at a 45° angle with the bevel up.
7. Pull the plunger back to aspirate tissue fluid.
8. If blood appears, the hypodermic needle is in a blood vessel and absorption will be too rapid. Start the procedure over with a new syringe.
9. If no blood appears, proceed with step 10.
10. Slowly inject the medication.
11. Remove the needle and dispose of it in a sharps container.
12. Place an adhesive bandage over the site; use the gauze for hemorrhage control if needed.
13. Monitor the patient.

After you give the injection, gently rubbing or massaging the site will help initiate systemic absorption.

Some authorities recommend using an air plug in the syringe. This is approximately 0.1 mL of air that follows the injection and pushes the medication further into the subcutaneous tissue, thus preventing leakage or medication loss. To place an air plug in the syringe, aspirate approximately 0.1 mL of air into the barrel after you have drawn up the medication. Pointing the needle downward and perpendicular to the ground, tap the syringe with your finger to dislodge the air pocket. It will float to the top of the plunger, and from there it will follow the medication into the subcutaneous tissue.

You can also deliver a subcutaneous injection into the sublingual region, or fleshy tissue below the tongue. To administer a subcutaneous injection, you place the hypodermic needle of a small, medication-filled syringe into the sublingual tissue and then inject the medication as appropriate. Epinephrine in severe cases of asthma or anaphylaxis can be administered in this manner.

Intramuscular Injection

Intramuscular injections deposit medication into muscle (*intra-,* within; *muscular,* muscle). Muscle is extremely vascular and permits systemic delivery at a moderate absorption rate. Medication absorption through muscle is also relatively predictable. To reach the muscle, a needle must penetrate the dermal and subcutaneous tissue (Figure 4-28 ●).

Several sites are used for intramuscular injections (Figure 4-29 ●). Depending on the site, varying quantities of medication can be delivered. These sites and their correlating volumes of medication include the following:

● *Deltoid.* The deltoid muscle is 3 to 4 fingerbreadths below the acromial process (the bony bump on the shoulder). It is highly vascular and permits easy access. You can deliver up to 2.0 mL into this muscle.

● *Dorsal gluteal.* The dorsal gluteal muscle, or buttock, is a common administration point for intramuscular injections. Injections here can deliver 5.0 mL of medication or more.

CONTENT REVIEW
▶ Intramuscular Injection Sites
- Deltoid
- Dorsal gluteal
- Vastus lateralis
- Rectus femoris

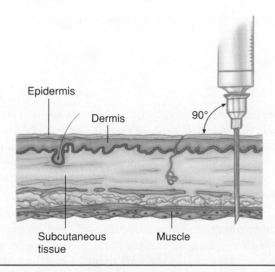

● **Figure 4-28** Intramuscular injection.

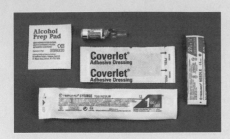

4-6a ● Prepare the equipment.

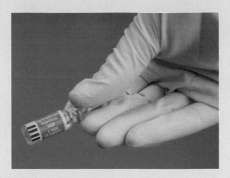

4-6b ● Check the medication.

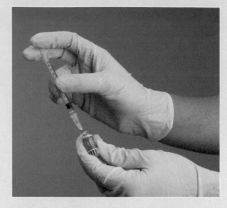

4-6c ● Draw up the medication.

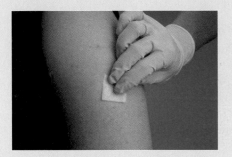

4-6d ● Prep the site.

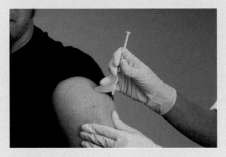

4-6e ● Insert the needle at a 45° angle.

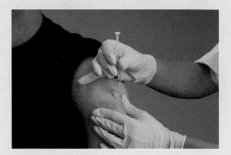

4-6f ● Remove the needle and cover the puncture site.

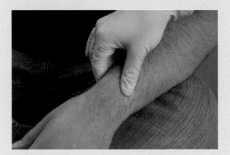

4-6g ● Monitor the patient.

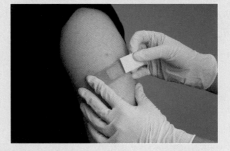

4-6h ● Apply an adhesive bandage to the injection site.

They cause little discomfort, but you must avoid the large sciatic nerve, which is the leg's major motor nerve. Damage to the sciatic nerve can decrease mobility or totally paralyze the leg. To help prevent neurologic complication, envision an imaginary quadrant over the buttock; administer all injections in the upper and outer quadrant.

● *Vastus lateralis.* The *vastus lateralis* muscle of the thigh is another common site for intramuscular injection, especially for pediatric patients. As at the dorsal gluteal muscle, injections here can deliver 5 mL of medication or more. To deliver medication at this site, imagine a grid of nine

boxes. Administer injections in the middle, outer box, or anterolateral part of the muscle.

● *Rectus femoris.* The *rectus femoris* lies over the femur and is closely associated with the *vastus lateralis* muscle. When utilizing the *rectus femoris* for intramuscular injection, place the medication into the center of the muscle at approximately midshaft of the femur. Up to 5 mL of medication volume can be administered into the *rectus femoris.*

When choosing a site, avoid bruised or scarred areas. Areas free of superficial blood vessels are most desirable.

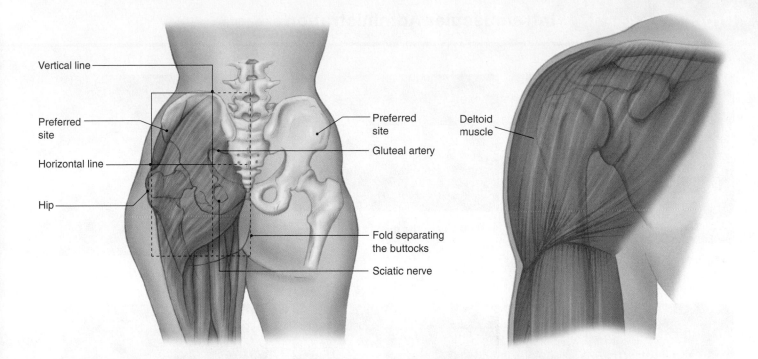

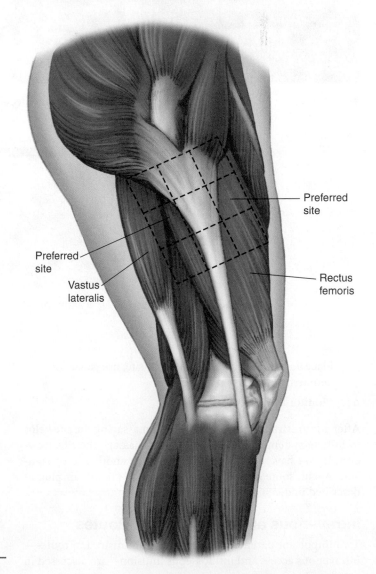

To perform an intramuscular injection, you will need the following equipment:

- Personal protective equipment
- Antiseptic preparation
- Packaged medication
- Syringe (1 to 5 mL, depending on dosage)
- 21- to 23-gauge hypodermic needle, 3/8 to 1 inch long
- Sterile gauze and adhesive bandage

Follow these steps to administer an intramuscular injection (Procedure 4-7):

1. Assemble and prepare the needed equipment.
2. Use Standard Precautions and confirm the medication, indication, dosage, and need for intramuscular injection.
3. Draw up medication as appropriate.
4. Prepare the site with antiseptic solution.
5. Stretch the skin taut over the injection site with your nondominant hand.
6. Insert the needle just into the skin at a 90° angle with the bevel up.
7. Pull back the plunger to aspirate tissue fluid.
   - If blood appears, the hypodermic needle is in a blood vessel, and absorption of the medication will be too rapid. Start the procedure over with a new syringe.
   - If no blood appears proceed with step 8.
8. Slowly inject the medication.
9. Remove the needle and dispose of it in the sharps container.

● **Figure 4-29** Intramuscular injection sites.

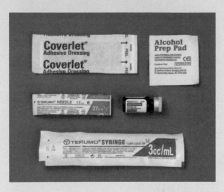

4-7a ● Prepare the equipment.

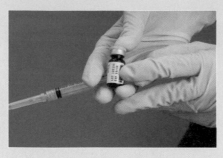

4-7b ● Check the medication.

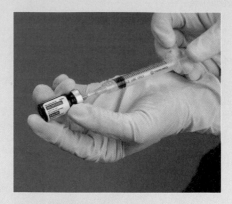

4-7c ● Draw up the medication.

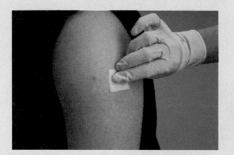

4-7d ● Prepare the site.

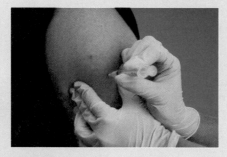

4-7e ● Insert the needle at a 90°
angle.

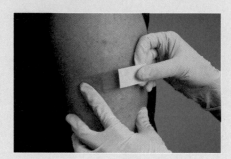

4-7f ● Remove the needle and cover
the puncture site.

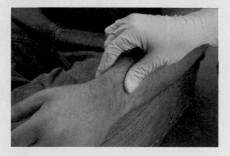

4-7g ● Monitor the patient.

10. Place an adhesive bandage over the site; use gauze for
hemorrhage control if needed.

11. Monitor the patient.

After administration, gently rubbing or massaging the site helps
to initiate systemic absorption. Do not massage the site, however, if you have administered heparin or another anticoagulant. Again, some authorities recommend a 0.1-mL air plug as
described under subcutaneous injection.

Intravenous and Intraosseous Routes

Two important parenteral medication administration routes—
intravenous access and intraosseous infusion—are discussed in
detail in Part 2.

PART 2: Intravenous Access, Blood Sampling, and Intraosseous Infusion

INTRAVENOUS ACCESS

Intravenous (IV) access (*intra-*, within; *venous*, vein), or **cannulation**, is a routine paramedic procedure. Circulating blood
transports chemicals, proteins, and fluids throughout the body.
Venous circulation can likewise deliver medications and fluids
into the body and provides an invaluable tool for treating the
sick and injured.

The following situations indicate intravenous access:

- Fluid and blood replacement
- Medication administration
- Obtaining venous blood specimens for laboratory analysis

Since veins are easier to locate and penetrate, venous access is preferable to arterial access. Additionally, venous circulation pressure is lower than arterial and presents fewer hemorrhage control complications.

Types of Intravenous Access

Medical care providers use two types of intravenous access, peripheral and central. As a paramedic, you will most often perform peripheral intravenous access. Central venous access is rarely, if ever, performed in the prehospital setting.

Peripheral Venous Access

Although challenging, **peripheral venous access** is relatively easy to master. As its name implies, it uses peripheral veins. Common sites include the arms and legs and, when necessary, the neck. Figure 4-30 ● illustrates the specific veins commonly accessed on the hand, forearm, and leg.

As some patients' veins may not be readily visible, you must know venous topography. In these cases, you will have to locate veins based on anatomic layout and palpation. Exhaust all possibilities on the arms before trying to locate the veins of the legs. Leg veins are more difficult to access and present complications more frequently. For neonates and infants, you may access veins in the scalp. Volume 6, Chapter 4 explains that technique.

When establishing a peripheral IV, start at the distal end of the extremity and work proximally. Once you have attempted cannulation, the disruption in blood flow hinders using veins distal to that site. However, the purpose of access also determines site selection. For example, rapid fluid administration requires larger veins like the antecubital fossa, as opposed to the smaller veins of the hand. The external jugular vein is considered a peripheral vein and can be accessed when other peripheral sites are not available.

The major advantage of peripheral venous access is that it is relatively simple to perform because visualizing and accessing the veins is usually easy. In addition, you can access peripheral veins while simultaneously doing other life-sustaining procedures such as CPR or endotracheal intubation. Conversely, peripheral veins collapse in hypovolemia or circulatory failure, thus becoming difficult to locate and access. Furthermore, the peripheral veins of geriatric patients, pediatric patients, or those with peripheral vascular disease may be fragile and difficult to cannulate. Finally, peripheral veins may roll and elude IV placement.

Central Venous Access

Central venous access utilizes veins located deep within the body. These include the internal jugular, subclavian, and femoral veins. They are larger than peripheral veins and will not collapse in shock. Central IV lines are placed near the heart for long-term use. Typically, they are used when medical conditions require repeated access for medication and/or fluid delivery. They also are used for transvenous pacing or for monitoring central venous pressure.

A special type of central line is the **peripherally inserted central catheter**, or **PICC**, line. PICC lines are smaller than those routinely used for central access and are threaded into the central

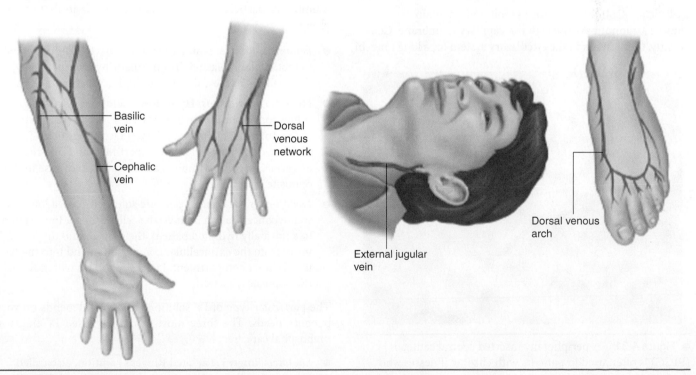

Basilic vein

Cephalic vein

Dorsal venous network

External jugular vein

Dorsal venous arch

● **Figure 4-30**   Peripheral IV access sites: veins of the arm, hand, neck, and foot.

circulation via a peripheral site (Figure 4-31 ●). PICC lines are most often used in infants and children requiring long-term care.

Central venous access is typically restricted to the hospital setting because of its invasive nature and high risk of complications such as arterial puncture, pneumothorax, and air embolism. Central veins cannot be accessed during procedures such as CPR, and they often require a chest X-ray for placement confirmation. You may nonetheless encounter a central line during interfacility transports or in a chronically ill homebound patient. Protocols in some EMS systems allow paramedics to access existing central lines during emergency care. Still other systems allow their paramedics to place certain central lines. Always follow local protocols regarding central line access and insertion. For more information about central venous access, consult a text on advanced venipuncture techniques.

Equipment and Supplies for Venous Access

To establish intravenous access, you will need the following specialized equipment and supplies.

Intravenous Fluids

Intravenous fluids are chemically prepared solutions tailored to the body's specific needs. They replace the body's lost fluids and/or aid the delivery of IV medications. They also can keep a vein patent when no fluid or medication therapy is required.

Intravenous fluids come in four different forms: colloids, crystalloids, blood, and oxygen-carrying fluids.

Colloids **Colloidal solutions** solutions contain large proteins that cannot pass through the capillary membrane. Consequently, they remain in the circulatory system for a long time. In addition, colloids have osmotic properties that attract water into the circulatory system. A small quantity of colloid can significantly increase intravascular volume (volume of blood and fluid contained within the blood vessels). Common colloids include the following:

● *Plasma protein fraction (Plasmanate).* Plasmanate is a protein-containing colloid. Its principal protein, albumin, is suspended with other proteins in a saline solvent.

● *Albumin.* Albumin contains only human albumin. Each gram of albumin will retain approximately 18 milliliters of water in the bloodstream.

● *Dextran.* Dextran is not a protein but a large sugar molecule with osmotic properties similar to those of albumin. It comes in two molecular weights: 40,000 and 70,000 Daltons. Dextran 40 has from two to two-and-a-half times the colloidal osmotic pressure of albumin. Anaphylactic reaction is a possible side effect.

● *Hetastarch (Hespan).* Like Dextran, hetastarch is a sugar molecule with osmotic properties similar to those of protein. Hetastarch does not appear to share Dextran's side effects.

Although colloids help maintain vascular volume, using them in the field is not practical. Their high cost, short shelf life, and specific storage requirements suit them better to the hospital setting. However, the paramedic who works in an emergency department, critical care transport, or at a mass-casualty incident may have to administer colloidal solutions.

Crystalloids **Crystalloids** are the primary prehospital IV solutions. Crystalloids contain electrolytes and water but lack colloids' larger proteins and larger molecules. The many preparations of crystalloid solutions are classified by their tonicity (number of particles per unit volume) relative to that of body plasma:

● *Isotonic solutions.* **Isotonic** solutions have a tonicity equal to that of blood plasma. In a normally hydrated patient, they will not cause a significant fluid or electrolyte shift.

● *Hypertonic solutions.* **Hypertonic** solutions have a higher solute concentration than do the cells. When administered to the normally hydrated patient, they cause fluid to shift out of the intracellular compartment and into the extracellular compartment. Later, solute will diffuse in the opposite direction.

● *Hypotonic solutions.* **Hypotonic** solutions have a lower solute concentration than do the cells. When administered to a normally hydrated patient, they cause fluid to move from the extracellular compartment and into the intracellular compartment. Later, the solutes will move in the opposite direction.

The particular type of IV solution you select depends on your patient's needs. The three most commonly used IV fluids in prehospital care are:

● *Lactated Ringer's.* Lactated Ringer's solution, also called Hartman's solution, is an isotonic electrolyte solution. It

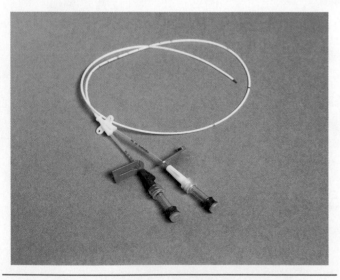

● **Figure 4-31** A peripherally inserted central catheter (PICC) is often used in patients with chronic illnesses who require repeated vascular access.

contains sodium chloride, potassium chloride, calcium chloride, and sodium lactate in water.

- **Normal saline solution.** Normal saline is an isotonic electrolyte solution containing 0.9 percent sodium chloride in water.

- **5 percent dextrose in water (D₅W).** D_5W is a hypotonic glucose solution used to keep a vein patent and to supply calories needed for cellular metabolism. While D_5W initially increases circulatory volume, glucose molecules rapidly diffuse across the vascular membrane and increase the free water.

Both lactated Ringer's and normal saline solution are used for fluid replacement because of their immediate ability to expand the circulating volume. However, due to the movement of electrolytes and water, two-thirds of either solution will be lost to the extravascular space within 1 hour. Crystalloids such as normal saline mixed with D_5W or half-strength normal saline (0.45 percent) are combinations or modifications of the previous solutions.

Occasionally, you will have to warm or cool the IV fluid. A hypothermic patient may benefit from having a crystalloid warmed before and during fluid administration. Warm fluids assist in elevating the patient's core temperature. Conversely, cool fluids may benefit the patient with an increased core temperature. With the introduction of **induced therapeutic hypothermia (ITH)**, prehospital providers now commonly administer cold IV fluids to cardiac arrest victims to minimize subsequent secondary injury. You can cool or warm fluids by storing them in a special temperature-controlled compartment or by using the heater or air conditioner in the ambulance, helicopter, or mobile intensive care unit. Commercial fluid heaters are available. Their use is detailed later in this chapter. Some fluids, such as blood and some colloids, require constant storage in a cool environment.

Blood The most desirable fluid for replacement is whole blood. Unlike colloids and crystalloids, the hemoglobin in blood carries oxygen. Blood, however, is a precious commodity and must be conserved so that it can be of benefit to the most people. Its use in the field is generally limited to aeromedical services or mass-casualty incidents. O-negative blood's universal compatibility makes it ideal for administration in the field. Volume 4, Chapter 9 discusses blood in detail.

Oxygen-Carrying Solutions Considerable research has been devoted to the development of solutions that carry oxygen. There are two general classes of oxygen-carrying solutions: perfluorocarbons and hemoglobin-based oxygen-carrying solutions (HBOCs). These agents provide a significant advantage over standard colloids and crystalloids because, as their name indicates, in addition to replacing volume they can transport oxygen.

- **Perfluorocarbons.** Perfluorocarbon compounds are in various stages of research and testing. These agents are denser than water and have a high capacity to dissolve large quantities of gases such as oxygen.

- **Hemoglobin-based oxygen-carrying solutions (HBOCs).** HBOCs represent a potential major development in the field

of emergency and critical care. These products differ from other intravenous fluids in that they have the capability to transport oxygen. HBOCs contain long chains of *polymerized hemoglobin*. This hemoglobin is obtained from either expired donated human blood or bovine (cow) blood. The hemoglobin is removed from the red blood cells and then repeatedly filtered to remove any infectious substances or antigenic proteins. Finally, the individual hemoglobin molecules are joined together in a large chain through a chemical process known as polymerization. HBOCs are compatible with all blood types and do not require blood typing, testing, or crossmatching. Unfortunately, the clinical trials to date have been disappointing.

Packaging of Intravenous Fluids Most intravenous fluids and blood are packaged in soft plastic or vinyl bags of various sizes (50, 100, 250, 500, 1,000, 2,000, and 3,000 mL) (Figure 4-32 ●). Some contain medication that is incompatible with plastic or vinyl and must be packaged in glass bottles.

The IV-fluid container provides important information.

- **Label.** A label on every IV bottle or bag lists the fluid type and expiration date. Like any other medication, intravenous solutions have a shelf life; do not use them after their expiration date. Discard any fluid that appears cloudy, discolored, or laced with particulate. In addition, avoid using any fluid whose sealed packaging has been opened or tampered with.

- **Medication administration port.** A medication port on IV-solution bags or bottles permits you to inject medication into the fluid for infusion.

- **Administration set port.** The administration set port is where you place the spike from the IV administration tubing.

Administration Tubing

Intravenous **administration tubing** connects the solution bag to the IV **cannula** that is inserted into the patient's vein. Administration tubing is made of very flexible clear plastic. You must

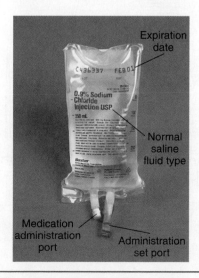

● **Figure 4-32** IV solution container.

select from several types of administration tubing according to your patient's need. All tubing is packaged in a sterile container. If the container is opened or appears damaged, select another administration set. Any pathogens on the tubing will enter the patient, possibly causing long-term complications.

Microdrip and Macrodrip Tubing **Microdrip** administration tubing delivers relatively small amounts of fluid to the patient. It is more appropriate when you need to restrict the overall fluid volume a patient will receive. **Macrodrip** administration tubing delivers relatively large amounts of fluid. It is more appropriate when volume replacement is necessary, as in shock, fluid replacement, or hypotension.

To effectively deliver intravenous fluids, you must be thoroughly familiar with the microdrip and macrodrip administration sets, their components, and their subtle differences (Figure 4-33 ●).

- *Spike.* The **spike** is a sharp-pointed plastic device that you insert into the administration set port on the IV solution bag. A plastic sheath covering the spike keeps it sterile. When the sheath is removed, you must use a medically clean technique to avoid contaminating the spike. If the spike becomes contaminated, discard the administration set and start over with new tubing.

- *Drip chamber.* The **drip chamber** is a clear plastic chamber that allows you to view the **drip rate**. The drip chamber is

squeezable; when compressed, it collects fluid from the IV solution bag and acts as a reservoir for administration. For optimal fluid delivery, the drip chamber should be about one-third full; a line on the chamber marks the correct fluid level.

- *Drop former.* Inside the drip chamber is a **drop former**. In microdrip administration tubing, the drop former is a hollow metal stylet. In macrodrip tubing, it is a large circular opening at the top of the drip chamber. The drop former regulates each drop's size. The narrow metal stylet in the microdrip tubing creates smaller drops; the wider opening in the macrodrip tubing creates larger drops. In either case, the drop former's precise calibration allows you to calculate fluid volumes by counting **drops**:

  ○ Microdrip 60 drops = 1 mL
  ○ Macrodrip 10 drops = 1 mL

Depending on the manufacturer, macrodrip sets may equate 15 or 20 drops to 1 mL. You must know drops per milliliter to calculate flow rates or medicated infusion dosages.

- *Tubing.* Intravenous administration tubing is clear and very flexible. Thus, you can watch the solution flow through the administration set, and you can manipulate the tubing in tight situations. Some medications such as intravenous nitroglycerin are chemically incompatible with regular tubing and require special tubing.

- *Clamp.* IV administration tubing has a simple plastic clamp. When slid over the tubing, the clamp completely stops the flow of solution from the IV bag to the patient. It prevents both the entrainment of air into the tubing when changing IV bags and the backflow of medication when administering medications. You can also use it to stop infusion without disturbing the flow-regulator setting.

- *Flow regulator.* The flow regulator is a dial enclosed in a triangular plastic casing. It allows infinite control of flow rates ranging from a continuous stream to completely stopped. Rolling the dial towards the IV solution bag increases the drip frequency; rolling the dial towards the patient decreases the drip frequency.

- *Medication injection ports.* The **medication injection ports** have a self-sealing membrane into which you can insert a hypodermic needle for medication administration. Many sets now contain "needleless" medication ports that decrease the possibility of needlestick injuries. Their design varies, depending on the manufacturer. When possible, use the medication port nearest the patient.

- *Needle adapter.* The **needle adapter** is a rigid plastic device at the administration tubing's distal end. It is specifically constructed to fit into the hub of an intravenous cannula. Similar to the spike, the needle adapter is sterile and covered by a protective cap. If it becomes contaminated at any time, start over with a new administration set.

IV Extension Tubing **Extension tubing** is IV tubing used to extend the original macrodrip or microdrip setup (Figure 4-34 ●). Its packaging clearly marks it as such. Like

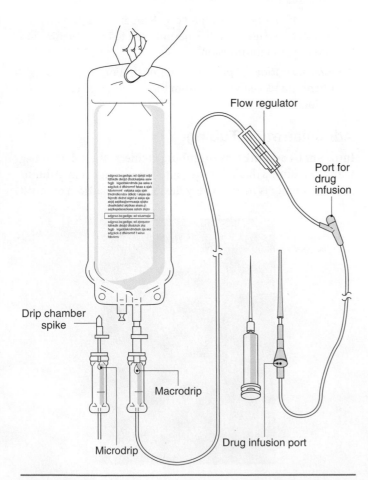

Flow regulator

Port for drug infusion

Drip chamber spike

Macrodrip

Microdrip

Drug infusion port

● **Figure 4-33** Macrodrip and microdrip administration sets.

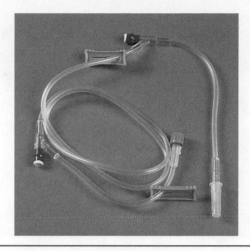

● **Figure 4-34** Extension tubing.

administration sets, extension tubing is sterile and must be handled accordingly.

Extension tubing also permits the paramedic to change the original administration tubing or the IV solution bag with little difficulty. For example, if you have to switch from a macrodrip set to a microdrip set, you can close the clamp on the extension and detach the primary tubing. Once you have flushed the new tubing with fluid, you place the needle adapter into the receiving port on the extension tubing and release the clamp. You can now resume fluid therapy without risking complications or having to painfully reinitiate a second IV line.

Electromechanical Pump Tubing   Mechanical infusion devices may require specially manufactured pump tubing (Figure 4-35 ●). Typically, pump tubing has special components that attach directly to the pump. Additionally, bladders and relief points permit you to void possible air bubbles. Many specific models of electromechanical infusion pumps require specific pump tubing. When using a mechanical infusion pump, be sure to have the appropriate tubing on hand. Consult the section on electromechanical infusion pumps for more information.

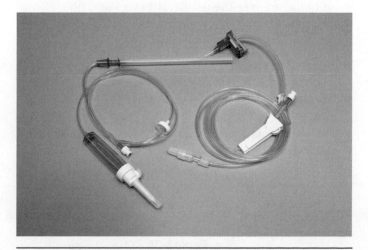

● **Figure 4-35**   IV pump tubing.

Measured Volume Administration Set   The **measured volume administration set** can deliver specific volumes of fluid with or without medication. It works well for patients who need specific or limited volumes of fluid, and it is especially advantageous for pediatrics, renal failure, or other patients who cannot tolerate fluid overload.

The measured volume administration set consists of either micro- or macrodrip tubing, with the addition of a large **burette chamber** marked in 1.0-mL increments (Figure 4-36 ●). The burette chamber holds between 120 and 150 mL of fluid. The components of the measured volume administration set include the following:

● Flanged spike
● Clamp
● Airway handle
● Medication injection port
● Burette chamber
● Float valve
● Drip chamber
● Flow regulator
● Medication injection port
● Needle adapter

When opened, the airway handle on top of the burette chamber permits air to be displaced or replaced as fluid enters or exits the chamber. If a medication must be mixed in a specific amount of IV solution, you can add it through the medication administration port after correctly filling the chamber.

Blood Tubing   Administering whole blood or blood components requires **blood tubing**, which contains a filter that prevents clots and other debris from entering the patient. Without

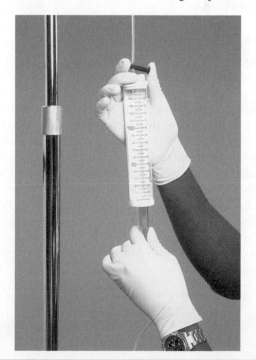

● **Figure 4-36**   Measured volume administration set.

exception, all blood must be filtered. Blood that is stored or delivered over an extended period is prone to form fibrin clots or to accumulate other debris. If these clots or debris enter the circulatory system, they can travel in the form of an embolus. Remember, once an embolus encounters a blood vessel too small for its passage, it will lodge and effectively block all blood flow distal to the point of occlusion.

Many aeromedical and facility-based paramedics administer blood and must be familiar with blood tubing. Although most ambulances do not carry blood, paramedics may initiate normal saline with blood tubing in anticipation that whole blood or blood products will be required immediately in the emergency department (Figure 4-37 ●).

Blood tubing comes in two configurations, straight and Y. Y tubing has two administration ports, one for blood and one for IV normal saline solution. Typically, blood is administered with normal saline. Fluids like lactated Ringer's increase the potential for blood coagulation. The two-port design permits immediate access to normal saline if the blood supply is exhausted or must be shut down, as for a transfusion reaction. When you use Y blood tubing, establish a traditional IV by connecting a bag of normal saline to the tubing. Attach the blood to the second port when needed, while maintaining strict medical asepsis. Using the flow regulator, discontinue the normal saline while opening the clamp regulating the flow of blood. Straight blood tubing has only one reservoir. Therefore, only blood is attached to the tubing. A medication administration port close to the needle adapter allows you to piggyback a secondary line of normal saline into the tubing.

Miscellaneous Administration Sets   Some tubing now has a manual dial that can set drops per minute or specific flow rates. Some manufacturers have created a single drip chamber that can create either microdrips or macrodrips, depending on the patient's need.

In-Line Intravenous Fluid Heaters

Technology now makes it possible to heat IV fluids to near body temperature in the field. Most EMS units store their IV fluids in the unit. These fluids, when opened, are at the same temperature as the ambient air. Thus, the temperature of IV fluids can vary significantly depending on where in the country (or world) you work. Many patients are very prone to the development of hypothermia following fluid administration. These include the elderly, children, the frail, and those suffering from fever or similar conditions. When indicated, it is prudent to use an in-line IV fluid heater to warm the IV fluid to body temperature. These devices are designed to shut down if the IV fluid temperature exceeds body temperature. Likewise, different devices are available in order to meet the various flow

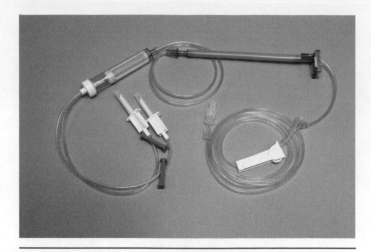

● **Figure 4-37**   Blood administration tubing.

requirements of, for example, trauma patients, pediatrics, or geriatrics.

Always use Standard Precautions. Open the unit and test the battery. Attach the in-line intravenous fluid heater between the end of the IV tubing and the extension tubing supplied with the unit. Turn the device on and monitor the indicator lights. The unit should remain with the patient on arrival at the hospital and throughout his hospital stay. It is switched to a direct current (DC) adapter on the patient's arrival at the floor.

Intravenous Cannulas

The intravenous cannula permits actual puncture and access into a patient's vein. The distal portion of the administration tubing connects to the IV cannula, thus completing the bridge between the solution bag and patient. The three basic types of IV cannulas are:

● Over-the-needle catheter
● Hollow-needle catheter
● Plastic catheter inserted through a hollow needle

Over-the-Needle Catheter   Often called an **IV catheter or cannula**, an **over-the-needle catheter** comprises a semi-flexible catheter enclosing a sharp metal stylet (needle) that is hollow and beveled at the distal end (Figure 4-38 ●).

● *Metal stylet (needle).* The metal stylet permits easy puncturing of the skin and blood vessel. Blood from the vein flows through the hollow stylet to the flashback chamber.
● *Flashback chamber.* The clear plastic flashback chamber allows you to see the blood after the metal stylet has punctured the vein. Blood in the flashback chamber confirms placement of the stylet in the vein.

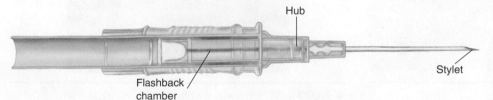

Hub

Flashback chamber

Stylet

● **Figure 4-38**   Over-the-needle catheter.

- *Teflon catheter.* The Teflon catheter slides over the metal stylet into a successfully punctured vein.
- *Hub.* Located on the back of the Teflon catheter, the hub receives the needle adapter of the administration tubing once removed from the metal stylet.

For peripheral venous access, the over-the-needle catheter is preferred since it is easy to place and anchor and permits freer movement of the patient. Most of these needles now have a needlestick protection mechanism that covers the exposed needle (Figure 4-39 ●).

Hollow-Needle Catheter

For pediatrics or other patients with tiny, delicate veins, use **hollow-needle catheters** (Figure 4-40 ●). These catheters do not have a Teflon tube; rather, the metal stylet itself is inserted into the vein and secured there. Because the sharp metal stylet can easily damage the vein, you must insert it very carefully. Some hollow-needle catheters have wings for guidance and securing into a vein. These hollow-needle catheters are referred to as winged catheters or butterfly catheters.

Catheter Inserted through the Needle

The **catheter inserted through the needle** is also called an **intracatheter**. It consists of a Teflon catheter inserted through a large metal stylet (Figure 4-41 ●). Used in the hospital setting to implement central lines, its proper placement requires great skill, as discussed previously.

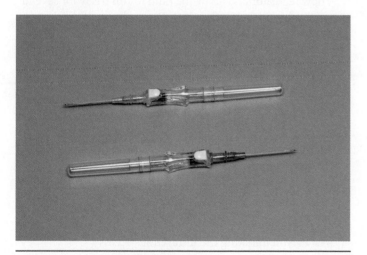

● **Figure 4-39** Safety IV catheters.

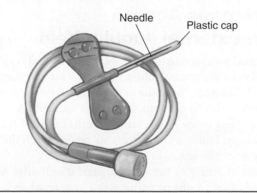

Needle

Plastic cap

● **Figure 4-40** Hollow-needle (butterfly) catheter.

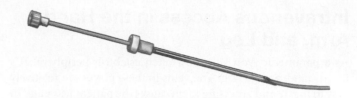

● **Figure 4-41** Catheter inserted through the needle.

The size of an intravenous cannula is expressed as its gauge. The *larger* the gauge, the *smaller* the diameter of the stylet and catheter. For example, a 22-gauge cannula is smaller than a 14-gauge cannula. The larger diameter, 14-gauge catheter allows greater flow rates than the smaller diameter 22-gauge cannula. When establishing venous access, choose the cannula size most appropriate for the patient's condition. Typical uses for the various sizes of cannulas are:

- *22-gauge.* Small gauges are used for *fragile* veins such as those of the elderly or children.
- *20-gauge.* Moderate gauges are used for the average adult who does not need fluid replacement.
- *18-gauge, 16-gauge, or 14-gauge.* Larger gauge cannulas are used to increase volume or to administer viscous medications such as dextrose. Blood can be administered only through a cannula that is 16 gauge or larger.

The largest gauge cannula that will fit into a vein is not always appropriate. A cardiac patient with large veins should not receive a 14-gauge cannula for medication administration, just as a multisystems trauma patient with good veins should not receive a 22-gauge cannula for fluid administration. Remember that intravenous access is painful and causes discomfort not only to those receiving it but also to family members watching a loved one in distress.

Miscellaneous Equipment

The **venous constricting band** is a flat rubber band applied proximal to the intended puncture site. It impedes venous return, thereby engorging veins and making them easier to see. This helps you to select the best site and makes venipuncture easier. Never restrict arterial blood flow with the constricting band, and never leave it in place longer than 2 minutes.

Intravenous access is an invasive procedure; therefore, you must use medically clean techniques, including antiseptic preparations, to prevent infection. Applying a sterile, impermeable dressing after venipuncture decreases the chance of infection.

Once you have established an IV, you must secure it to avoid losing the access. Medical tape and an adhesive bandage are inexpensive and easy to apply. You can also apply clear membranes over the site. Commercial devices manufactured specifically for this task are also available. Have gauze on hand for hemorrhage control if IV cannulation is unsuccessful or if blood leaks from around the site.

Obtaining a venous blood specimen at the time of venipuncture will save the patient from being stuck with a needle again later. This chapter's section on venous blood sampling discusses this technique in detail.

Intravenous Access in the Hand, Arm, and Leg

As a paramedic, you will most often establish peripheral IVs in the hand, arm, or leg. The veins in these places are relatively easy to locate and accessing them causes the patient less pain. In addition, the likelihood of complications is less with these veins than with the external jugular vein (discussed later) or central IV initiation. Therefore, the veins of the hand, arm, and leg are the primary sites for IV initiation.

To establish a peripheral IV in the hand, arm, or leg, use the following technique (Procedure 4-8):

1. Confirm indication and type of IV setup needed. Gather and arrange all supplies and equipment beforehand to make the process easy and accessible.
   - IV fluid
   - Administration set
   - Intravenous cannula
   - Tape or commercial securing device
   - Venous blood drawing equipment
   - Venous constricting band
   - Antiseptic solution

   When appropriate, explain the entire process to the patient. Apply the proper Standard Precautions—gloves, mask, and protective eyewear goggles, as IV access is invasive and presents the potential for blood exposure.

2. Prepare all needed equipment. Examine the IV fluid for clarity and expiration date. Insert the administration tubing spike in the IV solution bag's administration set port. Squeeze fluid from the IV fluid container into the drip chamber until it reaches the fill line. Open the clamp and/or flow regulator to flush the solution through the administration tubing and expel trapped air bubbles. Shut down the flow regulator and replace the cap over the needle adapter. Remember that the IV administration set is sterile; if any contamination occurs, you must replace the set with a new one.

3. Select the venipuncture site. Acceptable sites have clearly visible veins and are free of bruising or scarring. Straight veins are easier to cannulate than crooked ones.

4. Place the constricting band proximal to the intended site of puncture. Tighten it enough to impede venous blood flow without restricting arterial blood passage. Never leave the constricting band in place more than 2 minutes, as intrinsic changes will occur in the slowed venous blood.

5. Cleanse the venipuncture site. You must cleanse the intended site of pathogens to decrease the likelihood of infection. Alcohol and similar antiseptic solutions are the most commonly used. Start at the site itself and work outward in an expanding circle. This pushes pathogens away from the puncture site.

6. Insert the intravenous cannula into the vein. With your nondominant hand, pull all local skin taut to stabilize the vein and prevent it from rolling. With the distal bevel of the metal stylet up, insert the cannula into the vein at a 10° to 30° angle. Continue until you feel the cannula "pop" into the vein or see blood in the flashback chamber. The metal stylet is now in the vein; however, the Teflon catheter is not. To place the catheter into the vein, carefully advance the cannula approximately 0.5 cm further. (If you are using a butterfly cannula, it has no Teflon catheter, and you must carefully advance the needle itself.)

7. Holding the metal stylet stationary, slide the Teflon catheter over the needle into the vein. Place a finger over the vein at the catheter tip and tamponade (press gently downward to occlude the vein), thus preventing blood from flowing from the catheter and/or air from entraining into the circulatory system. Carefully remove the metal stylet, retract the needle, and promptly dispose of it in the sharps container. Remove the venous constricting band.

8. Obtain venous blood samples as discussed in the section on venous blood sampling.

9. Attach the administration tubing to the cannula. Remove the protective cap from the needle adapter and tightly secure the needle adapter into the cannula hub. Open the flow regulator and allow the fluid to run freely for several seconds. Adjust the flow rate. Do not let go of the cannula and administration tubing until you have secured them as explained in step 10.

10. Cover the catheter and puncture site with an adhesive bandage or other commercial device. Loop the distal tubing and secure with tape. This makes the medication administration port more accessible and attaches the device to the patient more securely. Continue by taping the administration tubing to the patient, proximal to the venipuncture site.

11. Label the intravenous solution bag with the following information:
    - Date and time initiated
    - Person initiating the intravenous access

12. Continually monitor the patient and flow rate.

Intravenous Access in the External Jugular Vein

The external jugular vein is a large peripheral blood vessel in the neck, between the angle of the jaw and the middle third of the clavicle. It connects into the central circulation's subclavian vein. Since it lies so close to the central circulation, cannulation here offers many of the same benefits afforded by central venous access. Fluids and medications rapidly reach the core of the body from this site.

Consider accessing the external jugular only after you have exhausted other means of peripheral access or when a patient requires immediate fluid administration. This is an extremely

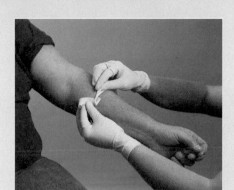

4-8a ● Place the constricting band.

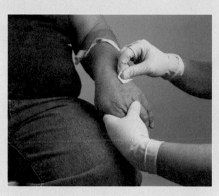

4-8b ● Cleanse the venipuncture site.

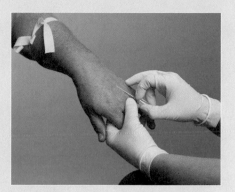

4-8c ● Insert the intravenous cannula into the vein.

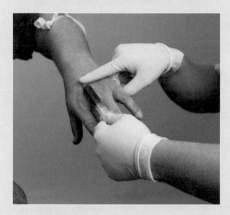

4-8d ● Withdraw any blood samples needed.

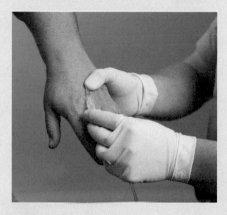

4-8e ● Connect the IV tubing.

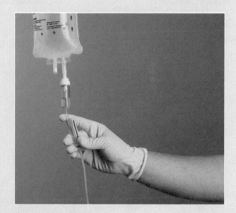

4-8f ● Turn on the IV and check the flow.

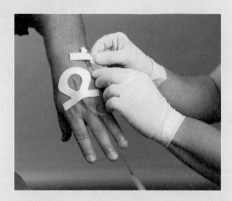

4-8g ● Secure the site.

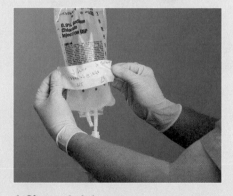

4-8h ● Label the intravenous solution bag.

painful site to access, so you typically will reserve its use for patients with a decreased or total loss of consciousness.

Cannulating the external jugular vein requires essentially the same equipment as other forms of peripheral IV access, plus a 10-mL syringe. You will not need a constricting band.

To access the external jugular, use the following technique (Procedure 4-9):

1. Prepare all equipment as for peripheral IV access in an arm, hand, or leg. In addition, fill the 10-mL syringe with

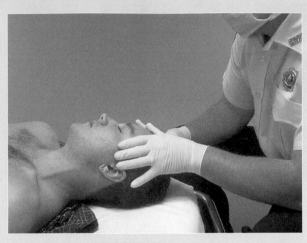

4-9a ● Place the patient supine or in the Trendelenburg position.

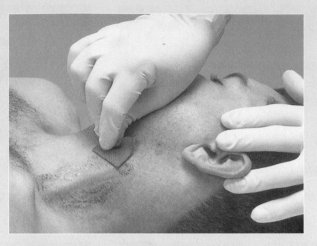

4-9b ● Turn the patient's head to the side opposite of access and cleanse the site.

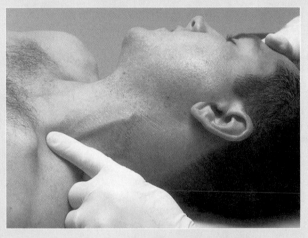

4-9c ● Occlude venous return by placing a finger on the external jugular just above the clavicle.

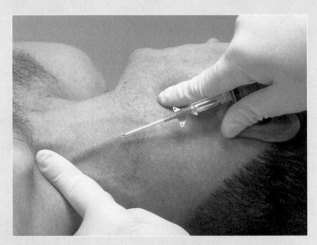

4-9d ● Point the catheter at the medial third of the clavicle and insert it, bevel up, at a 10° to 30° angle.

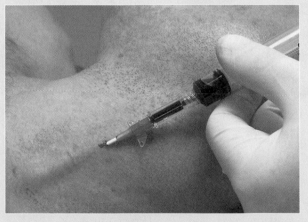

4-9e ● Enter the external jugular while withdrawing on the plunger of the attached syringe.

3 to 5 mL of sterile saline. Attach the distal part of the syringe to the flashback chamber of a large bore, over-the-needle catheter. Use Standard Precautions.

2. Place the patient supine and/or in the Trendelenburg position. This position will increase blood flow to the chest and neck, thus distending the vein and making it easier to see. In addition, the supine-Trendelenburg position decreases the chance of air entering the circulatory system during cannulation.

3. Turn the patient's head to the side opposite of access. This maneuver makes the site easier to see and reach; do not perform it if the patient has traumatic head and/or neck injuries.

4. Cleanse the site with antiseptic solution. Start at the site of intended puncture and work outward 1 to 2 inches in ever increasing circles.

5. Occlude venous return by placing a finger on the external jugular just above the clavicle. This should distend the vein, again allowing greater visualization and ease of puncture. Never apply a venous constricting band around the patient's neck.

6. Position the intravenous cannula parallel with the vein, midway between the angle of the jaw and the clavicle. Point the catheter at the medial third of the clavicle and insert it, bevel up, at a 10° to 30° angle.

7. Enter the external jugular while withdrawing on the plunger of the attached syringe. You will see blood in the syringe or feel a pop as the cannula enters the vein. Once inside the vein, advance the entire catheter another 0.5 cm so the tip of the Teflon catheter lies within the lumen of the vein. Then slide the Teflon catheter into the vein and remove the metal stylet as previously described and retract the needle. Immediately dispose of the metal stylet.

8. Obtain venous blood samples as discussed in the section on venous blood sampling.

9. Attach the administration tubing to the IV catheter. Allow the intravenous solution to run freely for several seconds. Set the flow rate and secure as appropriate.

10. Monitor the patient for complications.

While using the external jugular vein has advantages, it also has distinct drawbacks. You may inadvertently puncture the airway or damage the nearby arterial vessels. Additionally, this is a painful entry site for the conscious patient. To minimize risks, perform the procedure very carefully.

Intravenous Access with a Measured Volume Administration Set

When using a measured volume administration set, follow this procedure (Procedure 4-10):

1. Prepare the tubing by closing all clamps, and insert the flanged spike into the IV solution bag's spike port.

2. Open the airway handle. Open the uppermost clamp and fill the burette chamber with approximately 20 mL of fluid. Squeeze the drip chamber until the fluid reaches the fill line. Open the bottom flow regulator to purge air through the tubing. When all air is purged, close the bottom flow regulator.

3. Continue to fill the burette chamber with the designated amount of solution.

4. Close the uppermost clamp and open the flow regulator until you reach the desired drip rate. Leave the airway handle open, so that air replaces the displaced fluid.

To refill the burette chamber, open the uppermost clamp until you have delivered the desired volume; then repeat step 4.

You can also use measured volume administration sets for continuous fluid administration. Fill the burette chamber with at least 30 mL of solution and close the airway handle. Leave the uppermost clamp open and adjust the rate with the lower flow regulator.

Intravenous Access with Blood Tubing

To establish an IV with blood tubing, use the following procedure (Procedure 4-11):

1. Prepare the tubing by closing all clamps, and insert the flanged spike into the spike port of the blood and/or normal saline solution (Y-configured tubing).

2. Squeeze the drip chamber until it is one-third full and blood covers the filter. Repeat for the normal saline if you are using Y tubing.

3. If you are using straight tubing, piggyback a secondary line of normal saline into the blood tubing, unless you plan to piggyback the straight blood tubing into a large bore primary line.

4. Flush all tubing with normal saline and blood as appropriate.

5. Attach blood tubing to the intravenous cannula or into a previously established IV line.

6. Ensure patency by infusing a small amount of normal saline. Shut down when you have confirmed patency.

7. Open the clamp(s) and/or flow regulator(s) that allows blood to move from the bag to the patient. Adjust the flow rate accordingly.

8. When blood therapy is complete or must be discontinued, shut down the flow regulator from the blood supply and open the regulator(s) for the normal saline solution.

Factors Affecting Intravenous Flow Rates

If an IV does not flow properly, check for the following problems and correct them as appropriate.

- *Constricting band.* Has the venous constricting band been removed? This is probably the most common mistake both

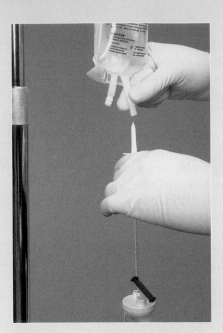

4-10a ● Spike the solution bag.

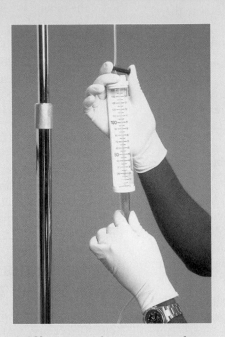

4-10b ● Open the uppermost clamp and fill the burette chamber with the desired volume of fluid.

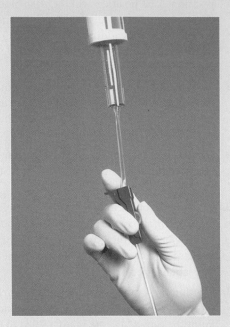

4-10c ● Close the uppermost clamp and open the flow regulator.

in and out of the hospital. Additionally, ensure that the patient is not wearing restrictive clothing that interferes with venous blood flow.

● *Edema at the puncture site.* Swelling at the IV site indicates fluid collection caused by infiltration. This **extravasation** occurs if you accidentally puncture the vein more than once, thus allowing IV solution and blood to escape from the second puncture and accumulate in the surrounding tissue. An infiltrated IV site is not usable.

● *Cannula abutting the vein wall or valve.* If the distal tip of the cannula butts against a wall or valve, carefully reposition it. You may have to untape and retape the cannula once you have achieved an adequate flow rate. Additionally, you may need to use an arm board to keep the patient's extremity straight, as flexion may kink the vein at the site and impede the solution's flow.

● *Administration set control valves.* Ensure that the flow regulator is open. Be sure to check the flow regulator and clamps of both the primary and any secondary or extension tubing.

● *IV bag height.* When you move the patient, you may raise the cannulation site above the IV solution bag. This interrupts the solution's gravitational flow from the bag into the patient.

● *Completely filled drip chamber.* Is the drip chamber completely filled? You can easily correct this by inverting the bag and squeezing the fluid from the drip chamber back into the bag.

● *Catheter patency.* A blood clot at the end of the Teflon catheter or needle may obstruct the flow of solution from the IV solution bag into the body. If the flow slows, increase the IV drip rate to keep the catheter or needle clear. If the flow stops completely, cleanse the medication administration port closest to the IV entry site with alcohol preparations and insert a syringe and hypodermic needle. Gently aspirate back on the syringe until the blood clot is pulled into the syringe. Never flush an IV that has stopped running because of a clot. Flushing will force the clot into the circulatory system and can cause occlusions in the heart or lungs.

If flow remains inadequate after you have eliminated all of these possible causes, lower the IV bag below the insertion site. If blood flows into the IV administration tubing, the site is patent and the problem lies elsewhere. If the problem persists, remove the IV and reestablish it on another extremity, using all new equipment. If you do not observe blood return, the site is inoperable.

Complications of Peripheral Intravenous Access

Even though it is a routine procedure, intravenous access is not trouble free. It can cause a number of complications.

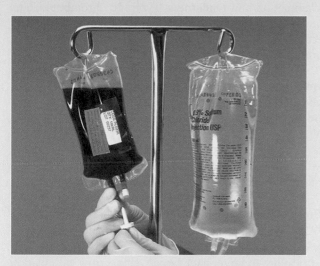

4-11a ● Insert the flanged spike into the spike port of the blood and/or normal saline solution.

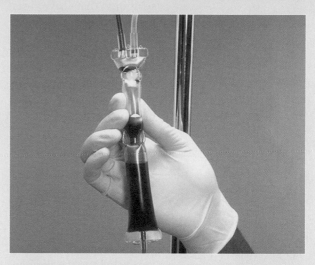

4-11b ● Squeeze the drip chamber until it is one-third full and blood covers the filter.

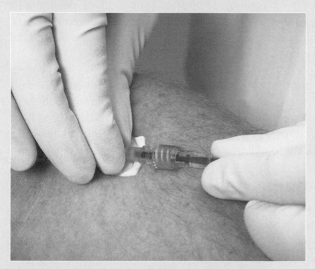

4-11c ● Attach blood tubing to the intravenous cannula or into a previously established IV line.

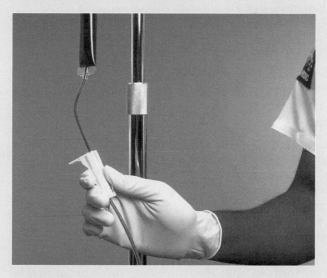

4-11d ● Open the clamp(s) and/or flow regulator(s) and adjust the flow rate.

Pain   Pain at the puncture site occurs during needle penetration or with extravasation. To minimize pain, use a smaller gauge catheter or use a 1 percent lidocaine solution (without epinephrine) to anesthetize the overlying skin before insertion.

Local Infection   Local infection occurs if you do not properly cleanse the site and thus introduce pathogens through the puncture. This complication does not become apparent until after the IV has been established for several hours.

Pyrogenic Reaction   **Pyrogens** (foreign proteins capable of producing fever) in the administration tubing or IV solution can cause a pyrogenic reaction. The abrupt onset of fever (100 °F to 106 °F), chills, backache, headache, nausea, and vomiting characterize these reactions. Cardiovascular collapse may also result.

Typically, a pyrogenic reaction will occur within one-half to one hour after you initiate an IV. If you suspect a pyrogenic reaction, immediately terminate the IV and reestablish access in the opposite side with new equipment and fluid.

Typically, pyrogenic reactions occur secondary to the use of intravenous solutions that have been contaminated with a microorganism or other foreign matter. Pyrogenic reactions underscore the need to discard any fluid that is cloudy or any equipment that has been opened.

Allergic Reaction A patient receiving IV therapy may develop an allergic reaction. Most often, allergic reactions accompany the administration of blood or colloidal (protein-containing) solutions. In addition, some patients may react to the latex in some types of IV administration tubing.

The sudden onset of hives (urticaria), itching (pruritus), localized or systemic edema, or shortness of breath may signify an allergic reaction. If you suspect an allergic reaction, stop the IV infusion and remove the IV catheter. Treat the patient as discussed in Volume 4, Chapter 5.

Catheter Shear A catheter shear can occur if you pull the Teflon catheter through or over the needle after you have advanced it into the vein. The soft plastic catheter will easily snag on the metal stylet's sharp point and shear off, thus forming a plastic **embolus**. Therefore, never draw the Teflon catheter over the metal stylet after you have advanced it.

Inadvertent Arterial Puncture Because arteries may lie close to veins, accidental arterial puncture may occur. Arterial blood is bright red and characteristically spurts with each contraction of the heart. When an arterial puncture occurs, immediately remove the catheter and apply direct pressure to the site for at least 5 minutes. Do not release the pressure until the hemorrhage has stopped.

Circulatory Overload **Circulatory overload** occurs if you administer too much fluid for the patient's condition. You must monitor flow rates carefully, especially for patients with medical conditions such as kidney failure or heart failure that are intolerant of excessive fluid. Continually examine the patient for signs of circulatory overload (crackles, tachypnea, dyspnea, and jugular venous distention, as discussed in Volume 3, Chapter 5). If you encounter circulatory overload, adjust the flow rate.

Thrombophlebitis **Thrombophlebitis**, or inflammation of the vein, is particularly common in long-term intravenous therapy. Redness and edema at the puncture site are typical signs of thrombophlebitis. This complication may also present as pain along the course of the vein, sometimes accompanied by inflammation and tenderness. Typically, thrombophlebitis does not occur until several hours after IV initiation. When you suspect thrombophlebitis, terminate the IV and apply a warm compress to the site.

Thrombus Formation A **thrombus**, or blood clot, can form if IV access injures the vessel wall. A thrombus may form around the catheter and occlude the movement of fluid between the IV and the blood vessel. If you suspect a thrombus, restart the IV using new equipment. Do not attempt to dislodge the clot with a fluid bolus, as this may create an embolus that causes neurologic or pulmonary complications.

Air Embolism **Air embolism** occurs when air enters the vein. Air embolus is most likely to occur during central venous access or when administration tubing has not been properly flushed. Failure to tamponade larger veins during cannulation may allow air into the vein.

Necrosis **Necrosis**, or the sloughing off of dead tissue, occurs later in IV therapy as medication (e.g., norepinephrine, epinephrine, dopamine, dobutamine) has extravasated into the interstitial space.

Anticoagulants **Anticoagulant** medications such as aspirin, platelet aggregate inhibitors, warfarin (Coumadin), or heparin increase the chance of bleeding and impede hemorrhage control during IV establishment. They drastically increase the complications of hematoma or infiltration.

Changing an IV Bag or Bottle

You may sometimes have to change an IV bag or bottle. This generally occurs when only 50 mL of solution remain and you must continue therapy after those 50 mL are depleted. Changing the solution bag or bottle is a sterile process. If the equipment becomes contaminated you should dispose of it.

To change the IV solution bag or bottle, use the following technique:

1. Prepare the new IV solution bag or bottle by removing the protective cover from the IV tubing port.
2. Occlude the flow of solution from the depleted bag or bottle by moving the roller clamp on the IV administration tubing.
3. Remove the spike from the depleted IV bag or bottle. Be careful not to drop or contaminate the spike in any way.
4. Insert the spike into the new IV bag or bottle. Ensure that the drip chamber is filled appropriately.
5. Open the roller clamp to the appropriate flow rate.

If air becomes entrained within the administration tubing during this process, cleanse the medication administration port below the trapped air and insert a hypodermic needle and syringe. Pull the plunger back to aspirate the trapped air into the syrine. After you have removed the air, adjust the IV flow rate as needed.

Intravenous Medication Administration

Medications can be delivered through an existing IV line. As the IV line is seated directly into a vein, the blood rapidly absorbs these medications and distributes them throughout the body. Intravenous administration avoids many of the barriers to medication absorption in other routes. For example, medications given via the gastrointestinal tract face enzymes and other chemicals that may deactivate, exacerbate, or in some other way alter the medication being administered. Likewise, local tissues can absorb medications administered via the subcutaneous or intramuscular routes, thus preventing the total dosage from reaching the bloodstream for delivery. The two methods for administering medications through an IV line are intravenous bolus and intravenous infusion.

Intravenous Bolus

An intravenous bolus involves injecting the circulatory system with a concentrated dose of medication through the medication administration port of an established IV. This procedure requires the following equipment:

- Personal protective equipment
- Antiseptic solution
- Packaged medication
- Syringe (size depends on the volume of medication you will administer)
- 18- to 20-gauge hypodermic needle, 1 to 1.5 inches long
- Existing intravenous line with medication port

To administer an intravenous medication bolus, use the following technique (Procedure 4-12):

1. Ensure that the primary IV line is patent.
2. Confirm the medication, indication, dosage, and need for an IV bolus. Confirm that the medication is compatible with the solution being infused.
3. Draw up the medication or prepare a prefilled syringe as appropriate.
4. Cleanse the medication port nearest the IV site with an antiseptic preparation.
5. Insert a hypodermic needle through the port membrane.

6. Pinch the IV line above the medication port. This prevents the medication from traveling toward the fluids bag, forcing it instead toward the patient.
7. Inject the medication as appropriate.
8. Remove the hypodermic needle and syringe and release the tubing.
9. Open the flow regulator to allow a 20-cc fluid flush. The fluid will push the medication into the patient's circulatory system.
10. Dispose of the hypodermic needle and syringe as appropriate. Monitor the patient for desired or undesired effects.

Intravenous Medication Infusion

Many cardiac medications and antibiotics are given as intravenous infusions (IV piggybacks). Intravenous medication infusions deliver a steady, continual dose of medication through an existing IV line. You may give them either as an initial dosage or to maintain medication levels after delivering an initial bolus.

Piggybacking IV infusions through an existing intravenous line gives you greater control over medication delivery and allows you to easily discontinue the infusion when therapy is complete or must be stopped. Never administer intravenous infusions as a primary IV line.

IV infusions are contained in bags or bottles of intravenous solution. If the IV infusion is premixed, read the label on the bag for the following information:

- Name of medication
- Total dosage in weight mixed in bag
- Concentration (weight per single cc)
- Expiration date

If the infusion is not premixed, make a label listing this information and attach it to the bag (Figure 4-42 ●). Additionally, note the date and time you mixed the infusion, and initial it.

Use the following technique to administer a medication as an IV infusion (Procedure 4-13):

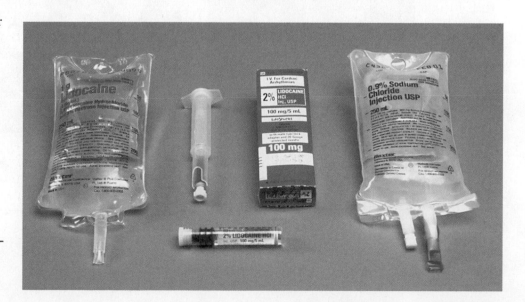

● **Figure 4-42** If an IV solution is not premixed, you will have to mix and label it yourself.

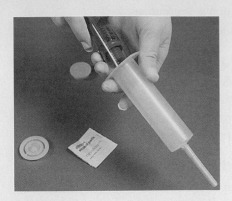

4-12a ● Prepare the equipment.

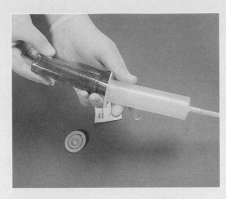

4-12b ● Prepare the medication.

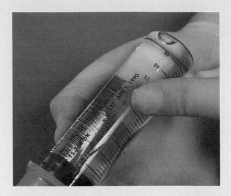

4-12c ● Check the label.

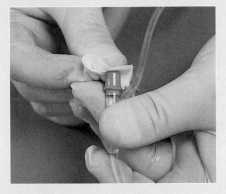

4-12d ● Select and clean an administration port.

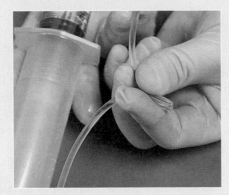

4-12e ● Pinch the line.

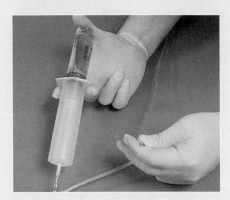

4-12f ● Administer the medication.

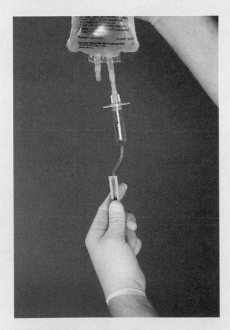

4-12g ● Adjust the IV flow rate.

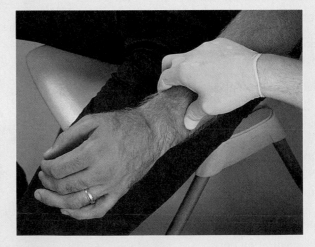

4-12h ● Monitor the patient.

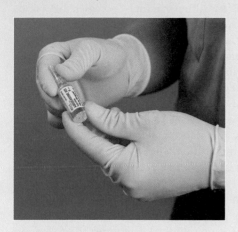

4-13a ● Select the drug.

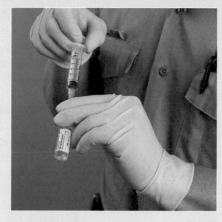

4-13b ● Draw up the drug.

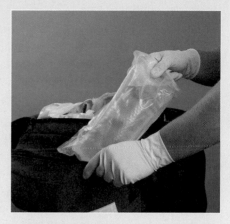

4-13c ● Select IV fluid for dilution.

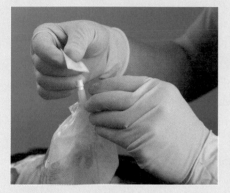

4-13d ● Clean the medication addition port.

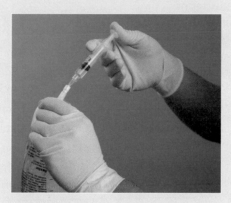

4-13e ● Inject the drug into the fluid.

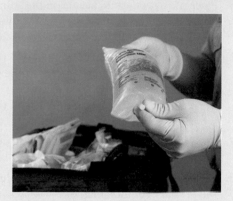

4-13f ● Mix the solution.

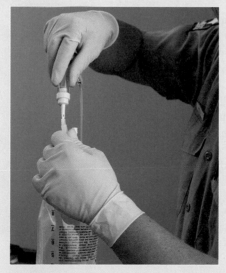

4-13g ● Insert an administration set and connect it to the main IV line with a needle.

1. Establish a primary IV line and ensure patency.

2. Confirm administration indications and patient allergies.

3. Prepare the infusion bag or bottle. (If the infusion is premixed, continue to step 4.)

    a. Draw up the appropriate quantity of medication from its source with a syringe.

    b. Cleanse the IV bag or bottle's medication port with an antiseptic wipe.

    c. Insert the hypodermic needle into the medication port and inject the medication.

    d. Gently agitate the bag or bottle to mix its contents.

    e. Label the bag or bottle.

4. Connect administration tubing to the medication bag or bottle and fill the drip chamber to the fluid line. Most infusions require microdrip tubing. If you use a mechanical infusion pump, you may need to use special tubing.

5. Place the hypodermic needle on the administration tubing's needle adapter and flush the tubing with solution. (The needle adapter typically accepts a 20-gauge needle.)

6. Cleanse the medication administration port on the primary line with alcohol and insert the secondary line's hypodermic needle. Secure the hypodermic needle and the secondary administration line with tape or another securing device.

7. Reconfirm the indication, medication, dose, and route of administration.

8. Shut down the primary line so that no fluid will flow from the primary solution bag.

9. Adjust the secondary line to the desired drip rate. If you are using a mechanical infusion pump, set it accordingly.

10. Properly dispose of the needle and syringe.

When the infusion is complete, shut down the secondary line with the flow regulator or a clamp. Open the primary line and adjust it to the indicated drip rate. Remove the hypodermic needle from the medication administration port and properly dispose of all contents. If required by your local protocols, retain the medication bag to verify administration and for quality assurance.

You can also use measured volume administration tubing to administer medicated infusions. First, fill the burette chamber of a measured volume administration device with a specific volume of fluid. Then you can inject the medication through the medication injection site on top of the burette chamber. You must adjust the flow rate to deliver the precise amount of medication required. In addition, you can mix the medication within the IV bag or bottles as previously described and use the measured volume administration tubing solely for administering the infusion rather than for mixing it.

Heparin Lock and Saline Lock

When a patient requires occasional IV medication drips or boluses but does not need continuous fluid, heparin locks are used. A **heparin lock** is a peripheral IV port that does not use a

bag of fluid. Like a typical IV start, it places an IV cannula into a peripheral vein; however, instead of IV administration tubing, it has attached short tubing with a clamp and a distal medication port (Figure 4-43 ●). A heparin lock decreases the risk of accidental fluid overload and electrolyte derangement. You also may withdraw blood samples from the lock if it is in a suitable vein. For short-term use, a **saline lock** may be used. Sterile saline is injected following the medication. Saline remains in the lock to keep it open. For long-term use, a heparin lock is preferred. Although it functions the same as a saline lock, a heparin lock is filled with a low-concentration solution of heparin, which aids in keeping any blood that gets into the device from clotting. Typically, a medication will be administered through the heparin lock. This is followed by a saline flush to ensure that no medication remains in the lock or hub. Then, the lock and hub are filled with a heparin solution. This aids in keeping the IV site open for a long period of time.

Initiating a heparin or saline lock requires the following equipment:

- IV cannula
- Heparin or saline lock
- Syringe with 3 to 5 cc sterile saline or commercial saline injection device
- Tape or commercial securing device
- Venous blood drawing equipment
- Venous constricting band
- Antiseptic solution
- Heparin for flush solution (if using heparin lock)—typically 10 or 100 units/mL

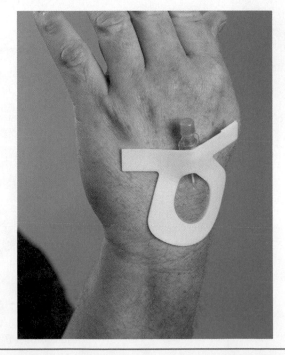

● **Figure 4-43** A saline or heparin lock can be used when a patient requires occasional medications or IV drips but does not need a continuous infusion.

To place a heparin lock, follow these steps:

1. Select the venipuncture site.
2. Place the constricting band proximal to the puncture site.
3. Cleanse the venipuncture site with antiseptic solution.
4. Insert the intravenous cannula into the vein.
5. Slide the Teflon catheter into the vein.
6. Carefully remove the metal stylet, retract or protect the stylet, and promptly dispose of it into the sharps container. Remove the venous constricting band.
7. Obtain venous blood samples, as explained under Venous Blood Sampling.
8. Attach the heparin lock tubing to the catheter hub.
9. Cleanse the medication port and inject 3 to 5 mL of sterile saline into the lock. Easy flow of the saline without edema at the puncture site indicates patency. If you encounter resistance or if edema forms, restart the procedure with new equipment. If a heparin lock is desired, fill the port with the designated heparin flush solution.
10. Apply an adhesive bandage or other commercial device. Secure the tubing to the patient.

To administer an IV medication bolus through a heparin lock, assemble the following equipment and supplies:

- Personal protective equipment
- Antiseptic solution
- Packaged medication
- Syringe (the size depends on the volume being administered)
- 18- to 20-gauge hypodermic needle 1 to 1½ inches long

After you have gathered all equipment and supplies, use the following technique to administer an IV medication bolus with a heparin or saline lock:

1. Confirm the medication, indication, dosage, and need for an IV bolus.
2. Draw up the medication or prepare a prefilled syringe as appropriate.
3. Cleanse the medication port nearest the IV site with an antiseptic solution.
4. Ensure that the plastic clamp is open.
5. Insert the hypodermic needle through the port membrane.
6. Inject the medication as appropriate.
7. Remove the hypodermic needle and dispose of it in the sharps container.
8. Follow the medication administration with a 10- to 20-mL saline flush from another syringe.
9. Properly dispose of the hypodermic needle and syringe. Monitor the patient for desired or undesired effects.

If fluid administration becomes necessary, you can unscrew the medication port and insert IV administration tubing. Periodically flush with sterile saline or heparin to prevent clot formation and occlusion at the Teflon catheter's distal end.

Venous Access Device

A **venous access device** is a surgically implanted port that permits repeated access to the central venous circulation. Implanted just under the skin, venous access devices are constructed of a plastic or stainless steel injection port and flexible catheter. The injection port, which lies just beneath the skin, contains a self-sealing septum that allows repeated penetration and access into the venous circulation. The self-sealing septum is connected to a flexible catheter that is placed within the lumen of a central vein, most often the superior vena cava (Figure 4-44 ●).

Typically, patients with venous access devices have chronic illnesses that require repeated intravenous access for medication administration, long-term intravenous therapy, or blood sampling. Generally, venous access devices are placed on the anterior chest near the third or fourth rib lateral to the sternum. A venous access device is apparent as a raised circle just beneath the skin.

Use of an indwelling central venous access device requires special training. Delivering a medication through the venous access device requires a special needle specific for the venous access device in question. A common needle, the **Huber needle**, has an opening on the side of its shaft instead of at the tip. When placed into the injection port, this configuration allows easy administration of medication into the venous access device. Never access a venous access device unless you have the specific needle unique for the particular device. Always ask the patient, family, or nursing staff about the type of venous access device. Often, they will have a supply of needles for the device.

To administer fluids, medication, or blood through a venous access device, you must first prepare the site using the following technique:

1. Use Standard Precautions.
2. Fill a 10-mL syringe with approximately 7 mL of normal saline.
3. Place a 21- or 22-gauge Huber needle (or other specialized needle) on the end of the syringe.

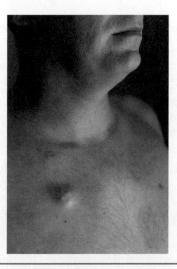

● **Figure 4-44** Example of a venous access device.

4. Cleanse the skin over the injection port with an antiseptic solution.

5. Stabilize the site with one hand while inserting the Huber needle at a 90° angle. Gently advance it until it meets resistance. This signals that the needle has contacted the floor of the injection port.

6. Pull back on the plunger and observe for blood return. The presence of blood confirms placement.

7. Slowly inject the normal saline to ensure patency.

To administer the medication by intravenous bolus, use the following technique:

1. Prepare the medication, fluid, or blood for administration.

2. Attach a 21- or 22-gauge Huber needle (or other specialized needle) to the end of the syringe.

3. Cleanse the skin over the injection port with antiseptic solutions.

4. Insert the needle into the injection port at a 90° angle until the needle cannot be further advanced. Pull back on the plunger of the syringe and observe for the return of blood. The presence of blood confirms proper placement.

5. Inject the medication as appropriate.

6. Remove and dispose of the syringe appropriately.

7. With another syringe and attached specialized needle, administer a bolus of heparinized saline to clear the catheter of any blood clots or other obstruction.

If the venous access device is not patent or access proves difficult, contact medical direction for further directives.

To administer IV fluids, use the following technique:

1. Prepare a primary IV line. Be sure to prime or flush the air from the administration tubing.

2. Attach a 21- or 22-gauge Huber needle (or other specialized needle) to the primary IV administration tubing. Insert a 10-mL syringe and hypodermic needle filled with 7 mL of normal saline solution into the tubing medication delivery port nearest the venous access device.

3. Cleanse the skin over the injection port with an antiseptic solution.

4. Insert the needle into the injection port at a 90° angle until it encounters resistance.

5. Pinch the administration tubing above the medication administration port and pull back on the syringe plunger. Observe for the return of blood. The presence of blood confirms proper placement.

6. Gently inject the 7 mL of normal saline solution.

7. Set the primary line to the appropriate flow rate.

If administering a secondary medicated infusion, continue as follows:

1. Prepare a secondary line containing the fluid, blood, or medicated solution for infusion.

2. Attach a hypodermic needle to the needle adapter of the secondary line. Insert the secondary line into a medication administration port on the primary tubing.

3. Shut down the primary line and infuse the medicated solution as appropriate. Look for ease of administration as a sign of patency.

4. When infusion is complete, administer a bolus of heparinized saline to clear the catheter of any blood clots or other obstruction.

Using a venous access device is a very sterile procedure. You must take care to clean the site before delivering medications. Other complications of using a venous access device include infection, thrombus formation, and dislodgment of the catheter tip from the vein.

Electromechanical Infusion Devices

Electromechanical infusion devices permit the precise delivery of fluid and/or medications through electronic regulation. Anytime that intravenous infusion occurs, electromechanical infusion pumps provide optimal delivery. Infusion devices are classified as either infusion controllers or infusion pumps.

Infusion Controllers Infusion controllers are gravity-flow devices that regulate the fluid's passage through the pump. Because infusion controllers do not use positive pressure, they will not force fluids into the extravascular space if you infiltrate the vein.

Infusion Pumps Infusion pumps deliver fluids and medications under positive pressure (Figure 4-45 ●). This pressure can cause complications such as hematoma or extravasation if you infiltrate the vein. Some infusion pumps contain a pressure monitor and will warn you if they encounter the increased resistance that occurs with infiltration.

Syringe-type infusion pumps are gaining popularity for medical transport. Syringe pumps deliver their medications from a medical syringe without a hypodermic needle instead of from IV solution bags, fluids, or liquid medications (Figure 4-46 ●). You place the syringe containing the medications in the pump, which uses computerized mechanics to gradually depress the plunger at the correct rate. These compact pumps prove advantageous during transport.

Manufacturers make many different electromechanical infusion pumps. Depending on the maker, pump compatibility may require specialized administration tubing. With some

LEGAL CONSIDERATIONS

Drawing Blood for Law Enforcement. *In some regions, paramedics may be asked to draw blood for law enforcement. If this is the case in your system, make sure that you have established protocols and medical director permission before performing the task. Be advised, you may well be called to court to testify about what you saw or what you did.*[10]

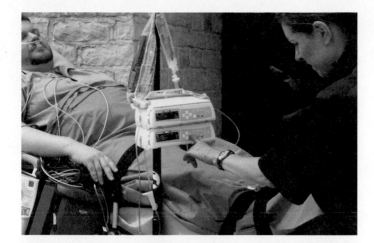

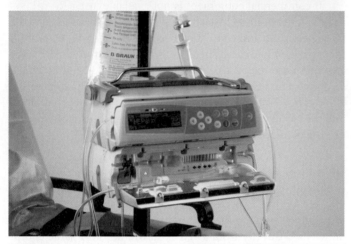

● **Figure 4-45** Modern infusion pump. (Both photos: © *Bound Tree Medical*)

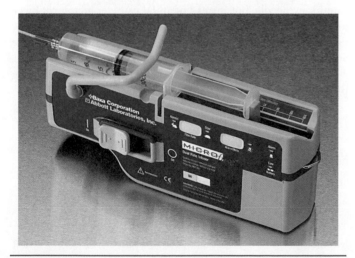

● **Figure 4-46** MicroFuse® Syringe Infuser. (*Photo courtesy of © Baxa Corporation*)

computerized pumps, you can enter the basic information and then the pump will perform all medical calculations internally and automatically set the drip rate. Most infusion pumps contain internal monitoring devices that sound an alarm for problems such as infiltration, occlusion, or fluid source depletion. Electronic devices are prone to malfunction, so you must be prepared to perform all calculations and set the drip rate manually.

Venous Blood Sampling

The laboratory analysis of blood can provide valuable information about the sick and/or injured patient. The concentrations of electrolytes, gases, hormones, or other chemicals in blood can often shed light on the underlying causes of vague complaints such as dizziness or generalized weakness. Additionally, blood evaluation can confirm suspected conditions. For example, elevated cardiac enzymes in a patient's blood can confirm a suspected myocardial infarction.

In the field, you often will be the first to assess and treat an ill or injured patient. Many of your interventions can alter the blood's composition and erase important information. If you obtain venous blood samples before performing those interventions, they will enable the physician to evaluate the patient's original status.

Venous blood is commonly obtained via venipuncture. Thus, paramedics, who routinely initiate intravenous access, can simultaneously obtain blood samples. Doing so saves considerable hospital time and avoids multiple needlesticks.

You should obtain venous blood in the following situations:

● During peripheral access

● Before medication administration

● When medication administration may be needed

Never stop to draw blood if it will delay critical measures such as medication administration in cardiac arrest or transport in a multisystem trauma.

Equipment for Drawing Blood

You will need the following equipment to obtain venous blood.

Blood Tubes **Blood tubes** are made of glass and have color-coded, self-sealing rubber tops. Blood tube sizes for adults generally range from 5 to 7 mL—for pediatrics, from 2 to 3 mL (Figure 4-47 ●). They are vacuum packed, and some contain a chemical anticoagulant. The different-colored tops correspond to specific anticoagulants. A label on every blood tube identifies the type of additive and its expiration date. Do not use a blood tube after its expiration date, as both the anticoagulant and the vacuum lose their effectiveness.

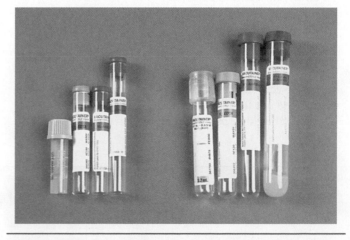

● **Figure 4-47** Blood tubes.

Using blood tubes in their correct order is essential. If you do not follow the proper sequence, the various anticoagulants will cause cross-contamination, skewing the results and rendering the blood useless. Your local EMS system and receiving hospitals can provide information about the appropriate order of tubes.

Miscellaneous Equipment Depending on the technique you use to obtain venous blood, you will also need syringes, hypodermic needles, and commercially manufactured plastic sleeves called vacutainers.

Obtaining Venous Blood

Obtaining venous blood is a simple process; however, if the blood is to remain usable, you must pay strict attention to detail. You can obtain blood either from an IV catheter or directly from the vein. Which technique you use will depend on the situation. In either case, venous blood samples are best obtained from sturdy veins such as the cephalic, basilic, or median. Smaller veins such as those on the back of the hand are more likely to collapse during retrieval, making the procedure difficult to complete.

Obtaining Venous Blood from an IV Catheter The most convenient way to obtain venous blood is through an IV catheter at the time of peripheral vascular access. In addition to blood tubes, you will need a tube holder (Figure 4-48 ●). The tube holder is commonly referred to as a **vacutainer**. A special adapter needle called a multidraw needle fits into the tube holder. The multidraw needle has a rubber-covered needle used to puncture the self-sealing top of the blood tube. The remaining portion of the multidraw needle protrudes from the tube holder and fits snugly into the hub of the IV catheter.

To obtain blood directly from the IV catheter, use the following procedure:

1. Assemble and prepare all equipment. Inspect the blood tubes for expiration or damage and insert the multidraw needle into the vacutainer.

   Note: Never place blood tubes into the assembled vacutainer and multidraw needle until you are ready to draw blood. This will destroy the vacuum and render the blood tube useless.

2. Establish IV access with the IV catheter. Do not connect IV administration tubing.

3. Attach the end of the multidraw needle adapter to the hub of the cannula.

4. In correct order, insert the blood tubes so that the rubber-covered needle punctures the self-sealing rubber top. Blood should be pulled into the blood tube.

5. Fill all blood tubes completely, as the amount of anticoagulant is proportional to the tube's volume. Gently agitate the tubes to mix the anticoagulant evenly with the blood.

6. Tamponade the vein and remove the vacutainer and multidraw needle. Attach the IV and ensure patency.

7. Properly dispose of all sharps.

8. Label all blood tubes with the following information:
   - Patient's first and last name
   - Patient's age and gender
   - Date and time drawn
   - Name of the person drawing the blood

If commercial equipment is not available, use a 20-mL syringe (Figure 4-49 ●). Attach the syringe's needle adapter to the IV catheter hub and gently pull back the plunger. Blood will fill the syringe. When the syringe is full, remove it from the IV catheter and place the IV line into the IV catheter. Carefully attach a hypodermic needle to the syringe to puncture the tops of the blood tubes. In the appropriate order, place the collected blood into the blood tubes and gently agitate. When finished, properly dispose of all sharps and label the blood tubes.

Obtaining Blood Directly from a Vein When IV access is difficult or unobtainable, you may draw blood directly from the vein with a hypodermic needle. This technique is useful for routine sampling that will not require further IV access. To draw blood directly from a vein, you will need the same equipment as for obtaining blood from an IV catheter, but instead of a standard needle and syringe you can use a **Luer sampling needle** (Figure 4-50 ●). A Luer sampling needle is similar to a multidraw needle, but instead of an IV catheter adapter it has a long, exposed needle. The Luer sampling needle screws into the vacutainer, and you insert the exposed needle directly into the vein. You will also need a constricting band and antiseptic wipes.

To obtain blood directly from a vein, use the following procedure:

1. Assemble and prepare all equipment. Inspect the blood tubes for expiration or damage, and insert the multidraw needle into the vacutainer.

2. Apply the constricting band and select an appropriate puncture site.

3. Cleanse the site with antiseptic solution.

4. Insert the end of the multi-sampling needle or the Luer sampling needle into the vein and remove the constricting band.

5. In the correct order, insert each blood tube so that the rubber-covered needle punctures the self-sealing rubber top. Blood should be pulled into the tube.

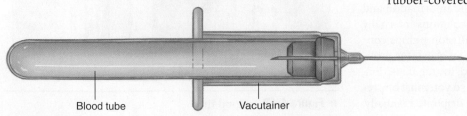

Blood tube   Vacutainer

● **Figure 4-48** Vacutainer with multi-sampling needle.

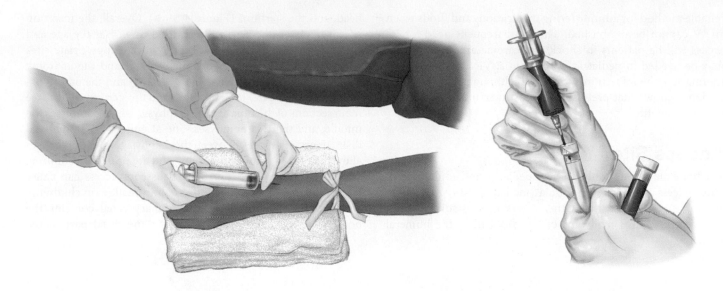

● **Figure 4-49**   Obtaining a blood sample with a 20-mL syringe.

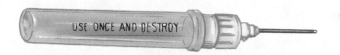

USE ONCE AND DESTROY

● **Figure 4-50**   Luer sampling needle.

6. Gently agitate the tube to evenly mix the anticoagulant with the blood. Completely fill all blood tubes, as the anticoagulant is proportional to the volume of the tube.

7. Place sterile gauze over the site and remove the sampling needle. Properly dispose of all sharps.

8. Cover the puncture site with gauze and tape or an adhesive bandage.

9. Label all blood tubes with the following information:
   ○ Patient's first and last name
   ○ Patient's age and gender
   ○ Date and time drawn
   ○ Person drawing the blood

Again, if commercial equipment is not available, you may use a 20-mL syringe. When using a syringe, attach an 18-gauge hypodermic needle to the end of the syringe and insert it into the vein. Gently pull back the plunger to fill the syringe with blood. When the syringe is full, remove the syringe and dress the puncture site. In the appropriate order, inject the collected blood into the blood tubes and gently agitate. When you have finished, properly dispose of all sharps and label the blood tubes.

Complications from drawing blood include damage to the vein wall, inadvertent removal of the IV catheter, and hemoconcentration and hemolysis of the blood sample. **Hemoconcentration** occurs when the constricting band is left in place too long, elevating the numbers of red and white blood cells in the sample. **Hemolysis** is the destruction of red blood cells. When red blood cells are destroyed, they release hemoglobin

and potassium, thus rendering the blood unusable. Causes of hemolysis include vigorously shaking the blood tubes after they are filled, using too small a needle for retrieval, or too forcefully aspirating blood into or out of a syringe.

Removing a Peripheral IV

You should remove any IV that will not flow or has fulfilled its need. To do so, completely occlude the tubing with the flow regulator and/or clamp. Remove all tape or other securing devices from the tubing and patient. Place a sterile gauze pad over the puncture site. Apply pressure to the gauze with the fingers or thumb of your nondominant hand. With your dominant hand, grasp the cannula at its hub and swiftly remove it, pulling straight back. The site may bleed, so apply direct pressure with the gauze for 5 minutes. Immediately dispose of all materials in the appropriate biohazard container. Apply an adhesive bandage or tape clean gauze over the site to protect against infection. Document that the catheter was removed intact.

INTRAOSSEOUS INFUSION

Intraosseous (IO) infusions involve inserting a rigid needle into the cavity of a long bone or into the sternum (*intra-*, within; *os*, bone). The bone marrow contains a network of venous sinusoids that drain into the nutrient and emissary veins. These sinusoids accept fluids and medications during intraosseous infusion and transport them to the venous system. Any solution or medication that can be administered intravenously, either bolus or infusion, can be administered by the intraosseous route.

The National Association of EMS Physicians (NAEMSP) has recommended that every EMS system should have at least one method of obtaining pediatric IO access and one method for obtaining adult IO access. While intravenous lines remain the preferred route of vascular access, IOs provide a rapid and reliable method for administering medications and fluids when an IV cannot be established. The most frequent need for IO access will be patients in shock and cardiac arrest. IO access may be needed in pediatric hypovolemia. Victims of multiple trauma may benefit from IO therapy although the prevailing evidence shows that prehospital fluids in trauma are of questionable benefit.[11–12]

Access Site

The bone most commonly used for pediatric and adult intraosseous access is the proximal tibia (medial and inferior to the anterior tibial tuberosity). Other insertion sites for the adult include the medial malleolus of the distal tibia, the humeral head, and the sternum (Figure 4-51 ●). Overall, the insertion site depends on the device being used as well as the age and condition of the patient. To properly locate appropriate sites and avoid complications, you must understand the anatomy and physiology of the tibia (Figure 4-52 ●) and the other possible (device-specific) insertion sites and the sternum. The three main sections of the tibia are the diaphysis, which comprises the middle, and the two epiphyses, one at either end. Epiphyseal disks, or growth plates, between the diaphysis and the epiphyses allow the tibia to grow and develop and are present in children. Damage to these disks during intraosseous access can cause long-term growth complications or abnormalities in children.

Within the diaphysis, the medullary canal contains the bone marrow. When placed correctly, the distal part of the

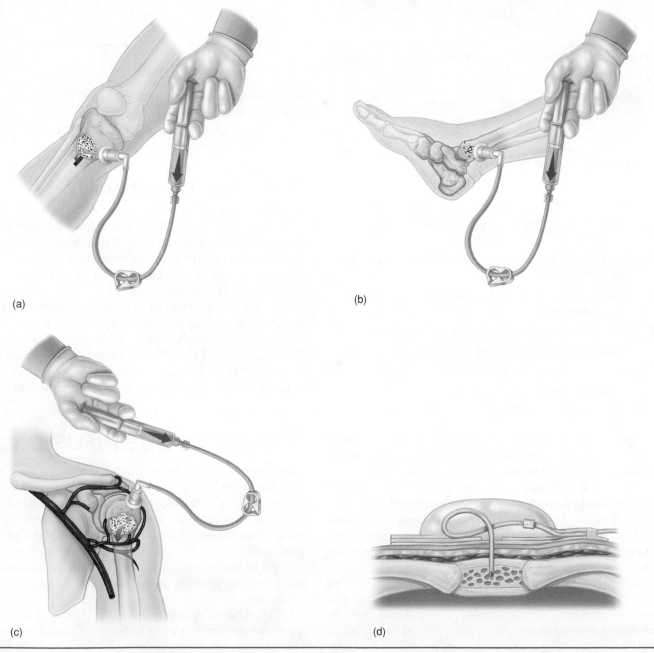

(a)

(b)

(c)

(d)

● **Figure 4-51**   Intraosseous needle placement sites depend on the device being used and include (a) the proximal tibia, (b) the medial malleolus of the distal tibia, (c) the humeral head, and (d) the sternum.

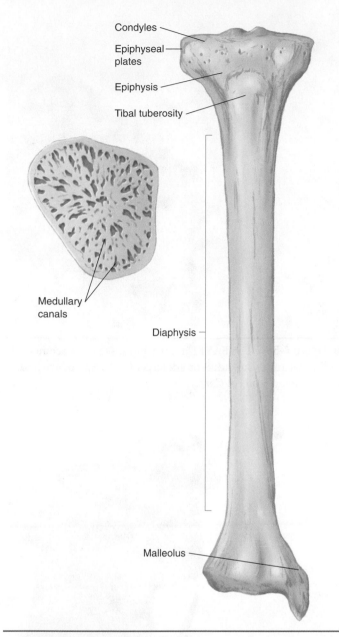

Figure 4-52 labels:
- Condyles
- Epiphyseal plates
- Epiphysis
- Tibal tuberosity
- Medullary canals
- Diaphysis
- Malleolus

● **Figure 4-52**   Anatomy of the tibia.

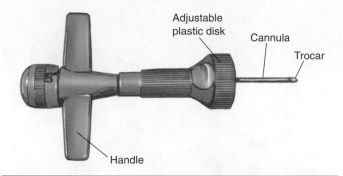

Figure 4-53 labels:
- Adjustable plastic disk
- Cannula
- Trocar
- Handle

● **Figure 4-53**   Intraosseous needle.

Equipment for Intraosseous Access

Intraosseous placement requires a specially designed needle and a 10-mL syringe. Manufactured specifically for IO access, an intraosseous needle is a 14- to 18-gauge hollow cannula with a sharp metal **trocar** inside (Figure 4-53 ●). The trocar gives strength for puncture and prevents occlusion during insertion. Upon placement, the trocar is removed. The intraosseous needle has a plastic handle for insertion and an adjustable plastic disk to stabilize the needle once it is in place. You will attach a 10-mL syringe containing 3 to 5 cc of sterile saline to the intraosseous needle. The syringe and saline are used similarly to IV access of the external jugular vein. A large-bore spinal needle with a trocar in place is an acceptable substitute for an intraosseous needle.

Other equipment for intraosseous placement is similar to that for a peripheral intravenous access line (fluid, administration tubing, tape, antiseptics, and gauze). However, you will not use a constricting band or traditional cannula. A pressure infuser is often needed for IO fluid administration. Some IO devices require a specialized adapter for flushing or using a pressure infuser. Depending on the specific intraosseous needle, you may need an adapter to connect the administration tubing and the needle.

Several commercial devices are available for both pediatric and adult intraosseous access. While these devices differ in their mechanism and location, they still must be placed through the cortex of a bone and into the marrow cavity where fluids and medications can be administered. Examples of commercial IO access devices include:

- **Bone Injection Gun (B.I.G.).** The Bone Injection Gun (B.I.G.) was developed in Israel and is available in an adult and a pediatric model (Figures 4-54a and 4-54b ●).
- **FAST1®.** The FAST1® allows adult intraosseous placement into the sternum. This site is easy to access, and the device is easy to insert. A special needle introducer guides insertion, and a dome protects the site after placement (Figure 4-55 ●).
- **EZ-IO™.** The EZ-IO™ uses a small drill to place the needle into the bone. The drill is reusable. The technique is based on the procedure routinely used by orthopedic surgeons. The manufacturer recommends placement in the proximal or distal tibia or the proximal humerus. The device is approved for both adults and children. Successful first-time placement of an intraosseous device with the EZ-IO™ is high (Figure 4-56 ●).

intraosseous needle will lie in the medullary canal. On either side of the proximal tibia are the medial and lateral condyles. You can identify the proximal epiphysis by palpating the condyles.

Between the condyles, on the top of the anterior tibial crest, is a palpable bump called the tibial tuberosity. The tibial tuberosity lies at the level of the epiphyseal growth plate. Consequently, the tibial tuberosity is extremely important in locating the appropriate pediatric intraosseous access site.

For the pediatric patient, you will establish intraosseous access on the medial aspect of the proximal tibia. This site is from two to three fingerbreadths below the tibial tuberosity. At this level, place the needle on the flat area medial to the anterior tibial crest. For adult or geriatric patients, place the needle at the distal part of the tibia, one to two fingerbreadths above the medial malleolus.

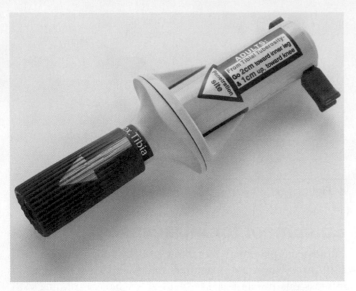

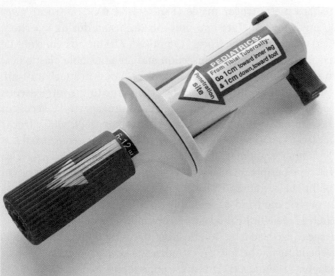

● **Figure 4-54** The Bone Injection Gun (B.I.G.): (a) adult model (b) pediatric model. (Both photos: *A.C.T.N.T. Healthcare Services www.bone-gun.com*)

Placing an Intraosseous Infusion

To place an intraosseous line, use the following technique (Procedure 4-14):

1. Determine the indication for intraosseous access.
2. Assemble and check all equipment.
3. Position the patient. Rotate the leg toward the outside to expose the medial, proximal aspect of the tibia.
4. Locate the access site. Palpate the tibia and use all landmarks.
   ○ *Pediatric.* Locate the tibial tuberosity. Move from one to two fingerbreadths below the tibial tuberosity and find the flat expanse medial to the anterior tibial crest.
   ○ *Adult or geriatric.* Find the medial locations (based on the device you are using). These can include the tibial tuberosity, sternum, or humeral head. Be familiar with

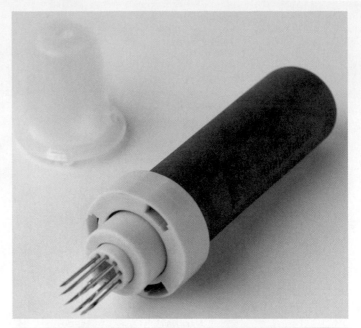

● **Figure 4-55** The FAST1® allows intraosseous placement in the sternum of an adult or adolescent (12 years of age and older). *(Pyng Medical Corp.)*

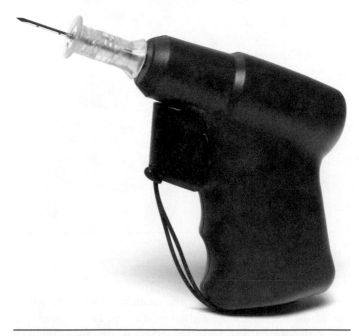

● **Figure 4-56** The EZ-IO™, which uses a small drill to place the needle into the bone, is approved for both adults and children. *(Vidacare.com)*

the accepted access sites as well as the operation of the particular IO device you are using.

5. Cleanse the site with an antiseptic solution. Start at the puncture site and work outward in an expanding circular motion.
6. Perform the puncture. Holding the needle perpendicular to the puncture site, insert it with a twisting motion until you feel a decrease in resistance or a "pop." When this occurs, the needle is in the medullary canal. Do not

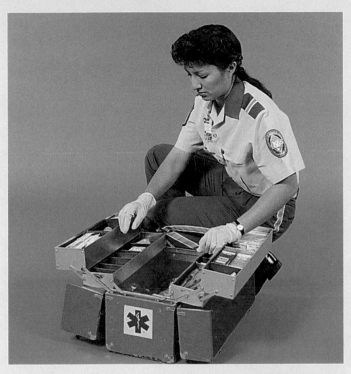

4-14a ● Select the medication and prepare equipment.

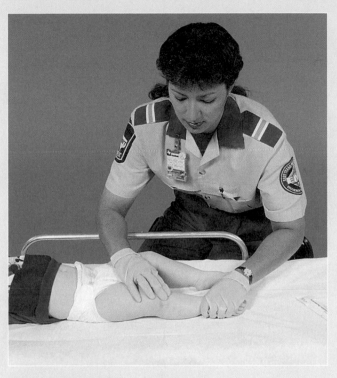

4-14b ● Palpate the puncture site and prep with an antiseptic solution.

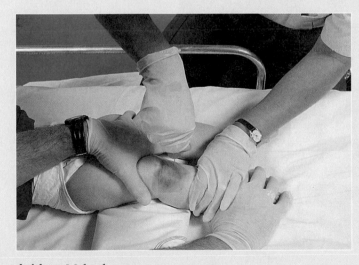

4-14c ● Make the puncture.

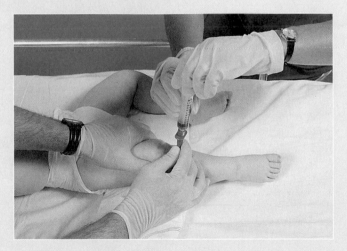

4-14d ● Aspirate to confirm proper placement.

(Continued)

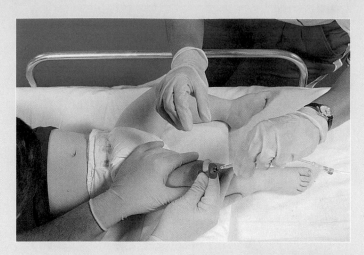

4-14e ● Connect the IV fluid tubing.

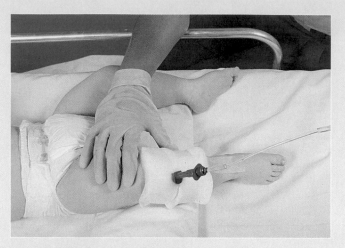

4-14f ● Secure the needle appropriately.

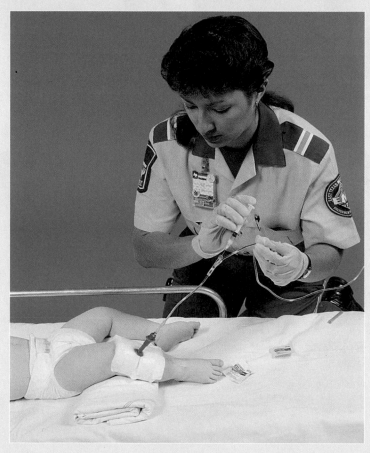

4-14g ● Administer the medication. Monitor the patient for effects.

advance it any further. Generally, you will need to insert the needle only 2 to 4 mm for entry.

7. Remove the trocar and attach the syringe. Slowly pull back the plunger to attempt aspiration into the syringe. Easy aspiration of bone marrow and blood confirms correct medullary placement.

8. Once you have confirmed placement, rotate the plastic disk toward the skin to secure the needle.

9. Remove the syringe and attach the prepared administration tubing and solution. Set the appropriate flow rate.

10. Secure the intraosseous needle as if securing an impaled object by surrounding it with bulky dressings and taping them securely in place. Commercial devices for securing an intraosseous needle are available.

After establishing intraosseous access, you must periodically flush the intraosseous needle to keep it patent. Failure to do so may allow the needle to become occluded, hindering medication administration.

Because the intraosseous needle is connected to the primary IV administration set and fluid, the intraosseous route can also deliver any solution or medication that can be administered by IV bolus or continuous infusion. To administer medications or solutions through the intraosseous route, use the medicinal administration port on the primary administration tubing with the techniques as described under Intravenous Medication Administration (Intravenous Medication Bolus and Intravenous Medication Infusion).

If an intraosseous infusion is complete or must be discontinued because of an adverse reaction, shut down the secondary line with the flow regulator or a clamp. Open the primary line and adjust it to the indicated drip rate. Remove the hypodermic needle from the medication administration port and properly dispose of all contents if the infusion has been exhausted.

Intraosseous Access Complications and Precautions

Intraosseous access poses serious potential complications:

- *Fracture.* Too large a needle or too forceful an insertion can fracture the tibia, particularly in very young children.

- *Infiltration.* Infiltration occurs when IV solution collects in the local tissues instead of in the intramedullary canal. Infiltration may occur if you run fluids through an incorrectly placed needle or if a fracture has occurred. An infusion that does not run freely or the formation of an edema at the puncture site indicates infiltration. If infiltration occurs, immediately discontinue infusion and restart on the other leg.

- *Growth plate damage.* An improperly located puncture may damage the growth plate and result in long-term growth complications. Locating the site with proper technique is the most effective way to avoid this complication.

- *Complete insertion.* Complete insertion occurs when the needle passes through both sides of the tibia, rendering the site useless. To avoid complete puncture, stop advancing the needle once you feel the pop. If complete puncture occurs, remove the intraosseous needle with a reverse twisting motion and start again on the other leg. Apply direct pressure and a sterile dressing over the site(s) for at least 5 minutes.

- *Pulmonary embolism.* If bone, fat, or marrow particles make their way into the circulatory system, pulmonary embolism may result. Proper technique and vigilance for signs associated with pulmonary embolism (sudden onset of chest pain or shortness of breath) are important to establishing and maintaining intraosseous access.

Other complications of intraosseous access are similar to those of peripheral intravenous access. They include local infection, thrombophlebitis, air embolism, circulatory overload, and allergic reaction.

Contraindications to Intraosseous Placement

Do not attempt intraosseous placement in the following situations:

- Fracture to the tibia or femur on the side of access
- *Osteogenesis imperfecta*—a congenital bone disease that results in fragile bones
- Osteoporosis
- Establishment of a peripheral IV line

Intraosseous placement is a relatively safe intervention that can be used for the critically ill patient. Its location allows access while you perform other interventions such as CPR or endotracheal intubation. Because you probably will use intraosseous access only infrequently, you must continually refresh this skill so that you can perform it properly when needed.

PART 3: Medical Mathematics

Proper medication administration requires basic mathematical proficiency. Because medication dosages are not always standardized, you may have to calculate amounts according to your patient's age, weight, or other medically related criteria. To properly prepare and administer medications, you must understand roman numerals and be proficient in the following mathematical skills:

- Multiplication
- Division
- Fractions
- Decimal fractions
- Proportions
- Percentages

If you are deficient in one or more of these areas, refer to any text on basic and intermediate math.[13]

METRIC SYSTEM

Medication doses are most often expressed and measured in metric units. Accepted worldwide, the metric system is pharmacology's principal system of measurement. Once you become familiar with it, the metric system is easy to use.

The metric system's three fundamental units are grams (mass), meters (distance), and liters (volume). In pharmacology, you will frequently encounter dosages greater or less than these fundamental units. To avoid long numbers with repetitive zeros when measurements are substantially less than or greater than the fundamental unit, the metric system adds prefixes to the fundamental units. Table 4–2 lists metric prefixes.

The most commonly used prefixes in pharmacology are *kilo-*, *centi-*, *milli-*, and *micro-* Prefixes above the fundamental units denote quantities larger than the standard gram, liter, or meter, while those below are smaller. The prefix *milli-* is smaller than the fundamental unit and *m* refers to 1/1,000. Thus, a *milliliter* equals 1/1,000 (one one-thousandth) of a liter. If you divided a liter into one thousand equal parts, a milliliter would equal one of those parts. Similarly, a milligram is 1/1,000 of a gram. If you divided a gram into one thousand equal parts, a milligram would equal one of those parts. The prefix *micro-* expresses 1/1,000,000. A *microgram* is 1/1,000,000 (one one-millionth) of a gram.

CULTURAL CONSIDERATIONS

The Metric System. *Although the United States has been slow to adopt the metric system, it is widely used in science and medicine. As a paramedic, you must be familiar with the metric system and be able to make calculations using it.*

Conversion between Prefixes

If you know the prefixes and their numeric equivalents, you can easily convert measurements to smaller or larger units. To convert a measurement to a smaller unit, multiply the original measurement by the numerical equivalent of the smaller measurement's prefix.

EXAMPLE 1. Convert 3 grams to milligrams.

Milligrams (1/1,000) are smaller than grams; therefore, multiply 3 by 1,000:

$$3 \text{ (grams)} \times 1,000 \text{ (milli)} = 3,000$$
$$3 \text{ grams} = 3,000 \text{ milligrams}$$

EXAMPLE 2. Convert 2.67 liters to milliliters.

Milliliters (1/1,000) are smaller than a liter; therefore, multiply 2.67 by 1,000:

$$2.67 \text{ liters} \times 1,000 \text{ (milli)} = 2,670$$
$$2.67 \text{ liters} = 2,670 \text{ milliliters}$$

To convert a measurement to a larger unit, divide the original measurement by the numerical equivalent of the smaller measurement's prefix.

TABLE 4–2 | Metric Prefixes

Prefix	Multiplier	Abbreviation
Kilo	1,000	(k)
Hecto	100	(h)
Deka	10	(D)
Deci	1/10 or 0.1	(d)
Centi	1/100 or 0.01	(c)
Milli	1/1,000 or 0.001	(m)
Micro	1/1,000,000 or 0.000001	(mcg or μg)

EXAMPLE 3. Convert 1,600 micrograms to grams.

A microgram is 1/1,000,000 the size of a gram; therefore, divide 1,600 by 1,000,000:

$$1,600/1,000,000 = 0.0016 \text{ grams}$$

$$1,600 \text{ micrograms} = 0.0016 \text{ grams}$$

When converting a measurement to or from a prefix that is not the fundamental unit, first convert the *existing* measurement to the *fundamental* measurement. Then convert the fundamental measurement to the desired unit.

EXAMPLE 4. Convert 5.6 milligrams to micrograms.

First, convert the 5.6 milligrams to grams:

$$5.6 \text{ milligrams}/1,000 = 0.0056 \text{ grams (g)}$$

$$5.6 \text{ milligrams} = 0.0056 \text{ grams}$$

Now, convert 0.0056 grams to micrograms as previously described:

$$0.0056 \text{ (grams)} \times 1,000,000 = 5,600 \text{ micrograms}$$

$$5.6 \text{ milligrams} = 5,600 \text{ micrograms}$$

For the beginner, this technique avoids confusion. The more experienced provider will be able to make a direct conversion from milligrams to micrograms.

TABLE 4–3	Metric Equivalents	
Household	**Apothecary**	**Metric**
1 gallon	4 quarts	3.785 liters
1 quart	1 quart	0.946 liters
16 ounces	approximately 1 pint	473 milliliters
1 cup	approximately 1/2 pint	approximately 250 milliliters
1 tablespoon		approximately 16 milliliters
1 teaspoon		approximately 4 to 5 milliliters

Household and Apothecary Systems of Measure

In the past, pharmacology traditionally used the household and apothecary systems to measure medication dosages. Gradually, the metric system has replaced those systems, but you may occasionally encounter their remnants. Table 4–3 gives the metric equivalents of the household and apothecary units you will most likely confront.

Weight Conversion

Some medications' dosages are calculated according to kilograms of body weight. To convert pounds to kilograms, use the following formula:

$$\text{kilograms} = \text{pounds}/2.2$$

EXAMPLE 5. How many kilograms does a 182-lb person weigh?

$$\text{kilograms} = 182 \text{ lb}/2.2$$

$$\text{kilograms} = 82.7$$

Temperature

The international thermometric scale measures temperature in degrees Celsius. While degrees Celsius is often cited interchangeably with degrees centigrade, the two scales are slightly different. For practical purposes, however, you can think of them both as dividing the interval between the freezing and boiling points of water into 100 equal parts, with 0° being the freezing point and 100° being the boiling point. The household measurement system, in contrast, divides the interval between the freezing and boiling points of water into 180 equal parts, with 32° being the freezing point and 212° being the boiling point. When taking a body temperature, use the following formulas to convert between degrees Fahrenheit and degrees Celsius:

$$°F = 9/5 \, °C + 32$$

$$°C = 5/9 \, (°F - 32)$$

EXAMPLE 6. Convert 98.2 °F to °C

$$°C = 5/9 \ (98.2 - 32)$$
$$°C = 5/9 \ (66.2)$$
$$°C = 36.8$$
$$98.2 \ °F = 36.8 \ °C$$

EXAMPLE 7. Convert 28.4 °C to °F

$$°F = 9/5 \ (28.4) + 32$$
$$°F = 51.12 + 32$$
$$°F = 83.1$$
$$28.4 \ °C = 83.1 \ °F$$

Converting between the different prefixes and between different systems of measurement is crucial in calculating medication dosages. You should continually practice all conversions, not only during your formal education but also throughout your career in the emergency medical services.

Units

Some medications are measured in **units**. Penicillin, heparin, and insulin are administered in units. Units, in pharmacology, are a measure of biological activity, not of weight, mass, or volume. Thus, units do not convert between the metric, household, and apothecary systems.

MEDICAL CALCULATIONS

Frequently you will have to apply basic mathematical principles to calculate specific quantities before administering medications and fluids. In prehospital care, the following forms of medications often require calculation:

- Oral medications
- Liquid parenteral medications
- Intravenous fluid administration
- Intravenous medication infusions

Most medications are provided in **stock solution**. Therefore, you must calculate the exact amount of medication to remove from the stock for administration. To calculate basic medication dosage, you will need three facts:

- Desired dose
- Dosage on hand
- Volume on hand

Desired Dose   The **desired dose** is the specific quantity of medication needed. Most dosages are expressed as a weight (grams, milligrams, or micrograms). Dosages may be standard or calculated according to body weight or age.

Dosage and Volume on Hand   All liquid medications are packaged as concentrations. **Concentration** refers to weight per volume. A liquid medication's concentration is the medication's weight (grams, milligrams, or micrograms) per volume of liquid (mL) in which it is dissolved. For example, 50 percent Dextrose (D_{50}) is packaged as a concentration of 25 grams (weight) dextrose in 50 mL (volume) of water. From the concentration, you can determine the **dosage on hand** (weight) and the **volume on hand**. For 50 percent Dextrose, the dosage on hand is 25 grams and the volume on hand is 50 mL. Concentrations are identified on all medication packaging and labels.

Because you cannot see the desired dose dissolved in liquid, you must convert its weight to volume, a readily visible measurement, using the following formula:

$$\text{volume to be administered} = \frac{\text{volume on hand} \ (\text{desired dose})}{\text{dosage on hand}}$$

To use this formula, you must express all weight and volume measurements with the same metric prefix. For example, if the desired dose is expressed in *milli*grams, the dosage on hand must also be expressed in *milli*grams, volume on hand in *milli*liters.

CALCULATING DOSAGES FOR ORAL MEDICATIONS

The following example illustrates how to calculate the volume of a specific medication dosage:

EXAMPLE 1. A physician orders you to administer 90 mg of acetaminophen to a pediatric patient. The liquid acetaminophen is packaged as a concentration of 500 mg in 8 mL of solution. How much of the medication will you administer?

Because you cannot see the 90 mg of acetaminophen, you must convert this weight to a volume. To do so you need these facts:

$$\text{desired dose} = 90 \text{ mg}$$
$$\text{dosage on hand} = 500 \text{ mg}$$
$$\text{volume on hand} = 8 \text{ mL}$$

Use the formula to calculate the dosage's volume:

$$\text{volume to be administered} = \frac{\text{volume on hand}\,(8 \text{ mL}) \times \text{desired dose}\,(90 \text{ mg})}{\text{dosage on hand}\,(500 \text{ mg})}$$

$$\text{volume to be administered} = (8 \text{ mL} \times 90)/500 \text{ mg}$$
$$\text{volume to be administered} = 720 \text{ mL}/500$$
$$\text{volume to be administered} = 1.44 \text{ mL}$$

Administer 1.44 mL of solution to deliver 90 mg of acetaminophen.

Another way to calculate medication dosages is the ratio (fraction) and proportion method. A ratio (fraction) illustrates a relationship between two numbers. A proportion is the comparison of two numerically equivalent ratios. Using the variable *x*, the previous problem can be stated:

$$8 \text{ mL}/500 \text{ mg} = x \text{ mL}/90 \text{ mg}$$

To solve the problem, cross-multiply the numerals:

$$\frac{8 \text{ mL}}{500 \text{ mg}} \times \frac{x}{90 \text{ mg}}$$

$$x = \frac{720 \text{ mL mg}}{500 \text{ mg}}$$

$$x = 1.44 \text{ mL}$$

Converting Prefixes

The following example shows how to calculate the volume to be administered when the desired dose, the dosage on hand, and the volume on hand are not all expressed in metric units with the same prefix.

EXAMPLE 2. A physician orders you to give 250 mg of a medication via IV bolus. The multidose vial contains 2 grams of the medication in 10 mL of solution. How much of the medication should you administer?

Because the desired dose is expressed as *milli*grams, the dosage on hand must be converted from grams to milligrams. In the metric system, 2 grams equal 2,000 milligrams. You now know:

$$\text{desired dose} = 250 \text{ mg}$$
$$\text{dosage on hand} = 2,000 \text{ mg}$$
$$\text{volume on hand} = 10 \text{ mL}$$

MATH SUMMARY 1

$$x = 8 \text{ mL} \times 90 \text{ mg}$$
$$x = 8 \text{ mL} \times 90 \text{ mg}$$
$$x = \frac{720 \text{ mL mg}}{500 \text{ mg}}$$
$$x = 1.44 \text{ mL}$$

MATH SUMMARY 2

$$\frac{8 \text{ mL}}{500 \text{ mg}} \times \frac{x}{90 \text{ mg}}$$
$$x = \frac{720 \text{ mL mg}}{500 \text{ mg}}$$
$$x = 1.44 \text{ mL}$$

Now you can use the formula to calculate the volume to be administered:

$$\text{volume to be administered} = \frac{\text{volume on hand (10 mL)} \times \text{desired dose (250 mg)}}{\text{dosage on hand (2,000 mg)}}$$

$$\text{volume to be administered} = (10 \text{ mL} \times 250 \text{ mg}) / 2,000 \text{ mg}$$

$$\text{volume to be administered} = 2,500 \text{ mL mg}) / 2,000 \text{ mg}$$

$$\text{volume to be administered} = 1.25 \text{ mL}$$

Administer 1.25 mL of solution to deliver 250 mg of medication.

You can also solve this problem using the ratio proportion as follows:

$$10 \text{ mL}/2,000 \text{ mg} = x/250 \text{ mg}$$

$$2,500 \text{ mL mg} = 2,000 \text{ mg } x$$

$$2,500 \text{ mL mg}/2,000 \text{ mg} = x$$

$$1.25 \text{ mL} = x$$

Tablets also come in stock doses. If the dosage of one tablet or pill is more than needed, divide the tablet or pill to make the correct dose. Do not divide enteric or time-release capsules.

Calculating Dosages for Parenteral Medications

You can use the same formula to calculate specific doses and volume for parenteral medication delivery.

EXAMPLE 3. A physician wants you to administer 5 milligrams of medication subcutaneously. The ampule contains 10 mg of the medication in 2 mL of solvent. How much medication should you use?

$$\text{desired dose} = 5 \text{ mg}$$

$$\text{dosage on hand} = 10 \text{ mg}$$

$$\text{volume on hand} = 2 \text{ mL}$$

$$\text{volume to be administered} = \frac{\text{volume on hand (2 mL)} \times \text{desired dose (5 mg)}}{\text{dosage on hand (10 mg)}}$$

$$\text{volume to be administered} = (2 \text{ mL} \times 5 \text{ mg}) / 10 \text{ mg}$$

$$\text{volume to be administered} = 10 \text{ mL mg} / 10 \text{ mg}$$

$$\text{volume to be administered} = 1.0 \text{ mL}$$

Using the ratio and proportion method, the problem is solved as follows:

$$2 \text{ mL}/10 \text{ mg} = x/5 \text{ mg}$$

$$10 \text{ mL mg}/10 \text{ mg} = x$$

$$1.0 \text{ mL} = x$$

Calculating Weight-Dependent Dosages

Occasionally, you will have to calculate the desired dose according to the patient's weight.

EXAMPLE 4. You must administer 1.5 mg/kg of lidocaine via IV bolus to a patient in stable ventricular tachycardia. The concentration of lidocaine is 100 mg in a prefilled syringe containing 10 mL of solution. The patient weighs 158 lb.

Start by converting the patient's weight to kilograms:

$$\text{kilograms} = \text{pounds}/2.2$$

$$\text{kilograms} = 158 \text{ lb}/2.2$$

$$\text{kilograms} = 71.82$$

The patient weighs approximately 72 kg.

Calculate the desired dose:

$$1.5 \text{ mg/kg} \times 72 \text{ kg} = 108 \text{ mg}$$

You now know these three facts:

$$\text{desired dose} = 108 \text{ mg}$$

$$\text{dosage on hand} = 100 \text{ mg}$$

$$\text{volume on hand} = 10 \text{ mL}$$

Use the same formula as before to calculate the volume to be administered:

$$\text{volume to be administered} = \frac{\text{volume on hand } (10 \text{ mL}) \times \text{desired dose } (108 \text{ mg})}{\text{dosage on hand } (100 \text{ mg})}$$

$$\text{volume to be administered} = (10 \text{ mL} \times 100 \text{ mg}) / 100 \text{ mg}$$

$$\text{volume to be administered} = 1{,}080 \text{ mL } \cancel{\text{mg}}) / 100 \cancel{\text{mg}}$$

$$\text{volume to be administered} = 10.8 \text{ mL}$$

Administer 10.8 mL of solution to deliver 108 mg of lidocaine.

After you have calculated the desired dose, you can solve this problem using the ratio and proportion method as previously illustrated.

Calculating Infusion Rates

To deliver fluid or medication through an IV infusion, you must calculate the correct infusion rate in drops per minute. To do so you must know the administration tubing's drip factor, as well as the volume on hand, desired dose, and dosage on hand.

Medicated Infusions

To calculate the correct IV infusion rate, use the following formula:

$$\text{drops / minute} = \frac{\text{volume on hand} \times \text{drip factor} \times \text{desired dose}}{\text{dosage on hand}}$$

EXAMPLE 5. A physician wants you to administer 2 mg per minute of lidocaine to a patient. To prepare the infusion, you mix 2 grams of lidocaine in an IV bag containing 500 milliliters of 5 percent dextrose in water (D_5W). You will use a microdrip administration set (60 drops/mL). Calculate the infusion rate.

$$\text{desired dose} = 2 \text{ mg/minute}$$

$$\text{dosage on hand} = 2{,}000 \text{ mg (2 grams)}$$

$$\text{volume on hand} = 500 \text{ mL}$$

$$\text{drip factor} = 60 \text{ drops/mL}$$

$$\text{drops/minute} = \frac{\text{volume on hand } (500 \text{ mL}) \times \text{drip factor } (60 \text{ drops / mL}) \times \text{desired dose } (2 \text{ mg})}{\text{dosage on hand } (2{,}000 \text{ mg})}$$

$$\text{drops/minute} = (500 \times 60 \times 2) / 2{,}000$$

$$\text{drops/minute} = (60{,}000) / 2{,}000$$

$$\text{drops/minute} = 30$$

Run the infusion at 30 drops/minute to infuse 2 mg of lidocaine per minute.

Fluid Volume over Time

Fluids with or without medications may require administration over a specific period of time. To deliver the fluid correctly, you must calculate volume/time. This calculation requires the following information:

- Volume to be administered
- Drip factor of the administration set (drops/mL)
- Total time of infusion (minutes)

To calculate the **infusion rate**, use this formula:

$$\text{drops / minute} = \frac{\text{volume to be administered } (\text{drip factor})}{\text{time in minutes}}$$

MATH SUMMARY 6

$$x = \frac{10 \text{ mL} \times 108 \text{ mg}}{100 \text{ mg}}$$

$$x = \frac{1{,}080 \text{ mL } \cancel{\text{mg}}}{100 \cancel{\text{mg}}}$$

$$x = 10.8 \text{ mL}$$

MATH SUMMARY 7

$$\frac{10 \text{ mL}}{100 \text{ mg}} = \frac{x}{108 \text{ mg}}$$

$$x = \frac{1{,}080 \text{ mL } \cancel{\text{mg}}}{100 \cancel{\text{mg}}}$$

$$x = 10.8 \text{ mL}$$

MATH SUMMARY 8

$$x = 500 \text{ mL} \times 60 \text{ drops/mL}$$

$$\frac{\times 2 \text{ mg / min}}{2{,}000 \text{ mg}}$$

$$x = \frac{60{,}000 \text{ } \cancel{\text{mL}} \text{ drops } \cancel{\text{mL}} \text{ } \cancel{\text{mg}} \text{ min}}{2{,}000 \cancel{\text{mg}}}$$

$$x = 30 \text{ drops/min}$$

EXAMPLE 6. A physician tells you to administer 500 milliliters of normal saline solution to a patient over 1 hour (60 minutes). The administration tubing is a macrodrip set with a drip factor of 10 drops/mL. At what drip rate would you run this infusion?

$$\text{volume to be administered} = 500 \text{ mL}$$

$$\text{administration set drip factor} = 10 \text{ drops/mL}$$

$$\text{total time of infusion} = 60 \text{ minutes}$$

Calculate the infusion rate:

$$\text{drops/minute} = (500 \times 10)/60$$

$$\text{drops/minute} = 5{,}000/60$$

$$\text{drops/minute} = 83.3$$

MATH SUMMARY 9

$$x = \frac{500 \text{ mL} \times 10 \text{ drops/mL}}{60 \text{ minutes}}$$

$$x = \frac{5{,}000 \text{ mL } 10 \text{ drops mL}}{60 \text{ min}}$$

$$x = 83.3 \text{ drops/min}$$

Set the flow rate at approximately 83 drops per minute to infuse 500 milliliters of normal saline in almost exactly 60 minutes.

You can use the same formula to determine how long it will take to use all the fluid in a container.

EXAMPLE 7. You are transporting a patient with an IV antibiotic. The infusion rate is 45 drops/minute and the administration tubing is a microdrip set (60 drops/mL). 150 milliliters remain in the 500 milliliter bag of D_5W. How long until the antibiotic will complete infusion?

Use the same formula as in example 6; however, in this instance you will find time in minutes.

$$45 \text{ drops/minute} = \frac{(150 \text{ mL})(60 \text{ drops/mL})}{x}$$

$$45 \text{ drops/minute} = \frac{9{,}000 \text{ mL drops mL}}{x}$$

$$x = \frac{9{,}000 \text{ mL drops mL}}{45 \text{ drops/minute}}$$

$$x = 200 \text{ minutes}$$

MATH SUMMARY 10

$$x = 9{,}000 \text{ mL}$$

$$\frac{\text{drops/mL}}{45 \text{ drops/min}}$$

$$x = 200 \text{ min}$$

The antibiotic will complete infusion in 200 minutes, or 3 hours and 20 minutes.

Calculating Dosages and Infusion Rates for Infants and Children

Infants and children cannot tolerate under- or overdoses of medication and fluids. When you administer infusions to pediatric patients, you must calculate exact flow rates. Because infants and children differ drastically from adults in size and internal development, their dosages often depend on weight. Most weight-dependent dosages express the patient's weight in kilograms, so you must make the appropriate conversion from pounds as discussed earlier. Occasionally, you may encounter a medication that is based on body surface area (BSA). Chemotherapeutic agents for children are often based on body surface area. While you will not initiate such medications, you may encounter them on critical care transports either by ground or air. Many aids for calculating pediatric medication doses and infusion rates are available, including charts, forms, and length-based resuscitation tapes. While these devices are helpful, you should not rely on them exclusively. They are no substitute for knowledge.[14]

▣ SUMMARY

Medication administration is a fundamental skill used in the treatment of the sick and injured. For medications to be effective, they must be *safely* delivered into the body by the *appropriate* route. Many different routes for medication delivery are available to the paramedic; however, specific medications require specific routes for administration. In addition, you must accurately calculate many medication dosages. Dosage errors and inappropriate medication administration can result in serious side effects or even death for the patient, not to mention casting serious doubt on your ability or causing loss of your certification.

Keep in mind that medication calculations can be completed by a variety of methods. What is important is to find a method that works for you and gets you the right answer every time you work a problem. Once you identify this method, stick with it and practice it, because you never know when you will need to do a calculation in less than favorable conditions.

Always remember that it is your responsibility to be familiar with all routes of medication delivery and the techniques for establishing and utilizing them. You will use some routes of medication administration infrequently, and they will quickly fade from memory, while you will use other routes almost daily. Nonetheless, someone's well-being may depend on your ability to utilize any one of the routes of administration in an emergency. Therefore, periodic review of all routes used in medication administration is highly recommended.

YOU MAKE THE CALL

You have been called for a 53-year-old male patient experiencing chest pain and shortness of breath. After assessing the patient, you find him to be alert and oriented, with a clear airway, and breathing adequately at a rate of 16 breaths per minute. His distal pulses are strong, and his skin is cool and slightly diaphoretic. Your partner obtains the following vital signs: blood pressure 142/88 mmHg, pulse 92 beats per minute, and respirations 16 and easy. The patient exhibits no jugular venous distention or peripheral edema, and breath sounds are clear bilaterally. The 12-lead cardiac monitor shows a sinus rhythm with ST segment elevation in leads V_1 through V_3. The patient has no medical allergies and is on no medications. He denies any previous medical history.

In addition to high-flow, high-concentration oxygen, you elect to administer nitroglycerin, morphine sulfate, and aspirin, based on your suspicion of an acute myocardial infarction. Accordingly, you quickly establish an IV line.

1. Before administering aspirin or any other medication orally (p.o.), what major consideration must you be sure of?

2. Of the following medications and routes of delivery, which will provide the fastest and most predictable rate of absorption?
- Aspirin—enteral tract
- Nitroglycerin—sublingual
- Morphine sulfate—IV bolus

3. When administered sublingually, how is the nitroglycerin absorbed into the body?

4. You elect to administer 3 mg of morphine sulfate to the patient. The medication is packaged as 10 mg in 5 mL of solution in a multidose vial. How many milliliters must you administer to give the 3 mg of morphine?

See Suggested Responses at the back of this book.

REVIEW QUESTIONS

1. The simplest and often the most neglected form of Standard Precautions is:
a. hand washing.
b. donning a gown.
c. wearing gloves.
d. wearing eye goggles.

2. A cleansing agent that is toxic to living tissue is:
a. sterile.
b. antiseptic.
c. disinfectant.
d. medically clean.

3. A drug administered through the mucous membranes of the ear and ear canal is a(n):
a. buccal medication.
b. nasal medication.
c. aural medication.
d. ocular medication.

4. "Within the dermal layer of the skin" defines:
a. buccal.
b. intradermal.
c. subcutaneous.
d. intramuscular.

5. The state in which solutions on opposite sides of a semipermeable membrane are in equal concentration describes a(n) _____ state.
a. colloid
b. isotonic
c. hypertonic
d. hypotonic

6. To minimize the chances of a catheter shear reaching the patient's central circulation, always leave the venous constricting band in place until you have completely removed the needle from the catheter. However, never leave the constricting band in place more than _____ minutes.

a. 1.5   c. 3

b. 2   d. 4

7. Medically clean techniques include:

a. hand washing.

b. glove changing.

c. discarding equipment in opened packages.

d. all of the above.

8. To minimize or eliminate the risk of an accidental needlestick, the paramedic must:

a. recap needles only as a last resort.

b. minimize the tasks performed in a moving ambulance.

c. immediately dispose of used sharps in a sharps container.

d. all of the above.

9. The abbreviation _____ designates the right eye.

a. o.u.   c. o.d.

b. o.p.   d. o.s.

10. In an acute respiratory emergency involving a patient with a metered dose inhaler, always use a(n) _____ instead of the MDI.

a. LMA

b. ET tube

c. nebulizer

d. nasal airway

11. When using an endotracheal tube, you must increase conventional IV dosages from _____ – _____ times.

a. 1, 2   c. 2, 3

b. 2, 2½   d. 3½, 4

12. A _____ is a liquid that contains small particles of solid medication.

a. syrup   c. emulsion

b. elixir   d. suspension

13. _____ denotes any drug administration outside the gastrointestinal tract.

a. Enema   c. Parenteral

b. Enteral   d. Suppository

14. Which of the following is not a parenteral drug delivery route?

a. sublingual route

b. intravenous access

c. intraosseous infusion

d. intramuscular injection

15. All of the following are examples of colloidal solutions except:

a. Dextran.   c. lactated Ringer's.

b. Hespan.   d. Albumin.

16. _____, or inflammation of the vein, is particularly common in long-term intravenous therapy.

a. Necrosis   c. Thrombus formation

b. Air embolism   d. Thrombophlebitis

17. Which of the following is not an enteral route of drug administration?

a. inhalational   c. rectal

b. oral   d. buccal

18. Advantages of saline and heparin locks include all of the following except:

a. provides a peripheral IV port.

b. does not need continuous fluid infusion.

c. blood samples cannot be withdrawn from the lock.

d. decreases the risk of accidental electrolyte derangement.

19. Causes of hemolysis include:

a. using too small a needle for retrieval.

b. vigorously shaking the blood tubes after they are filled.

c. too forcefully aspirating blood into or out of a syringe.

d. all of the above.

20. Which of the following is not considered a complication of intraosseous access?

a. local infection   c. fat embolism

b. air embolism   d. thrombophlebitis

21. The bone most commonly used for intraosseous access is the:

a. tibia.   c. fibula.

b. femur.   d. humerus.

22. The three fundamental units of the metric system are:

a. meters, liters, grains.

b. grams, meters, liters.

c. inches, pints, pounds.

d. grams, liters, ounces.

23. 1,000 milligrams equals:

a. 1 kilogram.   c. 0.001 gram.

b. 1 gram.   d. 10 grams.

24. A patient weighs 90 kg. What is his weight in pounds?

a. 180   c. 75

b. 41   d. 198

25. The metric prefix *hecto-* means:

a. 1.   c. 100.

b. 10.   d. 1,000.

26. The metric system is based on what number system?

a. ratios   c. fractions

b. decimals   d. percentages

27. Medical control orders you to administer Valium, 2.0 mg. The medication is in a prefilled syringe labeled 10 mg in 2 cc. You draw up the correct dose, which is:

a. 0.20 mL.   c. 0.4 cc.

b. 2.0 mL.   d. 4.0 cc.

28. To administer 35 mg of Benadryl from a syringe labeled 50 mg/cc you would give:

a. 1.5 cc.   c. 0.7 mL.

b. 0.8 cc.   d. 0.7 mg.

29. 0.75 liters converted to milliliters is:
- a. 1,075 mL.
- c. 75 mL.
- b. 1.075 mL.
- d. 750 mL.

30. Two grams is equal to:
- a. 1,000 mg.
- c. 3,000 mg.
- b. 2,000 mg.
- d. 2,000 mL.

31. 2.5 grams is equal to:
- a. 150 mg.
- c. 2,500 mg.
- b. 1,500 mg.
- d. 2,000 mg.

32. 1 kilogram is equal to:
- a. 2.0 pounds.
- c. 0.2 pounds.
- b. 2.2 pounds.
- d. 2.2 kilograms.

See Answers to Review Questions at the back of this book.

REFERENCES

1. Hobgood, C., J. B. Bowen, J. H. Brice, B. Overby, and J. H. Tamayo-Sarver. "Do EMS Personnel Identify, Report, and Disclose Medical Errors?" *Prehosp Emerg Care* 10 (2006): 21–27.

2. Vilke, G. M., S. V. Tornabene, B. Stepanski et al. "Paramedic Self-Reported Medication Errors." *Prehosp Emerg Care* 11 (2007): 80–84.

3. Harris, S. A. and L. A. Nicolai. "Occupational Exposures in Emergency Medical Service Providers and Knowledge of and Compliance with Universal Precautions." *Am J Infect Control* 38 (2010): 86–94.

4. Rickard, C., P. O'Meara, M. McGrail, D. Garner, A. McLean, and P. Le Lievre. "A Randomized Controlled Trial of Intranasal Fentanyl vs. Intravenous Morphine for Analgesia in the Prehospital Setting." *Am J Emerg Med* 25 (2007): 911–917.

5. Barton, E. D., C. B. Colwell, T. Wolfe et al. "Efficacy of Intranasal Naloxone as a Needleless Alternative for Treatment of Opioid Overdose in the Prehospital Setting." *J Emerg Med* 29 (2005): 265–271.

6. Holsti, M., B. L. Sill, S. D. Firth, F. M. Filloux, S. M. Joyce, and R. A. Furnival. "Prehospital Intranasal Midazolam for the Treatment of Pediatric Seizures." *Pediatr Emerg Care* 23 (2007): 148–153.

7. Kelly, A. M., D. Kerr, P. Dietze, I. Patrick, T. Walker, and Z. Koutsogiannis. "Randomised Trial of Intranasal versus Intramuscular Naloxone in Prehospital Treatment for Suspected Opioid Overdose." *Med J Aust* 182 (2005): 24–27.

8. Warner, G. S. "Evaluation of the Effect of Prehospital Application of Continuous Positive Airway Pressure Therapy in Acute Respiratory Distress." *Prehosp Disaster Med* 25 (2010): 87–91.

9. Niemann, J. T., S. J. Stratton, B. Cruz, and R. J. Lewis. "Endotracheal Drug Administration during Out-of-Hospital Resuscitation: Where Are the Survivors?" *Resuscitation* 53 (2002): 153–157.

10. Harrison, G., K. G. Speroni, L. Dugan, and M. G. Daniel. "A Comparison of the Quality of Blood Specimens Drawn in the Field by EMS versus Specimens Obtained in the Emergency Department." *J Emerg Nurs* 36 (2010): 16–20.

11. Fowler, R., J. V. Gallagher, S. M. Isaacs, E. Ossman, P. Pepe, and M. Wayne. "The Role of Intraosseous Vascular Access in the Out-of-Hospital Environment (resource document to NAEMSP position statement)." *Prehosp Emerg Care* 11 (2007): 63–66.

12. Leidel, B. A., C. Kirchhoff, V. Braunstein, V. Bogner, P. Biberthaler, and K. G. Kanz. "Comparison of Two Intraosseous Access Devices in Adult Patients under Resuscitation in the Emergency Department: A Prospective, Randomized Study." *Resuscitation* 81 (2010): 994–999.

13. Eastwood, K. J., M. J. Boyle, and B. Williams. "Paramedics' Ability to Perform Drug Calculations." *West J Emerg Med* 10 (2009): 240–243.

14. Bernius, M., B. Thibodeau, A. Jones, B. Clothier, and M. Witting. "Prevention of Pediatric Drug Calculation Errors by Prehospital Care Providers." *Prehosp Emerg Care* 12 (2008): 486–494.

FURTHER READING

Bledsoe, Bryan E. and Dwayne Clayden. *Prehospital Emergency Pharmacology.* 7th ed. Upper Saddle River, NJ: Pearson/Prentice Hall, 2012.

Campbell, John Emory and the Alabama Chapter of the American College of Emergency Physicians. *International Trauma Life Support for Prehospital Providers.* 6th ed. Upper Saddle River, NJ: Pearson/Prentice Hall, 2012.

Kee, Joyce L. and Evelyn R. Hayes. *Pharmacology: A Nursing Process Approach.* 6th ed. Philadelphia: W. B. Saunders Company, 2009.

Lesmeister, Michele B. *Math Basics for the Health Professional.* 3rd ed. Upper Saddle River, NJ: Pearson/Prentice Hall, 2009.

Martini, Frederic. *Fundamentals of Anatomy and Physiology.* 8th ed. San Francisco: Benjamin Cummings, 2008.

McKenry, Leda M., et al. *Pharmacology in Nursing.* 21st ed. St. Louis: Mosby, 2003.

McSwain, Norman E. and Scott Frame. *Prehospital Trauma Life Support.* 7th ed. St. Louis: Mosby, 2010.

Mikolaj, Alan A. *Drug Dosage Calculations for the Emergency Care Provider.* 2nd ed. Upper Saddle River, NJ: Pearson/Prentice Hall, 2003.

On the Web

Visit Brady's Paramedic website at www.bradybooks.com/paramedic.

5 Airway Management and Ventilation

Bryan Bledsoe, DO, FACEP, FAAEM, EMT-P
W. E. Gandy, JD, NREMTP
Darren Braude, MD, MPH, FACEP

STANDARD

Airway Management, Respiration, and Artificial Ventilation

COMPETENCY

Integrates comprehensive knowledge of anatomy, physiology, and pathophysiology into the assessment to develop and implement a treatment plan with the goal of ensuring a patent airway, adequate mechanical ventilation, and respiration for patients of all ages.

OBJECTIVES

Terminal Performance Objective

After reading this chapter you should be able to apply principles of airway management and ventilation to the assessment and management of patients.

Enabling Objectives

To accomplish the terminal performance objective, you should be able to:

1. Define key terms introduced in this chapter.

2. Explain the importance of immediate recognition and management of problems with a patient's airway, breathing, or oxygenation.

3. Explain the importance of nonlinear thinking and action in assessment and management of problems with the airway and ventilation.

4. Describe the legal liability associated with poor assessment and management of airway and ventilation.

5. Recognize the anatomical structures of the upper and lower airway.

6. Describe the functions of the upper and lower airway structures.

7. Apply knowledge of differences in pediatric airway and respiratory anatomy to managing a pediatric patient's airway and ventilation.

8. Explain the physiology of respiration and ventilation.

9. Describe the etiologies and pathophysiology of the upper airway and inadequate ventilation.

10. Recognize the signs and symptoms of upper airway obstruction and inadequate ventilation.

11. Demonstrate management of upper airway obstruction and inadequate ventilation.

12. Identify problems with the airway, breathing, and oxygenation through primary and secondary patient assessment and noninvasive respiratory monitoring.

13. Differentiate between patients for whom supplemental oxygen administration is indicated and those for whom it is not indicated.

14. Describe the risks and benefits of supplemental oxygen administration.

15. Recognize the indications and contraindications for basic airway interventions, including the following:
    a. various positioning techniques
    b. administering supplemental oxygen by a variety of devices
    c. manual airway maneuvers
    d. inserting basic airway adjuncts
16. Demonstrate techniques of basic airway management, including positioning, administering supplemental oxygen by a variety of devices, manual airway maneuvers, and inserting basic airway adjuncts.
17. Differentiate between adequate and inadequate breathing in a patient.
18. Recognize the need for artificial ventilation of a patient.
19. Demonstrate techniques of ventilation, including:
    a. mouth-to-mouth/mouth-to-nose ventilation (in an apneic patient in the absence of equipment)
    b. mouth-to-mask ventilation
    c. bag-valve-mask ventilation
    d. use of cricoid pressure in conjunction with techniques of ventilation
    e. demand valve device
    f. transport ventilator
20. Demonstrate modifications of ventilation techniques for pediatric patients.
21. Describe the indications, contraindications, advantages, disadvantages, complications, equipment, and techniques for the use of advanced airway devices and techniques, including various extraglottic airways, endotracheal intubation, and cricothyrotomy.
22. Under the supervision of a lab instructor or clinical preceptor and as allowed in your scope of practice, demonstrate effective techniques of advanced airway management, including the following:
    a. Insertion of extraglottic airways
    b. orotracheal intubation
    c. blind nasotracheal intubation
    d. digital intubation
    e. trauma patient airway management
    f. verification of endotracheal tube placement
    g. foreign body removal under direct laryngoscopy
    h. pediatric intubation
    i. needle cricothyrotomy
    j. open cricothyrotomy
23. Recognize complications of advanced airway management.
24. Take actions to correct complications of advanced airway management.
25. Discuss management of post-intubation agitation and field extubation.
26. Explain the considerations in medication-assisted intubation.
27. Describe procedures for medication-assisted intubation.
28. Describe the pharmacology of agents commonly used in medication-assisted intubation.
29. Given a variety of scenarios of patients requiring airway management, including patients with a difficult airway, intervene to establish an effective airway and ventilation without delay.
30. Recognize predictors of a difficult airway.
31. Defend your decision-making processes in scenarios involving airway management and ventilation.

32. Manage airway and ventilation in patients with stomas.

33. Demonstrate effective suctioning of the oropharynx and trachea (in an intubated patient).

34. Take steps to minimize and manage gastric distention.

35. Accurately and completely document relevant information about assessment and management of the airway, ventilation, and oxygenation in patient care reports.

KEY TERMS

CASE STUDY

Ellis County Unit 947, along with a Fire Engine, is dispatched to a motor vehicle collision on rural County Road 664, approximately eight miles from town. This particular stretch of road is well known to paramedics because of a number of serious crashes over the last several months. The road contains numerous sharp curves and is under construction in several locations. Today, Unit 947 is staffed by paramedic Kathy Mulligan and AEMT

William Benson. In addition, paramedic student Sharon Rodriquez is assigned to the unit for her paramedic field internship. There are three volunteer firefighter/EMTs on the engine.

On arrival at the scene, they find one vehicle that has apparently run off the road and struck a telephone pole. Witnesses to the crash estimate the vehicle was traveling at approximately 45 miles per hour before striking the pole. The lone 24-year-old male occupant was ejected from the vehicle and lies face down in a ditch approximately 50 feet from the car. After ensuring scene safety and donning the appropriate personal protective equipment, Kathy assesses the patient. She finds him to be unresponsive. William, Sharon, and the firefighters help her logroll the patient to a supine position while applying cervical-spine precautions. Sharon holds in-line cervical spine stabilization while Kathy opens the airway with the modified jaw-thrust technique.

The patient exhibits agonal respirations. In addition, gurgling noises are heard with each breath. After suctioning bloody secretions from his mouth, Kathy attempts to insert an oropharyngeal airway. However, the patient's teeth are tightly clenched, and the airway will not pass. Sharon places a nasal airway, and then the entire team provides three-person ventilatory support with a bag-valve-mask unit and 100-percent oxygen. The Glasgow Coma Score is 5.

They load the patient into 947 and initiate Code 3 transport to the closest Level 1 Trauma Center 31 minutes away. En route, they obtain a full set of vital signs, keep the patient warm, and start a large-bore IV. The patient's blood pressure is 167/92, HR 110, and oxygen saturation is only 88 percent despite optimal BVM ventilation. Kathy radios to have another paramedic meet them en route so they can perform rapid sequence intubation (RSI), as their protocols require that two medics be present for this procedure.

When they meet up with the second paramedic 23 minutes from the hospital, they are still having trouble maintaining adequate oxygenation, and there is no indication of tension pneumothorax or other treatable etiology. The two medics agree that RSI is indicated. One of the firefighters maintains in-line cervical stabilization as they remove the front of the collar. They give the 100-kg patient 30 mg of etomidate and 200 mg of succinylcholine. Forty-five seconds after succinylcholine was administered, the fasciculations (muscle twitches) have passed from head to toe, and the patient is flaccid.

Kathy attempts bimanual laryngoscopy but is unable to visualize the glottis or posterior cartilages. She makes one attempt with an endotracheal tube introducer under the epiglottis, which is unsuccessful, and the patient's oxygen saturations are noted to be falling. The two medics then elect to place an LMA-Supreme airway. They inflate the cuff and begin ventilations with high-concentration supplemental oxygen, using a self-inflating bag. The patient's oxygen saturation quickly rebounds, and they decompress the stomach with a gastric tube inserted through the dedicated channel on the device. They replace the cervical collar, connect the LMA-Supreme to the transport ventilator, and monitor capnography and other vitals. They adjust the ventilator to maintain a normal exhaled CO_2 and administer fentanyl and midazolam to keep the patient comfortable. They arrive at the trauma center 16 minutes later. The patient's blood pressure is 147/84, HR is 98, saturation is 93 percent, and exhaled CO_2 is 35.

The trauma team leaves the LMA-Supreme in place to obtain initial radiographs and CT scans that reveal a pulmonary contusion and a large subdural hematoma that requires emergent surgical drainage. In the operating room, the patient is intubated through the LMA-Supreme, using fiber-optic guidance. Following surgery, the patient begins to regain consciousness but requires continued intubation for 72 hours because of oxygenation and ventilation issues. On day four, he is successfully extubated and moved to a regular hospital room.

Kathy and her Unit 947 team stop by the hospital to visit after the patient is extubated. He has no recall of the crash at all. The last thing he remembers is looking on the floor of his car for a CD that he dropped. One week after the crash, he is discharged to rehabilitation with minimal neurologic deficits.

INTRODUCTION

Airway management and ventilation are the first and most critical steps in the primary assessment of every patient you will encounter (unless the patient is in cardiac arrest, when chest compressions will come first). Airway management and ventilation go hand in hand. You must immediately establish and maintain an open airway while providing adequate oxygen delivery and carbon dioxide elimination for all patients. Without adequate airway maintenance and ventilation, the patient will succumb to brain injury or even death in as little as 4 minutes. Early detection and intervention of airway and breathing problems, including dispatcher-guided interventions by bystanders, are vital to patient survival.

Airway management and ventilation have always been taught to occur in a stepwise (linear) process. Recommended sequences include the standard ABC (airway, breathing, circulation) sequence, as well as the CAB (compressions, airway, breathing) sequence recommended by the American Heart Association for a patient who appears to be in cardiac arrest when chest compression must come first. These established sequences (ABC and CAB) can help rescuers remember what to do in emergency situations.

With regard to airway and/or ventilation problems, paramedics should approach the patient more globally and consider the whole picture, rather than blindly following predetermined steps. You cannot assess an airway if the patient is not breathing. You cannot assess breathing if there is no airway. Therefore, airway and ventilation need to be considered and managed together. Ultimately, circulation also will depend on an intact airway and adequate ventilation and respiration. The respiratory, cardiovascular, and neurologic systems all play an important role in airway management and ventilation. Stated another way, airway and ventilation problems must be approached in a nonlinear fashion with a number of factors considered simultaneously.

Your deliberate and precise use of simple, basic airway skills is the key to successful airway management and good patient outcome. Once you have applied the basic airway techniques to properly provide oxygenation and ventilation for your patient, you can then use more sophisticated airway maneuvers and skills, if necessary, to further stabilize his airway. You must continually monitor and reassess the airway, being careful to watch for displacement of any placed airway devices, mucous plugging, equipment failure, or the development of a pneumothorax.

This chapter will provide the information and skills you will need to manage even the most difficult airway. It begins with a review of the respiratory system's anatomy and physiology and then explores the primary assessment and management of the airway and ventilation. Finally, it details enhanced airway management options for the more experienced paramedic.

The chapter is divided into four parts:

Part 1: Respiratory Anatomy, Physiology, and Assessment

Part 2: Basic Airway Management and Ventilation

Part 3: Advanced Airway Management and Ventilation

Part 4: Additional Airway and Ventilation Issues

PART 1: Respiratory Anatomy, Physiology, and Assessment

ANATOMY OF THE RESPIRATORY SYSTEM

The respiratory system provides a passage for **oxygen**, a gas necessary for energy production, to enter the body and for **carbon dioxide**, a waste product of the body's metabolism, to exit. This gas exchange, called *respiration*, requires a patent, open airway as well as adequate respiratory function. Many pathological processes can inhibit respiration. To understand the interventions that you will use to maintain adequate airway and ventilatory function, you must thoroughly understand the anatomy of the upper and lower airway.

Upper Airway Anatomy

The *upper airway* extends from the mouth and nose to the larynx (Figure 5-1 ●). It includes the nasal cavity, oral cavity, and pharynx. The larynx joins the upper and lower airways.

The Nasal Cavity

The nasal cavity is the most superior part of the airway. The maxillary, frontal, nasal, ethmoid, and sphenoid bones comprise the lateral and superior walls of the nasal cavity. The hard palate forms the floor of the nasal cavity. The cartilaginous and highly vascular nasal **septum** separates the right and left nasal cavities.

Several structures connect with the nasal cavity. These include the sinuses, the eustachian tubes, and the lacrimal ducts. The **sinuses** are air-filled cavities that are lined with a mucous membrane. There are four pairs of sinuses: the ethmoid sinuses, the frontal sinuses, the maxillary sinuses, and the sphenoid sinuses. The sinuses, named for the bone where they are contained, help reduce the overall weight of the head and are thought to assist in heating, purifying, and moistening the inhaled air. The sinuses help trap bacteria and other substances entering the nasal cavity. Because of this, they can become infected. Fractures of the upper sinuses (sphenoids) can occasionally cause cerebrospinal fluid (CSF) to leak from the cranial cavity into the nasal cavity. Clinically this presents with clear fluid draining from the nose (rhinorrhea) and can provide a direct route for the transmission of pathogens to the brain and associated structures. The **eustachian tubes**, or auditory tubes, connect the ear with the nasal cavity and allow for equalization of pressure on each side of the tympanic membrane. Swallowing can assist in equalizing this pressure. The **nasolacrimal ducts** drain tears and debris from the eyes into the nasal cavity. This can cause the nose to run when someone cries.

Air enters the nasal cavity through the external **nares** (nostrils). Nasal hairs just inside the external nares initially filter the incoming air. The air then proceeds into the nasal cavity, where it strikes three bony projections, the superior, middle, and inferior turbinates, or conchae. These shelflike structures, which are parallel to the nasal floor, serve as conduits into the sinuses, increase

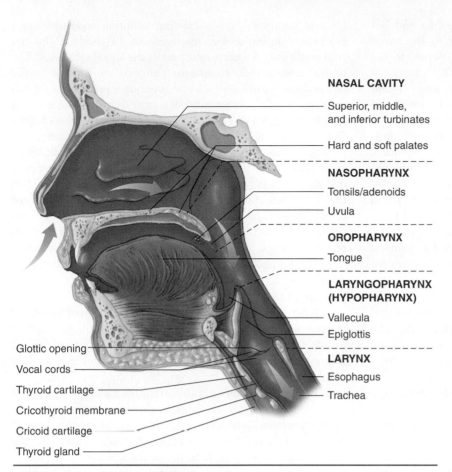

NASAL CAVITY

Superior, middle, and inferior turbinates

Hard and soft palates

NASOPHARYNX

Tonsils/adenoids

Uvula

OROPHARYNX

Tongue

LARYNGOPHARYNX (HYPOPHARYNX)

Vallecula

Epiglottis

LARYNX

Esophagus

Trachea

Glottic opening

Vocal cords

Thyroid cartilage

Cricothyroid membrane

Cricoid cartilage

Thyroid gland

● **Figure 5-1** Anatomy of the upper airway.

the surface area of the nasal cavity, and cause turbulent airflow. This turbulence helps to filter the air by depositing airborne particles on the **mucous membrane** lining the nasal cavity. Hair-like fibers called cilia propel those trapped particles to the back of the pharynx, where they are swallowed. Because the mucous membrane is covered with **mucus** and has a rich blood supply, it also immediately warms and humidifies the air entering the nose. By the time the air reaches the lower airway, it is at body temperature (37 °C), 100 percent humidified, and virtually free of airborne particles. Air proceeds from the nasal cavity through internal nares into the nasopharynx.

The tissue of the nasal cavity is extremely delicate and vascular. Because of this, it is susceptible to trauma. Always remember that improper or overly aggressive placement of tubes or mechanical airways can cause significant bleeding that direct pressure might not control.

The Oral Cavity

The cheeks, the hard and soft palates, and the tongue form the mouth, or oral cavity. The lips that surround the mouth's opening are fleshy folds of skin. Behind the lips lie the gums and teeth, normally numbering 32 in the adult. Significant force is required to avulse (dislodge) or fracture the teeth. Broken or dislodged teeth can potentially obstruct the airway. The hard palate anteriorly and the soft palate posteriorly form the top of the oral cavity and separate it from the nasal cavity. The tongue, a large muscle on the bottom of the oral cavity, is the most

common airway obstruction. It attaches to the mandible and the hyoid bone through a series of muscles and ligaments. The U-shaped hyoid bone is located just beneath the chin. The hyoid bone is unique. It is the only bone in the axial skeleton that does not articulate with any other bone. Instead, it is suspended by ligaments from the styloid process of the temporal bone and serves to anchor the tongue and larynx, as well as to support the trachea.

The Pharynx

The **pharynx** is a muscular tube that extends vertically from the back of the soft palate to the superior aspect of the esophagus. It allows the air to flow into and out of the respiratory tract and food and liquids to pass into the digestive system. It contains several openings, including the internal nares, the mouth, the larynx, and the esophagus.

The pharynx is divided into three regions: the nasopharynx, the oropharynx, and the laryngopharynx (hypopharynx). The nasopharynx is the uppermost region, extending from the back of the nasal opening to the plane of the soft palate. The oropharynx extends from the plane of the soft palate to the hyoid bone. The adenoids, lymphatic tissue in the mouth and nose, filter bacteria. Either hypertrophy or swelling of the adenoids from infection may make them large enough to obscure your view. The laryngopharynx extends posteriorly from the hyoid bone to the esophagus and anteriorly to the larynx. The laryngopharynx is especially important in airway management.

Because the mouth and pharynx serve dual purposes for respiration and digestion, a number of mechanisms help prevent accidental blockage. To prevent foreign material from entering the trachea and lungs, sensitive nerves activate the body's cough and swallowing mechanisms as well as the **gag reflex**.

Located anteriorly in the hypopharynx is the epiglottis, a leaf-shaped cartilage that prevents food from entering the respiratory tract during swallowing. Just anterior and superior to the epiglottis is the **vallecula**, a fold formed by the base of the tongue and the epiglottis. It is an important landmark for endotracheal **intubation**. A series of ligaments and muscles connect the epiglottis to the hyoid bone and mandible. Immediately behind the hypopharynx are the fourth and fifth cervical vertebral bodies.

The Larynx

The **larynx** is the complex structure that joins the pharynx with the trachea (Figure 5-2 ●). Lying midline in the neck,

CONTENT REVIEW

► Upper Airway Components
  • Nasal cavity
  • Oral cavity
  • Pharynx
► Regions of the Pharynx
  • Nasopharynx
  • Oropharynx
  • Laryngopharynx

it is attached to and lies just inferior to the hyoid bone and anterior to the esophagus. It consists of the thyroid and cricoid cartilage (both considered tracheal cartilage), glottic opening, vocal cords, arytenoid cartilage, pyriform fossae, and cricothyroid membrane.

The main laryngeal cartilage is the shield-shaped thyroid cartilage. Larger in males than in females, the thyroid cartilage forms the anterior prominence called the Adam's apple. The arytenoid cartilage, which forms a pyramid-shaped attachment for the vocal cords posteriorly, is an important landmark for endotracheal intubation. Posteriorly, smooth muscle closes a gap in the thyroid cartilage. Directly behind the Adam's apple, the thyroid cartilage houses the glottic opening, the narrowest part of the adult trachea, which is bordered by the vocal cords. The patency of the glottic opening, or **glottis**, depends heavily on muscle tone. On either side of the glottic opening are the pyriform fossae, recesses that form the lateral borders of the larynx. The thyrohyoid membrane attaches the upper end of the thyroid cartilage to the hyoid bone.

Within the laryngeal cavity lie the true vocal cords, white bands of cartilage that regulate the passage of air through the larynx and produce voice by contraction of the laryngeal muscles. The vocal cords can also close together to prevent foreign bodies from entering the airway. The passage of an endotracheal tube between the vocal cords interferes not only with the creation of sound, but also with the protective function of coughing. Beneath the thyroid cartilage is the cricoid cartilage, which forms the inferior border of the larynx. Often it is considered the first tracheal ring. Unlike the thyroid and other tracheal cartilages, whose posterior surfaces are open and not fused, the cricoid cartilage forms a complete ring. The esophagus lies behind the cricoid cartilage, so pressure applied in a posterior direction to the anterior cricoid cartilage is thought to occlude the esophagus

(**cricoid pressure**), thus inhibiting vomiting and subsequent **aspiration** during airway management. In children, the cricoid cartilage is the narrowest part of the laryngeal airway. The fibrous **cricothyroid membrane** connects the inferior border of the thyroid cartilage with the superior aspect of the cricoid cartilage. It is the site for surgical airway techniques. A mucous membrane lines most of the larynx. Rich with nerve endings from the vagus nerve, it is so sensitive that any irritation sparks a cough, or forceful exhalation of a large volume of air. First, air is drawn into the respiratory passageways. Next, the glottic opening shuts tightly, trapping the air within the lungs. Then the abdominal and thoracic muscles contract, pushing against the diaphragm and increasing intrathoracic pressure. The vocal cords suddenly open, and a burst of air forces foreign particles out of the lungs. The laryngeal mucous membrane is so sensitive that its stimulation by a laryngoscope or endotracheal tube can cause bradycardia (slow pulse rate), hypotension (low blood pressure), and decreased respiratory rate.

Other structures proximate to the larynx and of particular interest when you perform surgical airways are the thyroid gland, carotid arteries, and jugular veins. The thyroid gland is a "bow-tie" shaped endocrine gland located in the neck. It is highly vascular and lies inferior to the cricoid cartilage. It contains two lobes, one on each side of the trachea. These lobes are joined in the middle by the isthmus that extends across the trachea. The carotid arteries run closely along the trachea. Several branches of the carotid arteries cross the trachea. Likewise, the jugular veins lie very close to the trachea. Several branches of the jugular veins, such as the superior thyroid vein, cross the trachea.

Lower Airway Anatomy

The lower airway extends from below the larynx to the alveoli (Figure 5-3 ●). This is where the respiratory exchange of oxygen and carbon dioxide occurs. Helpful landmarks are the fourth cervical vertebra at the posterior superior border, and the xiphoid process anterior inferiorly, although the posterior lung extends beyond this inferiorly.

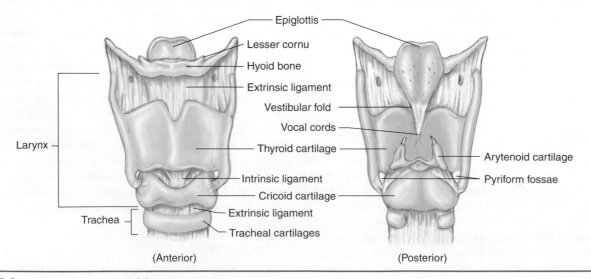

● **Figure 5-2**   Internal anatomy of the upper airway.

The Trachea

As air enters the lower airway from the upper airway, it first enters and then passes through the **trachea**. The trachea is a 10- to 12-centimeter-long tube that connects the larynx to the two mainstem bronchi. It contains cartilaginous, C-shaped, open rings that form a frame to keep it open. The trachea is lined with respiratory epithelium containing cilia and mucous-producing cells. The mucus traps particles that the upper airway did not filter. The cilia then move the trapped particulate matter up into the mouth where it is swallowed or expelled.

The Bronchi

At the carina, the trachea divides, or bifurcates, into the right and left mainstem **bronchi**. The right mainstem bronchus is almost straight, while the left mainstem bronchus angles more acutely to the left. Because of this, the right mainstem is often the site of aspirated foreign bodies. In addition, when an endotracheal tube is inserted too far, it tends to enter the right mainstem bronchus, thus ventilating only the right lung. Mainstem bronchi enter the lung tissue at the hilum and then divide into the secondary and tertiary bronchi. The secondary and tertiary bronchi ultimately branch into the bronchioles, or small airways.

The bronchioles are encircled with smooth muscle that contains beta-2 (β_2) adrenergic receptors. When stimulated, these beta-2 receptors relax the bronchial smooth muscle, thus increasing the airway's diameter. This bronchodilation can increase the amount of air transported through the bronchiole.

Conversely, parasympathetic receptors, when stimulated, cause the bronchial smooth muscles to contract, thus reducing the diameter of the bronchiole. This bronchoconstriction can inhibit the movement of air through the bronchiole.

After approximately 22 divisions, the bronchioles turn into the respiratory bronchioles. These structures contain only muscular connective tissue and have a limited capacity for gas exchange. The respiratory bronchioles terminate at the alveoli.

The Alveoli

The respiratory bronchioles divide into the alveolar ducts, which terminate in balloonlike clusters of **alveoli** called alveolar sacs (Figure 5-4 ●). The alveoli contain an alveolar membrane that is only one or two cell layers thick. Because of this, the alveoli comprise the key functional unit of the respiratory system. Most oxygen and carbon dioxide gas exchanges take place here, although limited gas exchange may occur in the alveolar ducts and respiratory bronchioles. The alveoli become thinner as they expand. This facilitates diffusion of oxygen and carbon dioxide. The alveoli's surface area is massive, totaling more than 40 square meters—enough to cover half of a tennis court. These hollow structures resist collapse largely because of the presence of surfactant, a chemical that decreases their surface tension and makes it easier for them to expand. Alveolar collapse (**atelectasis**) can occur if surfactant is insufficient or if the alveoli are not inflated. No gas exchange takes place in atelectatic alveoli.

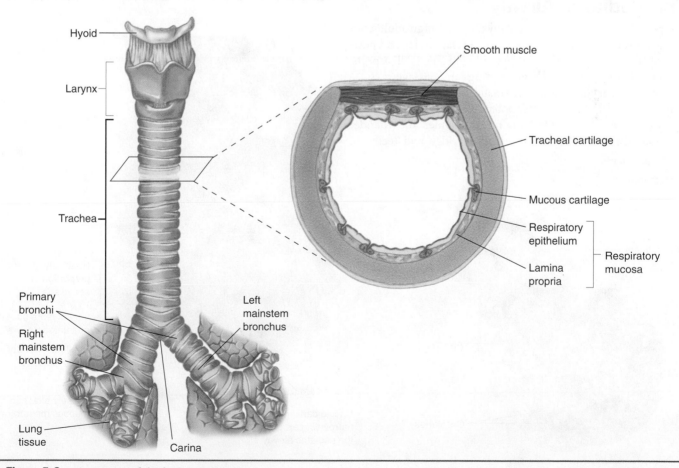

● **Figure 5-3**   Anatomy of the lower airway.

CONTENT REVIEW
▶ Lower Airway Components
  • Trachea
  • Bronchi
  • Alveoli
  • Lung parenchyma
  • Pleura

The Lung Parenchyma

The alveoli are the terminal ends of the respiratory tree and the functional units of the lungs. As such, they are the core of the lung **parenchyma**. The lung parenchyma is arranged in two pulmonary lobules that form the anatomic division of the lungs. These lobules are further organized into lobes. The right lung has three lobes, the upper lobe, the middle lobe, and the lower lobe. The left lung, which shares thoracic space with the heart, has only two lobes, the upper lobe and the lower lobe.

The Pleura

Membranous connective tissue, called **pleura**, covers the lungs. The pleura consists of two layers, visceral and parietal. The visceral pleura envelops the lungs and does not contain nerve fibers. In contrast, the parietal pleura lines the thoracic cavity and does contain nerve fibers. The potential space between these two layers, called the pleural space, usually holds a small amount of fluid that reduces friction between the pleural layers during respiration. Occasionally, the pleura can become inflamed, causing significant pain with respiration. This condition, called *pleurisy*, is a common cause of chest pain, particularly in cigarette smokers.

The Pediatric Airway

The pediatric airway is fundamentally the same as an adult's, but you will need to know the differences in relative size and position of some components. The airway is smaller in all aspects, particularly the diameters of the openings and passageways.

In the pharynx, the jaw is smaller and the tongue relatively larger, resulting in greater potential airway encroachment (Figure 5-5 ●). The epiglottis is much floppier and rounder ("omega" shaped). The dental (alveolar) ridge and teeth are softer and more fragile than an adult's and potentially more subject to damage from airway maneuvers.

The larynx lies more superior and anterior in children and is funnel-shaped because the cricoid cartilage is undeveloped. Before the age of 10, the cricoid cartilage is the narrowest part of the airway. Most significantly, even a small foreign body or a limited degree of swelling in the pediatric airway can be life threatening. Because of this, young children tend to suffer more problems related to the trachea than do older children. A common example is croup (laryngotracheobronchitis), a viral infection that causes the soft tissues below the glottis to swell. This can reduce the diameter of the airway, potentially causing serious problems.

The ribs and the cartilage of the pediatric thoracic cage are softer and more pliable. This lack of rigidity lessens the thoracic wall's and accessory muscles' ability to assist lung expansion during inspiration. As a result, infants and children tend to rely more on their diaphragms for breathing. Always pay close attention to these differences when treating pediatric patients, especially those with respiratory complaints.

PHYSIOLOGY OF THE RESPIRATORY SYSTEM

Just as successful airway management requires a firm understanding of airway anatomy, a good outcome for these patients requires a working knowledge of the mechanics of oxygenation and ventilation. Your knowledge of normal respiratory

Smooth muscle

Elastin fibers

Alveoli

Capillaries

● **Figure 5-4**   Anatomy of the alveoli.

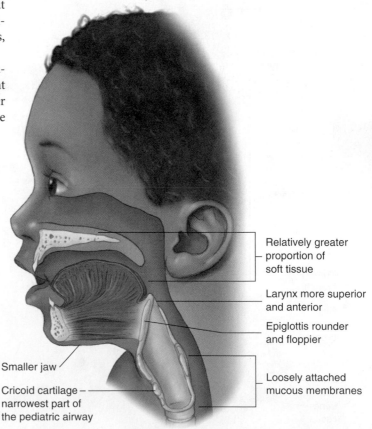

Relatively greater proportion of soft tissue

Larynx more superior and anterior

Epiglottis rounder and floppier

Loosely attached mucous membranes

Smaller jaw

Cricoid cartilage – narrowest part of the pediatric airway

● **Figure 5-5**   Anatomy of the pediatric airway.

physiology will lay the groundwork for your comprehension of important pathophysiology and will help you to determine which actions will ensure optimal patient care.

Respiration and Ventilation

Respiration, as noted earlier, is the exchange of gases between a living organism and its environment. Pulmonary, or external, respiration occurs in the lungs when the respiratory gases are exchanged between the alveoli and the red blood cells in the pulmonary capillaries through the capillary membranes (Figure 5-6 ●). Cellular, or internal, respiration, however, occurs in the peripheral capillaries. It is the exchange of the respiratory gases between the red blood cells and the various body tissues. Cellular respiration in the peripheral tissue produces carbon dioxide (CO_2). The blood picks up this waste product in the capillaries and transports it as bicarbonate ions through the venous system to the lungs. While respiration describes the process of gas exchange in the lungs and peripheral tissues, **ventilation** is the mechanical process that moves air into and out of the lungs. Ventilation is necessary for respiration to occur.

The Respiratory Cycle

Nothing within the lung parenchyma makes it contract or expand. Pulmonary ventilation, therefore, depends on changes in pressure within the thoracic cavity. These changes occur in a respiratory cycle involving coordinated interaction among the respiratory system, the central nervous system, and the musculoskeletal system.

The thoracic cavity is a closed space, opening to the external environment only through the trachea. The diaphragm separates the thoracic cavity from the abdomen. When the diaphragm contracts, it draws downward, away from the thoracic cavity, thus enlarging it. Likewise, when the muscles between the ribs, or intercostal muscles, contract, they draw the rib cage upward and outward, away from the thoracic cavity, further increasing its volume.

The respiratory cycle begins when the lungs have achieved a normal expiration and the pressure inside the thoracic cavity equals the atmospheric pressure. At this point, respiratory centers in the brain communicate with the diaphragm by way of the phrenic nerve, signaling it to contract and thus initiate the respiratory cycle. As the size of the thorax increases in relation to the volume of air it holds, pressure within the thorax decreases, becoming lower than atmospheric pressure. This negative intrathoracic pressure invites air into the thorax through the airway. Because the visceral and parietal pleura remain in contact with each other under normal circumstances, the highly elastic lungs immediately assume the thoracic cavity's internal contour. These combined factors move air into the lungs (inspiration). At the same time, the alveoli inflate with the lungs. They become thinner as they expand, allowing oxygen and carbon dioxide to diffuse across their membranes.

When the pressure in the thoracic cavity again reaches that of the atmosphere, the alveoli are maximally inflated. Pulmonary expansion stimulates microscopic stretch receptors in the bronchi and bronchioles. These receptors signal the respiratory center by way of the vagus nerve to inhibit inspiration, and the air influx stops. This process is primarily protective, as it prevents overinflation of the lungs.

At the end of inspiration, the respiratory muscles now relax, thus decreasing the size of the chest cavity, and in turn increasing the intrathoracic pressure. The naturally elastic lungs recoil, forcing air out through the airway (expiration) until intrathoracic and atmospheric pressure are equal once again. Normal expiration is a passive process, while inspiration is an active process, using energy. In respiratory inadequacy, when this process fails to provide satisfactory gas exchange, the patient may use accessory respiratory muscles such as the strap muscles of his neck and his abdominal muscles to augment his efforts to expand the thoracic cavity.

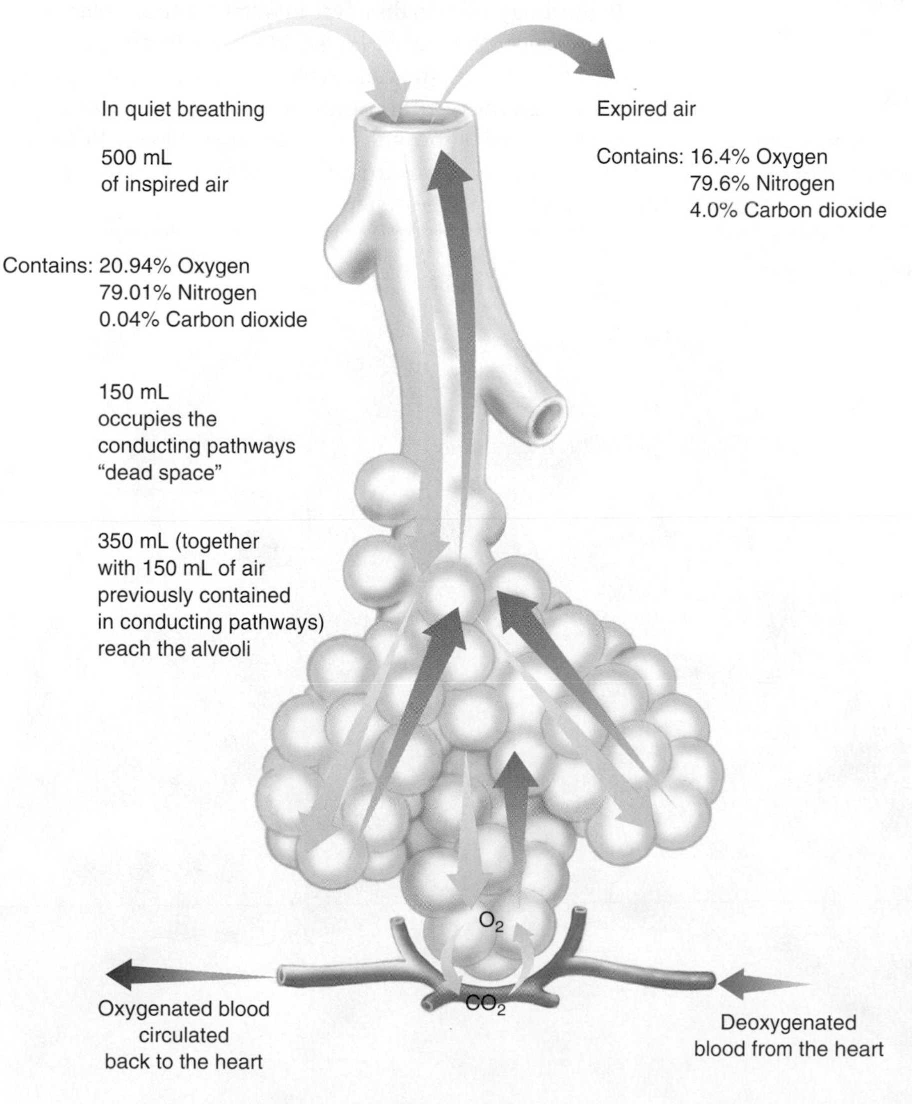

In quiet breathing

500 mL
of inspired air

Contains: 20.94% Oxygen
79.01% Nitrogen
0.04% Carbon dioxide

150 mL
occupies the
conducting pathways
"dead space"

350 mL (together
with 150 mL of air
previously contained
in conducting pathways)
reach the alveoli

Expired air

Contains: 16.4% Oxygen
79.6% Nitrogen
4.0% Carbon dioxide

O_2

CO_2

Oxygenated blood
circulated
back to the heart

Deoxygenated
blood from the heart

● **Figure 5-6** Diffusion of gases across an alveolar membrane.

Pulmonary Circulation

Respiration also requires an intact circulatory system. In fact, during each cardiac cycle, the heart pumps as much blood to the lungs as it pumps to the peripheral tissues. In the capillaries, these cells take oxygen from red blood cells coming from the arterial system and give up carbon dioxide to blood returning to the venous system. The venous system carries this deoxygenated blood to the right side of the heart, and the right ventricle pumps it into the pulmonary artery (Figure 5-7 ●). The pulmonary artery immediately branches into the right and the left pulmonary arteries, each supplying its respective lung. In turn, both branches quickly fan into smaller arteries that end in the pulmonary capillaries. These capillaries are spread over the surfaces of the alveoli, where the red blood cells exchange carbon dioxide for oxygen. The pulmonary capillaries recombine into larger veins, eventually terminating in the pulmonary vein. The pulmonary vein empties the oxygenated blood into the left atrium of the heart. Finally, the heart transports the oxygenated blood through the left ventricle and into the systemic arterial system via the aorta and its tributaries.

The lungs themselves receive little of their blood supply from the pulmonary arteries or veins. Instead, bronchial arteries that branch from the aorta supply most of their blood. Bronchial veins return this blood from the lungs to the superior vena cava.

Measuring Oxygen and Carbon Dioxide Levels

You can determine the amount of oxygen and carbon dioxide in the blood by measuring their partial pressures. **Partial pressure** is the pressure exerted by each component of a gas mixture. In other words, the partial pressure of a gas is its percentage of the mixture's total pressure. The partial pressure of oxygen at normal atmospheric pressure, for example, is the percentage of oxygen in atmospheric air (21 percent) multiplied by the atmospheric pressure at sea level (760 torr, or 14.7 pounds per square inch):

$$0.21 \times 760 \text{ torr} = 159.6 \text{ torr}$$

(Note that torr and mmHg are the same measures of pressure.) Earth's atmosphere consists of four major respiratory gases: nitrogen (N_2), oxygen (O_2), carbon dioxide (CO_2), and water (H_2O). Although nitrogen is metabolically inert, it is needed to inflate gas-filled body cavities such as the chest. Table 5–1 lists these four respiratory gases' partial pressures and concentrations in the environment and in the alveoli.

Since alveolar partial pressure and arterial partial pressure are essentially the same in the normal lung, normal arterial partial pressures for oxygen and carbon dioxide may be expressed:

Oxygen (PaO_2) = 100 torr (average = 80–100)

Carbon dioxide ($PaCO_2$) = 40 torr (average = 35–45)

Alveolar partial pressures are abbreviated **PA** (PAO_2 and $PACO_2$), whereas arterial partial pressures are abbreviated **Pa** (PaO_2 and $PaCO_2$). Because these values are usually the same, however, they typically appear as the shortened notations PO_2 and PCO_2.

Diffusion

Diffusion is the movement of a gas from an area of higher concentration (partial pressure) to an area of lower concentration, attempting to reach equilibrium. Diffusion transfers gases between the lungs and the blood and between the blood and the peripheral tissues. The rate of diffusion of a gas across the pulmonary membranes depends on the gas's solubility in water. For example, carbon dioxide is 21 times more soluble in water than oxygen and readily crosses the pulmonary capillary membranes. In the peripheral tissues, the gradient (direction of diffusion) for CO_2 is from the tissue, where its concentration is high, to the capillary blood, where its concentration is low.

In the lungs, oxygen dissolves in water at the alveolar membrane and leaves the area of higher PO_2, the alveoli, and enters the area of lower PO_2, the venous blood in the pulmonary capillaries. Concurrently, carbon dioxide leaves the area of higher PCO_2, the arterial blood, and enters the area of lower PCO_2, the alveoli. The blood returns from the pulmonary vein to the heart and then moves into the systemic circulation.

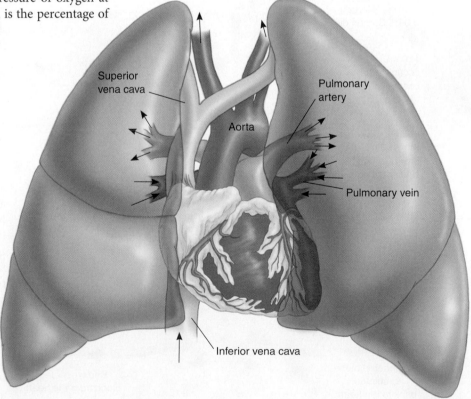

Superior vena cava

Aorta

Pulmonary artery

Pulmonary vein

Inferior vena cava

● **Figure 5-7**   Pulmonary circulation.

TABLE 5-1 | Partial Pressures and Concentrations of Gases

	Partial Pressure		Concentration	
	Atmospheric	Alveolar	Atmospheric	Alveolar
Nitrogen	597.0 torr	569.0 torr	78.62%	74.9%
Oxygen	159.0 torr	104.0 torr	20.84%	13.7%
Carbon dioxide	0.3 torr	40.0 torr	0.04%	5.2%
Water	3.7 torr	47.0 torr	0.50%	6.2%
TOTAL	760.0 torr	760.0 torr	100.00%	100.0%

pulmonary conditions such as emphysema, asthma, or pneumothorax

- Decreased diffusion across the pulmonary membrane when diffusion distance increases or the pulmonary membrane changes—for example, when fluid enters the space between the alveolar membrane and the pulmonary capillary membrane, as in pneumonia, chronic obstructive pulmonary disease (COPD), or pulmonary edema (swelling)

Oxygen Concentration in the Blood

Oxygen diffuses into the blood plasma, where most of it combines with hemoglobin and is measured as oxygen saturation (SaO_2). The remainder is dissolved in the blood and is measured as the PaO_2. Hemoglobin approaches 100 percent saturation when the PaO_2 of dissolved oxygen reaches 90 to 100 torr. Each gram of saturated hemoglobin carries 1.34 milliliters of oxygen. Oxygen saturation is the ratio of the blood's actual oxygen content to its total oxygen-carrying capacity:

$$\text{Oxygen saturation} = O_2 \text{ content}/O_2 \text{ capacity} \times 100(\%)$$

The hemoglobin molecule carries the vast majority of oxygen in the blood (approximately 97 percent). Very little oxygen dissolves in the plasma. Since partial pressure measurements detect only the amount of oxygen dissolved in the plasma and do not always reflect the total oxygen saturation of hemoglobin, they can be misleading. For example, a patient who has suffered carbon monoxide poisoning cannot transport enough oxygen to the essential tissues since carbon monoxide displaces oxygen from the hemoglobin molecule. But an arterial blood gas sample might reveal a normal or high PaO_2. This would indicate that adequate oxygen was reaching the blood. In fact, however, an inadequate amount of hemoglobin would be available to transport the oxygen to the peripheral tissues, thus resulting in peripheral hypoxia.

The oxygen content of the arterial blood can be calculated using the following standardized equation:

$$CaO_2 = (SaO_2 \times Hgb \times 1.34) + (0.003 \times PaO_2)$$

where CaO_2 is the **arterial oxygen concentration** (mL/dL), SaO_2 is **hemoglobin oxygen saturation** (%), **Hgb** indicates the amount of **hemoglobin** present (g/dL), 1.34 is a constant and represents the amount of oxygen bound to one gram of hemoglobin at one atmosphere pressure, 0.003 is the amount of oxygen dissolved in plasma (mL/g Hgb), and PaO_2 is the partial pressure of oxygen dissolved in the plasma (mmHg). Normal CaO_2 is 17–24 mL/dL.

Several factors can affect oxygen concentrations in the blood:

- Decreased hemoglobin concentration (anemia, hemorrhage)
- Inadequate alveolar ventilation due to low inspired-oxygen concentration, respiratory muscle paralysis, and

- Ventilation/perfusion mismatch occurs when a portion of the alveoli collapses, as in atelectasis. Blood travels past these collapsed alveoli without oxygenation (shunting), without carbon dioxide transfer, and without oxygen uptake. This can result from **hypoventilation**, which can occur secondary to pain or inability to inspire (traumatic asphyxia). When the lung collapses, as in **pneumothorax**, **hemothorax**, or a combination of the two, less surface area is available for gas exchange. Alternately, a ventilation/perfusion mismatch can occur when blood is prevented from reaching the alveolar capillary membranes but alveolar ventilation remains adequate. This occurs when a blood clot travels to or is formed in the pulmonary arterial system, a condition known as pulmonary thromboembolism.

You can correct oxygen derangements by increasing ventilation, administering supplemental oxygen, using intermittent positive-pressure ventilation (IPPV), or administering medications to correct underlying problems such as pulmonary edema, asthma, or **pulmonary embolism**. The emergency being treated determines the desired fractional concentration of oxygen (**FiO₂**) to be delivered. It is crucial to remember not to withhold oxygen from any patient whose clinical condition indicates its need.

Carbon Dioxide Concentrations in the Blood

The blood transports carbon dioxide mainly in the form of bicarbonate ion (HCO_3^-). It carries approximately 70 percent as bicarbonate and approximately 23 percent combined with **hemoglobin**. Less than 7 percent is dissolved in the plasma. Unlike oxygen, when carbon dioxide binds with hemoglobin, it binds to an amino acid and not to the iron-containing heme binding site where oxygen binds (Figure 5-8 ●). Several factors influence carbon dioxide's concentration in the blood, including increased CO_2 production and/or decreased CO_2 elimination:

- Hyperventilation lowers CO_2 levels and can be the result of an increased respiratory rate or deeper respiration, both of which increase the **minute volume**. (We discuss minute volume more completely later in this chapter.)

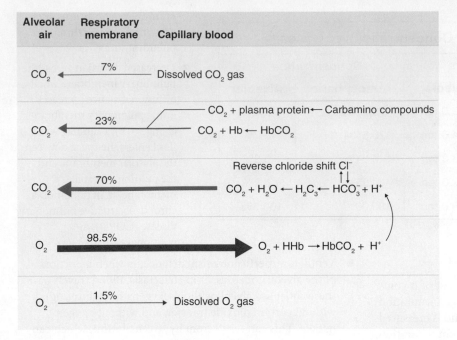

● **Figure 5-8** Respiratory gas exchange and transport at the alveolar/capillary membrane.

frequency decreases the respiratory rate. The medulla is connected to the respiratory muscles primarily via the vagus nerve. This is an involuntary pathway. If the medulla fails to initiate respiration, an additional control center in the pons, called the *apneustic center,* assumes respiratory control to ensure the continuation of respirations. A third center, the *pneumotaxic center,* also in the pons, controls expiration (Figure 5-9 ●).

Stretch Receptors   During inspiration, the lungs become distended, activating stretch receptors. As the degree of stretch increases, these receptors fire more frequently. The impulses they send to the brainstem inhibit the medullary cells, decreasing the inspiratory stimulus. Thus, the respiratory muscles relax, allowing the elastic lungs to recoil and expel air from the body. As the stretch decreases, the stretch receptors stop firing. This process, called the *Hering-Breuer reflex,* prevents overexpansion of the lungs.

Chemoreceptors   Other involuntary respiration controls include central chemical receptors in the medulla and peripheral chemoreceptors in the carotid bodies and in the arch of the aorta. These chemoreceptors are stimulated by decreased PaO_2, increased $PaCO_2$, and decreased pH. (The pH scale expresses the degree of acidity or alkalinity. A lower pH indicates greater acidity; a higher pH indicates greater alkalinity; Chapter 1 discusses pH in greater detail.) Cerebrospinal fluid (CSF) pH is the primary control of respiratory center stimulation. The CSF pH responds very quickly to changes in arterial PCO_2. Any increase in PCO_2 will decrease CSF pH, which will in turn stimulate the central chemoreceptors to increase respiration. Conversely, low $PaCO_2$ levels will raise CSF pH, in turn decreasing chemoreceptor stimulation and slowing respiratory activity. Because $PaCO_2$ is inversely related to CSF pH, $PaCO_2$ is seen as the normal neuroregulatory control of respirations. Additionally, any increase in the arterial PCO_2 stimulates the peripheral chemoreceptors to signal the brainstem to increase respiration, thus speeding CO_2 elimination from the body.

Hypoxic Drive   The body also constantly monitors the PaO_2 and the pH. In fact, **hypoxemia** (decreased partial pressure of oxygen in the blood) is a profound stimulus of respiration in a normal individual. People with chronic respiratory disease such as emphysema and chronic bronchitis tend to retain CO_2 and, therefore, have a chronically elevated $PaCO_2$. Chemoreceptors in the periphery eventually become accustomed to this chronic condition, and the central nervous system stops using $PaCO_2$ to regulate respiration. This activates a default mechanism called **hypoxic drive**, which increases respiratory stimulation when PaO_2 falls and inhibits respiratory stimulation when PaO_2 climbs. High-volume oxygen administration to people with this condition can cause respiratory arrest. Because high-concentration oxygen can quickly double or even triple the PaO_2, peripheral chemoreceptors stop stimulating the respiratory centers, causing **apnea** (cessation

- Causes of increased CO_2 production include:
  - Fever
  - Muscle exertion
  - Shivering
  - Metabolic processes resulting in the formation of metabolic acids.
- Decreased CO_2 elimination (increased CO_2 levels in the blood) results from decreased alveolar ventilation. Common causes include hypoventilation due to:
  - Respiratory depression by drugs
  - Airway obstruction
  - Impairment of the respiratory muscles
  - Obstructive diseases such as asthma and emphysema.

Increased CO_2 levels (**hypercarbia**) are usually treated by increasing the rate and/or volume of ventilation and by correcting the underlying cause.

Regulation of Respiration

Voluntary and Involuntary Respiratory Controls

The number of times a person breathes in 1 minute, the **respiratory rate**, is unique in that both voluntary and involuntary nervous system mechanisms control it. We do not ordinarily need to make a conscious effort to breathe; our brains automatically regulate this function. However, we can voluntarily override our involuntary respirations until physical and chemical mechanisms signal the nervous system's respiratory centers to provide involuntary impulses and correct any breathing irregularities.

Nervous Impulses from the Respiratory Center   The main respiratory center lies in the *medulla,* located in the brainstem. Various neurons within the medulla initiate impulses that result in respiration. A rise in the frequency of these impulses increases the respiratory rate. Conversely, a decrease in their

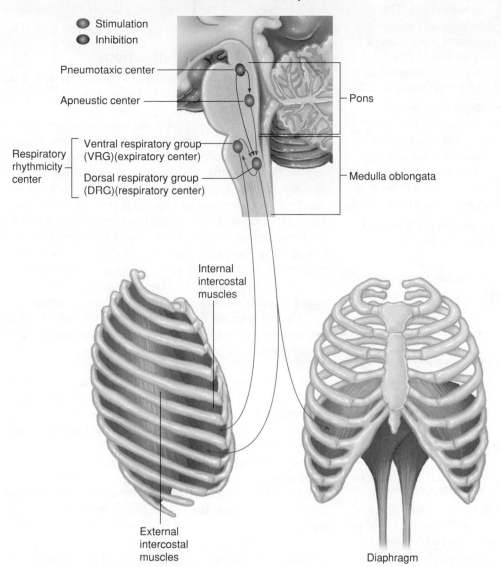

Nervous Control & Respiration

Stimulation
Inhibition

Pneumotaxic center

Apneustic center

Pons

Respiratory rhythmicity center
- Ventral respiratory group (VRG)(expiratory center)
- Dorsal respiratory group (DRG)(respiratory center)

Medulla oblongata

Internal intercostal muscles

External intercostal muscles

Diaphragm

● **Figure 5-9**   Nervous control of respiration.

This knowledge will enable you to adapt your mechanical ventilation techniques to your patient's size, lung compliance, need for hyperventilation, or other individual requirements. It is especially crucial in situations that call for advanced mechanical ventilator skills. Respiratory capacities and measurements with which you must be familiar include:

- **Total lung capacity (TLC).** **Total lung capacity** is the maximum lung capacity—the total amount of air contained in the lung at the end of maximal inspiration. In the average adult male, this volume is approximately 6 liters.

- **Tidal volume (V_T).** The **tidal volume** is the average volume of gas inhaled or exhaled in one respiratory cycle. In the adult male this is approximately 500 mL (5 to 7 cc/kg).

- **Dead space volume (V_D).** The dead space volume is the amount of gas in the tidal volume that remains in air passageways unavailable for gas exchange. It is approximately 150 mL in the adult male. Anatomic dead space includes the trachea and bronchi. Obstructions or diseases such as chronic obstructive pulmonary disease or atelectasis can cause physiologic dead space.

- **Alveolar volume (V_A).** The alveolar volume is the amount of gas in the tidal volume that reaches the alveoli for gas exchange. It is the difference between tidal volume and dead-space volume (approximately 350 mL in the adult male):

$$V_A = V_T - V_D$$

- **Minute volume (V_{min}).** The minute volume is the amount of gas moved in and out of the respiratory tract in 1 minute:

$$V_{min} = V_T \times \text{respiratory rate}$$

- **Alveolar minute volume ($V_{A\text{-}min}$).** The alveolar minute volume is the amount of gas that reaches the alveoli for gas exchange in 1 minute:

$$V_{A\text{-}min} = (V_T - V_D) \times \text{respiratory rate or}$$
$$V_{A\text{-}min} = V_A \times \text{respiratory rate}$$

of breathing). Although this is a potential threat, it is never appropriate to withhold oxygen from a patient for whom oxygen therapy is indicated. However, you must be prepared to assist with ventilations if the patient's respiratory effort becomes inadequate.

Measures of Respiratory Function

The respiratory rate is the number of respiratory cycles per minute, normally 12 to 20 breaths per minute in adults, 18 to 24 in children, and 40 to 60 in infants. Several factors affect respiratory rate:

- *Fever*—increases rate
- *Emotion*—increases rate
- *Pain*—increases rate
- *Hypoxia* (inadequate tissue oxygenation)—increases rate
- *Acidosis*—increases rate
- *Stimulant drugs*—increase rate
- *Depressant drugs*—decrease rate
- *Sleep*—decreases rate

Paramedics must fully understand ventilatory mechanics and capacities for the average adult's respiratory system.

CONTENT REVIEW

▶ Causes of Airway
Obstruction

• Tongue
• Foreign bodies
• Trauma
• Laryngeal spasm and
  edema
• Aspiration

▶ Blockage of the airway
is an immediate threat to
the patient's life and a true
emergency.

• *Inspiratory reserve volume (IRV).* The inspiratory reserve volume is the amount of air that can be maximally inhaled after a normal inspiration.

• *Expiratory reserve volume (ERV).* The expiratory reserve volume is the amount of air that can be maximally exhaled after a normal expiration.

• *Residual volume (RV).* The residual volume is the amount of air remaining in the lungs at the end of maximal expiration.

• *Functional residual capacity (FRC).* The functional residual capacity is the volume of gas that remains in the lungs at the end of normal expiration:

$$FRC = ERV + RV$$

• *Forced expiratory volume (FEV).* The forced expiratory volume is the amount of air that can be maximally expired after maximum inspiration.

RESPIRATORY PROBLEMS

Respiratory emergencies can pose an immediate life threat to the patient. You must calmly and quickly assess the severity of his illness or injury while considering the potential causes of and treatment for his respiratory distress. Often, he will give you little help, either because of anxiety or difficulty speaking. His respiratory difficulty may be due to airway obstruction, injury to upper or lower airway structures, inadequate ventilation caused by worsening of an underlying lung disease and fatigue, or central nervous system problems that threaten the airway or respiratory effort.

Airway Obstruction

Blockage of the airway is an immediate threat to the patient's life and a true emergency. **Upper airway obstruction** may be defined as an interference with air movement through the upper airway.

Airway obstruction may be either partial or complete. Partial obstruction allows either adequate or poor air exchange. Patients with adequate air exchange can cough effectively; those with poor air exchange cannot. They often emit a high-pitched noise while inhaling (stridor), and their skin may have a bluish appearance (cyanosis). They also may have increased breathing difficulty, which can manifest as choking, gagging dyspnea, or dysphonia (difficulty speaking). When you cannot feel or hear airflow from the nose and mouth, or when the patient cannot speak (aphonia), breathe, or cough, his airway is completely obstructed. He will quickly become unconscious and die if you

do not relieve the obstruction. In the absence of breathing, difficulty ventilating the patient will indicate complete airway obstruction.

Causes of Airway Obstruction

The tongue, foreign bodies, teeth, spasm or edema, vomitus, and blood can all obstruct the upper airway.

The Tongue The tongue is the most common cause of airway obstruction (Figure 5-10 ●). Normally, the submandibular muscles directly support the tongue and indirectly support the epiglottis. However, without sufficient muscle tone, the relaxed tongue falls back against the posterior pharynx, thus occluding the airway. This may produce snoring respiratory noises. At the same time, the epiglottis also may block the airway at the larynx. This at least diminishes airflow into the respiratory system, and the patient's breathing efforts may inadvertently suck the base of his tongue into an obstructing position. The patient's tongue can block his airway whether he is lateral, supine, or prone; however, the blockage depends on the position of the patient's head and jaw, so simple airway maneuvers such as the jaw-thrust can usually open his airway.

Foreign Bodies Large, poorly chewed pieces of food can obstruct the upper airway by becoming lodged in the hypopharynx. These cases often involve alcohol consumption and denture dislodgement. Because they frequently occur in restaurants and are mistaken for heart attacks, they are commonly called "café coronaries." The patient may clutch his neck between the thumb and fingers, a universal distress signal. Children, especially toddlers, often aspirate foreign objects, as they have the tendency to put objects into their mouths.

Trauma In trauma, particularly when the patient is unresponsive, loose teeth, facial bone fractures, and avulsed or swollen tissue may obstruct the airway. Secretions such as blood, saliva, and vomitus may compromise the airway and risk aspiration. Additionally, penetrating or blunt trauma may obstruct the airway by fracturing or displacing the larynx, allowing the vocal cords to collapse into the tracheal **lumen** (channel).

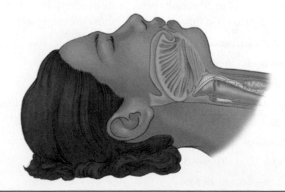

● **Figure 5-10** The tongue as airway obstruction. Note that the tongue has fallen backward, totally obstructing the airway.

Laryngeal Spasm and Edema Since the glottis is the narrowest part of an adult's airway, edema (swelling) or spasm (spasmotic closure) of the vocal cords is potentially lethal. Even moderate edema can severely obstruct airflow and cause asphyxia (the inability to move air into and out of the respiratory system). Just beneath the mucous membrane that covers the vocal cords is a layer of loose tissue where blood or other fluids can accumulate. This tissue may swell following injury, and the swelling will be slow to subside. Causes of laryngeal spasm and edema include trauma, anaphylaxis, epiglottitis, and inhalation of superheated air, smoke, or toxic substances. The most common cause of spasm is overly aggressive intubation. In addition, it often occurs immediately on **extubation**, especially when the patient is semiconscious. Some authors propose that laryngeal spasm can sometimes be partially overcome by strengthening ventilatory effort, forceful upward pull of the jaw, or the use of muscle relaxants, although the success of these maneuvers is quite variable.

Aspiration Vomitus is the most commonly aspirated material. Patients most at risk for this are those who are so obtunded (drowsy) that they cannot adequately protect their airways. This can occur with hypoxia, central nervous system toxins, or brain injury, among other causes. In addition to obstructing the airway, aspiration's other effects also significantly increase patient mortality. Vomitus consists of food particles, protein-dissolving enzymes, hydrochloric acid, and gastrointestinal bacteria that have been regurgitated from the stomach into the hypopharynx and oropharynx. If this mixture enters the lungs, it can result in increased interstitial fluid and pulmonary edema. The consequent marked increase in alveolar/capillary distance seriously impairs gas exchange, thus causing hypoxemia and hypercarbia. Aspirated materials can also severely damage the delicate bronchiolar tissue and alveoli. Gastrointestinal bacteria can produce overwhelming infections. These complications occur in 50 to 80 percent of patients who aspirate foreign matter.

Inadequate Ventilation

Insufficient minute volume respirations can compromise adequate oxygen intake and carbon dioxide removal. Additionally, oxygenation may be insufficient when conditions increase metabolic oxygen demand or decrease available oxygen. A reduction of either the rate or the volume of inhalation leads to a reduction in minute volume. In some cases, the respiratory rate may be rapid but so shallow that little air exchange takes place. Among the causes of such decreased ventilation are depressed respiratory function as from impairment of respiratory muscles or nervous system, bronchospasm from intrinsic disease, fractured ribs, pneumothorax, hemothorax, drug overdose, renal failure, spinal or brainstem injury, or head injury. In some conditions, such as sepsis, the body's metabolic demand for oxygen can exceed the patient's ability to supply it. Additionally, the environment may contain a decreased amount of oxygen, as in high-altitude conditions or a house fire, which also produces toxic gases such as cyanide and carbon monoxide. These situations of inadequate ventilation can lead to hypercarbia and hypoxia.

RESPIRATORY SYSTEM ASSESSMENT

Vigilance is the key to airway management in every patient. The trauma patient whose airway and breathing initially looked fine on exam may become symptomatic with the pneumothorax that was not initially evident. The asthma patient who initially responded to nebulizer treatment may have a sudden bronchospasm and worsen acutely. Minute-by-minute reassessment of the adequacy of every patient's airway and breathing is essential. The changes may be subtle increases in rate, worsening or onset of irregularity, or increased difficulty speaking. Assessment of the respiratory system begins with the primary assessment and should continue through the secondary assessment and the reassessment. (Volume 3 discusses the steps of patient assessment in detail.)

Primary Assessment

The purpose of the primary assessment is to identify any immediate threats to the patient's life, specifically **a**irway, **b**reathing, and **c**irculation problems (**ABCs**). For patients in cardiac arrest, compressions come before airway and breathing (CAB). However, as discussed in the introduction, airway assessment, management, and ventilation should be considered and can occur together.

First, assess the airway to ensure that it is patent. Snoring or gurgling may indicate potential airway problems. Next, determine the adequacy of breathing. If the patient is comfortable, with a normal respiratory rate, alert, and speaking without difficulty, you may generally assume that his airway is patent and breathing is adequate.

Patients with altered mental status warrant further evaluation. Feel for air movement with your hand or cheek (Figure 5-11 ●). Look for the chest to rise and fall normally with each respiratory cycle (Figure 5-12 ●). Listen for air movement and equal bilateral breath sounds (Figure 5-13 ●). The absence of breath sounds on one side may indicate a pneumothorax or hemothorax in the trauma patient. In an adult patient, the respiratory rate generally ranges between 12 and 20 breaths per minute. Breathing should be spontaneous, effortless, and regular. Irregular breathing suggests a significant problem and usually requires ventilatory support. Observe the chest wall for any asymmetrical movement. This condition, known as **paradoxical breathing**, may suggest a **flail chest**. Patients showing increased respiratory effort; insisting on upright, sniffing, or semi-Fowler's positioning; or refusing to lie supine should be considered to be in significant respiratory distress.

If the patient is not breathing, or if you suspect airway problems, open the airway using the head-tilt/chin-lift or jaw-thrust maneuver, as described later in this chapter. If trauma is possible, use the jaw-thrust maneuver while stabilizing the cervical spine in the neutral position. Once the airway is open, reevaluate the breathing status. If breathing is adequate, provide supplemental oxygen and assess circulation. Consider the use of airway adjuncts, as discussed later. If breathing is inadequate or absent, begin artificial ventilation (Figure 5-14 ●). When assisting a patient's breathing with a ventilatory device

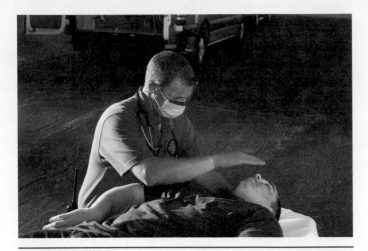

● **Figure 5-11**   Feel.

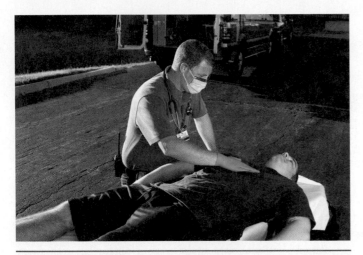

● **Figure 5-12**   Look.

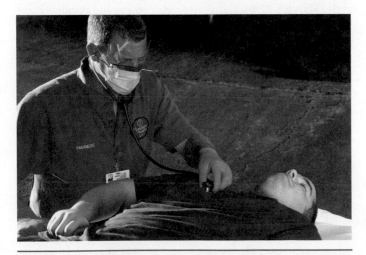

● **Figure 5-13**   Listen.

(bag-valve mask or other positive-pressure device), or after placing an airway adjunct (nasopharyngeal airway or oropharyngeal airway), or endotracheally intubating, monitor the chest's rise and fall to determine correct usage and placement.

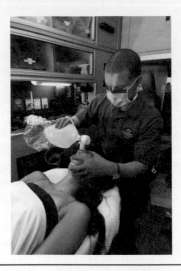

● **Figure 5-14**   Bag-valve-mask ventilation.

(We will discuss these ventilatory devices and mechanical airways in detail later in this chapter.)

Secondary Assessment

After you complete the primary assessment and correct any immediate life threats, conduct the secondary assessment while continuously monitoring the patient's airway, breathing, and circulation.

History

The time when the patient and his family noted the onset of symptoms is important information, as is whether the acute event occurred suddenly or gradually. Identifying possible triggers such as allergens or heat also can help the patient avoid them in the future. Additionally, the symptoms' course of development since onset will help direct diagnosis and treatment. Have they been progressively worsening, recurrent, or continuous? Associated symptoms will further help to assess the cause of the patient's problem. Has he had fever or chills, productive cough, chest pain, nausea or vomiting, or diaphoresis? Does he think his voice sounds normal?

The patient's past medical history will put his present complaints into perspective and help to identify the risk factors for a variety of likely diagnoses. Determine whether the present episode is similar to any past episodes of shortness of breath, what medical evaluations have been done, and what they have found. Has the patient ever been admitted to the hospital for his complaints? Has he ever been intubated?

The recent history leading to the onset of symptoms is also important. Did the patient run out of medication? Has he been noncompliant with (not taken) his medications? Did he drink too much fluid or alcohol? Did he have a seizure or vomit? Did he eat something that might induce an allergy? Did he receive any trauma? If an injury is involved, evaluate the mechanism of injury. Keep in mind that blunt trauma to the neck may have injured the larynx. Anything that makes the patient's condition better (ameliorates) or worse (exacerbates, aggravates) is also significant.

Physical Examination

Your physical examination of a patient with respiratory problems should continue the evaluation of his airway, breathing, and circulation begun during your primary assessment. Now you will use the physical examination techniques of inspection, auscultation, and palpation to evaluate his injury or illness in more detail and determine your plan of action. (Volume 2, Chapter 2, explains these techniques in detail.)

Inspection Begin the physical assessment by inspecting the patient. Evaluate the adequacy of his breathing. Note any obvious signs of trauma. Always remember to assess the skin color as an indicator of oxygenation status. Early in respiratory compromise, the sympathetic nervous system will be stimulated to help offset the lack of oxygen. When this happens, the skin will often appear pale and diaphoretic. **Cyanosis** (bluish discoloration) is another sign of respiratory distress. When oxygen binds with the hemoglobin, the blood appears bright red. Deoxygenated hemoglobin, however, is blue and gives the skin a bluish tint. This is not a reliable indicator, however, since severe tissue hypoxia is possible without cyanosis. In fact, cyanosis is considered a late sign of respiratory compromise. When it does appear, it usually affects the lips, fingernails, and skin. A red skin rash, especially if accompanied by hives, may indicate an allergic reaction. A cherry-red skin discoloration may on rare occasions be associated with carbon monoxide poisoning, as can bullae (large blisters).

Observe the patient's position. Tripod positioning (seated, leaning forward, with one arm forward to stabilize the body) may indicate COPD or asthma exacerbation; orthopnea (increased difficulty breathing while lying down) may indicate congestive heart failure, or asthma.

Next, inspecting for **dyspnea**—an abnormality of breathing rate, pattern, or effort—is essential. Dyspnea may cause or be caused by **hypoxia**. Prolonged dyspnea without successful intervention can lead to **anoxia** (the absence or near-absence of oxygen), which without intervention is a premorbid (occurring just before death) event, as the brain can survive only 4 to 6 minutes in this state. Remember that all interventions are useless if you do not establish a patent airway.

Also observe for the following modified forms of respiration:

- *Coughing*—forceful exhalation of a large volume of air from the lungs. This performs a protective function in expelling foreign material from the lungs.
- *Sneezing*—sudden, forceful exhalation from the nose. It is usually caused by nasal irritation.
- *Hiccoughing (hiccups)*—sudden inspiration caused by spasmodic contraction of the diaphragm with spastic closure of the glottis. It serves no known physiologic purpose. It has, occasionally, been associated with acute myocardial infarctions on the inferior (diaphragmatic) surface of the heart.
- *Sighing*—slow, deep, involuntary inspiration followed by a prolonged expiration. It hyperinflates the lungs and reexpands atelectatic alveoli. This normally occurs about once a minute.
- *Grunting*—a forceful expiration that occurs against a partially closed epiglottis. It is usually an indication of respiratory distress.

Note any decrease or increase in the respiratory rate, one of the earliest indicators of respiratory distress. Also, look for use of the accessory respiratory muscles—intercostal, suprasternal, supraclavicular, and subcostal retractions—and the abdominal muscles to assist breathing. This indicates increased respiratory effort secondary to respiratory distress. In infants and children, nasal flaring and grunting indicate respiratory distress. COPD patients having difficulty breathing will purse their lips during exhalation. Monitor the patient's blood pressure, including any differences noted during expiration versus inspiration. Patients with severe chronic obstructive pulmonary disease may sustain a drop in blood pressure during inspiration. This drop is due to increased pressure within the thoracic cavity that impairs the ability of the ventricles to fill. Thus, decreased ventricular filling leads to decreased blood pressure. A drop in blood pressure of greater than 10 torr is termed **pulsus paradoxus** and may be indicative of severe obstructive lung disease.

Determine if the pattern of respirations is abnormal—deep or shallow in combination with a fast or slow rate. Some common abnormal respiratory patterns include:

- *Kussmaul's respirations*—deep, slow or rapid, gasping breathing, commonly found in diabetic ketoacidosis
- *Cheyne-Stokes respirations*—progressively deeper, faster breathing alternating gradually with shallow, slower breathing, indicating brainstem injury
- *Biot's respirations*—irregular pattern of rate and depth with sudden, periodic episodes of apnea, indicating increased intracranial pressure
- *Central neurogenic hyperventilation*—deep, rapid respirations, indicating increased intracranial pressure
- *Agonal respirations*—shallow, slow, or infrequent breathing, indicating brain anoxia

Finally, observing altered mentation may be key in determining if breathing is adequate or if significant hypoxia may be present. If the patient's mental status is not normal, you must determine his usual baseline mental status before you can make this assessment.

Auscultation Following inspection, listen at the mouth and nose for adequate air movement. Then listen to the chest with a stethoscope (auscultate) (Figure 5-15 ●). In a prehospital setting, you should auscultate the right and left apex (just beneath the clavicle), the right and left base (eighth or ninth intercostal space, midclavicular line), and the right and left lower thoracic back or right and left midaxillary line (fourth or fifth intercostal space, on the lateral aspect of the chest). When the patient's condition permits, you can monitor six locations on the posterior chest, three right and three left. The posterior surface is preferable because heart sounds do not interfere with auscultation at this location. However, since patients are usually supine

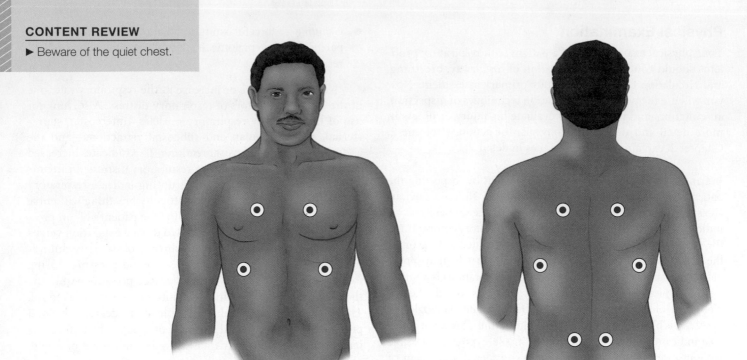

● **Figure 5-15** Positions for auscultating breath sounds.

during airway management, the anterior and lateral positions usually prove more accessible. Breath sounds should be equal bilaterally. Sounds that point to airflow compromise include:

● *Snoring*—results from partial obstruction of the upper airway by the tongue

● *Gurgling*—results from the accumulation of blood, vomitus, or other secretions in the upper airway

● *Stridor*—a harsh, high-pitched sound heard on inhalation, associated with laryngeal edema or constriction

● *Wheezing*—a musical, squeaking, or whistling sound heard in inspiration and/or expiration, associated with bronchiolar constriction

● *Quiet*—diminished or absent breath sounds are an ominous finding and indicate a serious problem with the airway, breathing, or both

Sounds that may indicate compromise of gas exchange include:

● *Crackles (rales)*—a fine, bubbling sound heard on inspiration, associated with fluid in the smaller bronchioles

● *Rhonchi*—a coarse, rattling noise heard on inspiration, associated with inflammation, mucus, or fluid in the bronchioles

When you assess the effectiveness of ventilatory support or the correct placement of an airway adjunct, remember that air movement into the epigastrium may sometimes mimic breath sounds. Thus, listening to the chest should be only one of several means that you use to assess air movement. Another method of checking correct placement of an airway adjunct is to auscultate over the epigastrium; it should be silent during ventilation.

When you provide ventilatory support, watch for signs of gastric distention. They suggest inadequate hyperextension of the neck, undue pressure generated by the ventilatory device, or improper placement of airway adjuncts.

Palpation Finally, palpate. First, using the back of your hand or your cheek, feel for air movement at the mouth and nose. (If an endotracheal tube is in place, you can check for air movement at the tube's adapter.) Next, palpate the chest for rise and fall. In addition, palpate the chest wall for tenderness, symmetry, abnormal motion, crepitus, and subcutaneous emphysema.

When ventilating with a bag-valve device, gauge airflow into the lungs by noting compliance. **Compliance** refers to the stiffness or flexibility of the lung tissue, and it is indicated by how easily air flows into the lungs. When compliance is good, airflow meets minimal resistance. When compliance is poor, ventilation is harder to achieve. Compliance is often poor in diseased lungs and in patients suffering from chest wall injuries or tension pneumothorax. If a patient shows poor compliance during ventilatory support, look for potential causes. Upper airway obstructions, which cause difficulty with mechanical ventilation, can mimic poor compliance. If ventilating the patient is initially easy but then becomes progressively more difficult, repeat the primary assessment and look for the development of a new problem, possibly related to the mechanical airway maneuvers. The following questions will aid this assessment:

● Is the airway open?

● Is the head properly positioned in extension (nontrauma patients)?

● Is the patient developing tension pneumothorax?

● Is the endotracheal tube occluded (a mucous plug or aspirated material)?

- Has the endotracheal tube been inadvertently pushed into the right or left mainstem bronchus?
- Has the endotracheal tube been displaced into the esophagus?
- Is the mechanical ventilatory equipment functioning properly?

Pulse rate abnormalities may also suggest respiratory compromise. Tachycardia (an abnormally fast pulse) usually accompanies hypoxemia in an adult, while bradycardia (an abnormally slow pulse) hints at anoxia with imminent cardiac arrest.

Noninvasive Respiratory Monitoring

Several available devices will help you measure the effectiveness of oxygenation and ventilation and maintain parameters at the appropriate levels. Those measurements used most commonly in prehospital care are pulse oximetry, CO-oximetry, and capnography. Peak expiratory flow testing can also be useful in the prehospital setting for some respiratory diseases, although it is not widely employed. These measurements use various devices and methodologies that, when used alone, have their limitations. However, when used together they can provide a fairly comprehensive and reliable picture of the patient's respiratory status. Table 5–2 details some of the advantages and limitations of pulse oximetry and capnography.

Pulse Oximetry

Pulse oximetry is widely used in prehospital emergency care and often referred to as the "fifth vital sign." A pulse oximeter measures hemoglobin oxygen saturation in peripheral tissues (Figure 5-16 ●). It is noninvasive (does not require entering the body), rapidly applied, and easy to operate. Pulse oximetry readings are generally accurate measures of arterial oxygen saturation and continually reflect any changes in peripheral oxygen delivery. In fact, pulse oximetry often detects problems with oxygenation faster than assessments of blood pressure, pulse, and respirations. When available, you should use it in virtually any situation to determine the patient's baseline value, to guide patient care, and to monitor the patient's responses to your interventions.

To determine peripheral oxygen saturation, you place a sensor probe over a peripheral capillary bed such as a fingertip, toe, or earlobe. In infants, you can wrap the sensor around the heel and secure it with tape. The sensor contains two light-emitting diodes and two sensors. One diode emits near-red light, a wavelength specific for oxygenated hemoglobin; the other emits infrared light, a wavelength specific for deoxygenated hemoglobin. Each hemoglobin state absorbs a certain amount of the emitted light, preventing it from reaching the corresponding sensor. Less light reaching the sensor means more of its type of hemoglobin is in the blood. The oximeter then calculates the ratio of the near-red and infrared light it has received to determine the **oxygen saturation percentage (SpO_2)**.

Pulse oximeters display the SpO_2 and the pulse rate as detected by the sensors. They show the SpO_2 either as a number or as a visual display that also shows the pulse's waveform and heart rate. The latter helps the provider ensure that the SpO_2

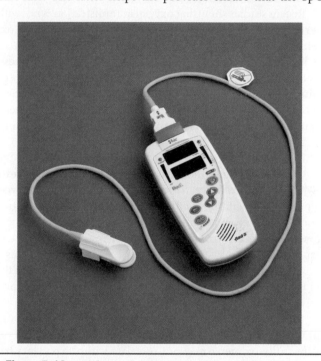

● **Figure 5-16**   Pulse oximeter.

TABLE 5–2 | Comparison of Pulse Oximetry and Capnography		
	Pulse Oximetry SpO$_2$	**Capnography ETCO$_2$**
Gas Measured	Oxygen (O$_2$)	Carbon dioxide (CO$_2$)
Parameter Evaluated	Oxygenation	Ventilation
Speed of Information Provided	● Reflects changes in oxygenation <5 minutes. ● Delayed detection of hypoventilation or apnea.	● Reflects changes in ventilation <10 seconds. ● Immediate detection of hypoventilation and apnea.
Compatibility	Should be used with capnography	Should be used with pulse oximetry

reading is based on good data. If the patient's pulse is 120 but the pulse oximetry waveform is only detecting 60, or the waveform is nearly flat, then the saturation reading is unlikely to be accurate. The relationship between SpO_2 and the partial pressure of oxygen in the blood (PaO_2) is very complex. However, the SpO_2 does correlate with the PaO_2. The greater the PaO_2, the greater will be the oxygen saturation. Since hemoglobin carries 98 percent of oxygen in the blood while plasma carries only 2 percent, pulse oximetry accurately analyzes peripheral oxygen delivery.

As a guide, normal SpO_2 varies between 96 and 99 percent at sea level. Readings between 91 and 95 percent indicate mild hypoxemia and warrant further evaluation and supplemental oxygen administration. Readings between 86 and 90 percent indicate moderate hypoxemia. You should generally give these patients high-concentration supplemental oxygen using a non-rebreather. Readings of 85 percent or lower indicate severe hypoxemia and warrant immediate intervention, including the administration of high-concentration oxygen, ventilatory assistance, or CPAP (discussed later). Your goal is to maintain the SpO_2 in the normal range (Table 5–3).

Recent studies show that oxygen administration is not without risk. Excess oxygen can cause the body to manufacture toxic chemicals called **free radicals**. (Free radicals were also discussed in Chapter 1.) These toxic chemicals can damage body tissues—especially in areas that are highly oxygen dependent, such as the brain and heart. Because of this, oxygen should be administered only to patients who are found to be hypoxic by pulse oximetry. Then, only enough supplemental oxygen should be administered to correct hypoxia and restore **normoxia** (increase it to within a normal range). Trying to fully saturate hemoglobin with oxygen can cause the formation of free radicals and result in what is called *oxidative stress*. Excess concentrations of oxygen (**hyperoxia**) should be avoided. The production of toxic free-radicals from oxygen administration has been associated with worsened outcomes in patients with brain trauma, stroke, and in post–cardiac arrest victims. It can cause numerous problems in neonates. Thus, always administer the lowest flow of oxygen that will restore normoxia (without causing hyperoxia) as evidenced by dynamic pulse oximetry readings.[1–3]

False readings with pulse oximetry are infrequent and vary with the type of device used. When they do occur, the heart rate on the pulse oximeter may not correlate with the patient's true heart rate, the waveform may be flat or nearly flat, and/or the oximeter will generate an error signal or a blank screen. Causes of false readings include carbon monoxide poisoning, high-intensity lighting, nail polish, poor perfusion, and certain hemoglobin abnormalities. Fortunately, second-generation pulse oximeters have eliminated many of these problems. In hypovolemia and in severely anemic patients, the pulse oximetry reading may be misleading. While the SpO_2 reading may be normal, the total amount of hemoglobin available to carry oxygen may be so markedly decreased that the patient will remain hypoxic at the cellular level.

Pulse oximetry provides key information about the patient and is an important part of emergency care, including prehospital care. However, it is only one assessment tool and does not replace other physical assessment or monitoring tools or skills. Do not depend solely on pulse oximetry readings to guide care. Always consider and treat the whole patient.

Pulse CO-Oximetry

Pulse CO-oximeters are devices that detect abnormal hemoglobins such as carboxyhemoglobin (from carbon monoxide poisoning) and methemoglobin (as seen in methemoglobinemia). Some devices can also detect total hemoglobin. Until recently, these devices were found only in hospital laboratories and required a blood sample. Recently, noninvasive CO-oximeters have been developed that will detect and measure carboxyhemoglobin in the same manner that standard pulse oximeters detect and report oxygen saturation. These devices may prove useful when screening patients with potential exposures or vague unexplained symptoms.

Pulse CO-oximeters use multiple wavelengths of light to detect various forms of hemoglobin found in humans (Figure 5-17 ●). Like a pulse oximeter, they detect hemoglobin with oxygen bound (oxyhemoglobin), and they detect hemoglobin without oxygen (deoxyhemoglobin). Depending on the device, they can also detect the following:

- *Carboxyhemoglobin.* When carbon monoxide (CO), a toxic gas, is inhaled, it will displace oxygen from the iron-containing heme molecules in hemoglobin. There are four heme binding sites on each hemoglobin molecule. CO will displace oxygen

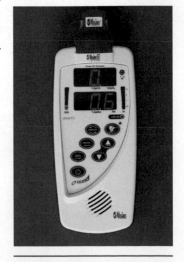

● **Figure 5-17** Pulse CO-oximetry. (© Dr. Bryan E. Bledsoe)

SpO₂ Reading (%)	Interpretation	Intervention
95–100	Normal	Change FiO_2 to maintain saturation.
91–94	Mild hypoxemia	Increase FiO_2 to increase saturation.
86–90	Moderate hypoxemia	Increase FiO_2 to increase saturation. Assess and increase ventilation.
<85	Severe hypoxemia	Increase FiO_2 to increase saturation. Increase ventilation.

TABLE 5–3 | Interpretation of Pulse Oximetry Readings and Recommended Actions

molecules that are already present on the heme, allowing the CO to bind and form carboxyhemoglobin. As the heme molecules are bound with CO, the oxygen-carrying capacity of the hemoglobin is reduced. Pulse CO-oximeters can detect increased carboxyhemoglobin. The amount of carboxyhemoglobin detected is reported as a percentage of total hemoglobin and abbreviated SpCO.[4–6]

- *Methemoglobin.* Methemoglobin is a form of hemoglobin in which the iron molecules in the heme units are in the ferric (Fe^{3+}) state. Thus, methemoglobin can neither bind nor transport oxygen. Methemoglobin has a bluish-brown color. Normally, there are enzyme systems (e.g., methemoglobin reductase) that can restore methemoglobin to the ferrous (Fe^{2+}) state, forming deoxyhemoglobin, so it can again transport oxygen. Typically, less than 2 percent of the hemoglobin in the body is in the form of methemoglobin, which cannot bind or transport oxygen. However, several conditions and drugs can cause abnormal elevations of methemoglobin (methemoglobinemia). Selected pulse CO-oximeters can measure methemoglobin and report it as a percentage of total hemoglobin (SpMET).[7, 8]

- *Total hemoglobin.* Pulse CO-oximetry now allows for noninvasive measurement of total hemoglobin in the prehospital setting (Figure 5-18 ●). This reading is reported as (SpHb). This now allows for the prehospital detection of anemia and blood loss and can serve as a surrogate indicator of the blood's oxygen-carrying content. When coupled with standard pulse oximetry readings (based on the arterial oxygen content formula discussed earlier), it is possible to noninvasively estimate oxygen content in the blood (SpOC).

Noninvasive monitoring technology is rapidly evolving. Many of the parameters discussed here are available on many of the popular commercial patient monitors used in EMS (Figure 5-19 ●). Like any other technology, prehospital personnel should not solely rely on monitoring technology. Instead, they should look at the entire patient picture and make treatment decisions based on multiple findings and parameters.

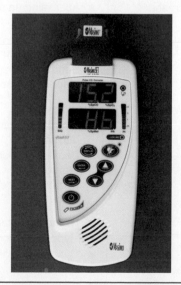

● **Figure 5-18** Total hemoglobin by pulse CO-oximetry. (© Dr. Bryan E. Bledsoe)

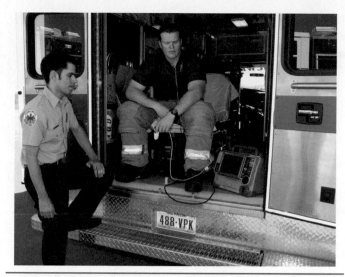

● **Figure 5-19** Multiple noninvasive parameters in a single display monitor. (© Dr. Bryan E. Bledsoe)

Capnography

Exhaled carbon dioxide (CO_2) monitoring, also called end-tidal carbon dioxide ($ETCO_2$) monitoring, or capnometry, is a noninvasive method of measuring the levels of carbon dioxide (CO_2) in the exhaled breath. **Capnography** is a recording or display of the exhaled carbon dioxide levels measured by capnometry. When first introduced into prehospital care, capnometry was used exclusively to verify proper endotracheal tube placement in the trachea. The detection of adequate levels of exhaled CO_2 following intubation confirms the tube is in the trachea (or above) and not in the esophagus. More robust technology provides accurate noninvasive measurements of exhaled CO_2 levels, thus providing medical personnel with information about the status of systemic metabolism, circulation, and ventilation. The use of capnometry and capnography has become commonplace in the operating room, in the emergency department, and in the prehospital setting.[9, 10]

Various terms have been applied to capnography, and a review of them may help you to understand the material in this section. These terms include:

- *Capnometry.* Capnometry is the measurement of expired CO_2. It typically provides a numeric display of the partial pressure of CO_2 (in Torr or mmHg) or the percentage of CO_2 present.

- *Capnography.* Capnography is a graphic recording or display of the capnometry reading over time.

- *Capnograph.* A capnograph is a device that measures expired CO_2 levels.

- *Capnogram.* A capnogram is the visual representation of the expired CO_2 waveform.

- *End-tidal CO_2 ($ETCO_2$).* End-tidal CO_2 is the measurement of the CO_2 concentration at the end of expiration (maximum CO_2).

- *$PETCO_2$.* $PETCO_2$ is the partial pressure of end-tidal CO_2 in a mixed gas solution.

- *PaCO₂.* The $PaCO_2$ represents the partial pressure of CO_2 in the arterial blood.
- *End-tidal gradient.* The end-tidal gradient is the difference between the partial pressure of arterial CO_2 ($PaCO_2$) and the end-tidal CO_2 ($ETCO_2$). It is calculated as:

$$PaCO_2 - ETCO_2 = \text{End-tidal gradient}$$

This value is normally less than 5 mmHg. However, an increase in dead space ventilation (ventilation of non-perfused lung tissue) reflects a ventilation/perfusion mismatch (V/Q mismatch). This occurs in pulmonary embolism and similar processes. As dead space ventilation increases, the $ETCO_2$ falls, thus widening the end-tidal gradient.

CO_2 is a normal end product of metabolism and is transported by the venous system to the right side of the heart and on to the lungs where it diffuses into the alveoli and is removed from the body through exhalation. When circulation is normal, exhaled CO_2 levels change proportionally with ventilation and are a very reliable estimate of the partial pressure of carbon dioxide in the arterial system ($PaCO_2$). Normal $PaCO_2$ is approximately 40 and a normal exhaled CO_2 is just 1 to 2 mm less, or 38 mmHg (Table 5–4).

When perfusion decreases, as occurs in shock or cardiac arrest, exhaled CO_2 levels reflect pulmonary blood flow and cardiac output, not ventilation. Decreased levels of exhaled CO_2 can be found in shock, cardiac arrest, pulmonary embolism, bronchospasm, and with incomplete airway obstruction (such as mucous plugging). Increased levels of exhaled CO_2 are found with hypoventilation, respiratory depression, and hyperthermia (Table 5–5).

CO_2 is detected by using either a colorimetric or an infrared device. It can be reported as a percentage (the amount of CO_2 in a given volume of gas) or as a partial pressure (mmHg).

Colorimetric Devices The colorimetric device is a disposable $ETCO_2$ detector that contains pH-sensitive, chemically impregnated paper encased within a plastic chamber (Figure 5-20 ●). It is placed in the airway circuit between the patient and the ventilation device. When the paper is exposed to CO_2, hydrogen ions (H^+) are generated, causing a color change in the paper. The color change is reversible and changes breath to breath. A color scale on the device estimates the $ETCO_2$ level. Colorimetric devices cannot detect hyper- or hypocarbia (increased or decreased CO_2 levels). If gastric contents or acidic drugs (e.g., endotracheal epinephrine) contact the paper in the device, subsequent readings may be unreliable.

Infrared Devices Electronic exhaled CO_2 detectors use an infrared technique to detect CO_2 in the exhaled breath (Figure 5-21 ●). A heated element in the sensor generates infrared radiation. The CO_2 molecules absorb infrared light at a very specific wavelength and can thus be measured. Electronic exhaled CO_2 detectors may be either qualitative (i.e., they simply

TABLE 5–4 | Comparison of PaCO₂ and ETCO₂

	Arterial CO_2 ($PaCO_2$) Arterial Blood Gases	End-Tidal CO_2 ($ETCO_2$) Capnography
Partial Pressure (mmHg)	35–45 mmHg	30–43 mmHg
Percentage (%)	4.6–5.9%	4.0–5.6%

TABLE 5–5 | Basic Rules of Capnography

Symptom	Possible Cause
Sudden drop of $ETCO_2$ to zero	• Esophageal intubation • Ventilator disconnection or defect in ventilator • Defect in CO_2 analyzer
Sudden decrease of $ETCO_2$ (not to zero)	• Leak in ventilator system; obstruction • Partial disconnect in ventilator circuit • Partial airway obstruction (secretions)
Exponential decrease of $ETCO_2$	• Pulmonary embolism • Cardiac arrest • Hypotension (sudden) • Severe hyperventilation
Change in CO_2 baseline	• Calibration error • Water droplet in analyzer • Mechanical failure (ventilator)
Sudden increase in $ETCO_2$	• Accessing an area of lung previously obstructed • Release of tourniquet • Sudden increase in blood pressure
Gradual lowering of $ETCO_2$	• Hypovolemia • Decreasing cardiac output • Decreasing body temperature; hypothermia; drop in metabolism
Gradual increase in $ETCO_2$	• Rising body temperature • Hypoventilation • CO_2 absorption • Partial airway obstruction (foreign body); reactive airway disease

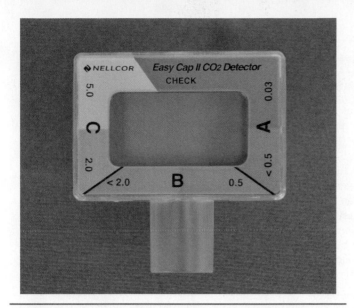

● **Figure 5-20** Colorimetric end-tidal CO_2 detector. *(© Edward T. Dickinson, MD)*

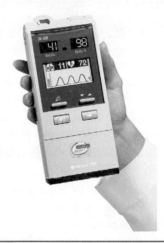

● **Figure 5-21** Handheld capnography unit. *(Image used by permission from Nellcor Puritan Bennett LLC, Boulder, Colorado, doing business as Covidien)*

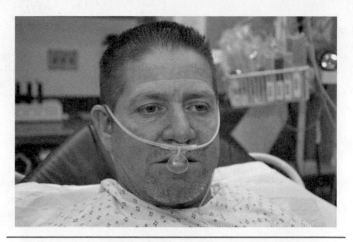

● **Figure 5-22** End-tidal carbon dioxide monitoring in a non-intubated patient. *(© Edward T. Dickinson, MD)*

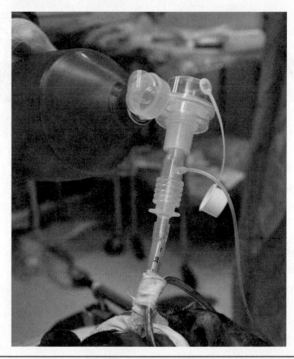

● **Figure 5-23** End-tidal carbon dioxide monitoring in an intubated patient. *(© Edward T. Dickinson, MD)*

detect the presence of CO_2) or quantitative (i.e., they determine how much CO_2 is present). Quantitative devices are now routinely used in prehospital care. Exhaled $ETCO_2$ readings can be monitored both in patients who are not intubated and in those who are intubated (Figures 5-22 ● and 5-23 ●). Most modern capnometers can both display a number and provide a digital waveform (capnogram) that reflects the entire respiratory cycle (Figure 5-24 ●).

There are two major types of capnography—mainstream and sidestream. Each has its advantages and disadvantages. With mainstream capnography, the infrared light is shone through the gas within the patient circuit. With sidestream capnography a sample of the gas is aspirated from the main gas flow circuit, using a separate sample line. This sample line is attached to a sensor unit that is typically housed in the patient monitor. The differences are illustrated in Table 5–6.

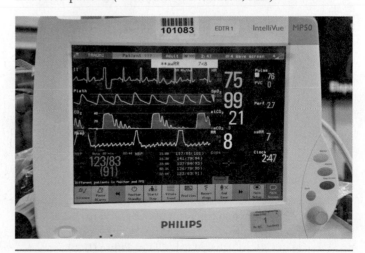

● **Figure 5-24** Some CO_2 detectors can display both a waveform and a number.

TABLE 5–6 | Comparison of Mainstream and Sidestream Capnography

Mainstream Capnography	Sidestream Capnography
CO_2 sensor located between ET tube and breathing circuit	CO_2 aspirated from a sampling tube and analyzed in an analyzer/sensor away from the patient
Advantages	
• Provides real-time information • More accurate • No sampling tube • Not affected by water vapor pressure changes	• Lightweight • Less expensive • Can be used in non-intubated patients (including CPAP) • Easy to connect • Disposable tubing • Can be used with simultaneous oxygen administration • Calibration automatic
Disadvantages	
• Bulkiness/weight of sensor • Can be used only in intubated patients • Expensive probe • Requires calibration	• Small sampling tube easily obstructed (e.g., by water vapor) • Slightly less accurate • Delay of several seconds analyzing sample • Water vapor may affect $ETCO_2$ reading • Pressure drop along sampling tube may affect $ETCO_2$ reading

Capnogram The capnogram reflects exhaled CO_2 concentrations over time. It is typically divided into four phases (Figure 5-25 ●).

- *Phase I.* Phase I (AB in Figure 5-25) is the respiratory baseline. It is flat when no CO_2 is present and corresponds to the late phase of inspiration and the early part of expiration (in which dead-space gases without CO_2 are released).

- *Phase II.* Phase II (BC in Figure 5-25) is the respiratory upstroke. This reflects the appearance of CO_2 in the alveoli.

- *Phase III.* Phase III (CD in Figure 5-25) is the respiratory plateau. It reflects the airflow through uniformly ventilated alveoli with a nearly constant CO_2 level. The highest level of the plateau (point D in Figure 5-25) is called the $ETCO_2$ and is recorded as such by the capnometer.

- *Phase IV.* Phase IV (DE in Figure 5-25) is the inspiratory phase. It is a sudden downstroke and ultimately returns to the baseline during inspiration. The respiratory pause restarts the cycle (EA in Figure 5-25).

Clinical Applications At its most basic, qualitative capnography may be used to assess correct initial and periodic endotracheal tube placement. Continuous quantitative capnography may be used in intubated patients to confirm initial tube placement and to constantly monitor for tube misplacement. Continuous waveform capnography may also be used to ensure proper exhaled CO_2 levels for head trauma and stroke patients. Continuous waveform capnography adds the ability to help troubleshoot hypoxemia and difficult ventilation and assess for bronchospasm, pulmonary embolus, and so on. Continuous waveform capnography also has utility in monitoring nonintubated patients. By following trends in the capnogram, prehospital personnel can continuously monitor the patient's condition, detect trends, and document the response to medications.

Several medical conditions and mechanical ventilation problems can be readily detected by capnography when compared to the normal capnogram (Figure 5-26 ●). These include:

- *Obstructive disease.* Obstructive pulmonary diseases, such as asthma and chronic obstructive pulmonary disease (COPD), obstruct air entry and alter the shape of the capnogram. These diseases give the typical "shark fin" shape to the capnogram (Figure 5-27 ●).

- *Rebreathing.* Rebreathing of gas can result in failure of the capnogram to reach the baseline. This can be due to

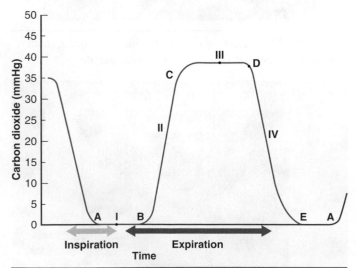

● **Figure 5-25** Normal capnogram. AB = *Phase I*: late inspiration, early expiration (no CO_2). BC = *Phase II*: appearance of CO_2 in exhaled gas. CD = *Phase III*: plateau (constant CO_2). D = highest point ($ETCO_2$). DE = *Phase IV*: rapid descent during inspiration. EA = respiratory pause.

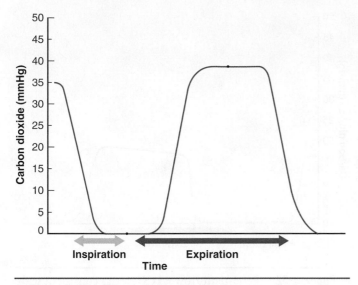

● **Figure 5-26** Normal capnogram. Capnography provides immediate information about the patient's ventilatory status.

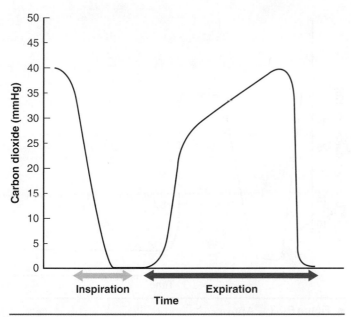

● **Figure 5-27** Capnogram pattern showing classic "shark fin" waveform consistent with obstructive pulmonary disease (asthma and COPD).

hyperventilation or to problems in the breathing circuit (Figure 5-28 ●).

● *Curare cleft.* Appears when neuromuscular blockers begin to subside. The depth of the cleft is inversely proportional to the degree of drug activity (Figure 5-29 ●).

● *Esophageal intubation.* The absence of a waveform, or the presence of a small disorganized waveform, is indicative of esophageal intubation (Figure 5-30 ●).

● *Endotracheal tube or circuit leak.* Waveform variations are seen when there is a leak in the endotracheal tube cuff or if the airway is too small for the patient (Figure 5-31 ●).

● *Ventilation/Perfusion (V/Q) mismatch.* With a ventilation/perfusion mismatch, as occurs in pulmonary embolism and similar conditions, the increase in dead space ventilation

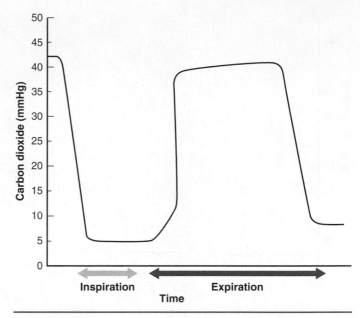

● **Figure 5-28** An elevation in the baseline indicates rebreathing of CO_2 and is generally seen with hyperventilation.

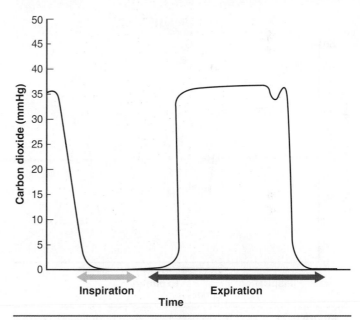

● **Figure 5-29** So-called "curare notch" or "curare cleft" seen in mechanically ventilated patients as neuromuscular blocker levels fall.

causes a decrease in $ETCO_2$ levels throughout the respiratory cycle (Figure 5-32 ●).

● *Apnea.* A fall of the waveform to the baseline indicates apnea (Figure 5-33 ●).

● *Hyperventilation.* Hyperventilation leads to elimination of CO_2 and a progressively lower exhaled CO_2 level (Figure 5-34 ●).

● *Hypoventilation.* Hypoventilation results in CO_2 retention and a progressive elevation in exhaled CO_2 levels (Figure 5-35 ●).

Exhaled CO_2 detection is also useful in CPR. During cardiac arrest, CO_2 levels fall abruptly following the onset of cardiac arrest. They begin to rise with the onset of effective CPR and return to near-normal levels with a return of spontaneous

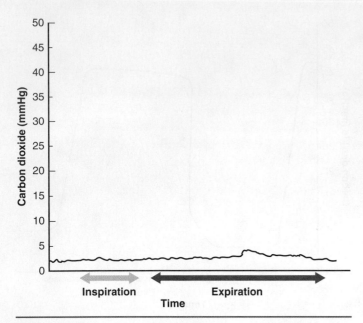

● **Figure 5-30** Capnogram showing absent waveform consistent with esophageal intubation.

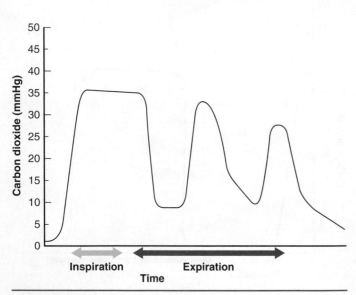

● **Figure 5-31** Waveform variations seen with leakage in the endotracheal tube cuff or in the breathing circuit.

circulation. During effective CPR, exhaled CO_2 levels have been found to correlate well with cardiac output, coronary perfusion pressure, and even with the effectiveness of CPR compressions.

Continuous waveform capnography is rapidly becoming a standard of care in EMS (Figure 5-36 ●). Misplaced endotracheal tubes represent a significant area of liability in EMS and the documentation provided by this technology can provide irrefutable evidence of proper endotracheal tube placement.

Peak Expiratory Flow Testing

Peak expiratory flow testing utilizes a disposable plastic chamber into which the patient exhales forcefully after maximal inhalation.

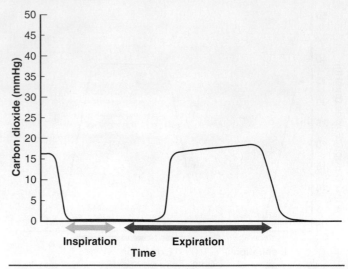

● **Figure 5-32** Persistently low $ETCO_2$ levels consistent with significant dead space ventilation (V/Q mismatch) as seen in pulmonary embolism.

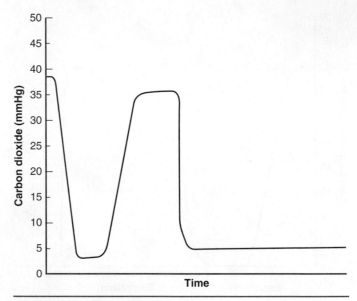

● **Figure 5-33** Apnea.

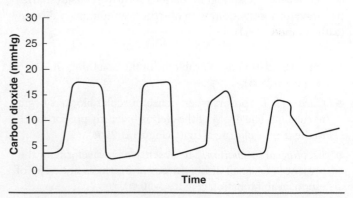

● **Figure 5-34** Progressive reduction in $ETCO_2$ levels consistent with hyperventilation.

It can be used as a crude measure of respiratory efficacy. Improving measurements can indicate good response to treatment of acute respiratory illness.

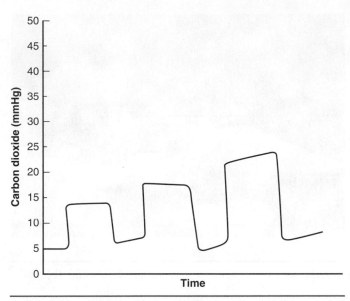

● **Figure 5-35** Progressive increase in $ETCO_2$ levels consistent with hypoventilation.

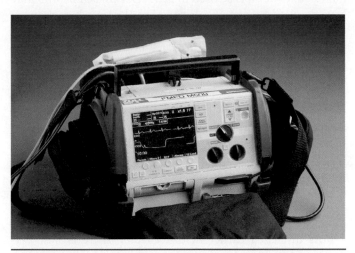

● **Figure 5-36** Most modern patient monitors allow the constant monitoring of numerous physiologic parameters.

PART 2: Basic Airway Management and Ventilation

Basic airway management and ventilation includes most airway maneuvers that have been shown to be lifesaving, including proper positioning, suctioning, oxygen administration, and bag-valve-mask (BVM) ventilation. Paramedics must continue to focus on these basic skills, despite their advanced training and techniques. It is easy to get tunnel vision when considering endotracheal intubation and other advanced procedures, yet these techniques are rarely lifesaving and are often worthless if not preceded by good basic management. As the senior member of most EMS teams, it is the responsibility of the paramedic to ensure that other providers on scene are performing optimal basic airway management. Lead by example whenever possible!

PROPER POSITIONING

Trauma patients are often confined to the supine position as a result of spinal immobilization. However, some circumstances may warrant flexibility, if permitted by local protocols. For example, the patient with facial and airway trauma who is able to maintain his airway as long as he is sitting up may be placed in a cervical collar in a seated position rather than restricted to a supine position.

Conscious medical patients should be maintained in their position of comfort if they are not placed in cervical immobilization. Unconscious medical patients who do not require other interventions, such as BVM ventilation, should be placed on their side with the head elevated (if not contraindicated) to minimize the risk of aspiration. Unconscious patients who do require airway and ventilation interventions, such as BVM ventilation or intubation, are usually best maintained in an **ear-to-sternal-notch position**, in which the supine patient's head is elevated to the point where the ear and the sternal notch are horizontally aligned (Figure 5-37 ●). This position is often referred to as the **sniffing position** in non-obese patients and the **ramped position** in obese patients. With both the sniffing and ramped positions, the ear-to-sternal notch alignment is maintained. This positioning maximizes upper airway patency allowing for effective ventilation and, if required, endotracheal intubation. It also improves the mechanics of ventilation, both with spontaneous breathing and with BVM ventilation.

Sniffing Position

To place non-obese patients in the sniffing position, first achieve an ear-to-sternal notch horizontal alignment by slightly flexing the patient's neck and extending the head (assuming no cervical spine injury is suspected). This can be maintained by placing a towel or small pillow under the head (Figure 5-38 ●).

Ramped Position

The strategy for positioning obese patients is different. It is often difficult or impossible to place them into the sniffing position by elevating just the head. Instead, you must elevate the entire upper portion of the body. This can be achieved with blankets, towels, and pillows or with a commercial wedge pillow (Figure 5-39 ●). When considering airway management in an obese patient, prepare a proper ramp (head and shoulder support) before transferring the patient. Lifting obese patients during airway management is often difficult.[11]

CONTENT REVIEW

▶ Ear-to-Sternal-Notch Positions
- Sniffing position (if patient is not obese)
- Ramped position (if patient is obese)

▶ Unconscious patients who require airway and ventilation interventions are usually best maintained in an ear-to-sternal-notch position (ear and sternal notch horizontally aligned).

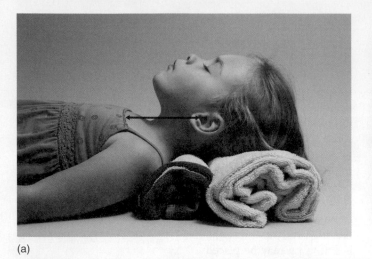

(a)

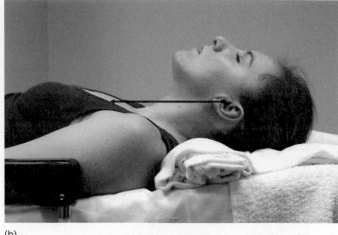

(b)

● **Figure 5-37**   Airway management and ventilation is improved when the ear-to-sternal notch axis is aligned. (a) child, (b) adult.

OXYGENATION

Oxygen is an important drug, and you must thoroughly understand its indications and precautions. Providing supplemental oxygen to patients who are frankly hypoxemic will diminish the hypoxia's secondary effects on organs such as the brain and the heart and lessen subjective respiratory distress.

In some circumstances, oxygen administration is also indicated even though the patient's oxygen saturation may be normal. Keep in mind that oxygen may be carried both on hemoglobin and dissolved in the blood. Under normal circumstances, the dissolved portion of oxygen is relatively insignificant. When supplemental oxygen is administered, the dissolved portion of oxygen may increase many fold. This relatively small amount of extra oxygen may be important to patients with tissue hypoxemia from any cause such as septic shock, myocardial infarction, cardiogenic shock, or severe trauma. Oxygen administration is also very important prior to intubation, regardless of the oxygen saturation. Finally, ill or injured pregnant patients may benefit from supplemental oxygen administration,

regardless of their oxygen saturation, to enhance oxygen delivery to the fetus.

Never withhold oxygen from any patient for whom it is indicated. Caution is advised in patients with COPD, who may have developed a hypoxic drive to breathe (in which reduced oxygen levels trigger breathing), as opposed to a normal hypercarbic drive to breathe (in which breathing is triggered by chronic hypercarbia, or elevated levels of carbon dioxide). In these patients there is a theoretical risk of depressing respirations as the body senses plentiful oxygen. This is rarely a clinical issue during all but the longest EMS transports. Thus, you should feel comfortable giving as much oxygen as necessary to maintain adequate oxygen saturations. Remember, however, that you do not necessarily need to return these patients to normal oxygen saturations, as their bodies are generally used to lower oxygen levels. Of course, you should monitor your patient closely for evidence of respiratory depression. You may also use capnography to assess for early signs of worsening hypercarbia.

As discussed earlier in this chapter, there is now evidence that high oxygen levels (hyperoxia) may be as dangerous as low levels (hypoxia) because of the possible formation of oxygen free radicals. This has been demonstrated in post–cardiac arrest patients, stroke patients, neonates, and head trauma patients. Therefore, oxygen saturation should always be maintained in the normal range, using the lowest necessary oxygen flow.

Oxygen Supply and Regulation

Oxygen is supplied either as a compressed gas or a liquid. Compressed

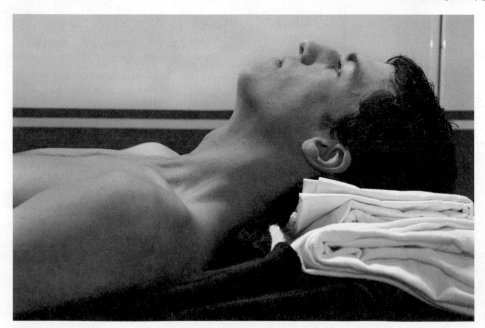

● **Figure 5-38**   The "sniffing position" provides adequate ear-to-sternal notch alignment in non-obese adults. (© *Edward T. Dickinson, MD*)

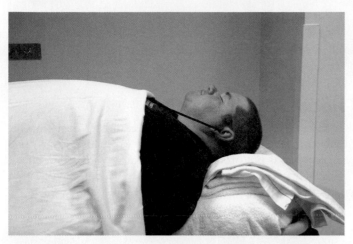

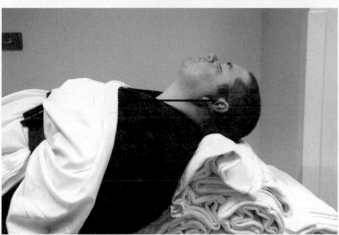

● **Figure 5-39** The "ramped position" allows adequate ear-to-sternal notch alignment in obese patients.

gaseous oxygen is stored in an aluminum or steel tank in 400-liter (D), 660-liter (E), or 3,450-liter (M) volumes. To calculate how long the oxygen will last, use the appropriate formula below—the same formula but with a different constant for each type of cylinder: 0.16 for a D cylinder, 0.28 for an E cylinder, and 1.56 for an M cylinder:

D cylinder tank life in minutes = (tank pressure in psi × 0.16) ÷ liters per minute

E cylinder tank life in minutes = (tank pressure in psi × 0.28) ÷ liters per minute

M cylinder tank life in minutes = (tank pressure in psi × 1.56) ÷ liters per minute

Liquid oxygen is cooled to aqueous form and warmed back to its gaseous state for delivery. Although liquid oxygen requires less storage space than an equal amount of compressed oxygen, you must keep it upright and accommodate other special requirements for its storage and transfer.

A regulator for an oxygen tank is either a **high-pressure regulator**, which is used to transfer oxygen at high pressures from tank to tank, or a **therapy regulator**, which is used for delivering oxygen to patients. The default pressure for therapy regulators is 50 psi, which is controlled within the regulator to allow for adjustable low-flow oxygen delivery.

Oxygen Delivery Devices

Oxygen delivery to patients is measured in liters of flow per minute (L/min). A number of delivery devices are available; the patient's condition will dictate which method you use. You must continually reassess the patient who requires oxygen therapy to be certain that the method of delivery and flow rate are adequate. Some patients may require positive pressure ventilation rather than a passive delivery device.

Nasal Cannula

The **nasal cannula** is a catheter placed at the nares. It provides an optimal oxygen supplementation of up to 40 percent when set at 6 L/min flow. At flow rates above 6 L/min, the nasal mucous membranes become very dry and easily break down. Patients generally tolerate the nasal cannula well. It is indicated for low-to-moderate oxygen requirements and long-term oxygen therapy.

Venturi Mask

The **Venturi mask** is a high-flow face mask that uses a Venturi system to deliver relatively precise oxygen concentrations, regardless of the patient's rate and depth of breathing. As oxygen passes into the mask through a jet orifice in the base of the mask, it entrains room air. The device then delivers the resulting mixture to the patient. Some Venturi masks have dial selectors to control the amount of ambient air taken in; others have interchangeable caps. Either type can deliver concentrations of 24 percent, 28 percent, 35 percent, or 40 percent oxygen. The liter flow depends on the oxygen concentration desired. The Venturi mask is particularly useful for COPD patients, who benefit from careful control of inspired oxygen concentration. These masks are rarely placed by EMS providers, but you will encounter them during transfers.

Simple Face Mask

The simple face mask is indicated for patients requiring moderate oxygen concentrations. Side ports allow room air to enter the mask and dilute the oxygen concentration during inspiration. Flow rates generally range from about 6 to 10 L/min, providing 40 to 60 percent oxygen at the maximum rate, depending on the patient's respiratory rate and depth. Delivery of volumes beyond 10 L/min does not enhance oxygen concentration. These devices are rarely carried by EMS providers but will be encountered during transfers.

Partial Rebreather Mask

The partial rebreather mask is indicated for patients requiring moderate-to-high oxygen concentrations when satisfactory clinical results are not obtained with the simple face mask. One-way discs that cover the partial rebreather mask's side ports prevent the inspiration of room air. Minimal dilution occurs with inspiration of residual expired air along with the supplemental oxygen. Maximal flow rate is 10 L/min.

Nonrebreather Mask

The nonrebreather mask has one-way side ports as well, but also has an attached reservoir bag to hold oxygen ready to inhale. It provides the highest oxygen concentration of all oxygen delivery devices available, or about 80 percent when set at 15 L/min of oxygen and the mask is fit tightly to the face. These masks are commonly used by EMS for initial management of patients with high oxygen requirements. Any patient who requires a nonrebreather should be closely monitored for refractory hypoxemia that requires invasive or noninvasive positive pressure ventilation.

Small-Volume Nebulizer

Nebulizer chambers containing 3 to 5 cc of fluid are attached to a face mask that allows for delivery of medications in aerosol form (nebulization) that is more likely to pass through the upper airway to the lower airways. Pressurized oxygen or air enters the chamber to create a mist, which the patient then inspires. Oxygen is the usual carrier but air is occasionally used in COPD patients, and a helium-oxygen mixture may be used in patients with upper airway obstruction.

Oxygen Humidifier

You can provide humidified oxygen to the patient by attaching a sterile water reservoir to the oxygen outlet. Humidified oxygen is often given to pediatric patients with upper airway problems such as croup, although there is no evidence that it improves outcomes. Humidification is also useful for patients receiving long-term oxygen therapy to prevent the complications of drying out the mucous membranes. Humidification is rarely necessary in the EMS setting.

Positive Airway Pressure

Positive airway pressure (PAP) is delivered via a face mask to maintain a constant level of pressure within the airway, which assists a patient in breathing by preventing collapse of the airway during inhalation. **Continuous positive airway pressure (CPAP)** maintains a steady level of pressure during both inhalation and exhalation. **Bilevel positive airway pressure (BiPAP)** maintains a higher level of pressure during inhalation and a lower level of pressure during exhalation. CPAP and BiPAP devices can be used to administer oxygen in conjunction with increased airway pressures.

MANUAL AIRWAY MANEUVERS

Manual maneuvers are the simplest airway management techniques. They require no specialized equipment, are safe, and are noninvasive. They are highly effective but are often neglected in prehospital care.

In the patient who is unconscious or has a decreased level of consciousness, posterior displacement of the tongue is often the cause of airway obstruction. The head-tilt/chin-lift and the jaw-thrust are safe and dependable maneuvers for relieving this obstruction. You should perform one of these techniques on all unconscious patients, but do not perform them on responsive patients.

If you suspect cervical spine injury, perform the modified jaw-thrust with in-line stabilization of the cervical spine. Always follow Standard Precautions and use a mask and face shield during airway management maneuvers.

Head-Tilt/Chin-Lift

In the absence of cervical spine trauma, the head-tilt/chin-lift is the best technique for opening the airway in an unresponsive patient who is not protecting his own airway (Figure 5-40 ●). This maneuver is potentially hazardous to patients with cervical spine injuries. To perform the head-tilt/chin-lift:

1. Place the patient supine and position yourself at the side of the patient's head.
2. Place one hand on the patient's forehead and, using firm downward pressure with your palm, tilt the head back.
3. Put two fingers of the other hand under the bony part of the chin and lift the jaw anteriorly to open the airway.

Caution: Avoid compressing the soft tissues of the neck and chin, which could cause airway obstruction.

Jaw-Thrust Maneuver without Head Extension

A jaw-thrust is acceptable for any unresponsive patient and recommended for any patient at risk for cervical spine injury who cannot protect his airway. It may be necessary to remove the cervical collar to advance the jaw sufficiently to open the airway; however, the provider performing the jaw-thrust is usually able to maintain manual in-line immobilization simultaneously. To perform the jaw-thrust:

● Lift the jaw using fingers behind the mandibular angles; do not tilt the head (Figure 5-41 ●). It usually helps to prop the thumbs on the cheekbones to provide some counter-force.

Although they are simple and effective, none of these manual airway maneuvers protects the airway from aspiration. Additionally, the jaw-thrust is difficult to maintain for an extended time. Placing an oral and/or nasopharyngeal airway, if

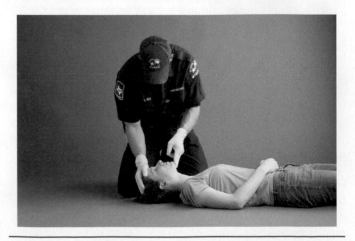

● **Figure 5-40**   Head-tilt/chin-lift maneuver.

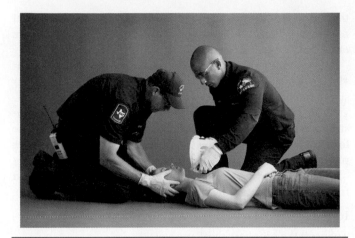

● **Figure 5-41** Modified jaw-thrust without head extension in trauma.

tolerated and not contraindicated, may open the airway sufficiently that a strong jaw-thrust is no longer required until the airway can be more definitively managed.

BASIC AIRWAY ADJUNCTS

In the absence of trauma, secretions, foreign bodies, and edema, basic manual airway maneuvers should succeed in clearing the tongue from the air passages. However, the tongue often falls back, subsequently, to block the airway again. Two available airway adjuncts, the nasopharyngeal airway and the oropharyngeal airway, prevent this. These adjuncts cannot replace good head positioning, but they do help to lift the base of the tongue forward and away from the posterior oropharynx, establishing and maintaining a patent airway.

Nasopharyngeal Airway

The **nasopharyngeal airway (NPA)**, or "nasal trumpet," is an uncuffed tube made of soft rubber or plastic. The nasopharyngeal airway follows the natural curvature of the nasopharynx, passing through the nose and extending from the nostril to the posterior pharynx just below the base of the tongue. It varies from 17 to 20 cm in length, and its diameter ranges from 20 to 36 F (**French**). A funnel-shaped projection at its proximal end helps prevent the tube from slipping inside a patient's nose and becoming lost or aspirated. The distal end is beveled to facilitate passage. Nasopharyngeal airways are generally underutilized. They are well tolerated in most patients and are very effective at maintaining the airway. Specific indications for the use of the nasopharyngeal airway include obtunded patients (those with reduced mental acuity, with or without a suppressed gag reflex) and unconscious patients. If the patient does not tolerate the nasopharyngeal airway, you should remove it.

Advantages of the Nasopharyngeal Airway

● It can be rapidly inserted and safely placed blindly.
● It bypasses the tongue, providing a patent airway.
● You may use it in the presence of a gag reflex.
● You may use it when the patient has suffered injury to his oral cavity.

● You may suction through it.
● You may use it when the patient's teeth are clenched.

Disadvantages of the Nasopharyngeal Airway

● It is smaller than the oropharyngeal airway.
● It does not isolate the trachea.
● It is difficult to suction through.
● It may cause severe nosebleeds if inserted too forcefully.
● It may cause pressure necrosis of the nasal mucosa.
● It may kink and clog, obstructing the airway.
● Inserting it is difficult if nasal damage (old or new) is present.
● You may not use it if the patient has or is suspected to have a basilar skull fracture, as the tube could inadvertently pass into the cranium.

The properly sized nasopharyngeal tube is slightly smaller in diameter than the patient's nostril, and in adults it is equal to or slightly longer than the distance from the patient's nose to his earlobe. Selecting the appropriate size is important. Too small a tube will not extend past the tongue; too long a tube may pass into the esophagus and result in hypoventilation of the lungs and distention of the stomach when positive pressure is applied (Figures 5-42 ● and 5-43 ●).

Inserting the Nasopharyngeal Airway

To insert a nasopharyngeal airway:

1. Ensure or maintain effective ventilation with supplemental oxygen.
2. Lubricate the exterior of the tube with a water-soluble gel to decrease trauma during insertion. Lidocaine gel may be used to increase tolerance of the device after insertion.
3. Select the naris that appears largest. Push gently up on the tip of the nose and pass the tube gently into the nostril

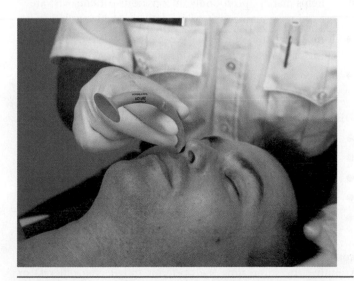

● **Figure 5-42** Nasopharyngeal airway.

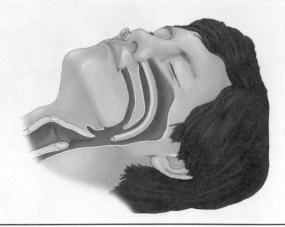

● **Figure 5-43**   Nasopharyngeal airway, inserted.

with the bevel oriented toward the septum and the airway directed straight back along the nasal floor, parallel to the mouth. Avoid pushing against any resistance, because this may cause tissue trauma and airway kinking.

4. Verify the appropriate position of the airway. Resolution of noisy breathing and improved compliance during bag-valve-mask ventilation support correct positioning. Also, feel at the airway's proximal end for airflow on expiration.

5. Provide supplemental oxygen and/or ventilate the patient as indicated.

Oropharyngeal Airway

The **oropharyngeal airway (OPA)** is a noninvasive semicircular plastic or rubber device designed to follow the palate's curvature. It holds the base of the tongue away from the posterior oropharynx, thus preventing it from obstructing the glottis. Its use is indicated in patients with no gag reflex.

Advantages of the Oropharyngeal Airway

● It is easy to place using proper technique.

● Air can pass around and through the device.

● It helps prevent obstruction by the teeth and lips.

● It helps manage profoundly unconscious patients who are breathing spontaneously or need mechanical ventilation.

● It makes suction of the pharynx easier, as a large suction catheter can pass on either side of the device.

● It serves as an effective bite block in case of seizures or to protect the endotracheal tube.

Disadvantages of the Oropharyngeal Airway

● It does not isolate the trachea or prevent aspiration.

● It cannot be inserted when the teeth are clenched.

● It may obstruct the airway if not inserted properly.

● It is easily dislodged.

● Return of the gag reflex may produce vomiting.

Do not use an oropharyngeal airway in conscious or semiconscious patients who have a gag reflex, because it may cause vomiting (by stimulating the posterior tongue gag reflexes) or laryngospasm. As is often said, "If a patient tolerates an oral airway,

then he needs an oral airway." The converse is also true: If a patient resists placement of the airway, then his gag reflex is intact and an oral airway is not indicated.

Oropharyngeal airways are available in sizes ranging from #0 (for neonates) to #6 (for large adults). Selecting the proper size is important. If the airway is too long, it can press the epiglottis against the entrance of the larynx, resulting in airway obstruction. If it is too small, it will not adequately hold the tongue forward. To measure for the appropriate oropharyngeal airway, place the flange beside the patient's cheek, parallel to the front of the teeth (Figure 5-44 ●). A properly sized airway will extend from the patient's mouth to the angle of his jaw (Figure 5-45 ●).

Inserting the Oropharyngeal Airway

To insert the oropharyngeal airway:

1. Open the mouth and remove any visible obstructions.

2. Ensure or maintain effective ventilation with supplemental oxygen.

3. Grasp the patient's jaw and lift anteriorly.

4. With your other hand, hold the airway device at its proximal end and insert it into the patient's mouth. Make sure the curve is reversed, with the tip pointing toward the roof of the mouth.

5. Once the tip reaches the level of the soft palate, gently rotate the airway 180° until it comes to rest over the tongue.

6. Verify appropriate position of the airway. Clear breath sounds and chest rise indicate correct placement.

7. Apply supplemental oxygen and/or positive pressure ventilation if indicated.

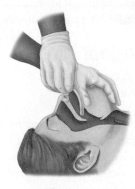

● **Figure 5-44a**   Insert the oropharyngeal airway with the tip facing the palate.

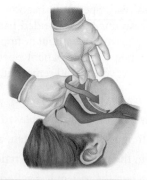

● **Figure 5-44b**   Rotate the airway 180° into position.

CONTENT REVIEW

▶ Remember that an unconscious patient's respiratory center may not function adequately.

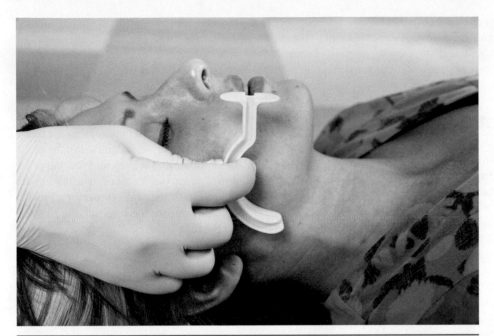

● **Figure 5-45** Measure the oropharyngeal airway externally to ensure proper sizing.

An alternative insertion method useful in both pediatric and adult patients is to press the tongue upward and forward with a tongue blade. Then, the airway can be advanced until the flange is seated at the teeth. This is the preferred method of airway insertion in infants and children.

Oral and/or nasal airways should be considered in all obtunded older pediatric and adult patients and are mandatory whenever the patient has signs of airway obstruction ("noisy breathing is obstructed breathing") or bag-valve-mask ventilation is difficult. These airways may also be used in combination such as two nasal airways, one nasal and one oral, or even two nasal and one oral airway in extreme circumstances.

VENTILATION

Many of your cases in the field will call for ventilatory support. These situations range from apneic (nonbreathing) patients to less obvious instances when patients are experiencing depressed respiratory function. Remember that an unconscious patient's respiratory center may not function adequately. A significant decrease in the patient's rate or depth of breathing will lead to decreased respiratory minute volume with subsequent hypercarbia and respiratory acidosis. This will result in further decreases in mental status, creating a vicious cycle. Hypoxemia may also result if the decrease in breathing is significant or oxygen demand is substantial. Acidosis and/or hypoxemia may eventually lead to respiratory or cardiac arrest.

Effective ventilatory support requires a tidal volume of 6 to 8 mL/kg of ideal body weight at a rate of 12 breaths per minute. Note that these volumes are significantly less than the 10 to 15 mL/kg that was formerly recommended.

When providing ventilatory support, you must generate enough force to overcome the elastic resistance of the lungs and chest wall, as well as the frictional resistance in the respiratory passageways, without overinflating the lungs. This is similar to blowing up a balloon; you must overcome the balloon's resistance in order to inflate it.

Keep in mind that air will travel the path of least resistance. If you do not maintain a tight seal between the ventilation mask and your patient's face, air will flow out of the gaps rather than through the respiratory passageways. If you do not keep the airway maximally open using proper positioning and airway adjuncts and keep the esophagus compressed with cricoid pressure, air will flow into the stomach rather than the lungs. Therefore, effective artificial ventilation requires a patent airway, an effective seal between the mask and the patient's face, and delivery of appropriate ventilatory volumes directed into the lungs and not into the stomach. Exercise care when you attempt to generate enough pressure to ventilate the lungs. Too much pressure may lead to gastric distention and regurgitation. Also, be certain that you allow the patient to exhale between delivered breaths.

Mouth-to-Mouth/Mouth-to-Nose Ventilation

Mouth-to-mouth and mouth-to-nose ventilation are the most basic methods of rescue ventilation, but their use is limited by exposure to body fluids and by limited oxygen delivery, as expired air contains only 17 percent oxygen. These methods are indicated only in the presence of apnea when no other ventilation devices are available. When using one of these methods, take care not to hyperinflate the patient's lungs nor to hyperventilate yourself.

Mouth-to-Mask Ventilation

The pocket mask is a clear plastic device with a one-way valve that you place over an apneic patient's mouth and nose. It prevents direct contact between you and your patient's mouth and expired air, thus reducing the risk of contamination and subsequent infection. A pocket mask also has an inlet for supplemental oxygen. Mouth-to-mask ventilation combined with an oxygen flow rate of 10 L/min can deliver an inspired oxygen concentration of approximately 50 percent. However, pocket masks are much less effective than bag-valve-mask devices and are very tiring for the rescuer.

To perform the mouth-to-mask technique, position the head to open the airway by one of the previously discussed methods (head-tilt/chin-lift or jaw-thrust), position the mask to obtain a good seal, and provide adequate ventilatory volumes. As with mouth-to-mouth and mouth-to-nose methods, hyperinflation of the patient's lungs, gastric distention in the patient, and hyperventilation in the rescuer are potential complications.

Bag-Valve-Mask Ventilation

The first technique employed for most patients who are not breathing or not breathing adequately is **bag-valve-mask (BVM)** ventilation with a self-inflating bag and reservoir attached to high-concentration oxygen. Many patients may be entirely managed with BVM ventilation while, in other cases, it is a bridge to more invasive techniques. BVM ventilation is one of the most important and challenging EMS skills and must be mastered. While the paramedic may need to delegate BVM ventilation to other providers, the paramedic is still responsible for ensuring good technique.

The bag-valve mask (BVM) consists of an oblong, self-inflating, silicone or rubber bag with two one-way valves (an air/oxygen-inlet valve and a patient valve), a detachable transparent plastic face mask, and an oxygen reservoir. Both the bags and the masks come in variable sizes to fit patients from neonates to large adults. The valve must be open for oxygen to flow to the patient. Some devices have a built-in colorimetric end-tidal CO_2 detector (Figure 5-46 ●) or positive-pressure valves. Because of the risk of transmitting infectious diseases, bag-valve masks should be disposable. Do not reuse them.

Some BVM devices have a pop-off valve to limit the risk of lung injury from overaggressive ventilation. However, some patients with high airway resistance and/or poor lung compliance require high pressures for ventilation, so a mechanism to override the pop-off valve is essential.

Another variety of BVM bag is the anesthesia bag, more commonly called a flow-inflating bag, which does not self-inflate but instead relies on an adequate flow of oxygen. Oxygen flow into the bag and flow out of the bag may be adjusted to maintain appropriate volumes in the bag so that the bag is neither over-inflated nor subject to collapsing entirely with each ventilation. Because they are more complicated to use, flow-inflating-bag devices are rarely used in EMS except in critical care transport of neonates and infants.

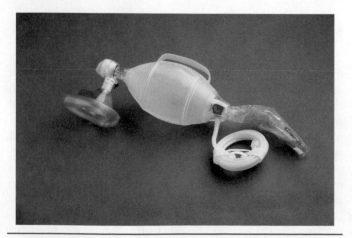

● **Figure 5-46** Bag-valve-mask unit.

Any patient who requires assisted ventilation needs supplemental oxygen, so high-flow (10 to 15 L/min) should always be used. Because of the attached reservoir, a bag-valve device can deliver 90 to 95 percent oxygen with these flow rates and a tight mask seal.

One, two, or three rescuers may perform bag-valve-mask ventilation. One-person BVM ventilation is the most difficult method to master, because obtaining and maintaining the mask seal while simultaneously delivering ventilations can be challenging, especially if there are secretions, facial hair, the need for high airway pressures, and/or the rescuer has small hands. Therefore, BVM ventilation should generally be performed with at least two providers, one to squeeze the bag and one to open the airway and maintain the mask seal.

Observe the patient for chest rise, development of gastric distention, and changes in compliance of the bag with ventilation. Complications of BVM ventilation include inadequate volume delivery if there is a poor mask seal or improper technique, barotrauma from overinflation of the lungs, and gastric distention.

Cricoid Pressure

Posterior pressure on the cricoid cartilage is referred to as cricoid pressure. Since the cricoid ring is the only complete ring in the trachea, posterior pressure on the front of the ring will be transmitted to the back of the ring and will hopefully compress the esophagus between the back of the cricoid ring and the front of the spinal column.

This maneuver became popular with the advent of **rapid sequence intubation (RSI)** as a means to limit regurgitation and subsequent aspiration. (RSI will be discussed in detail later in the chapter.) Recent evidence suggests that the risk-to-benefit ratio may not actually favor cricoid pressure during intubation, because cricoid pressure applied correctly to compress the esophagus often obscures the intubator's view of the larynx. Additionally, the esophagus does not always lie directly behind the cricoid ring, and the pressure itself causes a reflex decrease in lower-esophageal sphincter tone (actually working against the intended aspiration-sparing effect). However, cricoid pressure during BVM ventilation is likely to have a more favorable risk-to-benefit ratio and, as already noted, is recommended during optimal BVM ventilation if sufficient assistance is available.[12]

To locate the cricoid cartilage, palpate the thyroid cartilage (Adam's apple) and feel the depression just below it (cricothyroid membrane). The prominence just inferior to this depression is the ring of cricoid cartilage, which may be difficult to identify in female and obese patients. To perform cricoid pressure, apply firm downward pressure to the anterolateral aspect of the cartilage, using the thumb, index, and middle finger of one hand. If a lesser-trained provider is performing the maneuver, you should confirm that they are in the correct position (Figure 5-47 ●).

Use caution not to apply so much pressure as to deform and possibly obstruct the trachea; this is a particular danger in infants. The necessary pressure has been estimated as the amount of force that will compress a capped 50-cc syringe from 50 cc to the 30 cc marking. In the event that

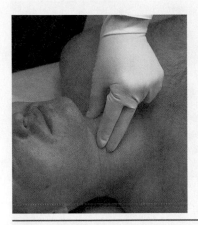

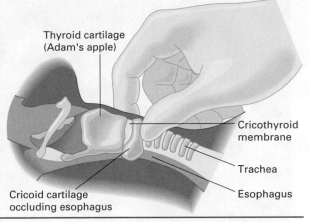

Thyroid cartilage
(Adam's apple)

Cricothyroid
membrane

Trachea

Esophagus

Cricoid cartilage
occluding esophagus

● **Figure 5-47**   Cricoid pressure.

CONTENT REVIEW

▶ The Rule of Threes for
Optimal BVM Ventilation

- Three providers
- Three inches
- Three fingers
- Three airways
- Three PSI
- Three PEEP

the patient actively vomits, it is imperative to release the pressure to avoid esophageal rupture. Similarly, if cricoid pressure is being performed during intubation, reduce or release the pressure if the intubator is having difficulty visualizing the vocal cords.

Optimal BVM Ventilation Using the Rule of Threes

The *rule of threes* was developed to help providers recall the components of optimal BVM ventilation. Many patients can be easily oxygenated and ventilated without using all components of the rule of threes. Whenever BVM ventilation is difficult, however, the rule of threes should be employed.

- *Three providers.* One provider on the mask, one on the bag, and one for cricoid pressure.

- *Three inches.* A reminder to place the patient in the sniffing position (elevate the head three inches) if not contraindicated.

- *Three fingers.* Three fingers on the cricoid cartilage to perform cricoid pressure.

- *Three airways.* In a worst-case scenario, the airway can be maintained, if necessary, with an orophraryngeal airway and two nasopharyngeal airways (one in each nostril).

- *Three PSI.* A gentle reminder to use the lowest pressure necessary to see the chest rise.

- *Three seconds.* A reminder to ventilate slowly and allow time for adequate exhalation.

- *Three PEEP.* Or up to 15 cm/H_2O positive-end expiratory pressure (PEEP) as needed to improve oxygen saturations.

Bag-Valve Ventilation of the Pediatric Patient

The differences in the pediatric patient's anatomy require some variation in ventilation technique. First, the child's relatively flat nasal bridge makes achieving a mask seal more difficult. Pressing the mask against the child's face to improve the seal can actually obstruct the airway, which is more compressible than an adult's. You can best achieve the mask seal with the two-person

BVM technique, using a jaw-thrust to maintain an open airway.

For BVM ventilation, the bag size depends on the child's age. Full-term neonates and infants will require a pediatric BVM with a capacity of at least 450 mL. For children up to 8 years of age, the pediatric BVM is preferred, although for patients in the upper portion of that age range you can use an adult BVM with a capacity of 1,500 mL if you do not maximally inflate it. Children older than 8 years require an adult BVM to achieve adequate tidal volumes. Additionally, be certain that the mask fits properly, from the bridge of the nose to the cleft of the chin. If a length-based resuscitation tape (Broselow tape) is available, you can use it to help determine the proper mask size.

To achieve a proper mask seal, place the mask over the patient's mouth and nose. Avoid compressing the eyes. Using one hand, place your thumb on the mask at the apex and your index finger on the mask at the chin (*C*-grip). Apply gentle pressure downward on the mask to establish an adequate seal. Maintain the airway by lifting the bony prominence of the chin with the remaining fingers forming an *E* under the jaw. Avoid placing pressure on the soft area under the chin. You may use the one-rescuer technique, although the two-rescuer technique will be more effective.

Ventilate according to current standards, obtaining chest rise with each breath. Begin the ventilation and say, "squeeze," providing just enough volume to initiate chest rise—being very careful not to overinflate the child's lungs. Allow adequate time for exhalation, saying, "release, release." Continue ventilations, maintaining the correct timing by saying, "squeeze, release, release." Use three criteria to assess adequacy of ventilations: (1) look for adequate chest rise; (2) listen for lung sounds at the third intercostal space, midaxillary line; and (3) assess for clinical improvement (skin color and heart rate).

Demand-Valve Device

The **demand-valve device**, also called the manually triggered, oxygen-powered ventilation device or flow-restricted, oxygen-powered ventilation device, will deliver 100 percent oxygen to a patient at its highest flow rates (40 liters per minute maximum). Flow is restricted to 30 cm H_2O or less to diminish gastric distention that can occur with its use (Figure 5-48 ●). Demand-valve devices have fallen out of favor because of the risks of gastric distension and barotrauma in unconscious patients.

► Extraglottic Airways

  • Retroglottic (dual-lumen)
    • ETC
    • PtL
  • Retroglottic (single lumen)
    • King LT
    • EGTA/EOA
  • Supraglottic
    • S.A.L.T.
    • LMA; LMA-Supreme; LMA-Fastrach
    • AirQ
    • Ambu Laryngeal Mask

► Since the majority of literature has failed to find a survival benefit to prehospital endotracheal intubation, and the procedure is associated with serious potential complications, many EMS systems are moving entirely to extraglottic airways or employing them earlier in the event of difficult intubation.

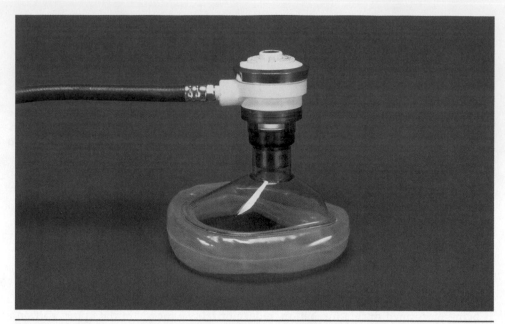

● **Figure 5-48**   Demand valve and mask.

PART 3: Advanced Airway Management and Ventilation

Advanced airway management has historically meant just endotracheal intubation and surgical airways (which will be discussed later in the chapter). However, it now includes placement of other invasive airways that do not pass through the vocal cords, such as extraglottic airways.[13–16]

EXTRAGLOTTIC AIRWAY DEVICES

Extraglottic airway (EGA) devices are inserted blindly into the airway to facilitate oxygenation and ventilation via a self-inflating bag or transport ventilator, but do not enter the glottis (the space between the vocal cords). Hence the term *extraglottic*, meaning "outside the glottis." Since EGAs do not enter the glottis, these devices do not require the use of a laryngoscope to visualize the glottic opening, although some of them permit it. Their insertion without laryngoscopy is described as "blind."

There are subcategories of EGAs, depending on where they actually "sit." Some sit in the esophagus, which places them behind the vocal cords (**retroglottic airways**); others sit above the vocal cords (**supraglottic airways**).[17]

EGAs may be used as a primary or secondary device depending on the provider's scope of practice and protocols and the clinical scenario. Use as a primary device means immediate use of the EGA without first trying to achieve endotracheal intubation; secondary use means use of the EGA only after an attempt at endotracheal intubation has failed. Accumulating evidence and experience suggest that EGAs are faster and easier to insert than an endotracheal tube and may be associated with fewer complications. It is very likely that these devices will play a growing role in prehospital airway management.

Retroglottic Airway Devices: Dual Lumen

Dual-lumen devices are designed to be inserted blindly into the esophagus but may still be used in the event of fortuitous tracheal placement. Clinical assessment is required to be sure that the correct port is used for ventilation. EGAs in this category include the Esophageal Tracheal Combitube (ETC) and the Pharyngeal Tracheal Lumen Airway (PTL).

Esophageal Tracheal Combitube (ETC)

The Esophageal Tracheal Combitube (ETC), also called simply the *Combitube,* is a dual-lumen retroglottic airway available in two sizes for patients over 4 feet tall. The ETC is inserted blindly through the mouth into the posterior oropharynx and then gently advanced—although directed esophageal placement using a laryngoscope is often employed in the operating room and may be employed by EMS providers if it is within their scope of practice. The tube may enter either the trachea or the esophagus (Figures 5-49 ● and 5-50 ●), but esophageal placement is most common. Since placement is nearly always esophageal, the port that ventilates in this position is longer, numbered 1, and is blue.[18, 19]

Advantages of the ETC

- ● Insertion is rapid and highly successful.
- ● It is time tested.
- ● Insertion does not require visualization.

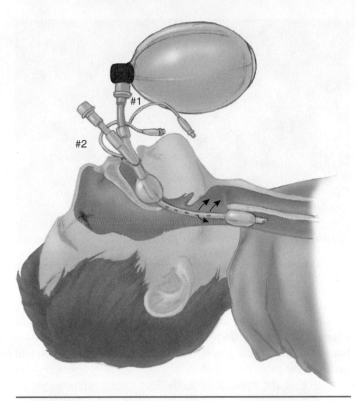

● **Figure 5-49** The Esophageal Tracheal Combitube (ETC) is a dual-lumen airway with a ventilation port for each lumen. The longer, blue port (#1) is the proximal port; the shorter, clear port (#2) is the distal port, which opens at the distal end of the tube. The ETC has two inflatable cuffs—a 100-mL cuff just proximal to the distal port and a 15-mL cuff just distal to the proximal port. First ventilate through the longer, blue port (#1). Ventilation will be successful if the tube has been placed (as is most common) in the esophagus.

● It will provide ventilation with either esophageal or tracheal placement.

● The large pharyngeal balloon may tamponade oral bleeding.

● It will generate high airway pressures for ventilation when necessary.

● It offers reasonable aspiration protection in either the esophageal or tracheal position.

● In the esophageal position, gastric decompression is possible through the #2 port.

● When intubating around the ETC, the proximal balloon may be deflated and the distal balloon left inflated to seal off the esophagus.

Disadvantages of the ETC

● Trauma, including esophageal perforation, has been reported.

● It cannot be placed with an intact gag reflex.

● High cuff volumes may result in tissue ischemia.

● It cannot be placed in patients under 4 feet tall.

● Clinical assessment is necessary to ensure ventilation through the correct port.

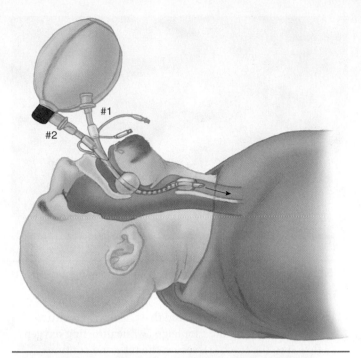

● **Figure 5-50** If ventilation through tube #1 is not successful, then ventilate through the shorter clear tube (#2). Ventilation will be successful if the tube has been placed in the trachea.

● It does not completely isolate the trachea in the esophageal position.

● Placement is not 100 percent foolproof.

Inserting the ETC

To place the ETC:

1. Perform optimal BVM ventilation with high-concentration oxygen.

2. Place the patient supine in a neutral position if possible.

3. Prepare and check equipment. Select a *Regular size* for patients 6 feet tall or taller. Select a *Small-Adult size* for patients less than 6 feet tall. Note that this sizing instruction is evidence-based but is different from the manufacturer's instructions.

4. Stabilize the cervical spine if cervical injury is possible.

5. Perform the **Lipp Maneuver** (or modified Lipp Maneuver) to preshape the ETC (Figure 5-51 ●).

6. Grab and lift the jaw or, if within your scope of practice, use a laryngoscope to create a channel and visualize the esophagus. Insert the ETC gently in midline and advance it past the hypopharynx to the depth indicated by the markings on the tube. The black rings on the tube should be between the patient's teeth.

7. Inflate the pharyngeal cuff with 100 mL of air and the distal cuff with 10 to 15 mL of air.

8. Ventilate through the longer, blue, #1, proximal port with a bag-valve device connected to 100 percent oxygen, while auscultating over the chest and stomach. If you hear bilateral breath sounds over the chest and none

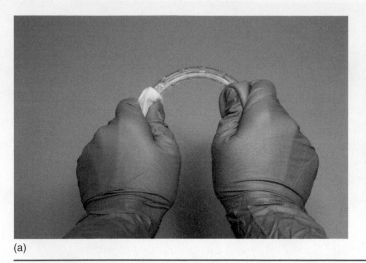

(a)

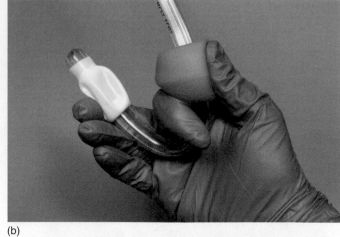

(b)

● **Figure 5-51** Lipp maneuver. (a) The Lipp maneuver and (b) the modified Lipp maneuver will aid in ETC placement and will help to minimize associated trauma to the airway.

over the stomach (indicating that the device is sitting in and occluding the esophagus while directing oxygen flow into the trachea), secure the tube and continue ventilating.

9. If you hear gastric sounds over the epigastrium and no breath sounds (indicating that the device is sitting in and occluding the trachea while directing oxygen flow into the esophagus), change ports and ventilate through the clear, shorter, #2, distal port to direct oxygen into the trachea. Confirm breath sounds over the chest with absent gastric sounds.

10. Use multiple confirmation techniques. End-tidal CO_2 is reliable with an ETC as long as the patient is producing CO_2. An esophageal detector device (EDD) may be used on an ETC by attaching it to the #2 port that is open on the distal end. Note that failure to inflate indicates appropriate esophageal positioning and you should continue ventilation through the #1 port. This is somewhat backwards compared to using an EDD to confirm endotracheal intubation. (The EDD will be explained in detail later.)

11. Secure the tube and continue ventilating with 100 percent oxygen.

12. Frequently reassess the airway and adequacy of ventilation.

Pharyngeo-Tracheal Lumen Airway (PtL)

The pharyngeo-tracheal lumen airway (PtL) is a two-tube system (Figure 5-52 ●). The first tube is short, with a large diameter; its proximal end is green. A large cuff encircles the tube's lower third. When inflated, the cuff seals the entire oropharynx. Air introduced at this tube's proximal end will enter the hypopharynx. The second tube is long, with a small diameter, and clear. It passes through and extends approximately 10 cm beyond the first tube. This second tube may be inserted

blindly into either the trachea or the esophagus. A distal cuff, when inflated, seals off whichever anatomical structure the tube has entered. When the second tube enters the trachea, you will ventilate the patient through it.

Each of the PtL's tubes has a 15/22-mm connector at its proximal end, allowing the attachment of a standard ventilatory device. A semirigid plastic stylet in the clear plastic tube allows redirection of the oropharyngeal cuff while the other cuff remains inflated. An adjustable, cloth neck strap holds the tube in place. When the long, clear tube is in the esophagus, deflating the cuff in the oropharynx allows you to move the device to the left side of the patient's mouth. This may permit endotracheal intubation while continuing esophageal occlusion. However, placement of an endotracheal tube with a PtL already in place is difficult at best.

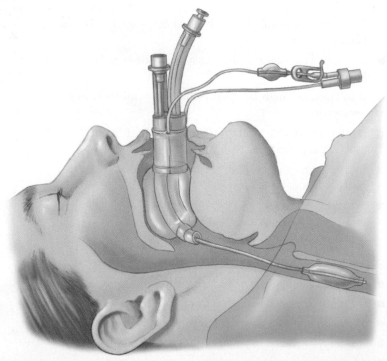

● **Figure 5-52** Pharyngo-tracheal lumen (PtL) airway.

Advantages of the PtL

- It can function in either the tracheal or esophageal position.
- It has no face mask to seal.
- It does not require direct visualization of the larynx and, thus, does not require the use of a laryngoscope or additional specialized equipment.
- It can be used in trauma patients, since the neck can remain in neutral position during insertion and use.
- It helps protect the trachea from upper airway bleeding and secretions.

Disadvantages of the PtL

- It does not isolate and completely protect the trachea from aspiration.
- The oropharyngeal balloon can migrate out of the mouth anteriorly, partially dislodging the airway.
- Intubation around the PtL is extremely difficult, even with the oropharyngeal balloon deflated.
- It cannot be used in conscious patients or those with a gag reflex.
- It cannot be used in pediatric patients.
- It can only be passed orally.

Inserting the PtL

To insert the pharyngeo-tracheal lumen airway:

1. Complete basic manual and adjunctive maneuvers and provide supplemental oxygen and ventilatory support with a BVM and hyperventilation.
2. Place the patient supine and kneel at the top of his head.
3. Prepare and check the equipment.
4. Place the patient's head in the appropriate position. Hyperextend the neck if there is no risk of cervical spine injury. Maintain neutral position with stabilization of the cervical spine if cervical spine injury is possible.
5. Insert the PtL gently, using the tongue-jaw-lift maneuver.
6. Inflate the distal cuffs on both PtL tubes simultaneously with a sustained breath into the inflation valve.
7. Deliver a breath into the green oropharyngeal tube. If the patient's chest rises and you auscultate bilateral breath sounds, the long clear tube is in the esophagus. Inflate the pharyngeal balloon and continue ventilations via the green tube.
8. If the chest does not rise and you auscultate no breath sounds, the long clear tube is in the trachea. Remove the stylet from the clear tube and ventilate the patient through that tube.
9. Attach the bag-valve device to the 15-mm connector, secure the tube, and continue ventilatory support with 100 percent oxygen.
10. Multiple placement confirmation techniques are again essential, as are good assessment skills. Misidentification of placement has been reported. Frequently reassess the airway and adequacy of ventilation.

If the patient regains consciousness or if the protective airway reflexes return, remove the PtL. It is best to remove the PtL before endotracheal intubation.

Complications of PtL placement include:

- Pharyngeal or esophageal trauma from poor technique
- Unrecognized displacement of the long tube from the trachea into the esophagus
- Displacement of the pharyngeal balloon

Retroglottic Airway Devices: Single Lumen

King LT Airway

The King LT airway is an airway with a large silicone cuff that disperses pressure over a large mucosal surface area (Figure 5-53 ●). This serves to stabilize the airway at the base of the tongue, thus minimizing the risk of injury to the vocal cords and trachea. The King LT airway allows up to 30 cm/H_2O ventilation pressures. It is supplied in three sizes: one for adults less than 61 inches (5 feet, 1 inch) in height, one for adults taller than 61 inches but less than 71 inches (5 feet, 11 inches) in height, and one for adults taller than 71 inches. The device can be cleaned, sterilized, and reused. A disposable latex-free version (King LT-D) is also available.[20–22]

The King LT-D is a disposable single-lumen retroglottic airway available in three adult and two pediatric sizes. (The "D" in LT-D means "disposable.") The adult sizes are also available in a King LTS-D model that has a channel to facilitate gastric decompression. The King has a large pharyngeal balloon and smaller esophageal balloon like other retroglottic airways, but both balloons are inflated through a single port with a single syringe. The King is able to generate significant airway pressures when needed and offers substantial aspiration reduction.

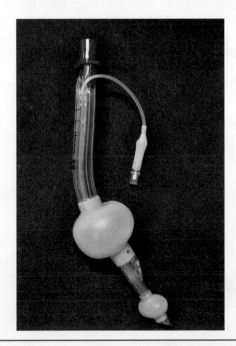

● **Figure 5-53** King LT Airway. (© *Edward T. Dickinson, MD*)

Esophageal Obturator Airway (EOA) and Esophageal Gastric Tube Airway (EGTA)

These devices were among the first extraglottic airways introduced. The Esophageal Obturator Airway (EOA) is a hollow, closed-ended tube with air holes at the level of the hypopharynx for ventilation, a distal cuff intended to block air from the esophagus, and a proximal end that fits into a mask. Ventilation, therefore, requires creation of a tight mask seal rather than relying on a large pharyngeal balloon. The Esophageal Gastric Tube Airway (EGTA) adds the ability to place a gastric tube through the distal port into the stomach for decompression of contents. These devices are now obsolete, since superior extraglottic airways have subsequently been introduced, although they still may be found in some areas.

Supraglottic Airway Devices

A number of supraglottic airway devices have been introduced, including the S.A.L.T. and various LMA devices.

Supraglottic Airway Laryngopharyngeal Tube (S.A.L.T.)

The supraglottic airway laryngopharyngeal tube (S.A.L.T.) is an extraglottic airway. It contains a central tube with a fenestrated (with an opening) end that overlies the larynx in the laryngopharynx (Figure 5-54 ●). It can serve two purposes. First, it can be used as a simple mechanical airway adjunct—much like an oropharyngeal airway. It has a collar on the proximal end and can be used with a BVM device. Alternatively, the S.A.L.T. can be used as a blind endotracheal tube introducer in situations where laryngoscopy is difficult or impossible.[23]

Laryngeal Airways

● Laryngeal airways are supraglottic airways. They are available in a variety of specific types, including the original LMA, the LMA-Supreme, the LMA-Fastrach, the CookGas AirQ, and the Ambu Laryngeal Mask.

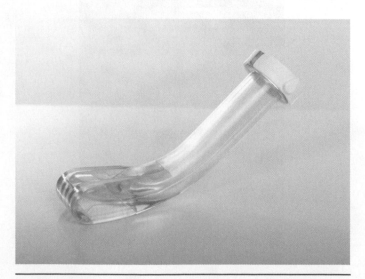

● **Figure 5-54**   S.A.L.T. Airway. (© *Microtek Medical, Inc.*)

Laryngeal Mask Airway

The Laryngeal Mask Airway (LMA) was the first laryngeal airway (Figure 5-55 ●). As this device is now off patent, there are multiple similar devices on the market. The LMA is commonly used in the operating-room (OR) setting for selected cases. EMS use was becoming widespread when this was the only supraglottic airway available. While the original LMA is easily inserted, EMS use of it is now limited because the LMA does not offer the features available in other, more recently introduced extraglottic devices.[24-26]

LMA-Supreme

The LMA-Supreme is an updated version of the LMA. The LMA-Supreme has several features that are very appealing for EMS use. The Supreme has a rigid design that makes for easy insertion without the need to place fingers in the mouth. The Supreme offers a very good seal against aspiration and facilitates gastric decompression through a separate channel. The Supreme can also generate high airway pressures when necessary to ventilate an obese patient or a patient with lung disease. Additionally, the Supreme has a built-in bite block and a fixation tab that makes it easy to secure the device with a single strip of tape (Figure 5-56 ●). The primary disadvantages of the Supreme are that the decompression channel will not accommodate a gastric tube larger than 14Fr, and blind intubation through the device is not possible.

LMA-Fastrach

The LMA-Fastrach was the first intubating laryngeal airway designed to facilitate blind endotracheal intubation with a special tube or a regular tube reverse loaded (i.e., with the curvature of the tube opposite to the curve of the device) (Figure 5-57 ●). The Fastrach is a rigid, anatomically curved airway tube that is wide

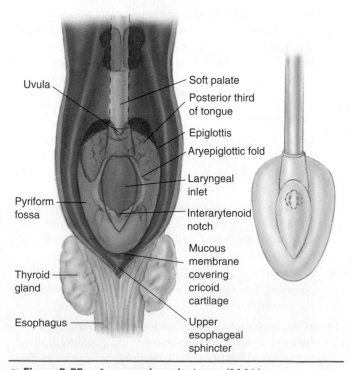

Uvula

Pyriform fossa

Thyroid gland

Esophagus

Soft palate

Posterior third of tongue

Epiglottis

Aryepiglottic fold

Laryngeal inlet

Interarytenoid notch

Mucous membrane covering cricoid cartilage

Upper esophageal sphincter

● **Figure 5-55**   Laryngeal mask airway (LMA).

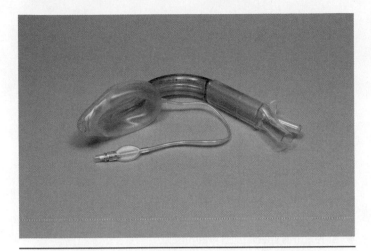

● **Figure 5-56**   LMA Supreme airway.

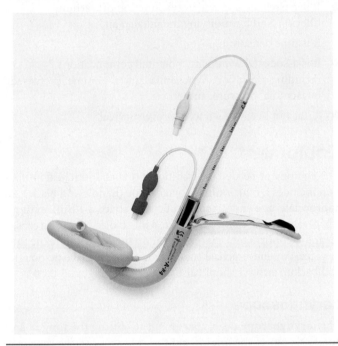

● **Figure 5-57**   LMA-Fastrach intubating laryngeal mask airway (LMA). *(Photo courtesy LMA North America, Inc.)*

CookGas AirQ

The AirQ is another intubating laryngeal airway (Figure 5-58 ●). In contrast to the Fastrach, the AirQ is available in pediatric sizes and looks much more like a traditional laryngeal airway. This shape allows intubation to be performed with an endotracheal tube introducer as well as with direct tube placement. The major disadvantages of the AirQ include the inability to decompress the stomach and the absence of literature validating the seal and success rates with blind intubation.

Ambu Laryngeal Mask

The Ambu laryngeal mask is a supraglottic, single-use, disposable airway (Figure 5-59 ●). It features a special curve that replicates the natural human airway anatomy. This curve is molded

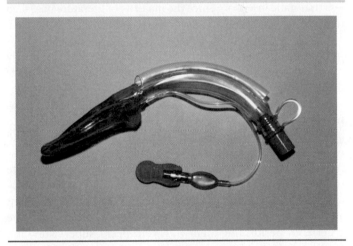

● **Figure 5-58**   CookGas AirQ airway. *(© Dr. Bryan E. Bledsoe)*

enough to accept an 8.0-mm cuffed endotracheal tube (ETT) and is short enough to ensure passage of the ETT cuff beyond the vocal cords. It has a rigid handle to facilitate insertion and adjustment of the device's position to enhance oxygenation and alignment with the glottis. There is an epiglottic elevating bar in the mask aperture that elevates the epiglottis as the ETT is passed through and a ramp that directs the tube centrally and anteriorly to reduce the risk of arytenoid trauma or esophageal placement. The Fastrach has been shown to have an excellent seal to protect against aspiration and generate high airway pressures when necessary. Extensive studies in the operating suite setting have demonstrated extremely high success rates with minimal training, even in obese patients and those with spinal precautions. Disadvantages include the inability to decompress the stomach, absence of sizes for patients less than 30 kg ideal body weight, and somewhat temperamental positioning for sustained bag-valve-device ventilation.

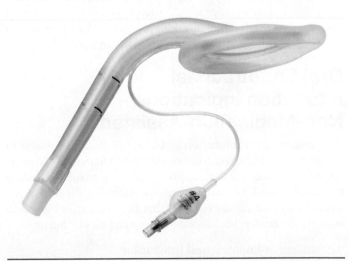

● **Figure 5-59**   Ambu laryngeal mask. *(© Ambu, Inc., Glen Burnie, MD)*

CONTENT REVIEW

▶ Endotracheal Intubation
Indicators

• Respiratory arrest
• Cardiac arrest
• Airway swelling
  (anaphylaxis; airway burns)

directly into the tube so that insertion is easy, without abrading the upper airway. The curve ensures that the patient's head remains in a neutral position when the mask is in use.

• It impedes gastric distention by channeling air directly into the trachea.
• It eliminates the need to maintain a mask seal.
• It offers a direct route for suctioning of the respiratory passages.
• It permits administration of the medications **l**idocaine, **e**pinephrine, **a**tropine, and **n**aloxone via the endotracheal tube. (Use the mnemonic LEAN or NAVEL [if vasopressin is added] to remember these medications.)

Disadvantages of Endotracheal Intubation

• The technique requires considerable training and experience.
• It requires specialized equipment.
• It requires direct visualization of the vocal cords.
• It bypasses the upper airway's function of warming, filtering, and humidifying the inhaled air.
• It is time consuming.
• It is associated with many potential complications including aspiration, hypoxemia, airway trauma, increased intracranial pressure, and others.
• It has not been shown to improve survival.

ENDOTRACHEAL INTUBATION

Endotracheal intubation involves inserting an endotracheal tube into the trachea, usually with direct visualization of the vocal cords—typically via direct laryngoscopy.

While endotracheal intubation provides optimal aspiration protection and ventilation, it comes at a high cost. These costs include prolonged scene times, potential airway trauma, and potential hypoxemia and aspiration. Furthermore, with this method you are bypassing important physiologic functions of the upper airway: warming, filtering, and humidifying the air before it enters the lower airway. As already noted, many extraglottic airways now provide excellent ventilation and significant aspiration protection with the benefit of much faster, easier, and less traumatic insertion. Since the majority of literature has failed to find a survival benefit to prehospital endotracheal intubation, and the procedure is associated with serious potential complications as discussed next, many EMS systems are moving entirely to extraglottic airways or employing them earlier in the event of difficult intubation.[27–30]

If you are performing endotracheal intubation, it is imperative that you select patients carefully (i.e., those most likely to benefit), perform the procedure correctly, practice regularly, and move early to a backup plan in the event of difficulty. Successfully accomplishing endotracheal intubation requires extensive training. Furthermore, you must maintain ongoing proficiency to ensure patient safety. To ensure the quality of your judgment and skill, you must continuously review field intubations and the criteria for performing them with your peers, supervisors, and medical director. Monitoring success rates for particular skills is not hard with an appropriate quality assurance program. Evaluating your ability to judge which patients you should intubate is considerably more difficult. Often it is better for the patient if you try other therapies before deciding to intubate.[31–33]

Oral Endotracheal Intubation Indications— Non-Medication-Assisted

Oral endotracheal intubation (OETI) is generally restricted to patients in cardiac or respiratory arrest or to patients in extreme respiratory failure that will allow such an invasive procedure to be performed. Intubation is particularly helpful in patients with anticipated airway swelling that may potentially go on to occlude the airway, such as anaphylaxis and airway burns.

Advantages of Endotracheal Intubation

• It isolates the trachea and permits complete control of the airway.

Equipment

The equipment needed for traditional oral endotracheal intubation includes a functioning laryngoscope (handle and blade), an appropriate-size endotracheal tube with stylet, a 10-mL syringe, a bag-valve mask, a suction device, a bite block, Magill forceps, a means to confirm tube placement, and a means to secure the tube in place. An endotracheal tube introducer (gum-elastic bougie) and backup airways should also be available (Figure 5-60 ●).

Laryngoscope

The **laryngoscope** is an instrument for lifting the tongue and epiglottis out of the line-of-sight so that you can see the vocal cords. You will typically use it to place an endotracheal tube, but you may also use it in conjunction with Magill forceps

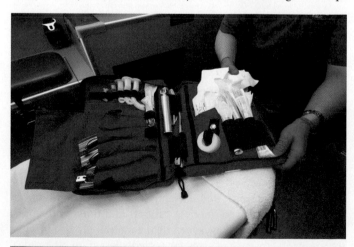

● **Figure 5-60** Airway roll and necessary airway management equipment and supplies.

to retrieve a foreign body obstructing the upper airway or to place retroglottic airways such as the Esophageal-Tracheal Combitube.

A laryngoscope consists of a handle and a blade. The handle may be either reusable or disposable. It houses batteries that power a light in the blade's distal tip. This light illuminates the airway, making it easier to see upper airway structures. The point attaching the handle and the blade is called the fitting; it locks the blade in place and provides electrical contact between the batteries and the bulb (Figure 5-61 ●). To prepare for intubation, attach the indentation on the proximal end of the laryngoscope's blade to the bar of the handle. It will click into place when properly seated. To determine if the laryngoscope is functional, raise the blade to a right angle with the handle until it clicks into place (Figure 5-62 ●). The light should turn on and be bright and steady. A yellow, flickering light will not sufficiently illuminate the anatomical structures. If the light fails to go on, the problem may be either dead batteries or a loose bulb. Every airway kit should include spare parts. Infrequently,

the contact points or the wire that runs through the blade to the bulb will fail.

Like the handle, the blade may be reusable or disposable. Blades may be divided into two types: curved and straight. The major variety of curved blades are called Macintosh, while there are several varieties of straight blades including, but not limited to, the Miller, Philips, and Wisconsin. Each has various advantages and proponents. Laryngoscope blades range in size from 00 for premature infants to 4 for large adults (Figure 5-63 ●).

The curved blade has a large flange for sweeping the tongue from the right side of the mouth to the left side and is generally inserted slowly, looking progressively for the base of the tongue and epiglottis. The curved blade is designed to fit into the vallecula (Figure 5-64 ●) and trigger a ligament that connects the epiglottis to the base of the tongue: the hyoepiglottic ligament. This will raise the epiglottis so that you can see the glottic opening.

The straight blades are designed to fit under the epiglottis and manually lift it out of the way (Figure 5-65 ●). The straight blade has no flange for sweeping the tongue and is best used by placing and maintaining it in the right side of the mouth, between the tongue and teeth (hence sometimes called "paraglossal" or "retromolar"), and directing the distal tip toward the midline. The straight blade may either be inserted progressively, as with a curved blade, or with a "hub technique," in which the entire blade is gently inserted into the esophagus all the way to the hub and then withdrawn slowly until the epiglottis pops into view. Because the blade and handle are on the right side of the mouth, there is limited working room, so an endotracheal tube introducer (described later) is often helpful to facilitate tube placement.

Several newer laryngoscope blades have been developed to aid in adequately visualizing the anterior airway, such as the ViewMax™, Grandview™, and articulating tip blades (Figures 5-66 ● and 5-67 ●).

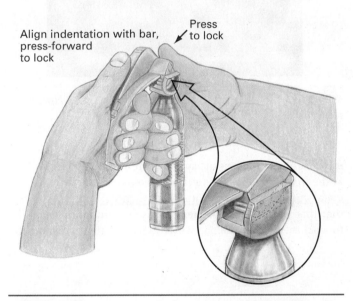

Align indentation with bar, press-forward to lock

Press to lock

● **Figure 5-61** Engaging the laryngoscope blade and handle.

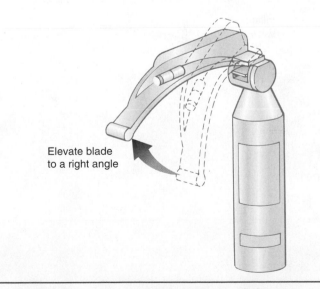

Elevate blade to a right angle

● **Figure 5-62** Activating the laryngoscope light source.

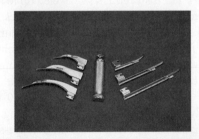

● **Figure 5-63** Laryngoscope blades in various sizes.

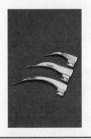

● **Figure 5-64** Curved blades in a variety of sizes.

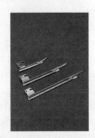

● **Figure 5-65** Straight blades in a variety of sizes.

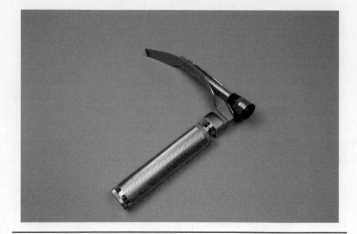

● **Figure 5-66**   ViewMax™ laryngoscope blade.

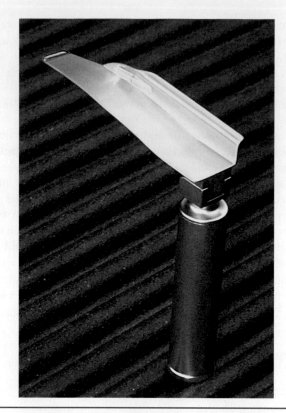

● **Figure 5-67**   Grandview laryngoscope blade. (© *Hartwell Medical*)

The choice of straight or curved blade is often a matter of experience and provider preference. In most patients, either will be adequate. Many providers find a curved blade easier to use, although this is often because straight-blade training has been limited. The straight-blade technique is worth mastering, however, as a straight blade combined with a bougie is often the "go-to technique" among experienced intubators for managing the difficult airway, particularly when only the epiglottis can be visualized. A straight blade is often better for endotracheal intubation in infants, because it helps to lift the relatively large and floppy epiglottis, although a curved blade may be useful to control a large infant tongue.

Endotracheal Tubes

The **endotracheal tube (ETT)** is a flexible translucent tube open at both ends and available in lengths ranging from 12 to 32 cm, with centimeter markings along its length (Figure 5-68 ●). The distal end has a beveled tip to facilitate smooth movement through airway passages. The proximal end has a standard 15-mm inside diameter and 22-mm outside diameter connector that attaches to the ventilatory device, usually either a self-inflating bag or a mechanical ventilator. The ETT is available with internal tube diameters ranging from 2.5 to 9.0 mm, which is clearly marked on the tube and packaging. The typical tube size is 7.0 to 7.5 mm for an average-sized female and 7.5 to 8.0 mm for average-sized adult males. (We discuss endotracheal intubation of children in detail later in this chapter.)

Adult tubes come with an inflatable cuff at the distal end to provide a seal between the tube and the trachea. Pediatric tubes are available with or without a cuff. Historically, only uncuffed tubes were placed in pediatric patients, but now it is common practice to use a cuffed tube in infants and older children. A thin inflation tube runs the length of the main tube from the distal cuff to a syringe. A one-way valve at the proximal end of the inflation tube permits the syringe to push air into the distal cuff or pull it out but prevents air from

escaping the cuff when the syringe is removed. A pilot balloon at the inflation tube's proximal end helps indicate whether the distal cuff is properly inflated, although evidence has shown that this is highly unreliable. Because overinflation may lead to tracheal mucosal damage, it is suggested that a manometer

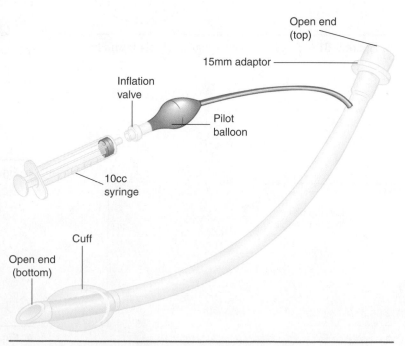

● **Figure 5-68**   ETT and syringe.

be used to ensure proper pressures, especially during longer transports. Alternatively, paramedics should learn to listen for air leakage and place only enough air in the cuff to inflate it without causing a leak. Always check the distal cuff for leaks before insertion.

Suppliers typically prewrap an ETT in a gently curved shape. This is because the trachea lies anteriorly in the neck, and the tube must be directed upward to enter the glottic opening. Stylets may be used to make further shape enhancements. Another variation is the Endotrol® ETT, which has a proximal O-shaped ring attached to a plastic wire that runs the length of the tube and terminates distally (Figure 5-69 ●). Pulling the ring bends the distal end of the tube upward and directs it into the glottic opening. This can facilitate placement of the tube without the need for a stylet, primarily during nasotracheal intubation.

Stylet

The malleable **stylet** is a plastic-covered metal wire that may be placed inside the ETT, stopping just short of the distal end, to allow the tube to be stiffened and maintained in the optimal shape for intubation (Figure 5-70 ●). Research has now shown that the optimal shape in most cases is "straight-to-cuff" with the distal tip angulated less than 35 degrees (Figure 5-71 ●). Anesthesiologists and anesthetists often avoid using stylets, as they may increase the chance of airway trauma. Stylets are

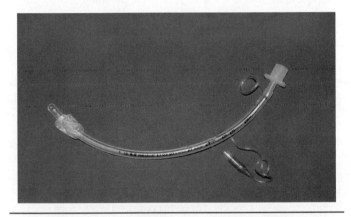

● **Figure 5-69**   Endotrol ETT.

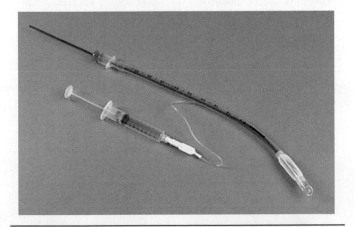

● **Figure 5-70**   ETT, stylet, and syringe, unassembled.
(© Dr. Bryan E. Bledsoe)

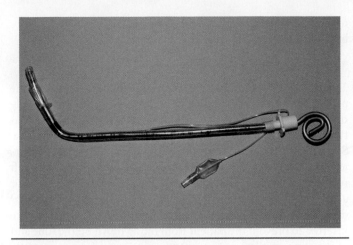

● **Figure 5-71**   ETT, stylet, and syringe, assembled for intubation with "straight-to-cuff" configuration of stylet and tube. (© Dr. Bryan E. Bledsoe)

frequently used in EMS and emergency medicine to enhance control of the ETT and potentially improve intubation success, particularly in patients with challenging anatomy, but you need to use the stylet gently to minimize the possibility of airway trauma. Alternatively, you may attempt intubation without a stylet and have a tracheal tube introducer at the ready in case you encounter difficulty.

Endotracheal Tube Introducer

The **endotracheal tube introducer**, commonly called a *gum-elastic bougie*, is a 60- or 70-cm straight, semi-rigid, stylet-like device with a distal bent tip that is covered with a protective resin (Figure 5-72 ●). It is used to facilitate endotracheal intubations when only the epiglottis may be visualized—that is, "semi-blind" intubations or Cormack-LeHane Class 3 views (discussed later in this chapter). Tactile feedback is used to determine the correct intratracheal positioning, and once that positioning is achieved, an endotracheal tube can be passed over the introducer into the trachea. This is discussed further under "Objective Techniques" later in this chapter.

10 mL Syringe

The syringe allows you to inflate the distal cuff to avoid air leaks around the tube. Although a 10 mL syringe is commonly used, this much air is rarely, if ever, necessary and may cause tracheal ischemia. Use a manometer to gauge the correct volume, or listen

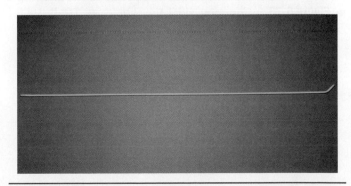

● **Figure 5-72**   Gum elastic Bougie. (© Dr. Bryan E. Bledsoe)

for air leakage with ventilation. Assessment of the pilot balloon has been shown to be inadequate for determining safe cuff volumes.

Tube-Holding Devices

The reasons for securing the ETT are twofold. First, moving the patient about during resuscitation or transportation can easily dislodge the tube and cause cardiovascular stimulation, an elevation in intracranial pressure, or injury to the tracheal mucosa. Second, the person providing ventilatory support may inadvertently push down on the ETT, forcing it into the right or left mainstem bronchus. The tube may be secured with tape, cloth, or a commercial device (Figure 5-73 ●). If not using a commercial device that has an integral bite block, an oral airway should be inserted to prevent the patient from biting down on the tube and obstructing ventilation. Note that the airway need not be correctly sized nor inserted in a rotary manner when used in this manner.

Magill Forceps

The **Magill forceps** are scissor-style clamps with circular tips used primarily to remove foreign bodies in the airway (Figure 5-74 ●).

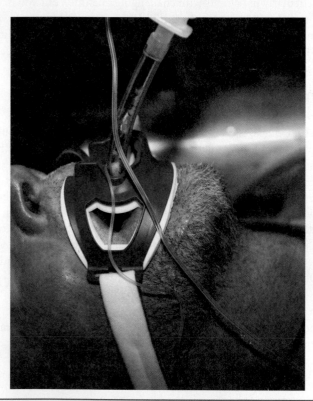

● **Figure 5-73**   Commercial ET tube holder. (© *Dr. Bryan E. Bledsoe*)

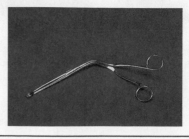

● **Figure 5-74**   Magill forceps.

Lubricant

Water-soluble lubricants facilitate inserting the ETT. Do not use petroleum-based lubricants; they may damage the ETT and cause tracheal inflammation.

Suction Unit

A suction unit helps to remove secretions and foreign materials from the oropharynx during intubation attempts. It is a vital

LEGAL CONSIDERATIONS

Negligence and Malpractice Suits. *Although negligence and malpractice lawsuits against EMS personnel are relatively uncommon, many of those that do arise involve airway management. Airway issues may result in death or serious disability, so paramedics must take great care to ensure that airway management procedures are properly performed. In systems not using medication-assisted intubation, the most common source of airway-related claims is unrecognized esophageal intubation. Systems performing medication-assisted intubation also expose themselves to claims related to inappropriate intubation and failed intubations in patients who arguably may have done better without intubation in the first place.*

Your best line of defense is to be highly competent in these procedures. This starts with your initial paramedic education but must continue after school is completed. If you work in a system where there is limited opportunity to use your airway skills, then you should increase your in-service education and arrange to spend some time in the operating suite if this is available. When there, do not overlook opportunities to place extraglottic airways and to practice bag-valve-mask ventilation.

Always make sure that all airway equipment is functioning properly at the beginning of each shift and after each call. After performing endotracheal intubation, it is essential to confirm and document proper tube placement by at least three methods, including at least one objective means such as an esophageal detector device or capnography. Following intubation, periodically and obsessively check and confirm continued proper tube placement, especially after any patient movement. If there is a doubt in regard to tube placement, the tube should be checked or removed and mechanical ventilation continued by other means.

You must have at least one extraglottic airway available at all times as a backup and have a clear plan of when to use it based on your experience, patient condition, service or regional protocols, and local convention. Persisting in attempts to intubate with resulting hypoxemia, airway trauma, and aspiration is a common source of EMS airway litigation. If you are using medication-assisted intubation, you should carefully weigh the risks and benefits, including any predicted difficulties in airway management, before proceeding, and consider calling medical control in borderline cases.

Finally, clear and accurate documentation is imperative. Be especially mindful of documenting your indication for airway management, other options considered, tube confirmation, and any noted complications.

element that you must never forget. (This will be discussed in more detail later in this chapter.)

End-Tidal CO$_2$ Detector or Esophageal Detector Device

It is imperative that all tube placements be confirmed objectively using an end-tidal CO$_2$ detector or an esophageal detector device. It is not adequate to rely on subjective measures such as direct visualization, misting, lung sounds, or an absence of epigastric sounds.

Protective Equipment

Endotracheal intubation, like many airway procedures, carries the risk of exposure to body substances. Because of this, it is essential to employ Standard Precautions. These include, but are not limited to, gloves, mask, protective eyewear, and possibly a gown. Remember, personal safety comes first! Always use Standard Precautions.

Complications of Endotracheal Intubation

Intubation presents a number of potential complications. Properly attending to detail and taking appropriate precautions will help you to avoid many of these problems.

Equipment Malfunction

Equipment malfunctions consume valuable time when you are establishing an airway. Having a preassembled airway kit that is checked regularly will lessen the chances of this occurring. Ideally, someone should check the airway kit daily to be sure that all needed supplies are present and that the laryngoscope bulb, batteries, and blade are in good working condition.

Tooth Breakage and Soft-Tissue Laceration

Endotracheal intubation can easily injure the lips and teeth, but you can eliminate this hazard by carefully using the laryngoscope as an instrument, not a tool. Guide the blade gently into the mouth and avoid pressure on the teeth. When manipulating the jaw anteriorly, keep your wrist straight while lifting with your shoulder, using gentle traction upward and toward the feet rather than rotating and flexing your wrist (i.e., levering). All levers require a fulcrum—and the only fulcrums available in your patient's mouth will be his upper incisors. Having an assistant apply a jaw-thrust during laryngoscopy and paying attention to precise triggering of the hyoepiglottic ligament in the vallecula when using a curved blade will also minimize trauma.

If you use the laryngoscope too roughly, you can also traumatize the patient's tongue, posterior pharynx, glottic structures, and trachea. This can also happen if you direct the tube away from the midline into the pyriform sinuses, allow the stylet to protrude from the distal end of the ETT, or merely apply too much pressure to a styletted tube. In some cases, the trauma may be so substantial that the patient can no longer be ventilated with an extraglottic airway device or bag-valve mask. A gentle technique, attention to detail, and moving early to

alternative strategies in the event of difficulty are the keys to avoiding these traumatic complications.

Aspiration

Aspiration is the entry of stomach contents, blood, or secretions into the lungs. A common cause of aspiration during non-medication-facilitated airway management is placing a laryngoscope (or tongue blade or oropharyngeal airway) into the mouth of a patient who has just enough gag reflex to vomit but is too obtunded to fully protect his airway. Therefore, you need to be very gentle in placing anything into the mouth when you are not sure if the patient has an intact gag reflex. Rapid sequence intubation, discussed later, is intended to minimize the risk of aspiration through the use of a neuromuscular blocking agent that eliminates the gag reflex and prevents active vomiting. Use of a sedative alone to facilitate intubation without a neuromuscular blocker potentially creates a high risk for aspiration, as these drugs will depress the patient's ability to protect his airway without eliminating the gag reflex.

Elevated Intracranial Pressure

Intracranial pressure (ICP) can become elevated during intubation from the reflex response to stimulation of the airway with a laryngoscope and endotracheal tube, whether or not the patient is sedated and/or paralyzed. In most patients, this elevation is of no clinical significance. In a few rare patients with intracranial bleeding or masses who are on the brink of brain herniation, this increase can have significant repercussions. In such patients you can either avoid the procedure altogether, use medications to attempt to blunt the reflex response, and/or use a very gentle technique. The possibility of increasing ICP is one of the reasons why nasotracheal intubation is relatively contraindicated in head injury and stroke.

Transport Delays

Whenever an airway procedure is performed on scene rather than en route, it will add to the total out-of-hospital time. In some cases there may be no choice, but in other cases it may be possible to defer the intubation until transport or to perform a bridge procedure, such as placing an extraglottic airway or providing BVM ventilation. The paramedic needs to look at the big picture and decide if the underlying problem can be adequately treated in the prehospital setting by airway management or whether the patient requires an emergency lifesaving procedure that is only available at the hospital, such as a catheterization or surgery.

Hypoxemia

Delays in oxygenation from prolonged intubation attempts can produce profound, life-threatening hypoxemia. If the patient has a measurable oxygen saturation, it is simple to monitor and abort

CONTENT REVIEW

► To avoid hypoxemia during intubation, limit each intubation attempt to no more than 20 seconds before reoxygenating the patient.

the attempt as soon as the saturation reaches a predetermined cut-off level, usually 90 percent for patients with head trauma or stroke. For patients without a detectable oxygen saturation, it is much more difficult to know when to abort the attempt, although it is safe to assume such patients have very little reserve. One basic rule is to limit each intubation attempt to no more than 20 seconds before stopping to reoxygenate the patient. To gauge this interval, some paramedics were once taught to hold their breath from the time they stop ventilating the patient until they start again; this is no longer recommended, as it is very difficult to perform a complex procedure while holding your breath.

If you cannot pass the tube through the vocal cords on the first attempt, at least identify your landmarks and note any unique or difficult features that may be modifiable. For example, if you can only identify the epiglottis, this will warrant use of a bougie, or a very anterior larynx will prompt use of external laryngeal manipulation or better positioning. The absence of any identifiable landmarks should prompt placement of an extraglottic airway.

Esophageal Intubation

Misplacement of the ETT into the esophagus deprives the patient of oxygenation and ventilation. It is potentially lethal, resulting in severe hypoxemia and brain death if you do not recognize it immediately. It also directs air into the stomach, encouraging regurgitation, which can lead to aspiration. Indicators of esophageal intubation include:

- An absence of chest rise and absence of breath sounds with mechanical ventilation
- Gurgling sounds over the epigastrium with each breath delivered
- Distention of the abdomen
- An absence of breath condensation in the endotracheal tube
- A persistent air leak, despite inflation of the tube's distal cuff
- Cyanosis and progressive worsening of the patient's condition
- Phonation (noise made by the vocal cords)
- No color change with colorimetric exhaled CO_2 detector
- An absent waveform on capnography
- A falling pulse oximetry reading

If you have any suspicion that the tube is in the esophagus, remove it immediately. Perform BVM ventilation with 100 percent oxygen and either initiate transport, place an extraglottic airway, or repeat endotracheal intubation with another tube.[34, 35]

Endobronchial Intubation

If you pass the endotracheal tube successfully through the vocal cords and advance it too far, it likely will enter either the right or left mainstem bronchus, although it is far more likely to pass into the right mainstem, which angles away from the trachea less acutely

than does the left. In either case, the ETT then ventilates only one lung, and the result is hypoventilation and hypoxia from inadequate gas exchange. Also, when the bag-valve device **insufflates** enough air for two lungs into the smaller area of only one lung, it can create enough pressure to cause barotrauma, such as a pneumothorax, worsening the patient's condition. Findings in endobronchial intubation include breath sounds present on one side of the chest but diminished or absent on the other, poor compliance (resistance to ventilations with the bag-valve device), and evidence of hypoxemia.

You may avoid inserting the ETT too far by following these guidelines:

1. Advance proximal end of the cuff no more than 1 to 2 cm past the vocal cords.
2. Once the tube is positioned, hold it in place with one hand to prevent it from being pushed any farther.
3. Inflate the cuff and firmly secure the tube in place with tape or a commercial tube-holding device.
4. Note the number marking on the side of the ETT where it emerges from the patient's mouth at the teeth, gums, or lips. This will allow you to quickly recognize any changes in tube placement. Approximate ETT depth for the average adult is 21 cm at the teeth for women and 23 cm at the teeth for men, although this will vary.

To resolve the problem, loosen or remove any securing devices and withdraw the ETT until breath sounds are present and equal bilaterally. Be certain to deflate the cuff when pulling back on the ETT.

Tension Pneumothorax

Any tear in the lung parenchyma can cause a pneumothorax. This may occur from excessive pressure being applied to a healthy lung or normal pressures applied to abnormal lungs such as occurs in COPD patients or patients who have suffered recent chest trauma. If this is allowed to progress untreated, a tension pneumothorax may develop. A tension pneumothorax will adversely affect the other lung, the heart, and the structures of the mediastinum. Tension pneumothorax is marked by progressively worsening compliance (more difficulty in ventilating), diminished unilateral breath sounds, hypoxemia with hypotension, and distended neck veins. If you suspect tension pneumothorax, needle decompression of the chest is indicated, as described in Volume 5, Chapter 8.

Orotracheal Intubation Technique

Two paths for intubation are the orotracheal path (through the mouth) and the nasotracheal path (through the nose). The most widely used path for endotracheal intubation is the orotracheal route (through the mouth), because it allows direct visualization of the vocal cords and a clear view of the ETT's passage through them. Nasotracheal intubation will be discussed later in the chapter.

To perform orotracheal intubation in the absence of suspected trauma (Procedure 5–1):

1. Use Standard Precautions.
2. Place the patient supine and properly position the patient's head and neck. To visualize the larynx, you must align the

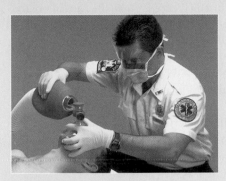

5-1a ● Ventilate the patient.

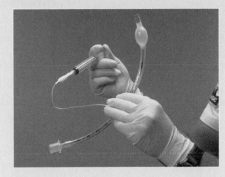

5-1b ● Prepare the equipment.

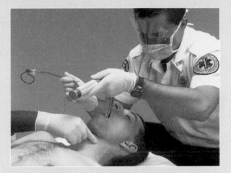

5-1c ● Apply the cricoid pressure and insert laryngoscope.

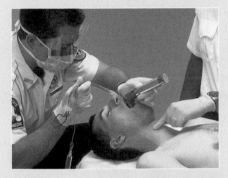

5-1d ● Visualize the larynx and insert the ETT.

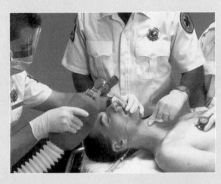

5-1e ● Inflate the cuff, ventilate, and auscultate.

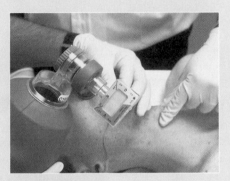

5-1f ● Confirm placement with an ETCO₂ detector.

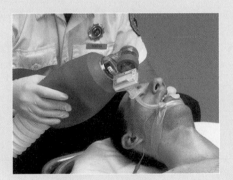

5-1g ● Secure the tube.

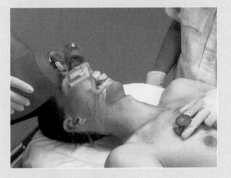

5-1h ● Reconfirm ETT placement.

three axes of the mouth, the pharynx, and the trachea. To do this, place the patient's head in a "sniffing position" by elevating the head and flexing the neck forward and the head backward. The ear and sternal notch should be on the same horizontal level. (Review Figure 5-38.) In obese patients it is necessary to place padding under the upper back, shoulders, and head to achieve the same position. This is called the "ramped position." (Review Figure 5-39.)

3. Perform BVM ventilation with 100 percent oxygen using the "rule of threes," as discussed earlier in the chapter under the discussion of BVM ventilation. Avoid aggressive

hyperventilation, as this is likely to fill the stomach with air and predispose to aspiration.

4. Prepare your intubation equipment as already discussed.

5. Turn on the suction and attach an appropriate tip.

6. Remove any dentures or partial dental plates.

7. Hold the laryngoscope in your left hand, whether you are right- or left-handed. Insert the laryngoscope blade gently into the right side of the patient's mouth. If using a curved blade, gently sweep the tongue to the left and work in the midline. If using a straight blade, remain on the right

side of the mouth. Your primary goal at this point is to visualize the epiglottis.

8. Advance the curved blade until the distal end is at the base of the tongue in the vallecula (Figure 5-75a ●). Advance the straight blade until the distal end is under the epiglottis (Figure 5-75b ●). Alternatively, with a straight blade, you may fully advance until the distal tip is in the esophagus and then visualize while slowly withdrawing the blade. If you cannot visualize the epiglottis, withdraw the blade, reposition the patient, and repeat.

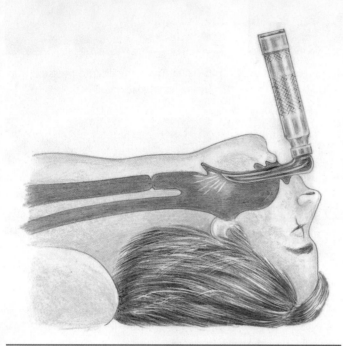

● **Figure 5-75a**   The curved blade is placed into the vallecula and indirectly lifts the epiglottis.

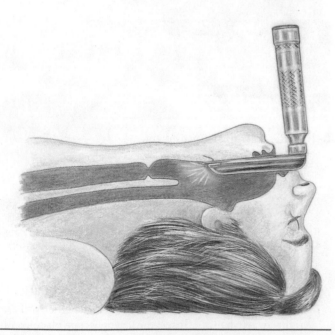

● **Figure 5-75b**   The straight blade is placed under the epiglottis and directly lifts the epiglottis upward to expose the vocal cords and glottic opening.

9. Keeping your left wrist straight, use your left shoulder and arm to continue lifting the mandible and tongue to a 45° angle to the ground (up and toward the feet) until landmarks are exposed (Figure 5-76 ●). Be careful not to put pressure on the teeth. Consider having an assistant perform the jaw-thrust simultaneously. At this point you may need to suction any large amounts of emesis, blood, or secretions in the posterior pharynx.

10. If you cannot see the landmarks clearly, have your partner release cricoid pressure. If you still cannot visualize the posterior cartilages, perform external laryngeal manipulation. You may not see the entire glottis or even part of it, but you should at least clearly visualize the posterior cartilages and interarytenoid notch.[36]

11. Hold the ETT in your right hand with your fingertips as you would a dart or a pencil. This gives you control to gently maneuver the ETT. Advance the tube through the right corner of the patient's mouth, and direct it toward the midline. Pass the ETT gently through the glottic opening until its distal cuff disappears beyond the vocal cords; then advance it another 1 to 2 cm. Hold the tube in place with your hand to prevent its displacement. Do not let go under any circumstance until it is taped or tied securely in place.

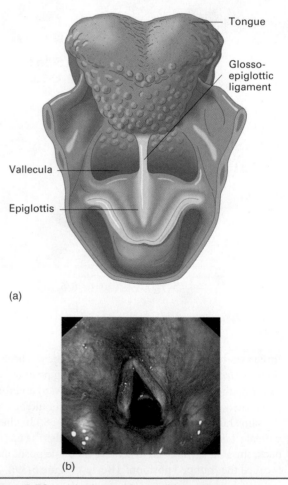

(a)

(b)

● **Figure 5-76**   (a) The epiglottis. (b) Laryngoscope view of the glottis, closed during the act of swallowing. (Photo b: © *Gastrolab/Photo Researchers, Inc.*)

12. Remove the stylet (if used) and attach a bag-valve device to the 15/22-mm connector on the tube.

13. Objectively confirm tube placement with capnography. In addition, check for equal breath sounds to be sure the tube is not too deep.

14. Ventilate the patient with 100 percent oxygen.

15. Gently insert an oropharyngeal airway to serve as a bite block, and secure the ETT with umbilical tape, adhesive tape, or a commercial tube-holding device.

16. Place the patient on the transport ventilator and monitor the continuous capnography waveform.

17. Reconfirm appropriate tube placement periodically, especially after any major patient movement or if there is any deterioration of patient status.

Verification of Proper Tube Placement

It is absolutely imperative that endotracheal placement of the tube be objectively confirmed immediately after placement and continuously throughout care, particularly if the patient is moved or deteriorates. You should employ a number of methods in the field to confirm correct ETT placement, but do not become overly reliant on technology. The patient's clinical condition should be the deciding factor in your patient management decisions. There have been countless EMS airway disasters related to unrecognized esophageal intubation. The common theme in these situations is excessive confidence and inappropriate reliance on subjective measures.

Subjective Techniques

Subjective methods of tube placement confirmation include direct visualization, tube misting, and auscultation for breath sounds. Well-performed EMS studies have demonstrated that reliance on subjective means alone results in a 10 to 20 percent rate of missed esophageal intubations. Therefore, subjective observations, although they are important, should not be relied on solely for confirmation of correct tube placement.

- *Direct visualization.* While seeing the tube pass through the cords should be considered the gold standard, this method of tube confirmation has failed. There are at least three possible explanations. First, in the emergency situation, visualization of the tube's passage through the cords is often unsatisfactory as a result of patient immobilization, positioning, or blood/vomit in the airway. Second, the tube itself often obscures visualization. Third, even if the tube is observed to pass through the cords, it may become dislodged when the stylet is removed and/or if the end-tidal CO_2 detector and BVM are attached before the tube has been secured. For these reasons direct visualization alone cannot be relied on to confirm tube placement.

- *Tube misting.* Observing mist or condensation in the tube, or a "vapor trail," has long been held out as a means of confirming tracheal placement of the tube, but it is not reliable. There have been many cases of a vapor trail noted with an esophageal intubation as well as cases when the vapor trail is missing with a correctly placed tracheal tube. Never make any decisions on tube placement based solely on tube misting.

- *Auscultation.* After intubation, breath sounds should be checked bilaterally and compared to pre-intubation breath sounds, unless ambient noise (e.g., in an aircraft) makes this impossible. Sounds should be present bilaterally if they were present bilaterally before intubation. Newly diminished sounds on the left with strong breath sounds on the right strongly suggest right mainstem intubation. Absence of sounds over the epigastrium should be confirmed. (Epigastric sounds suggest esophageal placement.) It is important to recognize that breath sounds have proved unreliable many times. This is particularly common in children (sounds are easily transmitted throughout the pediatric thorax), obese patients, and those with lung pathology. Like the other subjective means of tube confirmation, breath sounds should be neither relied on entirely nor ignored.

Objective Techniques

Objective methods of tube confirmation include capnography, esophageal detector device (EDD), endotracheal tube introducer, pulse oximetry, chest rise and fall, and presence or absence of gastric distention. Remember that objective methods such as these must be used, in addition to subjective observations, to confirm proper tube placement.

- *Capnography.* Detection of end-tidal CO_2 (capnography) is the gold standard for tube confirmation—if the patient is producing enough CO_2 to detect. As detailed previously, there are two types of end-tidal CO_2 detection: qualitative (indicating only if CO_2 is present or absent) and quantitative (providing a measure, usually with a waveform for analysis, of how much CO_2 is present). Either type is acceptable for initial tube verification. The quantitative detectors are better for ongoing monitoring, especially during air medical transport where clinical means are limited. There are virtually no false positive readings with these detectors. This means that if the detector says CO_2 is present, then you are not in the esophagus, but you may be above the trachea in the hypopharynx. On the other hand, false negatives may occur in the setting of cardiac arrest. During cardiac arrest, CO_2 production and transfer eventually cease. Therefore you may have the tube correctly in the trachea without evidence of CO_2 being present.

- *Esophageal detector device.* Use of an esophageal detector device (EDD) is another means of objective tube verification. A syringe device or bulb is placed on the end of the endotracheal tube to create suction (Figure 5-77 ●). If the tube is correctly placed in the trachea, the cartilaginous

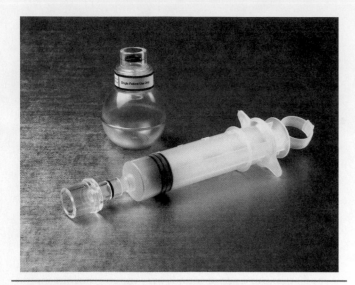

● **Figure 5-77** Bulb-type and syringe-type esophageal detector devices. *(Photo courtesy of LMA North America, Inc.)*

rings keep the trachea patent when suction is applied, so there is rapid air return into the device. If the tube is incorrectly placed in the esophagus, the soft distensible tissues occlude the end of the tube when suction is applied, so air return does not occur or occurs very slowly. These devices are inexpensive and are almost as accurate as capnography for detecting esophageal placements. In settings where most intubations are performed for cardiac arrest—that is, most EMS systems without rapid sequence intubation (RSI) capability—EDDs may be preferred to capnography since there is little point in measuring exhaled CO_2 in a cardiac arrest patient. These devices are FDA-approved down to 20-kg patients and have been well studied down to 10 kg. It is important, however, to use the "off-deflate" method in children: that is, squeeze the air out of the device before it is placed on the tube.

● *Endotracheal tube introducer.* While principally used to facilitate difficult intubations, an endotracheal tube introducer (bougie) may also be used to confirm tube placement. When a well-lubricated introducer is passed through an endotracheal tube that is correctly placed in the trachea, you should be able to feel it "hold up" (meet resistance) in the smaller airways within approximately 40 cm of the teeth or about 50 cm from tube end. (It has been said that you should also be able to feel "clicks" as the introducer passes over the tracheal rings. However, clicks may not be detectable because the tube bypasses most of the large rings of the trachea.) Absence of hold-ups at the depth where you would expect to feel them with a tracheal placement is an indication of incorrect esophageal placement.

● *Pulse oximetry and other findings.* As another objective finding, an increase in the oxygen saturation will help confirm proper placement of the endotracheal tube. Similarly, a rise and fall of the chest indicates correct endotracheal intubation. Worsening gastric distention may indicate esophageal placement. Any gastric distention should be investigated. Remember, though, that it is not uncommon for gastric distention to develop prior to

endotracheal intubation from mechanical ventilation. Even in experienced hands, it is very difficult to avoid gastric distention with mechanical ventilation until an endotracheal tube is placed.

Retrograde Intubation

Retrograde intubation is a technique in which a needle is inserted into the airway through the cricoid membrane from the outside, much like a needle cricothyrotomy, except it is directed superiorly rather than inferiorly. Once the needle is in the airway, a guidewire is passed through the needle and hopefully retrieved in the oral cavity and withdrawn through the mouth. An endotracheal tube is then passed over the wire into the airway.

One difficulty is that the guidewire must be withdrawn before the tube can be passed distal to the cricoid membrane, and that does not leave a lot of margin for error. Overall, the technique is not very rapid, so the patient must be quite stable. While some EMS services have embraced this technique over the years and used it successfully, there are not many cases where this would be the only viable approach. Retrograde intubation will probably be replaced by newer technology and simpler techniques, such as those making use of external laryngeal manipulation (ELM) and the gum-elastic bougie, which will be discussed under "Improving Endotracheal Intubation Success."

Optical Laryngoscopes

There are several devices that allow visualization of the glottic opening and associated anatomy using fiber-optic technology. Among these is the AirTraq®, a disposable device, available in a variety of adult and pediatric sizes, that transmits the view from the end of the device to a small attached screen via a prism mechanism (Figure 5-78 ●). The endotracheal tube is preloaded into a channel on the side of the device. Once the cords are visualized on the screen, the tube is advanced into the glottis through the channel. The tube is directable by redirecting the entire device rather than the tube itself. There is also an available video monitor that can be attached to project the obtained view onto a screen. Studies and clinical experience have found the AirTraq to be very successful, although the cost advantage of a disposable device is offset somewhat by having multiple sizes to stock with expiration dates and needing to use them regularly to maintain skills.

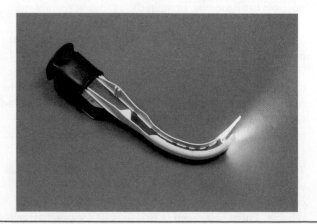

● **Figure 5-78** AirTraq.

Video Laryngoscopy

Video laryngoscopes have a camera on the distal end of the device that transmits a high-quality magnified image to a video screen that is either attached to the device directly or by a cable. The screen is held by an assistant, mounted in the ambulance, or placed on the patient's chest or bedside. The technique is considered indirect, in that the intubator looks at the screen while intubating, not directly in the patient's mouth, much like a video game. Studies with this technology demonstrate that it is superior to traditional direct laryngoscopy unless the pharynx is completely full of blood, emesis, or secretions. A number of devices are now available with a wide range of prices. None of these devices has been shown to be clearly superior to the others. This technology will likely replace traditional direct laryngoscopy in the years to come as prices come down (Figures 5-79 ● and 5-80 ●).[37]

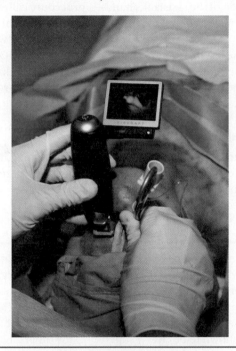

● **Figure 5-79**   McGrath video laryngoscope. (© *Dr. Bryan E. Bledsoe*)

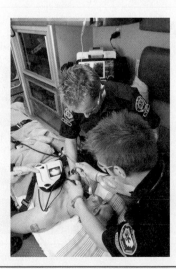

● **Figure 5-80**   GlideScope Ranger. (© *Kevin Link*)

Improving Endotracheal Intubation Success

Most studies of prehospital intubation show relatively poor success rates when using first-attempt and overall successful endotracheal tube placement as the marker of success. It is now clear, however, that physiologic parameters, such as maintenance of oxygen saturation and avoidance of aspiration and airway trauma during the intubation process, are far more important markers of success than the percentage of times an endotracheal tube is successfully placed within three attempts. It has also been demonstrated that success rates rapidly plateau after two or three attempts while complications go up exponentially. Therefore paramedics should strive to make their first attempt rapidly successful. How do we maximize the chance of rapid success on the first attempt? These include good initial training, ongoing practice, using the endotracheal tube introducer, managing neck pressure, optimal positioning, video laryngoscopy and other technology, and using rapid sequence intubation.

Good Initial Training

There is no substitute for being well trained from the beginning of your career. Bad habits are very difficult to break, and in times of stress we all naturally revert to what we learned first. Take your airway education very seriously and take advantage of every learning opportunity.

Ideally, you will be able to intubate a number of live patients under the watchful eye of an anesthesiologist or nurse anesthetist in the operating suite. Here you should focus on perfect technique and close observation of airway anatomy. You should also try to place as many extraglottic airways as possible if the opportunity presents itself.

During your field internship you will hopefully be able to intubate a number of patients under the supervision of an experienced paramedic where you can learn the ins and outs of managing airways in bad light, with lots of secretions, and with awkward positioning. The evidence suggests that at least 15 intubations are necessary for most providers to achieve at least 90 percent success in the operating suite, but more than 30 are necessary to achieve the same success in the field. Unfortunately, opportunities for operating suite practice for paramedics are very limited in some locales. You cannot expect optimal performance if you have not had sufficient experience, and your threshold for placing an extraglottic airway device should be lower, in that case, to avoid patient complications.

Ongoing Practice

Nearly as important as your initial training is the seriousness with which you maintain your skills. One study has demonstrated that patients cared for by a paramedic who had intubated more than 25 patients in the past 5 years did better than patients cared for by paramedics with lesser experience. If you do not intubate frequently in your practice setting, you should practice the basic motor skills and checklists routinely on a mannequin/simulator and visit the operating suite if possible.

Using the Endotracheal Tube Introducer

The endotracheal tube introducer (gum-elastic bougie) is a simple device that helps facilitate intubation when only the epiglottis is visible. It is a flexible device 60 to 70 cm in length that is stiff enough to be directable and to transmit tactile information (that is, you can feel its movements and responses) but flexible enough to allow a tube to be passed over it. There are disposable and nondisposable products of this kind, and each brand has a different balance of these properties, creating a unique feel and different performance for each, especially at temperature extremes. Some operators prefer to preshape the bougie, by holding it in a curved shape for several seconds before insertion.

Once the intubator identifies a difficult airway—despite optimal positioning, removal of the cervical collar with in-line immobilization and jaw-thrust maneuver, and external laryngeal manipulation—an introducer is placed into the pharynx with the *coude* tip (bent end) distal and anterior (Figure 5-81 ●). The introducer is then directed toward the likely location of the glottis.

If the introducer enters the airway, the operator may be able to feel "clicks" as the *coude* tip passes over each cartilaginous ring of the trachea. Since clicks cannot be felt in all cases, tracheal positioning should also be confirmed by hold-up, the resistance felt when the introducer passes into the smaller airways. If hold-up does not occur by the time the device has been inserted 40 cm beyond the teeth (introducers have a mark to indicate this distance), then it is safe to assume you are in the esophagus.

Once tracheal position is ensured, an endotracheal tube may be passed over the introducer while the intubator maintains an open channel with the laryngoscope. The scope is not removed until the tube is passed. A gentle counter-clockwise rotation of the tube over the introducer may be necessary to avoid its getting stuck on cartilages or cords. Once the tube is passed to the appropriate depth, the introducer is removed and the tube placement confirmed with the usual methods.

Many programs have introducers at the patient's side during all intubations. Some EMS programs have even adopted use of the introducer in place of a stylet for all intubations instead of waiting to use it only for difficult intubations. The introducer may also be used as a "place saver" if the glottic opening is swollen or smaller than anticipated, rather than withdrawing completely while preparing a smaller tube.

Managing Neck Pressure

As previously discussed, well-intended cricoid pressure can actually obscure the laryngeal view. If the intubator is having difficulty during laryngoscopy, he should direct the assistant performing cricoid pressure to reduce or completely release the pressure. If the view is still limited, the assistant should slide his hand up to the thyroid cartilage, and the intubator should move the larynx into an optimal position using his own right hand on top of the assistant's hand—a procedure called external laryngeal manipulation (ELM) (Figure 5-82 ●). A third option is to have the assistant apply backward, upward, rightward pressure on the larynx (the BURP maneuver) (Figure 5-83 ●). ELM affords the intubator the opportunity to use immediate hand-eye feedback to obtain the optimal view and is now generally preferred over the BURP maneuver.

Optimal Positioning

There is no substitute for a well-positioned patient. Unless contraindicated or impossible for reasons such as patient entrapment, all patients should be in a sniffing position or, if obese, in the ramped position.

Video Laryngoscopy

This technology is clearly changing how we intubate. Except in patients with excessive oral secretions, video laryngoscopy is superior to traditional direct laryngoscopy. As these devices become more affordable, they will likely take over EMS airway management. A number of devices are on the market, and none has been shown to be clearly superior to the others. Each device uses a different technique, but they are all very different from

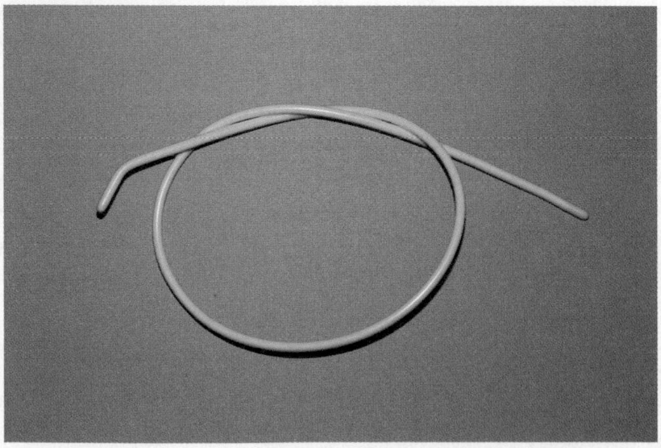

● **Figure 5-81**   Preshaping the bougie prior to use will improve insertion. Note the *coude* tip. (© *Dr. Bryan E. Bledsoe*)

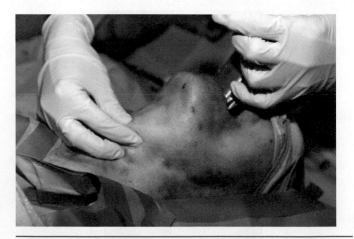

● **Figure 5-82**   External laryngeal manipulation (ELM) can assist with better visualization of the glottis and airway structures. (© *Dr. Bryan E. Bledsoe*)

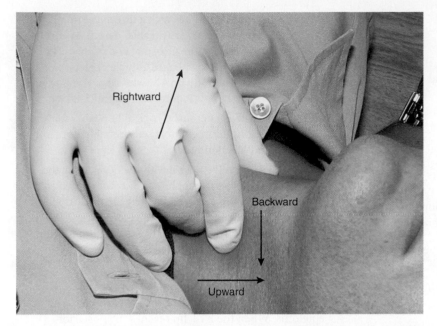

Intubating laryngeal airways allow for intubation with a high degree of success despite oral secretions, cervical precautions, and obesity.

Fiber-optic stylets combine the visualization common in flexible bronchoscopes seen in hospital operating suites and intensive care units with a rigid delivery device to simplify placement.

Most EMS services with a substantial budget are choosing video devices over fiber optics.

Using Rapid Sequence Intubation

Success rates with rapid sequence intubation (RSI) are routinely higher than success rates without RSI, although this may be offset by the increased potential for devastating complications. The balance of the literature to date has not shown improved survival with prehospital RSI. RSI is discussed in more detail later.

traditional direct laryngoscopy. If you have one of these devices, you will need specific training and regular practice in using it.

Other Technology

Other devices that may prove valuable in certain circumstances are specialized blades, lighted stylets, intubating laryngeal airways, and fiber-optic stylets. Most of these devices are much more affordable at this point than video laryngoscopes and will probably see greater use in EMS.

A number of different blades are available, including different shapes, different lighting mechanisms (e.g., IntuBrite), articulating tips, and attached prisms (Figure 5-84 ●).

Lighted stylets, such as the Trachlight, allow for intubation with a high degree of success despite oral secretions and cervical precautions (Figure 5-85 ●). The device is placed blindly into the airway with an endotracheal tube preloaded, and the intubator observes for a bright glow in the midline of the anterior neck, indicating tracheal placement. The tube is then slid over the device into the trachea. Unfortunately, this technique is more difficult in bright ambient light, with obese patients, and patients with very dark skin.

BLIND NASOTRACHEAL INTUBATION

As previously noted, the oral route is usually preferred over the nasal route for prehospital intubation. The **nasotracheal route** (through the nose and into the trachea) used to be very common in EMS, emergency medicine, and anesthesia but has generally fallen out of favor. In a few circumstances, however, the nasal route may be the best or only option, such as in the patient with trismus or with an anticipated difficult laryngoscopy, so this remains an important paramedic skill. When done by EMS, nasotracheal intubation is a "blind" procedure performed without direct visualization of the vocal cords; in the hospital setting it may be performed with direct visualization or fiber-optic guidance. It is important to remember that blind nasotracheal intubation (BNTI) requires a cooperative or unresponsive spontaneously breathing patient.

Relative Contraindications

● Suspected nasal fractures

● Suspected basilar skull fractures

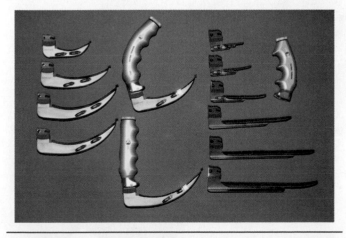

● **Figure 5-84**   Intubrite laryngoscope system. (© Dr. Bryan E. Bledsoe)

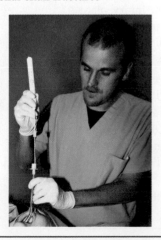

● **Figure 5-85**   Trachlight lighted stylet in use. (© Dr. Bryan E. Bledsoe)

- Suspected elevation of intracranial pressure
- Combative/uncooperative patient
- Coagulopathy, including therapeutic warfarin or heparin
- Significantly deviated nasal septum or other nasal obstruction
- Hypoxemia

Absolute Contraindications

- Cardiac or respiratory arrest

Disadvantages of Nasotracheal Intubation

The following disadvantages of nasotracheal intubation discourage its use unless clearly indicated by the patient's condition:

- It is often more difficult and time consuming to perform than orotracheal intubation.
- There is a significant risk of epistaxis (nosebleed).
- Smaller-diameter tubes must be placed, which makes ventilation more difficult.
- There is a significant risk of sinusitis, so these tubes must generally be changed out in the hospital.

The fact that there are so many contraindications and disadvantages means that many patients are not good candidates for this procedure.

Blind Nasotracheal Intubation Technique

To perform blind nasotracheal intubation (Figure 5-86 ●):

1. Use Standard Precautions.
2. Using basic manual and adjunctive maneuvers, open the airway and ventilate the patient with 100 percent oxygen.
3. Prepare your equipment.
4. Place the patient in his position of comfort. If the patient is unconscious or if you suspect cervical spine injury, place the patient supine and use manual in-line stabilization as appropriate.
5. Inspect the nose and select the larger nostril as your passageway.
6. Select the correct size endotracheal tube. Normally use a tube ½ to 1 full size smaller than for oral intubation. For an average adult male, a size 7 mm is appropriate. For an average adult female, a size

6.5 mm is appropriate. Tubes with a directable tip may make the procedure easier, if available. Attach an end-tidal CO_2 detection device to the proximal end of the tube. Alternatively, a device to enhance audible detection of breath sounds, such as the BAAM whistle or the Burden nasoscope, may be used (Figures 5-87 ● and 5-88 ●).

7. Lubricate the tube generously. Topical lidocaine may be preferred for long-term comfort but probably does not impact the initial attempt.
8. Insert the ETT into the nostril with the bevel along the floor of the nostril or facing the nasal septum, directed posteriorly. This will help avoid damage to the turbinates. There is some tendency to direct the tube upward, but recall that the nasopharynx runs directly anterior to posterior.
9. As you feel the tube drop into the posterior pharynx, listen closely at its proximal end for the patient's respiratory sounds, and observe for end-tidal CO_2. Sounds are loudest when the ETT is proximal to the epiglottis. When the ETT tip reaches the posterior pharyngeal wall, you must take care to direct it toward the glottic opening. This may be done with a directable-tip tube or by inflating the cuff, as the Endotrol tracheal tube. At this point, the tip of the ETT may catch in the pyriform sinus. If it does, you will feel resistance, and the skin on either side of the Adam's apple will tent. To resolve pyriform sinus placement, slightly withdraw the ETT and rotate it to the midline.
10. With the patient's next inhaled breath, advance the ETT gently but quickly into the glottic opening, observing exhaled CO_2. If you inflated the tube cuff to help with

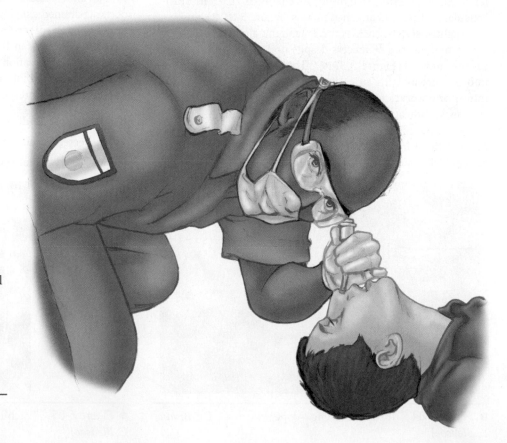

● **Figure 5-86** Blind nasotracheal intubation.

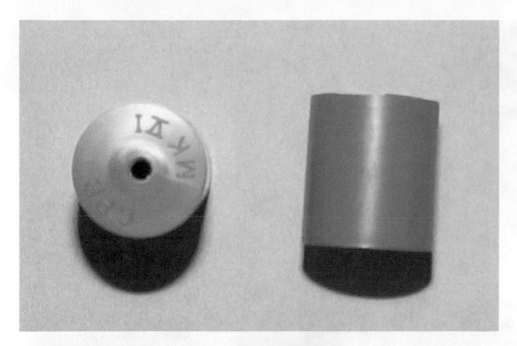

● **Figure 5-87** Beck Airway Airflow Monitor (BAAM) for blind nasotracheal intubations. (© *Great Plains Ballistics, Inc.*)

11. Holding the ETT with one hand to prevent displacement, inflate the distal cuff with enough air to eliminate any audible leak, connect a bag-valve device, ventilate the patient with 100 percent oxygen, and confirm proper placement of the ETT using multiple techniques, including bilateral breath sounds, absent epigastric sounds, and capnography.

12. Secure the ETT and reconfirm proper placement. Continue to observe the patient's condition, maintain ventilatory support, and frequently recheck ETT placement. Use continuous waveform capnography to monitor tube placement and ventilation.

DIGITAL INTUBATION

Digital intubation is another old technique that has largely been replaced by newer extraglottic airways and devices such as lighted stylets. However, digital intubation still may be a viable option in certain circumstances, such as a patient in a position that does not allow direct visualization, when there are copious secretions obscuring the airway, and in the event of equipment failure (Figure 5-89 ●). Digital intubation is risky for the paramedic; it may stimulate even a deeply comatose patient to clamp down and bite your finger. Do not use it with any patient who may have an intact gag reflex.

To perform digital intubation:

1. Use Standard Precautions.

2. Continue oxygenation with bag-valve mask and high-concentration oxygen.

3. Prepare and check your equipment. You will need the following items: an appropriately sized ETT, a malleable stylet, water-soluble lubricant, a 5- to 10-mL syringe, a bite block, and umbilical tape or a commercial anchoring device. Insert the stylet into the endotracheal tube and bend the ETT/stylet into a J shape.

4. Remove the front of the collar and have an assistant stabilize the neck as appropriate.

5. Place a bite block device between the patient's molars to help protect your fingers.

6. Insert your left middle and index fingers into the patient's mouth (Figure 5-90 ●). By alternating fingers, "walk" your hand down the midline while simultaneously tugging gently forward on the tongue.

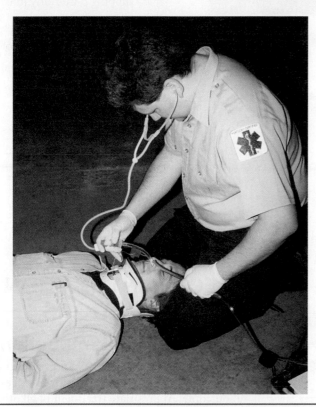

● **Figure 5-88** The Burden nasoscope, a commercial nasotracheal tube auscultation device. (© *Brant Burden, EMT-P*)

anterior displacement, the cuff must be deflated at this point. Continue passing the ETT until the distal cuff is just past the vocal cords, which should occur at a depth of approximately 26 cm in an average adult female and 28 cm in an average adult male. Coughing or bucking and anterior displacement of the larynx generally indicate tracheal placement, while gagging or vocal sounds indicate esophageal placement.

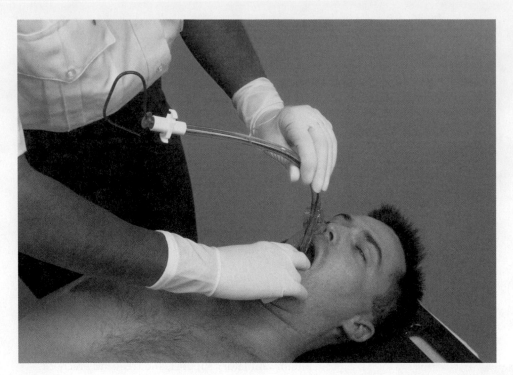

● **Figure 5-89** Blind orotracheal intubation by digital method.

8. Advance the tube, pushing it gently with your right hand. Use your left index finger to keep the tip of the ETT against your middle finger. This will direct the tip to the epiglottis.

9. Use your middle and index fingers to direct the tip of the ETT between the epiglottis (in front) and your fingers (behind). Then with your right hand advance the ETT through the cords while simultaneously maneuvering it forward with your left index and middle fingers. This will prevent it from slipping posteriorly into the esophagus.

10. Hold the tube in place with your hand to prevent its displacement, remove stylet, and inflate cuff.

11. Confirm placement with multiple techniques.

12. Ventilate the patient with 100 percent oxygen. Gently insert an oropharyngeal airway to serve as a bite block. Secure the ETT with umbilical tape. Repeat steps to confirm proper ETT placement and maintain ventilatory support. Continue your airway assessment periodically.

SPECIAL INTUBATION CONSIDERATIONS
Trauma Patient Intubation

Airway management and ventilatory support in the trauma patient are essential for a successful outcome. Appropriate treatment of all other injuries is meaningless if you do not ensure a patent airway and adequate oxygenation and ventilation.

The trauma patient, however, presents a number of obstacles to effective airway management and ventilation. These include difficult access, the need for extrication, blood in the oropharynx, distorted anatomy due to injury, and the need to protect the cervical spine. Getting an adequate seal on a mask is very difficult when the patient is being extricated or has significant facial trauma. You must keep the cervical spine in a neutral, in-line position throughout your management of all patients with known or suspected cervical spine trauma.

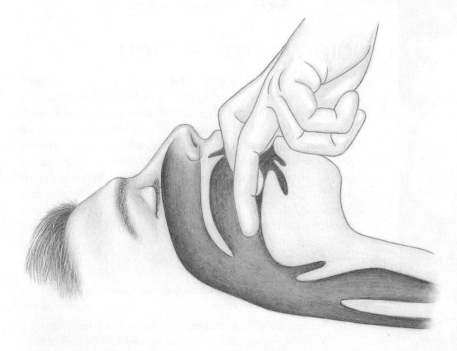

● **Figure 5-90** Digital intubation. Insert your middle and index fingers into the patient's mouth.

You may also use gauze to hold and extend the tongue more effectively, which lifts the epiglottis up and away from the glottic opening so that it is within reach of your probing fingers.

7. Palpate the arytenoid cartilage posterior to the glottis and the epiglottis anteriorly with your middle finger (Figure 5-91 ●). Press the epiglottis forward, and insert the endotracheal tube into the mouth, anterior to your fingers (Figure 5-92 ●).

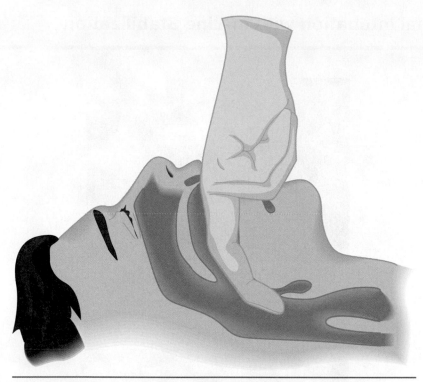

● **Figure 5-91** Digital intubation. Walk your fingers and palpate the patient's epiglottis.

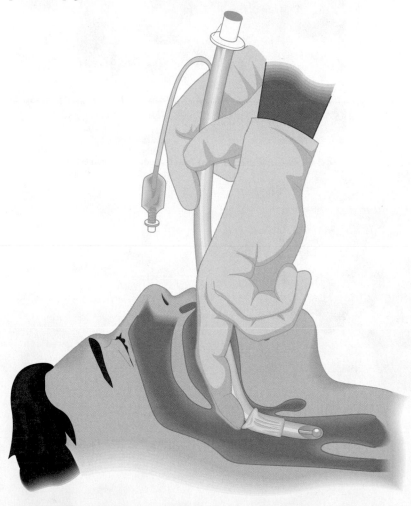

● **Figure 5-92** Digital intubation—insertion of the ETT.

Options for airway management include BVM ventilation, extraglottic devices, and intubation. Intubation may be performed with simple modifications of standard laryngoscopy techniques or others, using equipment such as lighted stylets or video laryngoscopy. Occasionally digital intubation or nasotracheal intubation may be employed.

To perform direct laryngoscopy with in-line stabilization (Procedure 5–2):

1. Use Standard Precautions.
2. Perform basic airway management including BVM ventilation with cricoid pressure.
3. Remove the front of the collar and have an assistant maintain in-line stabilization.
4. Immediately before laryngoscopy, have the assistant perform a jaw-thrust and release cricoid pressure.
5. Perform external laryngeal manipulation, and have the assistant who was performing cricoid pressure maintain optimal position of the larynx.

The trauma patient may present a number of obstacles to effective airway management and ventilation, including the need for extrication, blood in the oropharynx, distorted anatomy, and/or the need to protect the cervical spine. In addition, patients with nervous system trauma are very intolerant of hypoxemia. Therefore, you must have a plan to optimize your intubation attempts and must make early use of extraglottic airway devices.[38–42]

When a patient presents in a nontraditional position, the patient may still undergo direct laryngoscopy using an alternative approach such as a face-to-face technique. Alternatively, extraglottic airways may be used as a bridge until the patient can be positioned better, or they may be used all the way to the receiving hospital.

To perform orotracheal intubation on a trauma patient, you need an assistant who will both maintain in-line stabilization and simultaneously perform a jaw-thrust. Maintaining in-line stabilization of the cervical spine is, of course, critical for the trauma patient who may have suffered spinal injury. The jaw-thrust maneuver will not only open the airway but also will assist with direct laryngoscopy, since the patient cannot be placed into the optimal ear-to-sternal notch position.

It is imperative that the front of the cervical collar be removed during direct laryngoscopy to allow forward movement of the jaw. When using alternative techniques such as video laryngoscopy, intubating laryngeal airways, and lighted stylets, it may not be necessary to remove the front of the cervical collar.

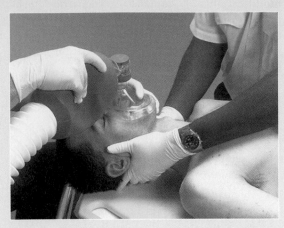

5-2a ● Ventilate the patient and apply manual C-spine stabilization.

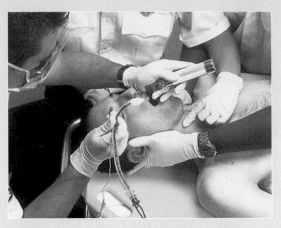

5-2b ● Apply cricoid pressure and intubate.

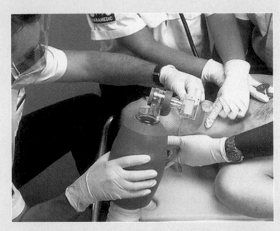

5-2c ● Ventilate the patient and confirm placement.

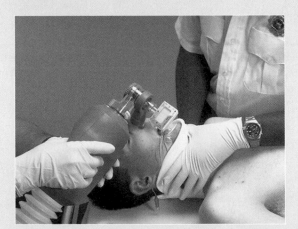

5-2d ● Secure the ETT and place a cervical collar.

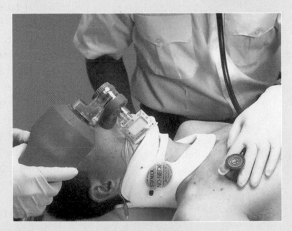

5-2e ● Reconfirm placement.

Foreign Body Removal under Direct Laryngoscopy

When confronted with a patient who has apparently choked, you should initially carry out basic maneuvers for airway obstruction that are appropriate to the patient's age and mental status, such as abdominal thrusts or chest thrusts. If these fail to alleviate the obstruction, direct visualization of the airway with a laryngoscope may enable you to remove an obstructing foreign body using Magill forceps or a suction device (Figure 5-93 ●). The procedure for visualizing the airway is identical to that used for orotracheal intubation.

Pediatric Intubation

Pediatric airway emergencies generally produce more anxiety than adult emergencies among both medical care providers and the family, although many airway procedures themselves are often easier to perform in this patient population. Historically, we have separated the parents and the child during resuscitation and critical procedures, but recent experience in the emergency department has shown it to be beneficial to have parents present. As difficult as it may be for the providers, children who are conscious usually benefit from having their parents present, and parents benefit from seeing all the efforts made to save their children, especially if these efforts are unsuccessful. The final decision on separation must be made on a case-by-case basis, by individual paramedics, in light of local protocols and customs.

A randomized controlled study in a large urban area comparing non-drug-facilitated intubation in children with BVM ventilation of children showed no improvement in outcomes with intubation over outcomes with BVM ventilation. Recent evidence also shows that extraglottic airway devices can be very effective in children. For now, the decision on whether pediatric intubation is part of the paramedic scope of practice and for what circumstances is determined locally.[43]

While airway management in children is similar to that for adults, there are a few important differences based on pediatric anatomy and physiology:

- *Structures are smaller.* The airway structures in children are proportionally smaller and more flexible than an adult's.
- *Nasal openings are small and adenoids are large.* Inserting any tube or device into a child's nose often causes trauma and bleeding because of the size and the presence of enlarged adenoid tissues.
- *Nasal airway diameters are inadequate.* Nasal pharyngeal airways and nasotracheal intubations are generally too large to be useful in the child.
- *Cricoid pressure can worsen the situation.* Because a child's cricoid is less rigid than an adult's, aggressive cricoid pressure can compress the cricoid and obstruct the airway.
- *Surgical airways are unavailable.* Surgical airway use is restricted to patients older than 6 to 10 years.
- *Tube size is critical.* Selecting the appropriate tube diameter for children is critical. Too large a tube can cause tracheal edema and/or damage to the vocal cords, while too small a tube may not allow exchange of adequate ventilatory volumes. Table 5–7 lists general guidelines for selecting ETT size according to the child's age, and many tables or devices based on the child's age, weight, or length are available. Another guide for children's sizes is this formula:

$$\text{ETT size (mm)} = (\text{Age in years} + 16) \div 4$$

Correct tube size for an 8-year-old, for instance, would be $(8 + 16) \div 4$, or 6 mm. You can also determine correct tube size by matching the diameter of the child's smallest finger.

- *Depth of ETT insertion is different.* The depth of insertion of the distal tip for pediatric endotracheal tubes should be 2 to 3 cm below the vocal cords, as deeper insertion may result in mainstem intubation or injury to the carina. The uncuffed ETT has a black glottic marker at its distal end that should be placed at the level of the vocal cords. The cuffed ETT should be placed so that the cuff is just below the vocal cords. For detailed guidelines regarding the depth of insertion for different age groups, refer to Table 5–7. Alternatively, you can use the formula described earlier.
- *The occiput is relatively large.* Infants will often require a towel roll behind the shoulders to maintain an open airway, much

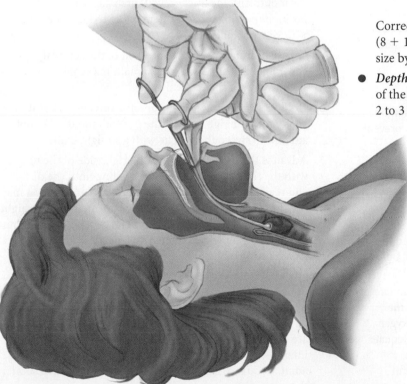

● **Figure 5-93** Foreign body removal with direct visualization and Magill forceps.

TABLE 5–7 | Approximate Size of ETT for Pediatrics

Patient's Age	ETT Size	Type	Depth of ETT Insertion	Laryngoscope Blade Size
Premature infant	2.5–3.0	Uncuffed	8 cm	0 straight
Full-term infant	3.0–3.5	Uncuffed	8–9.5 cm	1 straight
Infant to 1 year	3.5–4.0	Uncuffed	9.5–11 cm	1 straight
Toddler	4.0–5.0	Uncuffed	11–12.5 cm	1–2 straight
Preschool	5.0–5.5	Uncuffed	12.5–14 cm	2 straight
School age	5.5–6.5	Uncuffed	14–20 cm	2 straight
Adolescent	7.0–8.0	Cuffed	20–23 cm	3 straight or curved

the same way that older children and adults may require a towel roll behind the head.

- *The epiglottis is floppy and round ("omega" shaped).* A straight blade is usually preferred initially to control the epiglottis. An introducer may be useful if the glottis cannot be viewed.

- *The tongue is larger in relation to the oropharynx.* A curved blade may be useful to control the tongue during intubation.

- *The glottic opening is higher and more anterior in the neck.* Thus, it is easy to place the blade and tube too deep. External laryngeal manipulation (ELM) is useful to bring the glottis into view.

- *The narrowest part of the airway is the cricoid cartilage, not the glottic opening as in adults.* Uncuffed tubes were traditionally mandated on the theory that the narrow cricoid made the cuff unnecessary, although many current management protocols have changed, and cuffed tubes are being used more commonly. For now, most EMS services are still using uncuffed tubes for pediatric patients under the age of 8 years.

- *Greater vagal tone.* Infants and children are much more prone to bradycardia with hypotension during airway management, caused by hypoxemia or direct stimulation with the laryngoscope, or from succinylcholine. To prevent this complication, avoid long intubation attempts (see below) and be as gentle as possible during laryngoscopy. You must monitor heart rate throughout the procedure and stop the procedure to provide 100 percent oxygen by BVM ventilation or extraglottic airway device if the heart rate falls below 60 beats per minute in a child or below 80 beats per minute in an infant. You should also be prepared to give atropine (0.02 mg/kg, 0.1 mg minimum) by IV bolus, although this is never a substitute for oxygenation.

- *Higher basal metabolism combined with less functional residual capacity (smaller volume of air present in the lungs).* Children are more prone to a decrease in oxygen saturation during intubation attempts. Ensuring adequate preoxygenation, keeping intubation attempts short, and moving early to an extraglottic device are helpful precautions.

To perform endotracheal intubation on a pediatric patient (Procedure 5–3):

1. Use Standard Precautions.

2. Continue BVM ventilation with 100 percent oxygen while using a towel roll under the shoulders of an infant or towels under the head in older children (if not in cervical spine precautions) to achieve a sniffing position.

3. Prepare and check your equipment. As stated earlier, a straight blade is usually preferred in infants and small children, but it is suggested to have an age-appropriate curved blade available as well in case tongue control becomes critical. With children younger than 8 years, you will either use an uncuffed endotracheal tube or a cuffed tube that is a half size smaller than calculated with standard formulas. Because of the short distance between the mouth and the trachea, you rarely need a stylet to position the tube properly. Remember to lubricate the ETT with water-soluble gel.

4. In case of trauma, remove the front of the cervical collar and have an assistant maintain manual in-line stabilization of the cervical spine.

5. Hold the laryngoscope in your left hand and insert it gently into the right side of the patient's mouth. Do not attempt to sweep the tongue with a straight blade.

6. Advance the straight blade on the right side of the tongue with the tip directed toward the midline until the distal end reaches the base of the tongue. Alternatively, you may use the "hub technique" by initially advancing the straight blade gently into the esophagus as far as it will go without resistance, then withdrawing while performing ELM. If using a curved blade, sweep the tongue from right to left and advance in the midline.

7. Look for the tip of the epiglottis and gently lift with the tip of the blade while simultaneously performing ELM with an assistant's hand until the glottis or posterior cartilages are visualized. Keep in mind that a child—particularly an infant—has a shorter airway and a higher glottis than an adult. Because of this, you may see the cords much sooner than you expect.

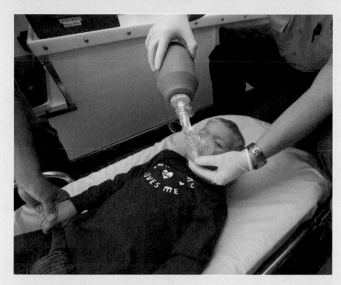

5-3a ● Ventilate the child.

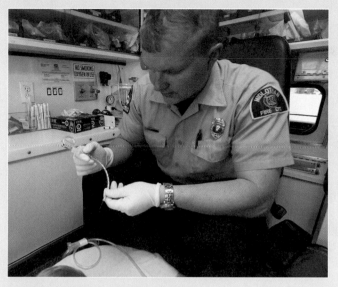

5-3b ● Prepare the equipment.

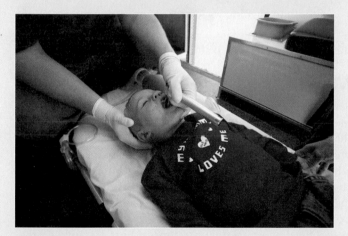

5-3c ● Insert the laryngoscope.

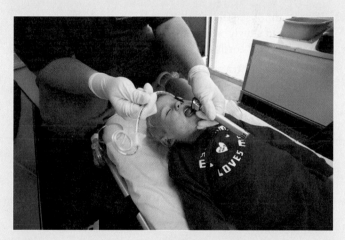

5-3d ● Visualize the child's larynx and insert the ETT.

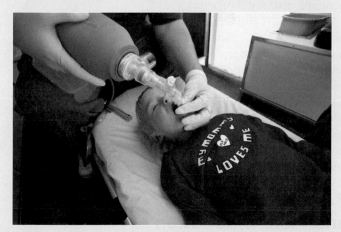

5-3e ● Ventilate, inflate the ETT cuff (if it is a cuffed tube), and auscultate.

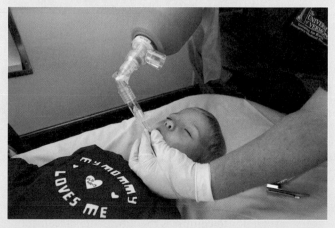

5-3f ● Confirm placement with an ETCO$_2$ detector or waveform capnography.

(Continued)

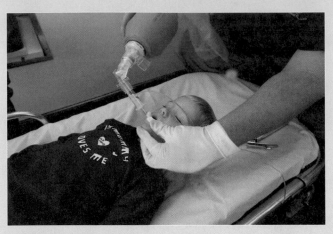

5-3g ● Secure the tube.

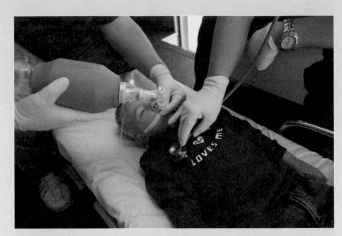

5-3h ● Reconfirm proper ETT placement.

8. If you cannot see the epiglottis, you are likely too deep. Gently and slowly withdraw while continuing to visualize until the vocal cords fall into view.

9. Grasp the endotracheal tube in your right hand and, under direct visualization of the vocal cords or posterior cartilages, insert it through the right corner of the patient's mouth into the glottic opening. Pass it through until the vocal cord marking on the tube is at the level of the cords or until the distal cuff of the ETT just disappears beyond the vocal cords. In some cases, advancing an endotracheal tube will be difficult at the level of the cricoid. Do not force the ETT through this region, as it may cause laryngeal edema and bleeding.

   Confirm correct placement of the ETT. Hold the tube in place with your left hand, attach an age-appropriate bag-valve device to the 15/22-mm connector, and deliver several breaths with an end-tidal CO_2 detector in-line. For additional confirmation, observe for symmetrical chest rise and fall with each ventilation. Also auscultate for equal, bilateral breath sounds at the lateral chest wall, high in the axilla, and absent breath sounds over the epigastrium. An esophageal detector device may also be used for patients over 10 kg as long as you squeeze the bulb before attaching it to the tube.

10. If the tube has a distal cuff, do not inflate it unless there is a detectable air leak. If a leak is audible, inflate the distal cuff with just enough air to stop the leak.

11. Secure the ETT with tape or a commercial device, being very careful not to compress the tube. Note placement of the distance marker at the teeth/gums, recheck for proper placement, and continue ventilatory support. Periodically reassess ETT placement and watch the patient carefully for any clinical signs of difficulty.

Continue ongoing waveform capnography monitoring if possible.

12. Place a gastric tube if allowed by protocol.

Monitoring Cuff Pressure

Several recent studies have shown that even experienced paramedics are unable to judge the pressure in an endotracheal tube cuff accurately by palpating the pilot balloon, and that cuff pressures may be way in excess of the recommended ranges. Similarly, we now know that excessive pressures can cause tracheal damage much sooner than previously thought. Combining these two pieces of information tells us that we must use extreme caution and vigilance regarding cuff pressures, because even if the prehospital transport time is short, it is unlikely that the hospital staff will assess cuff pressures in the initial management of a critically ill patient.

Ideally, cuff pressures would be assessed with a cuff manometer, but this is often not available. Second best is to place only enough air into the cuff to eliminate an audible leak. Providers may be surprised to find out that only 3 or 4 mL of air may be necessary to create an appropriate seal in some adults. A third option is to place only half of the cuff volume, but this may leave the patient at risk for both aspiration and tissue damage. Finally, some providers will inflate the cuff with 10 mL of air but leave the syringe attached for 10 to 20 seconds to allow any back-pressure to release.[44]

Post-Intubation Agitation and Field Extubation

Occasionally, an intubated patient will awaken and be intolerant of the ETT. This happens most often with patients who undergo rapid sequence intubation and then awaken from the sedative agent and paralytic. This occurrence usually indicates inadequate sedation/analgesia and/or inappropriate ventilator settings. Paralytics alone should never be given to treat agitation, as the patient will be fully aware of the paralysis (a harrowing feeling), even though his outward signs of agitation will resolve.

Only rarely should extubation be considered in the field, because this may be associated with serious complications such as aspiration, laryngospasm, and negative-pressure pulmonary edema—not to mention that the patient may deteriorate again and be difficult to reintubate. If the patient is clearly able to maintain and protect his airway, is intolerant of the tube and ventilator, no medications are available to make him comfortable, and reassessment indicates that the problem that led to endotracheal intubation is resolved (such as a narcotic overdose), extubation may be indicated.

To perform field extubation:

1. Use Standard Precautions.

2. Ensure adequate oxygenation. A crude method for accomplishing this in the field is to be certain that the patient's mental status, skin color, and pulse oximetry are optimal on room air with the ETT in place.

3. Prepare intubation equipment and suction.

4. Confirm patient responsiveness.

5. Position patient on his side if possible.

6. Suction the patient's oropharynx.

7. Deflate the ETT cuff.

8. Remove the ETT upon cough or expiration.

9. Provide supplemental oxygen as indicated.

10. Reassess the adequacy of the patient's ventilation and oxygenation.

CRICOTHYROTOMY

With proper training and frequent practice, including the use of rapid sequence procedures and newer technologies such as video laryngoscopy, you will be able to manage most airways in the field with BVM ventilation, an extraglottic airway device, or endotracheal intubation. Occasionally, however, extreme circumstances require a more invasive approach. In these situations, performing a cricothyrotomy may be the only way to ensure your patient's best chance for survival. Overall, however, the incidence of these procedures being performed in both the prehospital and hospital settings has fallen precipitously in the past five to ten years with the more widespread use of EGAs and RSI.

Two different techniques, **needle cricothyrotomy** (also called transtracheal jet ventilation or transtracheal jet insufflation) and **open cricothyrotomy**, both provide access to the airway through the cricothyroid membrane. A needle cricothyrotomy is generally the easier procedure but makes providing adequate ventilation more difficult; this approach is generally reserved for pediatric patients. The open cricothyrotomy technique is the more difficult procedure but allows for more effective oxygenation and ventilation. The open approach often takes longer than anticipated and has been associated with complications in up to 50 percent of cases. Therefore, you must master these techniques and reserve their use for situations in which you have exhausted your other options and have decided that no other means will establish an airway. Even when performed correctly, these procedures are highly invasive and prone to long-term complications, such as tracheal **stenosis**.

Indications that may warrant cricothyrotomy include situations that prevent adequate BVM ventilation, EGA placement, and endotracheal tube placement by the oral and nasal routes. An example is a patient with trismus (masseter muscle spasm that prevents opening the mouth), who cannot be oxygenated with a BVM ventilation, is also not a candidate for blind nasotracheal intubation, and presents in an EMS system that does not permit drug-facilitated airway management. Another example is a hypoxemic patient who has such severe facial trauma that BVM ventilation, EGA placement, and endotracheal intubation are not viable options. Other possible indications include total upper airway obstruction from epiglottitis or a foreign body, severe anaphylaxis, and burns to the face and respiratory tract.

Relative contraindications to performing cricothyrotomy in the field include inability to identify anatomical landmarks (including trauma and short, fat necks), crush injury to the larynx, suspected tracheal transection, and underlying anatomical abnormalities such as tumor or subglottic stenosis. There are no absolute contraindications to cricothyrotomy.

Needle Cricothyrotomy

Needle cricothyrotomy involves placing a large bore needle with plastic cannula, such as a 14-gauge intravenous catheter, through the cricothyroid membrane into the trachea. Oxygen must then be forced through this small-caliber device, using a bag-valve device or a high-pressure oxygen source. Ventilation by this route is called transtracheal jet ventilation or transtracheal jet insufflation. (*Insufflation* is blowing something into the body.)

Because very high pressures may insufflate large volumes of oxygen, **barotrauma**, including pneumothorax, is a potential complication. Exhalation is limited if it must take place through the same small-diameter catheter, which results in rising carbon dioxide levels. In some cases, the anatomy that required the needle cricothyrotomy for oxygenation does not impede normal exhalation.

In general, needle cricothyrotomy is considered a temporizing technique to be used for 30 minutes or less and restricted to pediatric patients in whom open cricothyrotomy is contraindicated. This technique has been removed from the paramedic scope of practice in some states because it is rarely used and there are few if any reports of it saving a life.

The potential complications of needle cricothyrotomy with jet ventilation include:

● Barotrauma from overinflation if using transtracheal jet insufflation

● Excessive bleeding due to improper catheter placement

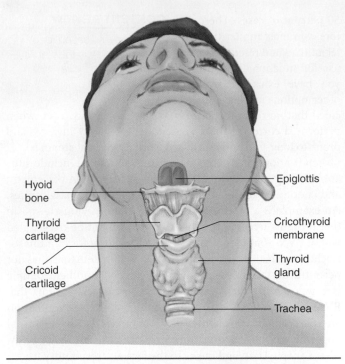

● **Figure 5-94** Anatomic landmarks for cricothyrotomy.

Hyoid bone
Thyroid cartilage
Cricoid cartilage
Epiglottis
Cricothyroid membrane
Thyroid gland
Trachea

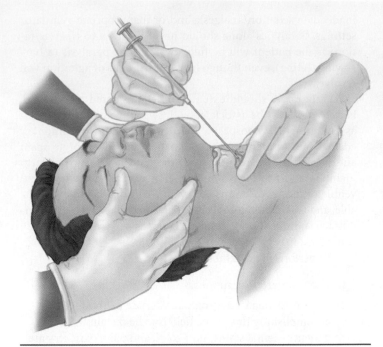

● **Figure 5-96** Proper positioning for cricothyroid puncture.

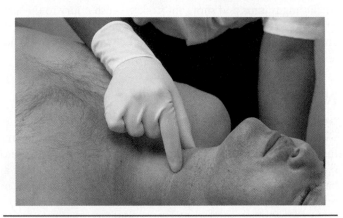

● **Figure 5-95** Locate/palpate the cricothyroid membrane.

- Subcutaneous emphysema from improper placement into the subcutaneous tissue, excessive air leak around the catheter, or laryngeal trauma

- Bleeding

- Hypoventilation and respiratory acidosis

- Aspiration as the airway is unprotected

Needle Cricothyrotomy with Jet Ventilation Technique

To perform needle cricothyrotomy with jet ventilation:

1. Use Standard Precautions, including face mask and shield.

2. Manage the patient's airway as well as possible with basic maneuvers and supplemental oxygen while you prepare your equipment. Attach a large-bore IV needle with a catheter (adults: 14- or 16-gauge; pediatrics: 18- or 20-gauge) to a 10- or 20-mL syringe. If time permits you

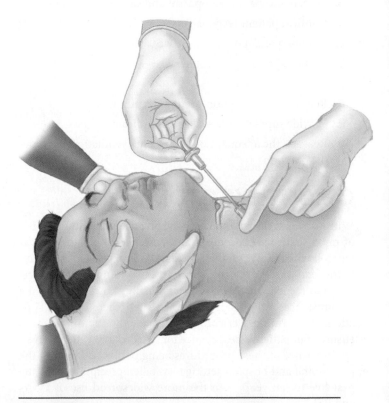

● **Figure 5-97** Advance the catheter with the needle.

may fill the syringe with sterile water or saline to facilitate detection of air when aspirating.

3. Place the patient supine and hyperextend the head and neck. (Maintain neutral position if you suspect cervical spine injury.) Position yourself at the patient's side.

4. Palpate the inferior portion of the thyroid cartilage and the cricoid cartilage. The indention between the two is the cricothyroid membrane (Figures 5-94 ● and 5-95 ●).

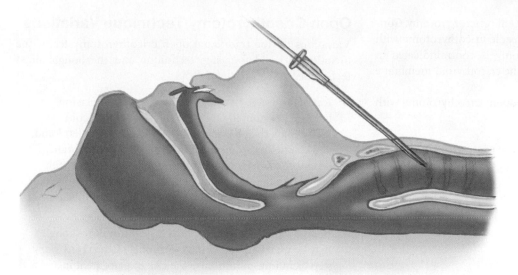

● **Figure 5-98** Cannula properly placed in the trachea.

5. Prepare the anterior neck with antiseptic solution.

6. Firmly grasp the laryngeal cartilages and reconfirm the site of the cricothyroid membrane.

7. Carefully insert the needle into the cricothyroid membrane at midline, directed 45° caudally (towards the feet) (Figure 5-96 ●). Often you will feel a pop as the needle penetrates the membrane.

8. Advance the needle while aspirating with the syringe. If air returns easily, the catheter is in the trachea. If blood returns or you feel resistance to return, reevaluate needle placement.

9. After you confirm proper placement, hold the needle steady and advance the catheter. Then withdraw the needle (Figure 5-97 ●).

10. Reconfirm placement by again withdrawing air from the catheter with the syringe. Secure the catheter in place (Figure 5-98 ●).

11. Attach the jet-ventilation device to the catheter and a 50-psi oxygen supply. If this is unavailable, you may connect a bag-valve device to the catheter using the inner adapter from a 7.5-mm endotracheal tube. The bag-valve device must be connected to oxygen.

12. Open the release valve to introduce an oxygen jet into the trachea (Figure 5-99 ●). Then adjust the pressure to allow adequate lung expansion (usually about 50 psi, compared with about 1 psi through a regulator).

13. Watch the chest carefully, turning off the release valve as soon as the chest rises. Exhalation then occurs passively through the glottis as a result of elastic recoil of the lungs and chest wall. Deliver at least 20 breaths per minute keeping the inflation-to-deflation time approximately 1:3. Keep in mind that you may need to adjust this to the patient's needs, particularly in COPD and asthma patients, who often require a longer expiration time.

14. Continue ventilatory support, assessing for adequacy of ventilations and looking for the development of any potential complications.

15. You should be anticipating the need for an alternative means of oxygenation and ventilation within approximately 30 minutes.

Open Cricothyrotomy

An open, or surgical, cricothyrotomy involves placing an endotracheal or tracheostomy tube directly into the trachea through a surgical incision at the cricothyroid membrane. Open cricothyrotomy is preferred to needle cricothyrotomy in older pediatric patients and adult patients, because it allows for enhanced oxygenation and ventilation and protects the airway against aspiration. The greater potential complications of open cricothyrotomy mandate even more training and skills monitoring than for the needle method.

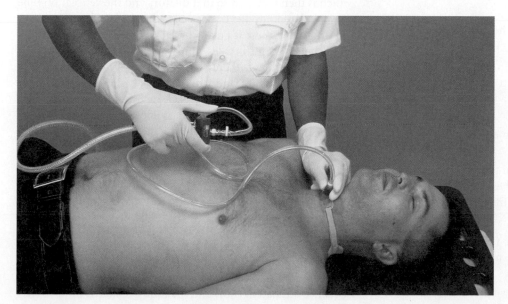

● **Figure 5-99** Jet ventilation with needle cricothryrotomy.

Indications are the same as for needle cricothyrotomy. Contraindications are the same as for needle cricothyrotomy with the addition that open cricothyrotomy is contraindicated in children under the age of 8 because the cricothyroid membrane is small and underdeveloped.

The potential complications of open cricothyrotomy with jet ventilation include:

- Incorrect tube placement into a false passage
- Cricoid and/or thyroid cartilage damage
- Thyroid gland damage
- Severe bleeding
- Laryngeal nerve damage
- Subcutaneous emphysema
- Vocal cord damage
- Infection

Open Cricothyrotomy Traditional Technique

To perform open cricothyrotomy by the traditional technique (Procedure 5–4):

1. Use Standard Precautions, including face mask and shield.
2. Use BVM ventilation and supplemental oxygen to maintain oxygenation and ventilation as well as possible while preparing supplies.
3. Locate the thyroid cartilage and the cricoid cartilage. Identify the cricothyroid membrane between these two cartilages.
4. Clean the area with antiseptic solution.
5. Stabilize the cartilages with one hand, while using a scalpel in the other hand to make a 2- to 4-cm vertical skin incision in the midline over the membrane.
6. Locate the cricothyroid membrane again, using blunt dissection if necessary.
7. Make a 1- to 2-cm incision in the horizontal plane through the membrane.
8. Insert a tracheal hook on the inferior portion of the thyroid cartilage to help maintain the opening. This may also be improvised with an adult or pediatric stylet.
9. Insert curved hemostats into the membrane incision and spread it open.
10. Insert either a cuffed endotracheal tube or a tracheostomy tube into the opening, directing the tube distally into the trachea. Ideally a 6-mm tube will fit, although smaller patients may require a smaller size.
11. Inflate the cuff and ventilate.
12. Confirm placement with multiple methods as available and appropriate.
13. Secure the tube in place.

Open Cricothyrotomy Technique Variations

Variations on the traditional open cricothyrotomy technique include the rapid four-step technique and the bougie-aided technique.

- *Rapid four-step.* In this technique, a single incision is made horizontally through the skin and cricoid membrane, then a tracheal hook is held in the left hand and traction is applied against the cricoid membrane, directed toward the feet, and the tube is inserted with the right hand, mimicking endotracheal intubation. This technique has been associated with more complications in some studies.
- *Bougie-aided.* An endotracheal tube introducer (bougie) may be used with either the traditional or the rapid four-step technique to minimize the risk of placement in a false passage, to allow the operator to let go without losing critical landmarks, and to ease threading of the tube. In the simplest version of this technique, an adult bougie is passed into the trachea through the incision in the cricothyroid membrane, directed distally, and intratracheal placement is confirmed with palpation of clicks as the bougie passes over the cartilage rings and/or palpation of hold-up within 20 cm. Note that the distance to hold-up is much shorter than when using the introducer/bougie through the mouth. Once placement is confirmed, the endotracheal or tracheostomy tube is threaded over the bougie into the trachea.

Minimally Invasive Percutaneous Cricothyrotomy

A number of hybrid techniques are available to perform a cricothyrotomy using a needle but allowing for a much larger diameter ventilation catheter. Some of these techniques involve devices that are placed blindly and that consist of the needle, a dilator, and a catheter, all in one. Other methods are based on Seldinger-technique (the same technique used for central line insertion) in which a guidewire is placed through a needle, which is then removed so that dilators and the ventilation tube may be placed into the trachea over the guidewire.

In general there is no advantage to these needle techniques over the open techniques, and complications may actually be higher, although there is substantial variation among devices and techniques. Individual agencies should consult their medical director and evaluate each device and technique on a case-by-case basis. We cannot stress enough that you must continuously practice this skill with the medical director's involvement to maintain proficiency.

MEDICATION-ASSISTED INTUBATION

Medication-assisted intubation (MAI), which is also called drug-assisted or pharmacologically assisted intubation, is becoming more common. MAI may take several forms, including rapid sequence intubation (RSI) and sedation-facilitated intubation.

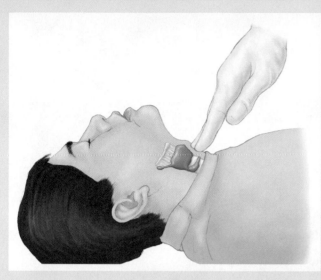

5-4a ● Locate the cricothyroid membrane.

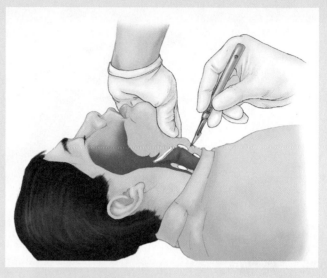

5-4b ● Stabilize the larynx and make a 1- to 2-cm skin incision over the cricothyroid membrane.

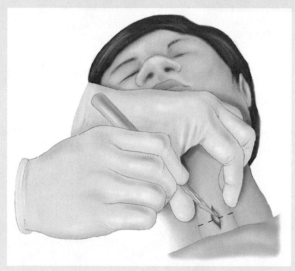

5-4c ● Make a 1-cm horizontal incision through the cricothyroid membrane.

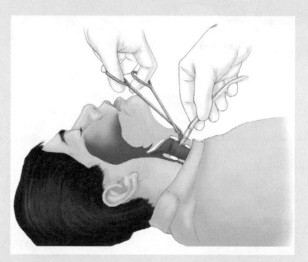

5-4d ● Using a curved hemostat, spread the membrane incision open.

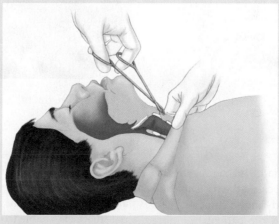

5-4e ● Insert an ETT (6.0 or 7.0) or Shiley (6.0 or 8.0).

(Continued)

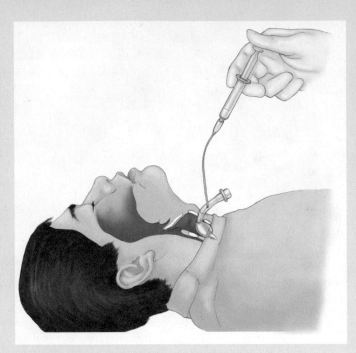

5-4f ● Inflate the cuff.

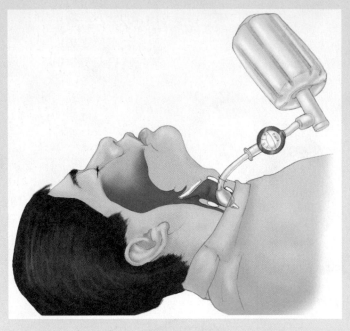

5-4g ● Confirm placement.

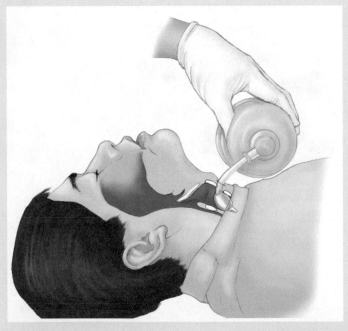

5-4h ● Ventilate.

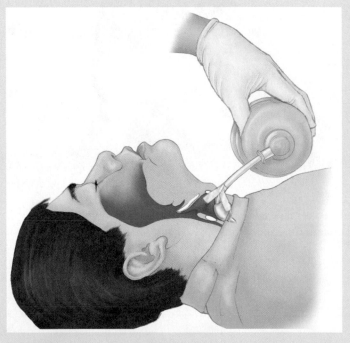

5-4i ● Secure the tube, reconfirm placement, and evaluate the patient.

MAI techniques give you the option of managing airways that you could not otherwise manage because the patient is too awake or has trismus, and they do it early in the clinical course when the procedure may be easier and the patient has more reserve to tolerate complications.

The flip side is that these procedures come with great risk, as you are employing very powerful medications that may result—and have resulted—in severe morbidity and death when the paramedic is unable to intubate and cannot maintain adequate oxygenation through other means. In the setting of cardiac arrest, of course, you cannot realistically make the situation any worse. MAI, however, is employed in patients who are alive and sometimes conscious, when both the potential benefits and the potential harms are greater.[45–51]

The current evidence has not found a survival benefit to prehospital RSI outside the air-medical setting, and in some cases survival rates are notably worse with RSI. Despite this literature, some EMS services have been able to employ these techniques safely and with apparent advantage to their patients, but it takes a lot of initial and ongoing training, active medical director involvement, a thorough quality assurance program, and the maturity to select patients carefully and move early to backup devices.

Rapid Sequence Intubation

Your immediate concern with every patient you treat is to maintain a patent airway and adequate oxygenation and ventilation (except for patients in cardiac arrest in whom chest compressions would come first). Clearly, if a patient is in cardiac arrest (once circulation has been attended to) or is in respiratory arrest, or is unconscious or obtunded and not protecting his airway, airway management with BVM ventilation, an EGA, or intubation is indicated.

Occasionally, however, you may encounter an awake patient with an airway disorder who is hypoxemic despite high-concentration oxygen via a nonrebreather or CPAP and therapy directed at the underlying problem. This patient is working hard to breathe but does not have adequate gas exchange to support life. Subtle altered mental status may indicate that some level of significant hypoxemia is putting essential brain functions at risk.

Assisting respirations with a BVM on such a patient is challenging because of patient anxiety. Nasal intubation is difficult and often exacerbates hypoxemia. You cannot perform oral intubation on this patient until he fatigues enough to have respiratory failure, with resultant unconsciousness and decreased muscle tone leading to loss of a gag reflex. By then, however, the patient will have suffered prolonged hypoxemia, possibly accompanied by myocardial infarction, brain or kidney damage, or vomiting with aspiration.

If a patient clearly is precipitously failing maximal aggressive medical management, or if the history of his problem clearly indicates that he will not be able to, or already cannot, protect his airway, then active intervention is appropriate to control the airway and provide adequate ventilation.

One potential solution to this problem is rapid sequence intubation (RSI). Classic rapid sequence *induction* is a procedure borrowed from anesthesia and modified in emergency medicine and EMS to become rapid sequence *intubation*.

RSI involves a series of steps that includes administration of a neuromuscular blocking drug to a critically ill or injured patient, who is presumed to have a full stomach, in order to facilitate oral intubation without aspiration or other complications. The procedure is called "rapid" because the individual steps are performed in "rapid succession," one right after the other, not because the entire procedure is fast. In fact, RSI can take quite a bit of time in some cases.

The entire RSI procedure is intended to minimize the risk of aspiration in a high-risk population. This requires preoxygenation

and avoiding positive pressure ventilation when possible. The risks of RSI are very substantial, since a patient undergoing the procedure is, by definition, breathing, yet you are giving the patient medications that will eliminate his respiratory drive and his ability to protect his own airway from aspiration.

Potential indications include those listed next. Note, however, that the fact that a patient meets a stated indication for RSI does not mean that this is the best thing to do for that individual patient.

Indications

● Impending or actual respiratory failure from any cause

● Impending or actual inability to protect the airway from any cause

● Combativeness secondary to presumed head trauma

● Hypoxemia despite maximal therapy

Relative Contraindications

● Predicted difficult airway

● Short ETA to hospital or more experienced providers

● Only one paramedic on scene

● Ability to manage the patient with less risky procedures

● When the only indication is airway protection

Absolute Contraindications

● Respiratory arrest

● Cardiac arrest

Preoxygenation

The air we are all breathing at this very moment is only 21 percent oxygen, regardless of your location or altitude; the remaining 79 percent is nearly all nitrogen. If all the nitrogen in your lungs were replaced with oxygen, you would have nearly five times the oxygen present now. This is what occurs with preoxygenation. Hence, preoxygenation is sometimes called "denitrogenation" or "nitrogen washout." This fivefold increase in oxygen in the lungs creates an oxygen reserve that the body can draw on once a patient has been administered a paralytic agent and ceases to breathe.

Patients with healthy lungs and adequate functional residual capacity may develop enough reserve from preoxygenation to survive up to 8 minutes of medication-induced apnea without desaturation (loss of blood oxygen saturation). Thus, preoxygenation allows us to chemically paralyze a patient yet withhold positive pressure ventilation, thereby limiting the risk of gastric insufflation and subsequent aspiration, without the patient becoming hypoxemic.

Unfortunately, many critically ill or injured patients cannot tolerate 8 minutes of apnea. Common clinical variables that impact the amount of apnea time a patient can withstand before becoming hypoxic include age, obesity, pregnancy, lung disease, baseline saturations, acute illness, and more (Table 5–8). Children, for instance, have shorter apnea times in large part

TABLE 5–8 | High-Risk Characteristics That Decrease Oxygen Reserve

Characteristics That Decrease Oxygen Reserve

Decreased Oxygen Storage Capacity

- Elderly
- Obesity
- Pregnancy
- Lung disease: acute, chronic, acute-on-chronic
- Chest trauma
- Baseline hypoxemia

Increased Oxygen Consumption

- Fever/sepsis
- Severe pain
- Alcohol withdrawal
- Cocaine/methamphetamine intoxication
- Tachycardia
- Shock
- Children

TABLE 5–9 | Patient Categorization and Preparations Following Preoxygenation

Preoxygenation Categories and Preparations

Adequate Reserve—Oxygen Saturation Near 100%

- Positive pressure ventilation usually not necessary
- Potential false sense of security if patients have high-risk characteristics

Limited Reserve—Oxygen Saturation 90–97%

- Some patients will require careful BMV ventilation
- Be prepared to abort intubation attempt
- Have rescue airway immediately available: not necessary to remove from package in advance

No Reserve—Oxygen Saturation Below 90%

- Positive pressure ventilation is unavoidable
- Consider CPAP/BiPAP or assisted respirations <u>before</u> medication
- Consider planned PPV with BVM or SGA after medication and before intubation
- Have rescue airway immediately ready for insertion: out of package and lubricated

because of their increased basal metabolism. Some patients, such as those with fever, shock, alcohol withdrawal, and cocaine/amphetamine intoxication, have substantially increased oxygen demand and "chew through" their reserve very quickly. Obese and pregnant patients have less reserve in large part because of limited functional residual capacity.[52]

In most cases, preoxygenation will be accomplished with a tight-fitting nonrebreather mask with 10–15 lpm flow for at least 3 minutes. Such a system delivers 70–90 percent oxygen and is sufficient for most patients. A bag-valve mask may be used *without* positive pressure to deliver 100 percent oxygen if desired. If positive pressure must be used due to patient hypoxia, concentrate on good technique to minimize air entry into the stomach.

After preoxygenation, patients may be roughly categorized as having "adequate," "limited," or "no" reserve, which generally dictates the preoxygenation preparations that should be made (Table 5–9). Patients with underlying lung disease, especially acute or acute-on-chronic disease resulting in hypoxemia, are a particularly scary group to intubate because they are hypoxic to

PATHO PEARL

Importance of Head Elevation. *Research has demonstrated that preoxygenation is more successful for most patients with at least 20 degrees of head elevation; this is especially true for obese patients. This is yet another reason that all trauma patients in spinal precautions should be considered difficult intubations. The inability to elevate the patient's head limits preoxygenation, and that in turn limits the amount of time you will have to perform the procedure. This also emphasizes the importance of keeping patients, particularly those with respiratory distress, in their position of comfort as long as their mental status allows.*

begin with, and they are prone to very rapid desaturation after medication.

Patients with a saturation of 100 percent after preoxygenation have an "adequate reserve," those less than 100 percent but above 90 percent have "limited reserve," and those less than 90 percent have "no reserve." In the first group (adequate reserve), the goal should be no positive pressure ventilation, although some patients, particularly those with any of the high-risk characteristics that were listed in Table 5–8, may still desaturate quickly.

In the second group (limited reserve), the clinician should plan to optimize first-pass success and anticipate that some patients will require careful positive pressure ventilation if the intubation attempt is prolonged.

In the last group (no reserve), positive pressure ventilation is unavoidable; the clinician should consider CPAP/BiPAP or assisted respirations before medication and be prepared to provide immediate optimal BVM ventilation and to place a rescue airway if saturations cannot be maintained. Many inexperienced providers faced with a patient who is desaturating make the mistake of waiting too long to abort the procedure, trying even harder or trying "just one more time," only to face critical hypoxia and cardiac arrest.

Airway Pharmacology

Premedications Premedications are drugs given early in the course of RSI to mitigate anticipated complications. Examples are lidocaine (to blunt the rise in intracranial pressure (ICP) associated with succinylcholine and laryngoscopy) and atropine (to prevent the bradycardia associated with succinylcholine in children).

As it turns out, none of these agents are required. Few have been proven to do what they were hoped to do, and all are associated with some potential adverse effects. The movement in the last few years has been away from the routine use of premedications.

Agents that might still be considered if time and protocols permit are:

- *Fentanyl.* At routine doses, fentanyl is an excellent analgesic (pain reliever) that may keep a patient more comfortable during a painful procedure such as intubation. At higher doses, fentanyl is a sympatholytic agent that blunts the hypertension, tachycardia, and ICP elevation associated with laryngoscopy. It is reasonable to consider giving all patients analgesic doses of fentanyl at least 3 minutes before the procedure and higher doses to patients at risk for life-threatening elevations of ICP. While fentanyl is highly regarded for its hemodynamic (blood flow/blood pressure) stability, it may occasionally cause hypotension (a drop in blood pressure) in patients who are dependent on their sympathetic drive for blood pressure maintenance, especially at higher doses.

- *Atropine.* Succinylcholine is associated with bradycardia (slow heartbeat) in younger children and in any patient receiving a second dose. Historically, atropine was recommended routinely 2 to 3 minutes before administration of succinylcholine to children less than 6 to

8 years of age to reduce the risk of bradycardia. Evidence now shows that this is optional, although atropine must always be at the bedside.

- *Lidocaine.* While commonly used in head injury patients to blunt an increase in ICP, there has been a movement away from this practice in some circles because of limited evidence for benefit and the potential risk of hypotension as well as time delays. There is evidence that lidocaine is useful in asthmatic patients to avoid or lessen bronchospasm triggered by airway manipulation.[53]

Induction Agents The purpose of an induction agent is to render the patient unaware during the procedure. Some EMS RSI protocols call for the use of induction agents only in awake patients. Since it is impossible to know how aware an unconscious patient might be, we recommend routine use for any patient who requires RSI (Table 5–10). Common induction agents used in EMS include:

- *Etomidate.* Etomidate is a great agent for induction since it rarely causes any rise or drop in blood pressure or pulse. It also works extremely fast with a relatively consistent dose response. There has been concern about suppression of adrenal gland function in septic patients, but thus far there is no evidence that this is a significant enough safety concern to cause EMS to avoid it.

TABLE 5–10 | Guidelines for Sedative (Induction) Agents

Guidelines for Sedative (Induction) Agents

Induction Agent	Dose	Onset	Duration (min)	Advantages	Disadvantages
Midazolam (Versed)	0.1–0.3 mg/kg	1–3 min	20–30 min	Amnesia effects, good sedative	Hypotension
Diazepam (Valium)	0.2–0.5 mg/kg	2–3 min	30–40 min	Amnesia effects	Hypotension, respiratory depression
Etomidate (Amidate)	0.3 mg/kg	1–2 min	5 min	Little effect on blood pressure, decreases intracranial pressure (ICP)	Suppresses cortisol, not good for head-injured patients
Ketamine (Ketalar)	1–2 mg/kg	1 min	10–20 min	Decreases bronchospasm, little hypotension, amnesia	Increases ICP
Sodium thiopental	3–5 mg/kg	1 min	5 min	Blunts ICP changes	Significant hypotension, bronchospasm
Propofol (Diprivan)	1–1.5 mg/kg	1 min	3–5 min	Rapid onset, good sedative effects	Significant hypotension
Fentanyl	3–5 mcg/kg	1–2 min	30–40 min	Little effect on blood pressure; blunts ICP changes	Can cause muscle rigidity in chest wall

- **Midazolam.** Midazolam is a benzodiazepine sedative/ hypnotic. The major advantage of midazolam is amnesia. That is, the patient is unlikely to recall the procedure. The major disadvantage is that the dose required for induction is commonly associated with hypotension. It is also hard to predict the dose that will make any particular patient unaware.

- **Ketamine.** Ketamine is a dissociative agent that is being used more in emergency medicine and critical care transport with some use in EMS as well. The advantages of ketamine are that it has a predictable dose response, does not cause hypotension, and provides analgesia as well as sedation. The major disadvantage is hypertension and tachycardia in some patients. There used to be concern about using ketamine in patients with head trauma and stroke, but that has largely been disproved as long as the patient is not hypertensive.

- **Propofol.** Propofol is commonly used in the hospital for induction, but its use is limited in EMS by potentially profound hypotension.

Neuromuscular Blocking Agents (Paralytics) Paralytics, or neuromuscular blocking agents, are drugs that temporarily stop skeletal muscle function without affecting cardiac or smooth muscle. The two primary categories are competitive and noncompetitive agents. The competitive agents have a dose response such that the higher the dose the quicker the paralysis takes place but the longer it lasts. Competitive agents are nondepolarizing; that is, they do not cause fasciculations (muscle twitches) and generally have fewer adverse effects and contraindications. Noncompetitive agents have a much more limited dose response such that the onset time and duration are somewhat fixed as long as a reasonable dose is used. The noncompetitive agents are also called depolarizing agents because they cause fasciculations before the onset of paralysis.[54–56]

- **Succinylcholine.** Succinylcholine is the prototype noncompetitive depolarizing neuromuscular blocker. Because of its fast onset (about 45 seconds) and short duration (about 8 minutes) this is the preferred agent for most EMS services. Unfortunately, succinylcholine has a host of potential adverse effects (Table 5–11) that result in a number of contraindications that must be considered in all patients. Succinylcholine is not routinely recommended for maintaining paralysis, so a second competitive agent must usually be carried as well.

- **Rocuronium.** Rocuronium is now the most commonly used competitive agent in emergency medicine and EMS. The onset time with rocuronium is only slightly longer than with succinylcholine (60 seconds) as long as higher doses are used. At the recommended intubation doses, rocuronium may last 30 minutes or longer. While this is often used as an argument against rocuronium for EMS use, it is used successfully by many services that argue that even 8 minutes is too long with succinylcholine before moving on to a rescue airway. Rocuronium has few adverse effects and may be used for initial and ongoing paralysis.

TABLE 5–11 | Contraindications to Succinylcholine

Contraindications to Succinylcholine (may exaggerate hyperkalemia)

Disease/Injury

Neuromuscular diseases
- Muscular dystrophies
- Myopathies
- Guillain-Barré

Stroke

Parkinson's disease (severe)

Tetanus

Botulism

Rhabdomyolysis

Burns >24–28 hours old

Spinal cord injury (>72 hours and <9 months old)

Prolonged immobility/paralysis

Severe infection (abdominal and neurologic)

Severe trauma (especially musculoskeletal)

- **Vecuronium.** Vecuronium is a competitive agent that is commonly used to maintain paralysis after succinylcholine. Vecuronium is a second- or third-line agent for RSI because of its long onset time. While there are tricks that may be used to shorten the onset time, they add complexity and a very long duration of action.

Sedatives and Analgesics Sedatives and analgesics are essential for keeping a patient comfortable after intubation. Both analgesia and sedation should be provided to every patient who is chemically paralyzed, unless contraindicated by hypotension, and to all other patients, unless you are confident that the patient is comfortable, such as an un-paralyzed post–cardiac arrest patient who is completely unresponsive.

- **Narcotics.** Narcotics are critical to provide analgesia. Fentanyl is used most commonly because it has a rapid onset and minimal effects on blood pressure unless the patient is sympathetic dependent. Other narcotics such as morphine may also be used cautiously.

- **Benzodiazepines.** Benzodiazepines are optimal for keeping patients sedated while intubated. Midazolam is a favorite among critical care transport crews because of its rapid onset and short duration. Lorazepam and diazepam may also be used. All benzodiazepines must be used cautiously in volume depleted and hypotensive patients.

- **Propofol.** Propofol infusions are commonly used in the intensive care unit and during critical care transport to maintain sedation. The very short duration of action facilitates neurologic examination when the infusion is stopped. Propofol is even more prone to cause hypotension than the benzodiazepines and must be used cautiously.

RSI Procedure

To perform a typical rapid sequence intubation, there are 10 steps, as listed next. As with other airway procedures, be sure to begin with Standard Precautions:

1. *Preoxygenate* to achieve nitrogen washout and create an oxygen reserve (as discussed earlier). Use a nonrebreather mask with high-concentration oxygen for at least 3 minutes if possible. Consider CPAP, assisted respiration, and BVM ventilation as indicated. Avoid positive pressure if the patient is not hypoxemic.

2. *Protect the C-spine* if indicated. The front of the cervical collar should be removed and manual in-line stabilization performed by an assistant who is also ready to perform a jaw-thrust maneuver.

3. *Position optimally* if possible. Patients not in cervical precautions should be placed in sniffing or ramped position.

4. *Apply pressure to the cricoid* if there is sufficient assistance available. The individual providing pressure should be prepared to release pressure and assist with external laryngeal manipulation (ELM) as directed by the intubator.

5. *Ponder* if intubation is really necessary. Are there other management options, if this is likely to be a difficult airway? Use a checklist if possible.

6. *Premedicate* if time permits and allowed by protocol and scope of practice. Consider regular-dose fentanyl for most patients, high-dose fentanyl for suspected critical ICP, and lidocaine for severe asthmatics.

7. *Prepare equipment,* using a checklist to ensure that all supplies are ready. This includes intubation, BVM ventilation, rescue, and post-intubation supplies.

8. *Sedate and paralyze,* using appropriate medications and doses. Most patients should receive both an induction agent and paralytic. The induction agent should routinely be given before the paralytic.

9. *Pass the tube* with direct or indirect visualization or an endotracheal tube introducer. Use all available adjunctive techniques including external laryngeal manipulation (ELM). Monitor oxygenation and be ready to abort the attempt *before* the oxygen level reaches critical point. In most cases, where the patient is adequately preoxygenated and has a saturation of 100 percent beforehand, the attempt should be stopped when the saturation reaches about 93 percent.

10. *Post-intubation management* begins with objective tube confirmation, using capnography. Lung sounds should be used to help guide tube depth. A bite block should be inserted, and the tube should be secured in place and the cervical collar replaced if indicated. The patient should be placed on the transport ventilator including in-line continuous capnography. The patient should then receive analgesia and sedation. Ongoing paralysis should be administered only if absolutely necessary to manage the patient on the ventilator and never without analgesia and sedation. Monitor oxygen saturation (SpO_2), end-tidal CO_2, blood pressure, clinical exam, and ventilator parameters.

Rapid Sequence Airway

Rapid sequence airway (RSA) is a new airway management technique in which the preparation and pharmacology of rapid sequence intubation (RSI) is paired with intentional placement of an extraglottic airway device, without prior attempt at direct laryngoscopy, in selected patients. The theoretical advantages to RSA over RSI include less hypoxemia, less airway trauma, and no risk of tube misplacement. The major risks are aspiration and ineffective ventilation. The risk of aspiration is offset by fewer airway attempts and new gastric-isolation EADs that achieve an excellent seal pressure and also allow for gastric decompression. The risk of ineffective ventilation is offset through careful patient and device selection.

RSA Indications
- Same as RSI

Absolute RSA Contraindications
- Upper airway pathology known or suspected
- Blunt or penetrating anterior neck trauma
- Inhalation injury
- Angioedema
- Anaphylaxis
- Upper airway tumor
- Obstructing upper airway infection—croup, epiglottitis, parapharyngeal abscess
- Caustic ingestion

Relative RSA Contraindications
- Patient's airway may be managed by other means
- Anticipated inability to ventilate by BVM
- Anticipated need for very high airway pressures
- Very high aspiration risk
- Short ETA to hospital or arrival of help with more resources
- Only one paramedic on scene

THE DIFFICULT AIRWAY

As a paramedic, you will be expected to be able to effectively manage patients where establishing and maintaining an airway may be difficult. It has been estimated that 1 out of 10 endotracheal intubations can be classified as "difficult," and intubation may be impossible in 1 out of 100 patients when conventional techniques (including straight-blade, ELM, and introducers) are attempted.[57, 58]

It is important, however, to think globally in terms of the difficult airway rather than considering only difficult intubation. The concept of the difficult airway includes difficult BVM ventilation, difficult extraglottic airway placement and ventilation, difficult intubation, and difficult cricothyrotomy.

CONTENT REVIEW

▶ The Difficult Airway

- Difficult BVM ventilation
- Difficult extraglottic airway placement
- Difficult intubation
- Difficult cricothyrotomy

- *Difficult bag-valve-mask ventilation*: a clinical situation in which a paramedic anticipates or experiences difficulty maintaining an adequate saturation (usually >90%) using high-concentration oxygen, basic airway adjuncts, and two-person technique.

- *Difficult extraglottic airway*: a clinical situation in which a paramedic anticipates or experiences difficult inserting or ventilating with an extraglottic airway device.

- *Difficult intubation*: a clinical situation in which a paramedic anticipates or experiences difficulty visualizing the vocal cords or posterior cartilages within one optimal attempt and without the patient developing hypoxemia.

- *Difficult cricothyrotomy*: a clinical situation in which a paramedic anticipates or experiences difficulty obtaining a surgical airway in less than 60 seconds.

- *Difficult airway*: a clinical situation in which a paramedic anticipates or experiences difficulty with any critical portion of airway management, including BVM ventilation, extraglottic airway placement, endotracheal intubation, or surgical cricothyrotomy.

Predictors of a Difficult Airway or Ventilation

It would be useful if we could reliably predict which airways are likely to cause difficulty and which will not (Table 5–12). This is particularly important if you are considering a medication-facilitated airway procedure. For those patients for whom we anticipate difficulty, we could call for help in advance, consider deferring the procedure, consider managing the airway with BVM ventilation or an extraglottic device, or simply be better prepared, such as having different blades or devices, an introducer, a backup airway, and cricothyrotomy supplies immediately available. In most emergency situations, however, a detailed airway assessment may not be practical. In many such cases, management must proceed, even when airway assessment predicts difficulty, because of patient acuity and a favorable risk-to-benefit analysis.

Predictors of difficult BVM ventilation include facial trauma, facial hair, obesity, and lack of teeth (assuming you don't have the dentures to replace during BVM ventilation). Other risk factors for difficult BVM ventilation demonstrated in the anesthesia literature include age over 55, history of snoring, Mallampati class 3 or 4 (discussed later), severely limited jaw protrusion, and thyromental distance (the distance between the thyroid notch and the bony point of the chin) less than 6 cm.

Predictors of difficult extraglottic airway (EGA) device placement include limited mouth opening. Situations in which an EGA may be inserted easily but where it may be difficult to ventilate the patient include massive secretions, morbid obesity, severe pulmonary disease, and pathology below the device, such as inhalation burns, laryngeal trauma, and angioedema.

TABLE 5–12	Predictors of Difficult Airway and Ventilation

Predictors of Difficult Airway and Ventilation

Difficult Bag-Valve-Mask Ventilation Predictors

- Facial trauma
- Facial hair
- Obesity
- Lack of teeth (and without dentures)
- History of snoring
- Mallampati grade 3 or 4
- Severely limited jaw protrusion
- Thyromental distance less than 6 cm

Difficult Extraglottic Airway Insertion or Ventilation Predictors

- Limited mouth opening
- Massive secretions
- Morbid obesity
- Severe pulmonary disease
- Pathology below the device (e.g., inhalation burns, laryngeal trauma, angioedema)

Difficult Laryngoscopy and Orotracheal Intubation Predictors

- Facial trauma or anomalies
- Increasing Mallampati grade
- Short thyromental distance
- Short sternomental distance
- Limited mouth opening
- Limited neck mobility
- Obesity
- Buckteeth

Difficult Surgical Airway (Cricothyrotomy) Placement

- Cricothyroid membrane cannot be located:
  - Morbid obesity
  - Anterior neck trauma
  - Prior radiation therapy
  - Ludwig's angina (skin infection to anterior neck)
- Tube insertion prevented by conditions within airway lumen:
  - Tumor
  - Infection
  - Swelling
  - Foreign body

Commonly used predictors of difficult laryngoscopy and intubation include facial trauma/anomalies, increasing Mallampati class (discussed later), short thyromental distance, short sternomental distance (distance between the suprasternal notch and the bony point of the chin), limited mouth opening, limited neck mobility, obesity, and buckteeth.

Predictors of difficult surgical airway placement include situations in which the cricothyroid membrane cannot be located—such as morbid obesity, anterior neck trauma, prior radiation

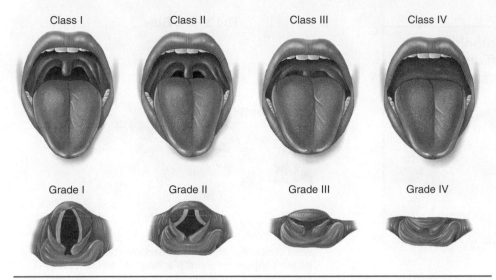

Class I   Class II   Class III   Class IV

Grade I   Grade II   Grade III   Grade IV

● **Figure 5-100** Airway scoring systems. Mallampati classification system (top); Cormack and LeHane classification system (bottom).

therapy, and infection such as Ludwig's angina (a very serious skin infection that tracks down into the anterior neck, usually from a dental infection)—and situations in which a tumor, infection, swelling, or foreign body within the airway lumen prevents tube insertion, even when the membrane can be located.

Difficult Airway Scoring Systems

Various difficult airway scoring systems have been developed to aid the clinician in detecting and managing the difficult airway. The most frequently used system of pre-intubation airway assessment is the **Mallampati classification system** (Figure 5-100 ●). With this system, the tonsillar pillars and the uvula are assessed. The more concealed the tonsillar pillars and the uvula, the more difficult the intubation. Based on these features, the patient's airway is classified into four classes. The higher the class, the more difficult the airway is expected to be.

Class I: Entire tonsil clearly visible

Class II: Upper half of tonsil fossa visible

Class III: Soft and hard palate clearly visible

Class IV: Only hard palate visible

Rarely will a paramedic have time to assess the Mallampati class prior to intubation attempts. The Mallampati assessment is done with the patient awake and sitting up. The patient opens his mouth and sticks his tongue out. Recognizing that the Mallampati system is of little use in the unconscious patient, Cormack and LeHane adapted the system to classify the view one sees with a laryngoscope. The **Cormack and LeHane grading system** is similar to Mallampati's (see Figure 5-100).

Grade 1: Entire glottic opening and vocal cords may be seen.

Grade 2: Epiglottis and posterior portion of glottic opening may be seen with a partial view of vocal cords.

Grade 3: Only epiglottis and (sometimes) posterior cartilages seen.

Grade 4: Neither epiglottis nor glottis seen.

A similar system used in EMS is the percentage of glottic opening (POGO) system. With the **POGO scoring system**, the percentage of the glottis that can be visualized is scored. The score ranges from 0 (none of the glottis visualized) to 100 (vocal cords fully visualized). This system also helps to predict the difficulty of endotracheal intubation (Figure 5-101 ●).

As you may already have figured out, airway classification systems like Mallampati, Cormack and LeHane, and POGO, while very helpful in more controlled or leisurely environments, have little application to emergency medicine. This is especially so in the case of the austere prehospital environment. However, knowing the features of these classification systems can help you to better anticipate the difficult airway.

"LEMONS"

"LEMONS" is an acronym that can be used to remember assessments and findings associated with a difficult airway. Factors that have been assembled into the LEMONS mnemonic can encompass the entire difficult airway assessment, including difficult bag-valve-mask ventilation, EGA insertion and ventilation, endotracheal intubation, and cricothyrotomy (Table 5–13). Unfortunately, most of these clinical assessments cannot be realistically performed in the austere prehospital environment. For example, the Mallampati score, as already noted, relies on having a cooperative patient sit up, open his mouth fully, and stick out

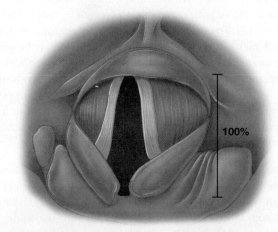

100%

Percentage of glottic opening (POGO) scale.

● **Figure 5-101** POGO scoring system.

TABLE 5–13 | LEMONS Mnemonic Used to Evaluate Difficult Airway

LEMONS	
L	Look externally
E	Evaluate 3-3-2 rule
M	Mallampati score
O	Obstruction
N	Neck mobility
S	Saturations

his tongue so the hard palate, uvula, and posterior pharynx can be visualized. The astute paramedic will still look into the mouth before committing to intubation in order to assess overall working room—a modified Mallampati score.

Look Externally   Look for factors that will make BVM ventilation, EGA, intubation, or surgical airway difficult. This includes facial hair, secretions, massive obesity, facial trauma, upper airway pathology, and gross face/neck anatomic deformities.

Evaluate 3-3-2 Rule   The 3-3-2 rule is one tool to help estimate the difficulty of laryngoscopy by assessing anatomic limitations to visualizing the larynx—for example, small mouth opening, short chin (no room to displace the tongue), and superior/anterior location (Figure 5-102 ●). Criteria evaluated are as follows (using the patient's finger measurements):

- Check that the mouth opening is at least **3** patient-sized fingers.
- Check that there is room for **3** patient-sized fingers between the tip of the chin and the hyoid bone.
- Check that there is room for **2** patient-sized fingers between the hyoid bone and the top of the thyroid cartilage.

Mallampati Score   The Mallampati score assesses the working space available within the mouth (review Figure 5-100 and see Table 5–14). To be done correctly, the patient must be able to sit up and stick out his tongue. A crude estimate may be substituted by manually opening the mouth and looking, although this technique has never been validated. A tongue blade may be used cautiously to avoid stimulating a gag reflex. The most important thing is to make sure you look into the mouth before committing to intubation to assess mouth opening, size of tongue, dentures/dentition, edema, trauma, and secretions.

Obstruction   The airway may be obstructed by a foreign body, the tongue, secretions, blood, or vomitus and/or edema. Edema may result from trauma, infectious causes such as epiglottitis and abscess, or from allergic reactions. Consider the age and history to predict possible obstruction. Intubating a pediatric patient with retropharyngeal abscess or an adult with Ludwig's angina is a scary proposition.

The 3–3–2 Rule

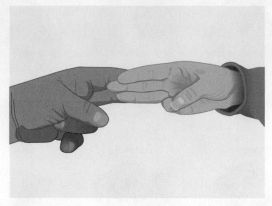

Keep in mind that the measurements are based on the *patient's* fingers, not yours! (For example, two of your fingers might equal three of the patient's.)

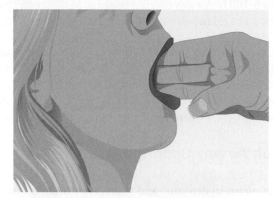

Check that the mouth opening equals at least 3 patient-sized fingers.

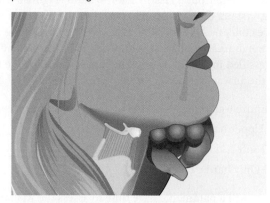

Check that there is room for 3 patient-sized fingers between the tip of the chin and the hyoid bone.

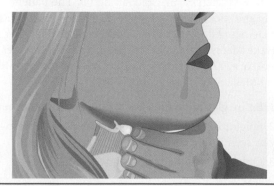

● **Figure 5-102**   The 3-3-2 rule.

Neck Mobility Neck mobility is most often limited by cervical spine immobilization, although patients with rheumatoid arthritis, spinal fusions, and elderly patients with severe degenerative disease may also have restricted range of motion. This is another reminder that any patient in spinal precautions should be considered to have a difficult airway. It is important in these cases that the front of the cervical collar is removed and manual stabilization with a jaw-thrust be applied during intubation to allow forward movement of the chin.

Saturations One of the most critical elements in airway management is the time allowed to successfully complete the procedure. The primary determinant of time in these procedures is the oxygen saturation and, in turn, your ability to preoxygenate and create an oxygen reserve. As noted earlier, a patient whose oxygen saturation is near 100 percent following preoxygenation has "adequate reserve," above 90 percent but less than 100 percent has "limited reserve," and less than 90 percent despite appropriate preoxygenation has "no reserve."

Effects of Obesity

The airway effects of obesity are complex but overall negative. Much of the anatomic problem with intubation in the morbidly obese may be overcome with proper positioning—that is, the ramped position, which was described earlier in the chapter.

Obesity also limits the effects of preoxygenation due to reduced functional residual capacity as well as increased oxygen demand so that time to perform the intubation before critical hypoxemia may be limited. Obesity definitely makes BVM ventilation more difficult, and some extraglottic rescue devices may not generate enough airway pressure to lift a very heavy chest. Finally, obesity may make identification of landmarks for a surgical airway very difficult.

Predicting Difficulty: An Imperfect Science

Prediction of difficult intubation is an imperfect science at best with limited applicability to most patients undergoing emergency airway management (Figure 5-103 ●). Prediction of difficult BVM ventilation is somewhat more reliable. Nonetheless,

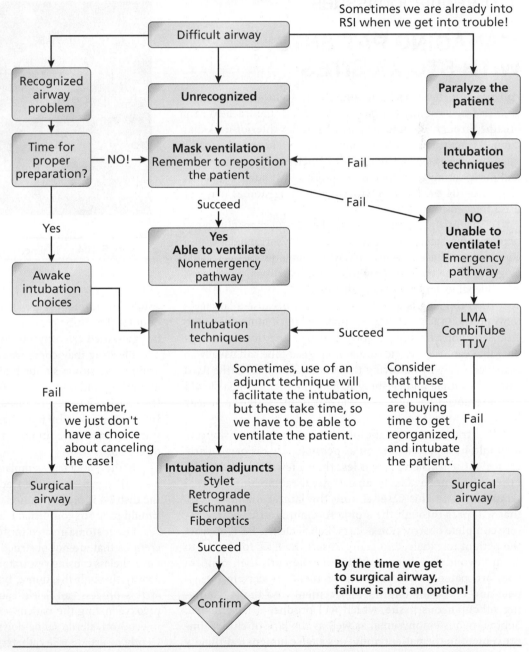

● **Figure 5-103**   Difficult airway management algorithm. (*From Stewart, C. E. Advanced Airway Management, Upper Saddle River, NJ; Pearson/Prentice Hall, 2002*)

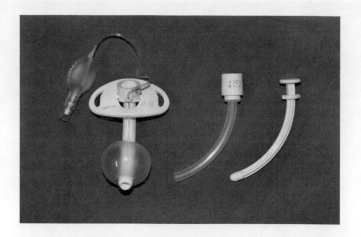

providers should look for and heed obvious warning signs of a difficult intubation or BVM ventilation and prepare accordingly. Do not, however, let the absence of any predicted difficulties create a sense of complacency. Any patient, no matter how favorable his airway appears, may prove difficult or impossible to intubate. If you have not encountered such a patient you have not yet intubated enough!

PART 4: Additional Airway and Ventilation Issues

MANAGING PATIENTS WITH STOMA SITES

Patients who have had a laryngectomy (removal of the larynx) or tracheostomy (surgical opening into the trachea) may breathe through a **stoma**, an opening in the anterior neck that connects the trachea with the ambient air. These patients frequently have tracheostomy tubes, which consist of an inner and outer cannula, in place to keep the soft-tissue stoma open (Figure 5-104 ●). Patients with longstanding stomas may not use a tracheostomy tube.

While providers often have anxiety about managing a patient with a stoma, this anxiety is usually unwarranted, because these patients have a secure airway. Potential problems include clogging of the tracheostomy tube with secretions, a dislodged tube, bleeding, and respiratory distress.

Tube clogging is a common problem because a laryngectomy produces a less-effective cough, making it more difficult to clear secretions. If these secretions organize, they form a mucous plug that can occlude the stoma. A clogged tube can usually be managed easily by removing the inner cannula from the fixed external cannula and cleaning it. The external cannula should not be removed, because the stoma may begin closing and it may be difficult to replace.

If a tracheostomy tube becomes completely dislodged, it should be replaced as soon as possible. This is particularly critical if the tracheostomy is less than a few weeks old. If another tube is not available, an endotracheal tube may be used temporarily. In this case, choose the largest diameter ETT that will pass through the stoma to maintain the airway before complete obstruction occurs. Lubricate the ETT, instruct the patient to exhale, and gently insert the ETT to about 1 to 2 cm beyond the distal cuff. Inflate the cuff, then confirm comfort, patency, and proper placement. Be certain to suspect and check for improper placement into the surrounding subcutaneous tissue, which will produce a false lumen. Subcutaneous emphysema, as well as the lack of clinical improvement in the patient, indicates a false lumen. If difficulty persists and the patient is in extremis, an endotracheal tube introducer may be passed into the stoma to gently confirm

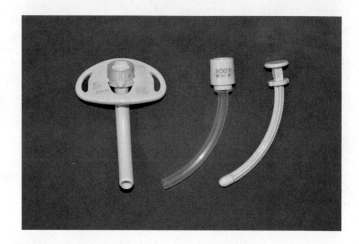

● **Figure 5-104**   Tracheostomy cannulae.

proper intratracheal positioning and the tracheostomy or endotracheal tube passed over the introducer, much as with a bougie-aided cricothyrotomy.

Bleeding may come from irritation of the skin externally around the stoma site or internally. External bleeding is usually minor, although it may scare the patient, especially if the tracheostomy is new or bleeding has not occurred previously. Internal bleeding, on the other hand, may be catastrophic. This warrants very expeditious transport and contact with medical direction.

If the patient is complaining of respiratory distress, you must first make sure the tracheostomy is patent. If it is, then the distress is probably unrelated to the tracheostomy, and you should perform your usual history and physical exam.

Other stoma-related problems to consider are excessive secretions that are not obstructing the lumen of the tube but are nevertheless causing respiratory problems. You may suction the airway through the stoma, but you must use extreme caution as this process can, itself, cause soft-tissue swelling. Begin by preoxygenating the patient with 100 percent oxygen and then inject 3 mL sterile saline down the trachea through the stoma. Gently insert a sterile catheter until resistance is met. While the patient coughs or exhales, suction the airway during withdrawal of the catheter.

TABLE 5–15 | Advantages and Disadvantages of Various Suction Types

Type	Advantages	Disadvantages
Hand-powered	Lightweight, portable, inexpensive, simple to operate	Limited volume, manually powered, fluid contact components are not disposable
Oxygen-powered	Small, lightweight	Limited suction power, uses a lot of oxygen
Battery-operated	Lightweight, portable, excellent suction power, simple to operate and troubleshoot in the field	Battery memory decreases with time; mechanically more complicated than hand-powered, some fluid contact components are not disposable
Mounted	Strong suction, adjustable vacuum power, disposable fluid contact components	Not portable, cannot be serviced in the field, no substitute power source

Supplemental oxygen may be delivered by placing an oxygen mask over the stoma or tracheostomy tube. If this is insufficient or if the patient requires positive pressure ventilation, it is very easy to attach a bag-valve device to the tracheostomy tube. If the patient has a stoma but no tracheostomy tube, then gently insert a lubricated endotracheal or tracheostomy tube to perform ventilation.

SUCTIONING

Anticipating and being prepared for complications when managing airways is the key for successful outcomes. You must anticipate that a patient may vomit and be prepared to turn the patient and **suction** in order to remove blood, mucus, and emesis. The first line of defense against aspiration should be gravity: turning the patient or just his head to the side (if not in cervical precautions) is faster and more effective than any suction device. However, suctioning equipment still must be readily available for all patients in case repositioning is not possible or as an adjunct to rotation.

Suctioning Equipment

Many kinds of suctioning devices are available. They may be handheld, oxygen-powered, battery-operated, or mounted (nonportable). Table 5–15 details the advantages and disadvantages of each.

To suit the prehospital environment, your equipment should be lightweight, portable, durable, generate a vacuum level of at least 300 mmHg when the distal end is occluded, and allow a flow rate of at least 30 liters per minute when the tube is open.

In addition to a portable device, the ambulance should have a mounted, vacuum-powered suction device that can generate stronger suction and that can be a backup device in case of equipment failure (Figure 5-105 ●).

The most commonly used suction catheters are hard/rigid catheters ("Yankauer" or "tonsil tip") and soft catheters ("whistle tip"). Table 5–16 summarizes their differences.

Because suctioning also removes oxygen, and because you must interrupt oxygen delivery in order to suction, you should limit each suctioning attempt to 10 seconds. If possible, hyperventilate the patient with 100 percent oxygen before and after each effort. Do not apply suction while inserting the catheter. Apply suction only as you withdraw the catheter after properly positioning it.

Complications of suctioning are usually related to hypoxemia from prolonged suctioning attempts without proper ventilation. The decrease in myocardial oxygen supply can cause cardiac dysrhythmias. Suctioning can also stimulate the vagus

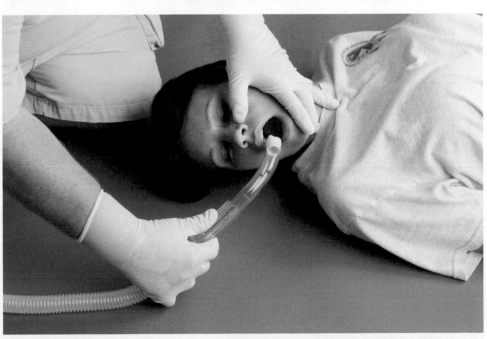

● **Figure 5-105** Oropharyngeal suctioning.

TABLE 5–16 | Types of Suctioning Catheters

Hard/Rigid Catheter	Soft Catheters
A large tube with multiple holes at the distal end	Long, flexible tube; smaller diameter than hard-tip catheters
Suctions larger volumes of fluid rapidly	Cannot remove large volumes of fluid rapidly
Standard size	Various sizes
Used in oropharyngeal airway only	Can be placed in the oropharynx, nasopharynx, or down the endotracheal tube
Removes larger particles	Suction tubing without catheter (facilitates suctioning of large debris)

nerve, causing bradycardia and hypotension, or the anxiety of being suctioned can cause hypertension and tachycardia. Stimulation of the cough reflex will cause a patient to cough, causing an increase in intracranial pressure and reducing cerebral blood flow.

Suctioning Techniques

You must have suction equipment by any patient who has airway compromise and will need airway management. Do not forget this basic and important skill. To suction a patient:

1. Use Standard Precautions, including protective eyewear, gloves, and face mask.

2. Preoxygenate the patient; this may require brief hyperventilation.

3. Determine the depth of catheter insertion by measuring from the patient's earlobe to his lips.

4. With the suction turned off, insert the catheter into your patient's pharynx to the predetermined depth.

5. Turn on the suction unit and place your thumb over the suction control orifice; limit suction to 10 seconds.

6. Continue to suction while withdrawing the catheter. When using a whistle-tip catheter, rotate it between your fingertips.

7. While maintaining ventilatory support, hyperventilate the patient with 100 percent oxygen.

In many cases you will suction extremely viscous, or thick, secretions that can obstruct the flow of fluid through the tubing. To reduce this problem, suction water through the tubing between suctioning attempts. This dilutes the secretions and facilitates flow to the suction canister. Most suction units have small water canisters for this purpose.

Tracheobronchial Suctioning

Suctioning is normally applied to the oropharynx. However, you may occasionally need to suction a patient through an endotracheal tube or a tracheostomy tube to remove secretions or mucous plugs from the tracheobronchial airway that can cause respiratory distress. Tracheobronchial suctioning risks hypoxemia, so ensuring adequate oxygenation before and after the procedure is essential. Sterile technique should be used to avoid contaminating the pulmonary system. Use only the soft-tip catheter intended for endotracheal use to avoid damaging any structures, and be certain to lubricate well. Once you have preoxygenated the patient with 100 percent oxygen, gently insert the lubricated tube, using sterile gloves, until you feel resistance (Figure 5-106 ●). Then apply suction for only about 10 seconds

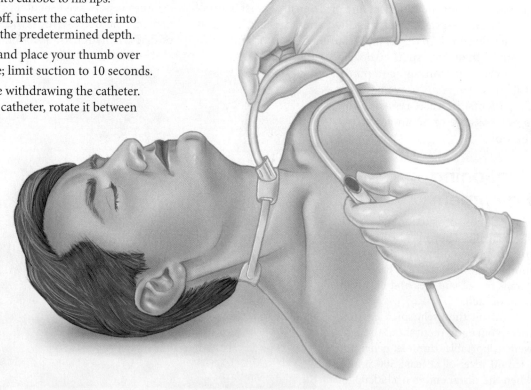

● **Figure 5-106** Tracheostomy suction technique.

while withdrawing the catheter. You may need to inject 3 to 5 cc of sterile water or saline down the endotracheal tube before suctioning to help loosen thick secretions.

GASTRIC DISTENTION AND DECOMPRESSION

A common problem during BVM ventilation is the entry of air into the stomach (gastric insufflation), which increases the risk of vomiting and regurgitation with subsequent aspiration. The enlarged stomach also pushes against the diaphragm, inhibiting the lungs' expansion and increasing resistance to ventilation. Pediatric patients are prone to bradycardia from vagal stimulation that may result. Ideally, gastric insufflation will be prevented rather than treated, as it is much less likely to occur with optimal BVM ventilation technique as discussed earlier in this chapter. Gastric insufflation is even less likely to occur with an extraglottic airway (EGA) device.

Unfortunately, even with optimal BVM ventilation technique, gastric insufflation is inevitable with prolonged ventilation, and poor BVM ventilation technique is still rampant in prehospital care. Therefore, paramedics will need to be able to treat this condition with gastric decompression, which involves the placement of a gastric tube into the stomach via the mouth (orogastric) or the nose (nasogastric) or through an EGA.

Nasogastric tube placement is generally preferred in awake patients, as it is more comfortable than orogastric placement and does not interfere with speech. However, placement in an awake patient is rarely necessary in prehospital care, except during some air medical transports, and is not discussed here.

Orogastric tube placement is recommended in most unconscious patients to minimize the risk of epistaxis and sinusitis. It is also recommended with facial fractures, to avoid placing the tube through a skull fracture into the brain, and in patients who are at increased risk for nasal bleeding. If the patient has an EGA in place that has a dedicated channel for gastric tube insertion, this should be used.

Contrary to popular belief, gastric tubes may be gently placed in patients who have gastric or esophageal varices unless they have undergone a banding or cautery procedure within the past two weeks. However, gastric intubation should be avoided if esophageal obstruction or perforation is suspected.

All three routes—nasogastric, orogastric, and EGA—carry the risk of misplacement into the lungs, although this is much less likely using an EGA. Both the oral and nasal routes put the patient at risk for vomiting and bleeding during insertion. For this reason, gastric tubes should not be placed in obtunded patients unless they are already intubated or have an EGA in place.

As for any other invasive procedure, you should always wear protective eyewear, gloves, and a face shield whenever you place a gastric tube. To place an orogastric tube in the unconscious patient:

1. Take Standard Precautions.
2. Place the patient's head in a neutral position while ventilating via the endotracheal tube or EGA.
3. Select the correct size gastric tube. Most adults take a 16 Fr when placed orally. Some EGAs will accommodate only larger or only smaller sizes, and this should be checked in advance.
4. Determine the approximate length of tube insertion by measuring from the epigastrium to the angle of the jaw, then to the mouth opening or to the proximal end of the EGA.
5. Generously lubricate the distal tip of the gastric tube and gently insert it into the oral cavity at midline.
6. Advance the tube gently to the length you determined prior to insertion.
7. Check that the tube has not curled in the mouth.
8. Confirm placement by injecting 30 to 50 mL of air while listening to the epigastric region for air entry into the stomach. In addition, end-tidal CO_2 detectors are now available that will attach to a gastric tube. In this case the detection of CO_2 indicates incorrect placement in the lungs, rather than correct placement in the stomach. Coughing also suggests malposition in the lungs, although this is unreliable in unconscious patients.
9. Apply gentle suction to the tube to evacuate gastric fluids and gas.
10. Secure the tube in place.
11. Document the indication for gastric decompression, the size tube placed, the technique, means of confirmation, any complications incurred, the type and volume of gastric contents evacuated, and the clinical response.

TRANSPORT VENTILATORS

Mechanical ventilation, as by a transport ventilator mounted in the ambulance, is designed to assist or replace the patient's own breathing. In a patient who is not breathing spontaneously, the mechanical ventilator provides "controlled" ventilations. Some mechanical ventilators are designed to provide intermittent "mandatory" ventilation; that is, the ventilator will assist a patient's own spontaneous breaths but will revert to controlled ventilations if the patient stops breathing.

There is accumulating evidence that mechanical ventilation is superior to manual ventilation except in the crashing patient where assessment of compliance and elimination of the ventilator as a source of the problem becomes essential. Mechanical

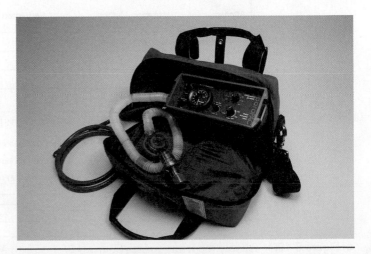

● **Figure 5-107**   Transport ventilators.

ventilation frees up provider hands and, when used correctly, is less likely to cause hemodynamic impairment or CO_2 fluctuations that have been associated with worse outcomes in head trauma patients. It is recommended that all patients with an invasive airway (ETT or EGA) be maintained on a ventilator all the way to patient turnover in the hospital when a ventilator is available and not contraindicated.

There are two general varieties of ventilators for prehospital use: simple compact devices with a minimum of options for general use and more complicated devices for critical care transport.

The simple out-of-hospital ventilator devices are designed for convenience and ease of use during short transports of relatively uncomplicated adult and older pediatric patients. These devices generally allow for control of ventilatory rate and tidal volume only.

AMERICAN MEDICAL RESPONSE OF EL PASO COUNTY
AIRWAY REPORTING FORM

Turn in this form attached to a copy of your PCR to CES mailbox immediately

DEMOGRAPHICS

PCR #:_____ Date:_____ Time called:_____ Time arrived:_____

Pt. Age:_____ Gender:_____ Patient Initials:_____ Pt. Weight:_____Kg

Attending Emp ID#_____ Attending Emp Name:_____

Hosp MR #:_____ Receiving ED Physician:_____

INDICATIONS FOR AIRWAY MANAGEMENT
- ☐ Apnea or agonal respiration
- ☐ Airway reflexes compromised
- ☐ Ventilation Compromised
- ☐ Injury or illness involving airway
- ☐ Anticipated compromise or decompensation
- ☐ Other: (describe)_____

ALL PROCEDURES PERFORMED (select all performed)
- ☐ BVM
- ☐ OPA
- ☐ NPA
- ☐ OETT (no medications)
- ☐ OETT (awake)
- ☐ OETT (RSI)
- ☐ NETT
- ☐ Digital Intubation
- ☐ Combitube
- ☐ LMA
- ☐ Cricothyrotomy (surgical)
- ☐ Cricothyrotomy (needle)

STATE OF AIRWAY PRIOR TO INTERVENTION
- ☐ Clear
- ☐ Emesis
- ☐ Sputum/Secretions
- ☐ Blood
- ☐ Teeth/Foreign objects
- ☐ Trismus -OR- Biting
- ☐ Gag Reflex: ABSENT
- ☐ Gag Reflex: PARTIAL
- ☐ Gag Reflex: PRESENT
- ☐ Combative/Resistive
- ☐ Burns
- ☐ Other:_____

BASIC INTERVENTIONS

Procedure	Size:	Done By:(emp # or agency)	Time
☐ NPA			
☐ OPA			
☐ BVM Vent	--- N/A ---		

INTUBATION INTERVENTIONS

AN ETI ATTEMPT IS DEFINED AS INSERTING THE TUBE INTO THE NOSTRIL OR INSERTING THE BLADE PAST THE TEETH/GUMS AMR PROTOCOL IS A MAXIMUM TOTAL OF THREE ATTEMPTS.

Pulsox pre-attempt: [____]

Pulsox drop < 90 during attempt? ☐ Yes ☐ No ☐ N/A (unable to get pulsox > 90 pre-attempt)

Cricoid pressure used: ☐ Yes ☐ No   Was Surevent used: ☐ Yes ☐ No

Attempt	Intubation Method: nett, oett,digital,RSI, etc.	Performed By (emp#)	Successful: (yes/no)	Time Performed:
# 1				
# 2				
# 3				
# 4				

PLACEMENT CONFIRMATION STEPS PERFORMED (Check only those actually performed)

YES/NO		YES/NO		YES/NO	
☐ ☐	Visualized Through Cords	☐ ☐	ETCO2 Colormetric Used (color):_____	☐ ☐	Lung Sounds PRESENT
☐ ☐	Negative EDD (In Trachea)	☐ ☐	ETCO2 Capnography Used (peak #)_____	☐ ☐	Gastric Sounds ABSENT
☐ ☐	Positive EDD (In Esophagus)	☐ ☐	Capnography Waveform Present	☐ ☐	Chest Rise/Fall
☐	Equivocal EDD (unsure placement)				

Tube Size: [____]   Tube Depth: [____]   How Secured: [____]

● **Figure 5-108** Airway reporting form. (*Courtesy of American Medical Response of El Paso County, Colorado and David Ross, DO, FACEP*)

MEDICATIONS USED: (check mark all meds used)

Medication	Dosage	Given By	Time Given	Medication	Dosage	Given By	Time Given
☐ Etomidate				☐ Fentanyl			
☐ Succinylcholine				☐ Morphine			
☐ Vecuronium				☐ Valium			
☐ Atropine				☐ Neosyn.			
☐ Lidocaine				☐ Viscous			
☐ Topical Spray				☐ Other			

IF FAILED INTUBATION, INDICATE SECONDARY (RESCUE) AIRWAY / VENTILATION TECHNIQUE USED (check all that apply)

Procedure	Done By:	Ventilation Yes/No	Time	Procedure	Done By:	Ventilation Yes/No	Time
☐ BVM (rescue)				☐ Cric (surgical)			
☐ Combitube				☐ Cric (needle)			
☐ LMA				☐ Other			

IF COMBITUBE WAS USED:

☐ Ventilation successful with # 1 blue tube (esophageal placement)   **Peak ETCO2:** [____] (from the tube used)

☐ Ventilation successful with #2 white tube (tracheal placement)

IF ALL ATTEMPTS AT INTUBATION FAILED, INDICATE SUSPECTED REASONS FOR FAILURE (check all that apply)

☐ Unable to visualize glottic opening   ☐ Difficult anatomy: (anterior, overbite, obesity, edema, tumor, etc.)

☐ Unable to pass vocal cords ·   ☐ Secretions / Blood / Vomit

☐ Complete obstruction; unable to clear   ☐ Unable to locate anatomical landmarks

☐ Inadequate patient or muscular relaxation   ☐ Poor patient access: (extrication, spinal immob., confined space, etc.)

☐ Poor jaw/ neck mobility   ☐ Arrival at hospital prior to completion of procedure

☐ Severe trauma   ☐ Other: _____

ED PHYSICIAN CONFIRMATION OF PROPER ETT / CRICOTHYROIDOTOMY PLACEMENT:

☐ Correct Placement   ☐ Incorrect Placement

Comments: _____
_____
_____

PHYSICIAN SIGNATURE: _____

MEDICAL DIRECTOR EVALUATION:

☐ Appropriate Intervention   ☐ Confirmation criteria MET

☐ Inappropriate Intervention   ☐ Confirmation criteria NOT met

MEDICAL DIRECTOR COMMENTS:
_____
_____
_____

MEDICAL DIRECTOR SIGNATURE: _____ **DATE REVIEWED:** _____

TURN IN THIS FORM ATTACHED TO A COPY OF YOUR PCR TO CES MAILBOX IMMEDIATELY

● **Figure 5-108** *(Continued)*

Most of these units deliver controlled ventilation only (will only breathe for patients who are not breathing on their own), while other units will function as intermittent mandatory ventilators (assisting spontaneously breathing patients), which revert to controlled mechanical ventilation in patients who are not breathing.

The inspired oxygen concentration is usually fixed at 100 percent, but it may be adjustable. Oxygen consumption on longer transports may be substantial. Most of these devices do not provide CPAP. These devices also offer little ability to monitor airway pressures or delivered volumes and usually do not have warning alarms but instead have a pop-off valve that prevents pressure-related injury. When airway pressure exceeds a preset level (typically 60 cm/H_2O), the valve opens, venting some of the tidal volume. This safety feature may actually hinder ventilation in patients who require greater positive pressure, such as those with significant lung pathology (e.g., cardiogenic pulmonary edema, adult respiratory distress syndrome [ARDS], pulmonary contusion, and bronchospasm). Consider using a bag-valve device if this problem occurs.

Critical care transport ventilators, in contrast to the simple units just described, offer a host of features such as different ventilator modes, enhanced monitoring, alarms, and more (Figure 5-107 ●). The increased adjustability allows for keeping the patient more comfortable with less sedation, analgesia, and paralysis. Some of these devices can be used to provide mask CPAP as well. Inspired oxygen concentration can usually be adjusted. These critical transport devices can be used on most pediatric patients and some neonates. The trade-off for these features is much higher cost, and their greater complexity requires much more extensive training. These advanced ventilators are worth considering if you have long transports, do a lot of interfacility transports, or have a large pediatric population.

DOCUMENTATION

Accurate and thorough documentation of airway management is critical for clinical care after the patient is transported, for quality assurance, and for medical/legal defense. Documentation should include not only what was done but also the thought process of why it was done and any complications that occurred. A significant percentage of claims and lawsuits that are filed against prehospital providers involve airway issues, and often these cases are won or lost based on the field documentation. Therefore, it is crucial that the provider learn to document in medically correct and legally sufficient terms exactly what was done in managing the airway.

The documentation sample shown in Figure 5-108 ● is by no means the only way to document airway management. It is, however, provided as an example. One may be tempted to say that the example is "over-documentation." However, few practitioners who have been called to testify under oath about their airway management would agree. Since patients who require prehospital airway management are at high risk for a bad outcome from the outset, and because airway management literally determines whether the patient lives or dies, it stands to reason that the greatest emphasis should be placed on detailed documentation of these issues.

SUMMARY

Airway assessment and maintenance is the most critical step in managing any patient. If you do not promptly establish a definitive airway and provide proper ventilation, the patient's outcome will be poor. Frequently reassessing the airway is mandatory to ensure that the patient has not decompensated, requiring additional airway procedures. Successful management of all airways requires the paramedic to follow the proper management sequence.

Basic airway and management skills can make the difference between a successful outcome and a poor patient prognosis. Once you have mastered these basic skills and made them a part of airway management in every patient, you should learn and use advanced skills such as intubation, RSI, and cricothyrotomy. You must maintain proficiency in all airway skills, especially the more advanced techniques, through ongoing continuing education, physician medical direction, and testing with each EMS service. If you cannot do this, it is in the patient's best interest to focus on less sophisticated airway skills. If you anticipate that every airway will be complicated, apply basic airway skills before using advanced procedures, and perform frequent reassessments, you will give the patient his best chance for meaningful survival.

YOU MAKE THE CALL

You and your paramedic partner, Preston Connelly, are assigned to District 4, a quiet suburban neighborhood, on a warm Saturday in June. At 2:00 P.M., you are dispatched to care for a choking child at the Happy Hotdog Restaurant on Main Street. On your way to the location, the dispatcher advises you that they are currently giving prearrival choking instructions to the bystanders at the scene. On arrival, you find a frantic mother who tells you that her 6-year-old son was eating a hotdog and drinking a soda when he started coughing and gasping for air. She keeps yelling for you to do something. Bystanders surround the child and are attempting to perform the Heimlich maneuver without success. On your primary assessment, you find a 6-year-old male lying on the floor, unconscious and apneic, with a pulse rate of 130. There is cyanosis surrounding his lips and fingernail beds, with a moderate amount of secretions coming from his mouth. There are no signs of trauma. You and Preston immediately start management of this child.

1. What is your primary assessment and management of this child?

2. What are your first actions?

3. What are your options for managing the airway after the obstruction is relieved?

4. What are the major anatomic differences between pediatric and adult patients in terms of airway management?

See Suggested Responses at the back of this book.

 REVIEW QUESTIONS

1. The depression between the epiglottis and the base of the tongue is called the:
   a. nare.
   c. larynx.
   b. glottis.
   d. vallecula.

2. The average volume of gas inhaled or exhaled in one respiratory cycle is the:
   a. minute volume.
   b. tidal volume.
   c. respiratory rate.
   d. total lung capacity.

3. A drop in blood pressure of greater than 10 torr during inspiration is called:
   a. compliance.
   b. laryngeal spasm.
   c. pulsus paradoxus.
   d. paradoxical breathing.

4. To avoid hypoxia during intubation, limit each intubation attempt to no more than _____ seconds before reoxygenating the patient.
   a. 10
   c. 30
   b. 20
   d. 40

5. _____ is NOT a preferred neuro-muscular blocking agent for emergency RSI.
   a. Atracurium
   b. Vecuronium
   c. Pancuronium
   d. Succinylcholine

6. The _____ is the most superior part of the airway.
   a. pharynx
   b. larynx
   c. oral cavity
   d. nasal cavity

7. The _____ is the only bone in the axial skeleton that does not articulate with any other bone.
   a. femur
   c. stapes
   b. hyoid
   d. patella

8. The _____ comprise(s) the key functional unit of the respiratory system.
   a. hilum
   b. alveoli
   c. bronchi
   d. respiratory bronchioles

9. The paramedic can correct oxygen derangements by:
   a. increasing ventilation.
   b. administering supplemental oxygen.
   c. using intermittent positive pressure ventilation.
   d. all of the above.

10. The _____ is the amount of gas in the tidal volume that remains in air passageways unavailable for gas exchange.
    a. base tidal volume
    b. minute volume
    c. dead-space volume
    d. total lung capacity

11. "Difficulty speaking" defines:
    a. aphagia.
    c. dysphonia.
    b. aphonia.
    d. dysphagia.

12. "An irregular pattern of rate and depth with sudden, periodic episodes of apnea, indicating increased intracranial pressure" describes:
    a. agonal respirations.
    b. Biot's respirations.
    c. Kussmaul's respirations.
    d. Cheyne-Stokes respirations.

13. _____ is often called the "fifth vital sign."
    a. Heart rate
    b. Blood pressure
    c. Pulse oximetry
    d. Blood glucose level

14. The visual representation of the expired CO_2 waveform is:
    a. capnogram.
    c. capnometry.
    b. capnograph.
    d. capnography.

15. Which of the following is NOT a disadvantage of the nasopharyngeal airway?
    a. It isolates the trachea.
    b. It is difficult to suction through.
    c. It is smaller than the oropharyngeal airway.
    d. It may cause severe nosebleeds if inserted too forcefully.

16. Advantages of endotracheal intubation include:
   a. It eliminates the need to maintain a mask seal.
   b. It isolates the trachea and permits complete control of the airway.
   c. It impedes gastric distention by channeling air directly into the trachea.
   d. All of the above.

17. _____ is generally the second-line paralytic when succinylcholine is contraindicated, because it has fewer cardiac and hypotensive side effects than other nondepolarizing agents.
   a. Atracurium
   b. Fentanyl
   c. Vecuronium
   d. Pancuronium

18. Relative contraindications for blind nasotracheal intubation include:
   a. suspected elevation of intracranial pressure.
   b. suspected basilar skull fracture.
   c. combative patient.
   d. all of the above.

19. The _____ can function in either the tracheal or esophageal position.
   a. ET   c. LMA
   b. PtL   d. PLA

20. Open cricothyrotomy is contraindicated in children under the age of _____ because the cricothyroid membrane is small and underdeveloped.
   a. 6   c. 10
   b. 8   d. 12

See Answers to Review Questions at the back of this book.

REFERENCES

1. Austin, M. A., K. E. Wills, L. Blizzard, E. H. Walters, and R. Wood-Baker. "Effect of High Flow Oxygen on Mortality in Chronic Obstructive Pulmonary Disease Patients in Prehospital Setting: Randomised Controlled Trial." *BMJ* 341 (2010): c5462.

2. Body, R. and K. Hogg. "Best Evidence Topic Reports. Oxygen in Acute Uncomplicated Myocardial Infarction." *Emerg Med J* 21 (2004): 75.

3. Moradkhan, R. and L. I. Sinoway. "Revisiting the Role of Oxygen Therapy in Cardiac Patients." *J Am Coll Cardiol* 56 (2010): 1013–1016.

4. Barker, S. J., J. Curry, D. Redford, and S. Morgan. "Measurement of Carboxyhemoglobin and Methemoglobin by Pulse Oximetry: A Human Volunteer Study." *Anesthesiology* 105 (2006): 892–897.

5. Bledsoe, B. E., K. Nowicki, J. H. Creel, D. Carrison, and H. W. Severance. "Use of Pulse CO-Oximetry as a Screening and Monitoring Tool in Mass Carbon Monoxide Poisoning." *Prehosp Emerg Care* 14 (2010): 131–133.

6. Rucker, J., J. Tesler, L. Fedorko et al. "Normocapnia Improves Cerebral Oxygen Delivery during Conventional Oxygen Therapy in Carbon Monoxide-Exposed Research Subjects." *Ann Emerg Med* 40 (2002): 611–618.

7. Camp, N. E. "Methemoglobinemia." *J Emerg Nurs* 33 (2007): 172–174.

8. Abu-Laban, R. B., P. J. Zed, R. A. Purssell, and K. G. Evans. "Severe Methemoglobinemia from Topical Anesthetic Spray: Case Report, Discussion and Qualitative Systematic Review." *CJEM* 3 (2001): 51–56.

9. Kupnik, D. and P. Skok. "Capnometry in the Prehospital Setting: Are We Using Its Potential?" *Emerg Med J* 24 (2007): 614–617.

10. Silvestri, S., G. A. Ralls, B. Krauss et al. "The effectiveness of Out-of-Hospital Use of Continuous End-Tidal Carbon Dioxide Monitoring on the Rate of Unrecognized Misplaced Intubation within a Regional Emergency Medical Services System." *Ann Emerg Med* 45 (2005): 497–503.

11. Collin, J. S., H. J. Lemmens, J. B. Brodsky et al., "Laryngoscopy and Morbid Obesity: A Comparison of the "Sniff" and "Ramped" Position." *Obes Surg* 14 (2004): 1171–1175.

12. Ellis, D. Y., T. Harris, and D. Zideman. "Cricoid Pressure in Emergency Department Rapid Sequence Tracheal Intubations: A Risk-Benefit Analysis." *Ann Emerg Med* 50 (2007): 653–665.

13. Hubble, M. W., L. Brown, D. A. Wilfong, A. Hertelendy, R. W. Benner, and M. E. Richards. "A Meta-Analysis of Prehospital Airway Control Techniques Part I: Orotracheal and Nasotracheal Intubation Success Rates." *Prehosp Emerg Care* 14 (2010): 377–401.

14. Hubble, M. W., D. A. Wilfong, L. H. Brown, A. Hertelendy, and R. W. Benner. "A Meta-Analysis of Prehospital Airway Control Techniques Part II: Alternative Airway Devices and Cricothyrotomy Success Rates." *Prehosp Emerg Care* 14 (2010): 515–530.

15. Colwell, C. B., K. E. McVaney, J. S. Haukoos et al. "An Evaluation of Out-of-Hospital Advanced Airway Management in an Urban Setting." *Acad Emerg Med* 12 (2005): 417–422.

16. Guyette, F. X., M. J. Greenwood, D. Neubecker, R. Roth, and H. E. Wang. "Alternate Airways in the Prehospital Setting (Resource Document to NAEMSP Position Statement)." *Prehosp Emerg Care* 11 (2007): 56–61.

17. Bercker, S., W. Schmidbauer, T. Volk et al. "A Comparison of Seal in Seven Supraglottic Airway Devices Using a Cadaver Model of Elevated Esophageal Pressure." *Anesth Analg* 106 (2008): 445–448, Table of Contents.

18. Cady, C. E. and R. G. Pirrallo. "The Effect of Combitube Use on Paramedic Experience in Endotracheal Intubation." *Am J Emerg Med* 23 (2005): 868–871.

19. Cady, C. E., M. D. Weaver, R. G. Pirrallo, and H. E. Wang. "Effect of Emergency Medical Technician-Placed Combitubes on Outcomes after Out-of-Hospital Cardiopulmonary Arrest." *Prehosp Emerg Care* 13 (2009): 495–499.

20. Russi, C. S., L. Miller, and M. J. Hartley. "A Comparison of the King-LT to Endotracheal Intubation and Combitube in a Simulated Difficult Airway." *Prehosp Emerg Care* 12 (2008): 35–41.

21. Gaither, J. B., J. Matheson, A. Eberhardt, and C. B. Colwell. "Tongue Engorgement Associated with Prolonged Use of the King-LT Laryngeal Tube Device." *Ann Emerg Med* 55(4) (2010): 367–369.

22. Guyette, F. X., H. Wang, and J. S. Cole. "King Airway Use by Air Medical Providers." *Prehosp Emerg Care* 11 (2007): 473–476.

23. Bledsoe, B. E., D. Slattery, R. Lauver, W. Forred, L. Johnson, and G. Rigo. "Can Emergency Medical Services Personnel Effectively Place and Use the S.A.L.T. Airway?" *Prehosp Emerg Care* 15 (2011): 359–365.

24. Murray, M. J., M. J. Vermeulen, L. J. Morrison, and T. Waite. "Evaluation of Prehospital Insertion of the Laryngeal Mask Airway by Primary Care Paramedics with Only Classroom Mannequin Training." *CJEM* 4 (2002): 338–343.

25. Chen, L. and A. L. Hsiao. "Randomized Trial of Endotracheal Tube versus Laryngeal Mask Airway in Simulated Prehospital Pediatric Arrest." *Pediatrics* 122 (2008): e294–e297.

26. Choyce, A., M. S. Avidan, C. Patel et al. "Comparison of Laryngeal Mask and Intubating Laryngeal Mask Insertion by the Naïve Intubator." *Br J Anaesth* 84 (2000): 103–105.

27. Davis, D. P. "Should Invasive Airway Management Be Done in the Field?" *CMAJ* 178 (2008): 1171–1173.

28. Bochicchio, G. V. and T. M. Scalea. "Is Field Intubation Useful?" *Curr Opin Crit Care* 9 (2003): 524–529.

29. Wang H. E. and D. M. Yealy. "Out-of-Hospital Endotracheal Intubation: Where Are We?" *Ann Emerg Med* 47 (2006): 532–541.

30. Wang, H. E., G. K. Balasubramani, L. J. Cook, J. R. Lave, and D. M. Yealy. "Out-of-Hospital Endotracheal Intubation Experience and Patient Outcomes." *Ann Emerg Med* 55(6) (2010): 527–537.e6.

31. Wang, H. E. and D. M. Yealy. "How Many Attempts Are Required to Accomplish Out-of-Hospital Endotracheal Intubation?" *Acad Emerg Med* 13 (2006): 372–377.

32. Warner, K. J., D. Carlbom, C. R. Cooke, E. M. Bulger, M. K. Copass, and S. R. Sharar. "Paramedic Training for Proficient Prehospital Endotracheal Intubation." *Prehosp Emerg Care* 14 (2010): 103–108.

33. Wang, H. E., B. N. Abo, J. R. Lave, and D. M. Yealy. "How Would Minimum Experience Standards Affect the Distribution of Out-of-Hospital Endotracheal Intubations?" *Ann Emerg Med* 50 (2007): 246–252.

34. Katz, S. H. and J. L. Falk. "Misplaced Endotracheal Tubes by Paramedics in an Urban Emergency Medical Services System." *Ann Emerg Med* 37 (2001): 32–37.

35. Jones, J. H., M. P. Murphy, R. L. Dickson, G. G. Somerville, and E. J. Brizendine. "Emergency Physician-Verified Out-of-Hospital Intubation: Miss Rates by Paramedics." *Acad Emerg Med* 11 (2004): 707–709.

36. Levitan, R. M., W. C. Kinkle, W. J. Levin, and W. W. Everett. "Laryngeal View during Laryngoscopy: A Randomized Trial Comparing Cricoid Pressure, Backward-Upward-Rightward Pressure, and Bimanual Laryngoscopy." *Ann Emerg Med* 47 (2006): 548–555.

37. Wayne, M. A. and M. McDonnell. "Comparison of Traditional versus Video Laryngoscopy in Out-of-Hospital Tracheal Intubation." *Prehosp Emerg Care* 14 (2010): 278–282.

38. Cobas, M. A., M. A. De la Peña, R. Manning, K. Candiotti, and A. J. Varon. "Prehospital Intubations and Mortality: A Level 1 Trauma Center Perspective." *Anesth Analg* 109 (2009): 489–493.

39. Davis, D. P., J. Peay, M. J. Sise et al. "The Impact of Prehospital Endotracheal Intubation on Outcome in Moderate to Severe Traumatic Brain Injury." *J Trauma* 58 (2005): 933–939.

40. Shafi, S. and L. Gentilello. "Pre-Hospital Endotracheal Intubation and Positive Pressure Ventilation Is Associated with Hypotension and Decreased Survival in Hypovolemic Trauma Patients: An Analysis of the National Trauma Data Bank." *J Trauma* 59 (2005): 1140–1145; discussion 1145–1147.

41. Zink, B. J. and R. F. Maio. "Out-of-Hospital Endotracheal Intubation in Traumatic Brain Injury: Outcomes Research Provides Us with an Unexpected Outcome." *Ann Emerg Med* 44 (2004): 451–453.

42. Stockinger, Z. T. and N. E. McSwain. "Prehospital Endotracheal Intubation for Trauma Does Not Improve Survival over Bag-Valve-Mask Ventilation." *J Trauma* 56 (2004): 531–536.

43. Gausche, M., R. J. Lewis, S. J. Stratton et al. "Effect of Out-of-Hospital Pediatric Endotracheal Intubation on Survival and Neurological Outcome: A Controlled Clinical Trial." *JAMA* 283 (2000): 783–790.

44. Henning, J., P. Sharley, and R. Young. "Pressures within Air-Filled Tracheal Cuffs at Altitude—An In Vivo Study." *Anaesthesia* 59 (2004): 252–254.

45. Mizelle, H. L., S. G. Rothrock, S. Silvestri, and J. Pagane. "Preventable Morbidity and Mortality from Prehospital Paralytic Assisted Intubation: Can We Expect Outcomes Comparable to Hospital-Based Practice?" *Prehosp Emerg Care* 6 (2002): 472–475.

46. Bernard, S. A., V. Nguyen, P. Cameron et al. "Prehospital Rapid Sequence Intubation Improves Functional Outcome for Patients with Severe Traumatic Brain Injury: A Randomized Controlled Trial." *Ann Surg* 252 (2010): 959–965.

47. Bulger, E. M., M. K. Copass, D. R. Sabath, R. V. Maier, and G. J. Jurkovich. "The Use of Neuromuscular Blocking Agents to Facilitate Prehospital Intubation Does Not Impair Outcome after Traumatic Brain Injury." *J Trauma* 58 (2005): 718–723; discussion 723–724.

48. Cudnik, M. T., C. D. Newgard, M. Daya, and J. Jui. "The Impact of Rapid Sequence Intubation on Trauma Patient Mortality in Attempted Prehospital Intubation." *J Emerg Med* 38 (2010): 175–181.

49. Davis, D. P., J. V. Dunford, J. C. Poste et al. "The Impact of Hypoxia and Hyperventilation on Outcome after Paramedic Rapid Sequence Intubation of Severely Head-Injured Patients." *J Trauma* 57 (2004): 1–8; discussion 8–10.

50. Davis, D. P., D. B. Hoyt, M. Ochs et al. "The Effect of Paramedic Rapid Sequence Intubation on Outcome in Patients with Severe Traumatic Brain Injury." *J Trauma* 54 (2003): 444–453.

51. Davis, D. P., M. Ochs, D. B. Hoyt, D. Bailey, L. K. Marshall, and P. Rosen. "Paramedic-Administered

Neuromuscular Blockade Improves Prehospital Intubation Success in Severely Head-Injured Patients." *J Trauma* 55 (2003): 713–719.

52. Dunford, J. V., D. P. Davis, M. Ochs, M. Doney, and D. B. Hoyt. "Incidence of Transient Hypoxia and Pulse Rate Reactivity during Paramedic Rapid Sequence Intubation." *Ann Emerg Med* 42 (2003): 721–728.

53. Butler, J. and R. Jackson. "Towards Evidence Based Emergency Medicine: Best BETs from Manchester Royal Infirmary. Lignocaine Premedication before Rapid Sequence Induction in Head Injuries." *Emerg Med J* 19 (2002): 554.

54. Reid, C., L. Chan, and M. Tweeddale. "The Who, Where, and What of Rapid Sequence Intubation: Prospective Observational Study of Emergency RSI outside the Operating Theatre." *Emerg Med J* 21 (2004): 296–301.

55. Walls, R. M., C. A. Brown, A. E. Bair, and D. J. Pallin, of the NEAR II Investigators. "Emergency Airway Management: A Multi-Center Report of 8937 Emergency Department Intubations." *J Emerg Med* 41(4) (2010): 347–354.

56. Wang, H. E., D. P. Davis, M. A. Wayne, and T. Delbridge. "Prehospital Rapid-Sequence Intubation; What Does the Evidence Show?" *Prehosp Emerg Care* 8 (2004): 366–377.

57. Kheterpal, S., L. Martin, A. M. Shanks, and K. K. Tremper. "Prediction and Outcomes of Impossible Mask Ventilation: A Review of 50,000 Anesthetics." *Anesthesiology* 110 (2009): 891–897.

58. Vadeboncoeur, T. F., D. P. Davis, M. Ochs, J. C. Poste, D. B. Hoyt, and G. M. Vilke. "The Ability of Paramedics to Predict Aspiration in Patients Undergoing Prehospital Rapid Sequence Intubation." *J Emerg Med* 30 (2006): 131–136.

FURTHER READING

American College of Surgeons, Committee on Trauma. *Advanced Trauma Life Support Course: Student Manual.* 8th ed. Chicago, IL: American College of Surgeons, 2008.

Bledsoe, Bryan E. and Dwayne Clayden. *Prehospital Emergency Pharmacology.* 7th ed. Upper Saddle River, NJ: Pearson/Prentice Hall, 2012.

Braude, D. *Rapid Sequence Intubation & Rapid Sequence Airway,* 2nd ed. Albuquerque, NM: University of New Mexico Press, 2009.

Stewart, Charles E. *Advanced Airway Management.* Upper Saddle River, NJ: Pearson/Prentice Hall, 2002.

PRECAUTIONS ON BLOODBORNE PATHOGENS AND INFECTIOUS DISEASES

Prehospital emergency personnel, like all health care workers, are at risk for exposure to blood-borne pathogens and infectious diseases. In emergency situations it is often difficult to take or enforce proper infection control measures. However, as a paramedic, you must recognize your high-risk status. Study the following information on infection control carefully.

Infection control is designed to protect emergency personnel, their families, and their patients from unnecessary exposure to communicable diseases. Laws, regulations, and standards regarding infection control include:

- *Centers for Disease Control and Prevention (CDC) Guidelines.* The CDC has published extensive guidelines on infection control. Proper equipment and techniques that should be used by emergency response personnel to prevent or minimize risk of exposure are defined.
- *The Ryan White Act.* The Ryan White Act of 1990 allows emergency personnel to find out if they were exposed to an infectious disease while rendering patient care. Employers are required to name a "designated officer" to coordinate communications with the treating hospital.
- *Americans with Disabilities Act.* This act prohibits discrimination against individuals with disabilities, including those with contagious diseases. It guarantees equal employment opportunities and job protection if the infected individual can perform essential job functions and does not pose a threat to the safety and health of patients and coworkers.
- *Occupational Safety and Health Administration (OSHA) Regulations.* OSHA has enacted a regulation entitled Occupational Exposure to Bloodborne Pathogens that classifies emergency response personnel as being at the greatest risk of occupational exposure to communicable diseases. This regulation requires employers to provide hepatitis B (HBV) vaccinations free of charge, maintain a written exposure control plan, and provide personal protective equipment. These requirements primarily apply to private employers. Applicability to local and state governmental employees varies by locality. Many states have developed their own OSHA plans.
- *National Fire Protection Association (NFPA) Guidelines.* This is a national organization that has established specific guidelines and requirements regarding infection control for emergency response agencies, particularly fire departments and EMS services.

STANDARD PRECAUTIONS AND PERSONAL PROTECTIVE EQUIPMENT

Emergency response personnel should practice Standard Precautions by which ALL body substances are considered to be potentially infectious. To practice Standard Precautions, all emergency personnel should utilize personal protective equipment (PPE). Appropriate PPE should be available on every emergency vehicle. The minimum recommended PPE includes the following:

- *Gloves.* Disposable gloves should be donned by all emergency response personnel BEFORE initiating any emergency care. When an emergency incident involves more than one patient, you should attempt to change gloves between patients. When gloves have been contaminated, they should be removed as soon as possible. To properly remove contaminated gloves, grasp one glove approximately 1 inch from the wrist. Without touching the inside of the glove, pull the glove halfway off and stop. With that half-gloved hand, pull the glove on the opposite hand completely off. Place the removed glove in the palm of the other glove, with the inside of the removed glove exposed. Pull the second glove completely off with the ungloved hand, only touching the inside of the glove. Always wash hands after gloves are removed, even when the gloves appear intact.
- *Masks and Protective Eyewear.* Masks and protective eyewear should be present on all emergency vehicles and used in accordance with the level of exposure encountered. Masks and protective eyewear should be worn together whenever blood spatter is likely to occur, such as during arterial bleeding, childbirth, endotracheal intubation, invasive procedures, oral

suctioning, and cleanup of equipment that requires heavy scrubbing or brushing. Both you and the patient should wear masks whenever the potential for airborne transmission of disease exists.

- *HEPA and N-95 Respirators.* Due to the resurgence of tuberculosis (TB), prehospital person-nel should protect themselves from TB infection through use of an N-95 or a high-efficiency particulate air (HEPA) respirator, as approved by the National Institute of Occupational Safety and Health (NIOSH). It should fit snugly and be capable of filtering out the tuberculo-sis bacillus. An N-95 or HEPA respirator should be worn when caring for patients with con-firmed or suspected TB. This is especially true when performing "high-hazard" procedures such as administration of nebulized medications, endotracheal intubation, or suctioning on such a patient.
- *Gowns.* Gowns protect clothing from blood splashes. If large splashes of blood are expected, such as with childbirth, wear impervious gowns.
- *Resuscitation Equipment.* Disposable resuscitation equipment should be the primary means of artificial ventilation in emergency care. Such items should be used once, then disposed of.

Remember, the proper use of personal protective equipment ensures effective infection con-trol and minimizes risk. Use ALL protective equipment recommended for any particular situation to ensure maximum protection.

Consider ALL body substances potentially infectious and ALWAYS practice Standard Precautions.

The following are suggested responses to the "You Make the Call" scenarios presented in each chapter of Volume 2, Paramedicine Fundamentals. Each represents an acceptable response to the scenario but should not be interpreted as the only correct response.

Chapter 1—Pathophysiology

1. Explain the physiologic basis for the patient's apparent dehydration.

As blood glucose levels start to rise, glucose is lost into the urine through the kidneys. This typically occurs when the blood glucose level exceeds 180 mg/dL. The glucose molecules have osmotic properties. Thus, they take water molecules with them into the urine. This phenomenon, called osmotic diuresis, ultimately causes a decrease in intravascular fluid volume resulting in dehydration. This causes tachycardia and ultimately a fall in blood pressure. Also, it is the pathophysiologic basis for the polyuria (excessive urination) and polydipsia (excessive thirst) associated with untreated diabetes.

2. Describe the role of insulin in glucose transport into the cell.

Insulin is necessary for the transport of the glucose molecule into the cell (except for cells in the brain). Insulin activates specialized glucose transport proteins present on the surface of the cell. If insulin levels are inadequate, then glucose cannot enter the cell to fuel the various metabolic processes. This causes the cells to shift to a less-effective form of metabolism (anaerobic metabolism and lipid metabolism), ultimately resulting in the accumulation of acids and ketones. As ketones rise, they are eliminated through the urine and the respiratory tract. When this occurs, the characteristic odor of ketones can often be detected on the breath and in the urine.

3. Prepare a prehospital treatment plan given the information provided.

Prehospital treatment should first address the airway and breathing. If necessary, provide airway and respiratory support. In most cases, the airway will be patent. Supplemental oxygen should be administered via a nonrebreather mask if the patient is hypoxic. Then, an IV should be started with an isotonic crystalloid solution such as normal saline. Often the patient will require several liters of fluid to replace lost volume. Later, the patient will require intravenous insulin to move the glucose into the cells for normal metabolic processes. This is often administered in the form of an insulin drip. Blood glucose levels must be constantly monitored to prevent iatrogenic hypoglycemia.

Chapter 2—Human Life Span Development

1. Do you believe that this is normal behavior for a patient of this age and in this particular situation?

Yes, it is exactly the type of behavior that should be expected from a patient this age and in this situation.

2. What is a likely reason for this behavior?

Adolescents are very concerned with modesty and privacy. The reason for her behavior is likely that her parents and younger sister are in the room with her. Additionally, the patient may have been hiding something from her parents, such as sexual activity, drug or alcohol use, birth control pills, or another issue, that she does not want to reveal to them or her sister.

3. What might you do to make this patient more cooperative?

If possible, have a "same sex" provider perform the patient assessment. If this is possible, then you might ask the parents and sister to leave the room. If there is no "same sex" provider available, then have the mother stay in the room for the protection of both the patient and the provider, but have her move to a point away from the bed so that answers to your questions cannot be heard. If possible, palpate the abdomen through a thin sheet to further protect the patient's modesty.

Chapter 3—Emergency Pharmacology

1. What is dopamine and what is its mechanism of action?

It is a catecholamine that stimulates alpha, beta, and, supposedly, dopaminergic receptors. It was given in moderate dosage, which stimulates the beta receptors more than the others. This increases the force of cardiac contraction, which may increase cardiac output and, subsequently, blood pressure.

2. *What was the purpose of the dopamine infusion?*

Dopamine was given to increase cardiac output. The patient is suffering from cardiogenic shock with pulmonary edema and needs to have his blood pressure increased. Raising his cardiac output with dopamine is preferable to increasing his peripheral vascular resistance (afterload), because his obvious difficulty overcoming existing afterload is causing the pulmonary edema.

3. *What is atropine's mechanism of action?*

Atropine is a parasympatholytic that blocks the effects of acetylcholine at the muscarinic receptors, specifically those at the heart's SA and AV nodes, which regulate heart rate. A side effect of succinylcholine administration is bradycardia (the physical act of intubation may also cause bradycardia). Atropine is therefore given as a prophylactic treatment against expected bradycardia. This bradycardic side effect is most notable in pediatric patients.

4. *What is the purpose of giving lidocaine to this patient?*

Succinylcholine may also lead to an increase in intracranial pressure. Lidocaine can preemptively block that increase by the same mechanism that decreases ventricular ectopy. However, usage of lidocaine in RSI remains controversial and is falling out of favor.

5. *Why was midazolam administered before succinylcholine?*

Midazolam is a sedative with amnesic properties. Succinylcholine is a neuromuscular blocker that induces muscular paralysis without affecting consciousness. This would be a very unpleasant sensation, so some type of sedation or anesthesia is given before any neuromuscular blockade.

6. *What are succinylcholine's classification and mechanism of action?*

Succinylcholine is a depolarizing (fasciculating) neuromuscular blocker that is given to induce paralysis. This is most frequently done to facilitate intubation in rapid sequence intubation. It acts by competing with acetylcholine at the nicotinic$_M$ receptors. When succinylcholine binds with these receptors, it causes depolarization much like acetylcholine; however, it remains bound to the receptor and prevents repolarization and subsequent depolarization of the muscle. This in turn prevents muscle contraction and causes paralysis. Pseudocholinesterase, an enzyme similar to acetylcholinesterase, eventually breaks down succinylcholine.

Chapter 4—Intravenous Access and Medication Administration

1. *Before administering aspirin or any other medication orally (p.o.), what major consideration must you be sure of?*

When administering a medication orally, or by way of the mouth and enteral tract, you must make sure that the patient has an adequate level of consciousness and can support his airway. Administering a medication orally to a semiconscious or unresponsive patient who cannot support his airway can cause an airway occlusion and/or aspiration into the lungs. If aspiration occurs, the patient is at risk for an inflammatory response and deadly aspiration pneumonia.

2. *Of the following medications and routes of delivery, which will provide the fastest and most predictable rate of absorption?*
   • *aspirin—enteral tract*
   • *nitroglycerin—sublingual*
   • *morphine sulfate—IV bolus*

The morphine sulfate delivered as an intravenous bolus will provide the most predictable and fastest rate of drug absorption. Any medication delivered directly into the venous circulation will be carried by the blood and quickly reach its target site.

Drug absorption in the enteral tract (aspirin given orally) can be affected adversely by physical activity, emotion, and the presence of food. Absorption via the sublingual route involves passage of the medication (nitroglycerin) through the mucous membranes beneath the tongue. Once it passes through these membranes, the drug can then be circulated via the venous circulation throughout the body. Even though passage is relatively fast, overall absorption does not occur as quickly as when the medication is injected directly into the venous circulation.

3. *When administered sublingually, how is the nitroglycerin absorbed into the body?*

When administering nitroglycerin via the sublingual route, the medication must be absorbed through the mucous membranes beneath the tongue. The area beneath the tongue is extremely rich with blood vessels. Once through the mucous membranes, the nitroglycerin is carried by the venous circulation and systemically distributed throughout the body.

4. *You elect to administer 3 mg of morphine sulfate to the patient. The medication is packaged as 10 mg in 5 mL of solution in a multidose vial. How many milliliters must you administer to give the 3 mg of morphine?*

Using the formula as discussed in the chapter, the drug dosage can be calculated as follows:

$$\frac{5 \text{ mL (volume on hand)} \times 3 \text{ mg (desired dose)}}{10 \text{ mg (dosage on hand)}} = 1.5 \text{ mL}$$

To deliver 3 mg of morphine sulfate, you must administer 1.5 mL of the medication solution.

Using the ratio and proportion method, the amount of drug to administer is calculated as follows:

$$5 \text{ mL}/10 \text{ mg} = x \text{ mL}/3 \text{ mg}$$
$$15/10 = x$$
$$x = 1.5 \text{ mL}$$

Chapter 5—Airway Management and Ventilation

1. *What is your primary assessment and management of this child?*

Your initial assessment always begins with making sure the scene is safe and donning PPE. Your next step is to determine if there is any suspected trauma and assess the child's LOC by gently tapping and calling the child's name. Quickly follow this with opening the airway (head-tilt/chin-lift if no trauma is suspected and jaw-thrust if trauma is suspected) and determine if the child is breathing. If the child is not breathing, give positive pressure ventilations ([times]2) by either BVM, FROPVD, or pocket mask and begin chest compressions. (Remember, these are done in lieu of abdominal thrusts for pediatric patients.) If you are the only ALS person on scene, these BLS maneuvers should be performed by your basic partner or another BLS-trained person while you prepare your equipment. Approximately every 2 minutes, you should stop the BLS compressions, assess the airway for a visible obstruction, and begin the compressions again.

Note: Even though the patient is not breathing, placing a nonrebreather mask over the patient's mouth and nose may help provide some oxygenation during the compressions. (If the airway is completely obstructed, this is less likely to help. However, if there is any air movement, no matter how small, the increased oxygenation provided by the NRB can do nothing but help.) Remember to remove the mask prior to attempting any type of ventilations.

If the airway obstruction is not relieved by BLS maneuvers within the first 2 minutes of your arrival, you should begin advanced airway procedures including the use of an appropriately sized extraglottic airway, direct laryngoscopy, and retrieving the occlusion with Magill forceps or placing an endotracheal tube. If the obstruction is still unrelieved, your last resort would be use of a surgical airway (cricothyrotomy) to create an airway until hospital doctors can remove the obstruction.

2. *What are your first actions?*

Your first actions are to gain control of the scene and call for any needed additional assistance, such as Emergency Medical Responders or other EMS units or law enforcement, to help with maintaining order. Additionally, you will want to attempt to determine the extent of the child's airway obstruction by opening the airway; listening, looking, and feeling for air movement and chest rise; and giving positive pressure ventilations with a BVM or pocket mask.

3. *What are your options for managing the airway after the obstruction is relieved?*

Upon relieving the airway obstruction, your first priority is to ventilate the patient and check for circulatory function or pulses. If pulses are present, you should proceed with securing the airway with whatever means necessary and available to maintain a secure, open airway. Options for this will include (in order from least invasive to most invasive):

- Oxygen delivery via nonrebreather mask
- Nasopharyngeal airway
- Oropharyngeal airway
- Blind insertion airway device
- Endotracheal tube

In addition to the airway device just mentioned, the patient should be placed on supplemental oxygen to maintain pulse oximetry levels of at least 90 percent. This may include nasal cannula, nonrebreather mask, or bag-valve mask.

4. *What are the major anatomic differences between pediatric and adult patients in terms of airway management?*

- Pediatric structures are smaller and more difficult to navigate.
- Pediatric tongues are larger in proportion.
- Nasal openings are smaller and adenoids are large on pediatric patients.
- The pediatric cricoid rings are pliable and may be compressed with overaggressive cricoid pressure.
- Distance from the vocal cords to the carina is closer in pediatrics, requiring the tube to be inserted only 2–3 cm below the cords.
- Large occiput in pediatrics makes positioning difficult.
- The pediatric epiglottis is floppy and round ("omega"-shaped), making use of the straight (Miller) blades more popular for pediatric intubation.
- The pediatric glottic opening is higher and more anterior in the neck, making it easier to insert the laryngoscope blade too deeply.
- The narrowest part of the pediatric airway is the cricoid cartilage, not the glottic opening.
- Children will desaturate (oxygen) faster than an adult.

ANSWERS TO REVIEW QUESTIONS

Below are the answers to the Review Questions presented in each chapter of Volume 2.

CHAPTER 1—
PATHOPHYSIOLOGY

1. a
2. b
3. c
4. b
5. d
6. a
7. d
8. a
9. c
10. c
11. b
12. d
13. b
14. b
15. d
16. d
17. b
18. c
19. a
20. d
21. b
22. c
23. c
24. b
25. c

CHAPTER 2—
HUMAN LIFE SPAN
DEVELOPMENT

1. c
2. d
3. c
4. a
5. c
6. b
7. c
8. c

CHAPTER 3—
EMERGENCY
PHARMACOLOGY

1. c
2. b
3. b
4. c
5. b
6. a

7. a
8. b
9. d
10. c
11. c
12. d
13. a
14. c
15. b
16. d
17. d
18. b
19. b
20. b

CHAPTER 4—
INTRAVENOUS
ACCESS AND
MEDICATION
ADMINISTRATION

1. a
2. c
3. c
4. b
5. b
6. b
7. d
8. d
9. c
10. c
11. b
12. d
13. c
14. a
15. c
16. d
17. a
18. c
19. d
20. d
21. a
22. b
23. b
24. d
25. c
26. b
27. c
28. c

29. d
30. b
31. c
32. b

CHAPTER 5—AIRWAY
MANAGEMENT AND
VENTILATION

1. d
2. b
3. c
4. b
5. b
6. d
7. b
8. b
9. d
10. c
11. c
12. b
13. c
14. a
15. a
16. d
17. c
18. d
19. b
20. b

GLOSSARY

ABCs   airway, breathing, and circulation.

ABO blood groups   four blood groups formed by the presence or absence of two antigens known as A and B. A person may have either (type A or type B), both (type AB), or neither (type O). An immune response will be activated whenever a person receives blood containing A or B antigen if this antigen is not already present in his own blood.

acid-base reaction   any chemical reaction that results in the transfer of protons.

acidosis   a high concentration of hydrogen ions; a pH below 7.35; an excess of acids in the body.

acids   substances that give up protons during chemical reactions.

acquired immunity   protection from infection or disease that is (1) developed by the body after exposure to an antigen (active acquired immunity) or (2) transferred to the person from an outside source such as from the mother through the placenta or as a serum (passive acquired immunity).

active transport   movement of a substance through a cell membrane against the osmotic gradient; that is, from an area of lesser concentration to an area of greater concentration, opposite to the normal direction of diffusion; requires the use of energy to move a substance.

acute   of sudden onset, as an acute disease.

adenosine triphosphate (ATP)   a high-energy compound present in all cells, especially muscle cells; when split by enzyme action, it yields energy. Energy is stored in ATP.

adipocytes   fat cells.

adipose tissue   fat.

adjunct medication   agent that enhances the effects of other medications.

administration tubing   flexible, clear plastic tubing that connects the solution bag to the IV cannula.

adrenergic   pertaining to the neurotransmitter norepinephrine.

aerobic metabolism   the second stage of metabolism, requiring the presence of oxygen, in which the breakdown of glucose (in a process called the Krebs or citric acid cycle) yields a high amount of energy. *Aerobic* means "with oxygen."

affinity   force of attraction between a medication and a receptor.

afterload   the resistance a contraction of the heart must overcome in order to eject blood; in cardiac physiology, defined as the tension of cardiac muscle during systole (contraction).

agonist   medication that binds to a receptor and causes it to initiate the expected response.

agonist-antagonist (partial agonist)   medication that binds to a receptor and stimulates some of its effects but blocks others.

AIDS (acquired immunodeficiency syndrome)   a group of signs, symptoms, and disorders that often develop as a consequence of HIV infection.

air embolism   air in the vein.

albumin   a protein commonly present in plant and animal tissues. In the blood, albumin works to maintain blood volume and blood pressure and provides colloid osmotic pressure, which prevents plasma loss from the capillaries.

alkalosis   a low concentration of hydrogen ions; a pH above 7.45; an excess of base in the body.

allergy   exaggerated immune response to an environmental antigen.

alveoli   microscopic air sacs where most oxygen and carbon dioxide gas exchanges take place.

amino acids   molecules containing an amine group, a carboxylic acid group, and varying side chains; among other functions, amino acids are the building blocks of proteins.

ampule   breakable glass vessel containing liquid medication.

amylopectin   a highly branched polymer of glucose; one of two types of starch, the other being amylose.

amylose   a linear, unbranched polymer of glucose; one of two types of starch, the other being amylopectin.

anabolism   the constructive phase of metabolism in which cells convert nonliving substances into living cytoplasm; the synthesis of steroid compounds by the body.

anaerobic metabolism   the first stage of metabolism, which does not require oxygen, in which the breakdown of glucose (in a process called glycolysis) produces pyruvic acid and yields very little energy. *Anaerobic* means "without oxygen."

analgesia   the absence of the sensation of pain.

analgesic   medication that relieves the sensation of pain.

anaphylaxis   a life-threatening allergic reaction; also called *anaphylactic shock.*

anencephaly   a birth defect in which a baby is born without parts of the brain and skull.

anesthesia   the absence of all sensations.

anesthetic   medication that induces a loss of sensation to touch or pain.

anion   an ion with a negative charge—so called because it will be attracted to an anode, or positive pole.

anoxia   the absence or near-absence of oxygen in certain tissues or in the body as a whole.

antacid   alkalotic compound used to increase the gastric environment's pH.

antagonist   medication that binds to a receptor but does not cause it to initiate the expected response.

antiarrhythmic   medication used to treat and prevent abnormal cardiac rhythms.

antibiotic   agent that kills or decreases the growth of bacteria.

antibody   a substance produced by B lymphocytes in response to the presence of a foreign antigen that will combine with and control or destroy the antigen, thus preventing infection.

anticoagulant   medication that inhibits blood clotting.

antiemetic   medication used to prevent vomiting.

antigen   a marker on the surface of a cell that identifies it as "self" or "non-self."

antigen-antibody complex   the substance formed when an antibody combines with an antigen to deactivate or destroy it; also called *immune complex.*

antigen-presenting cells (APCs)   cells, such as macrophages, that present (express onto their surfaces) portions of the antigens they have digested.

antigen processing   the recognition, ingestion, and breakdown of a foreign antigen, culminating in production of an antibody to the antigen or in a direct cytotoxic response to the antigen.

antihistamine   medication that arrests the effects of histamine by blocking its receptors.

antihyperlipidemic   medication used to treat high blood cholesterol.

antihypertensive   medication used to treat hypertension.

antineoplastic agent   medication used to treat cancer.

antiplatelet   medication that decreases the formation of platelet plugs.

antiseptic   cleansing agent that is not toxic to living tissue.

antitussive   medication that suppresses the stimulus to cough in the central nervous system.

anxious avoidant attachment   a type of bonding that occurs when an infant learns that his caregivers will not be responsive or helpful when needed.

anxious resistant attachment   a type of bonding that occurs when an infant is uncertain about whether or not his caregivers will be responsive or helpful when needed.

apnea   temporary stop in breathing.

apoptosis   response in which an injured cell releases enzymes that engulf and destroy itself; one way the body rids itself of damaged and dead cells.

arterial oxygen concentration (CaO_2)   a measure of oxygen content in the arterial blood.

asepsis   a condition free of pathogens.

aspiration   inhaling foreign material such as vomitus into the lungs.

assay   test that determines the amount and purity of a given chemical in a preparation in the laboratory.

atelectasis   alveolar collapse.

atom   the fundamental chemical unit, which contains subatomic particles, including electrons, protons, and neutrons.

atomic number   the number of protons in the nucleus of an atom; an element is defined by its atomic number.

atrophy   a decrease in cell size resulting from a decreased workload.

aural medication   medication administered through the mucous membranes of the ear and ear canal.

authoritarian   a parenting style that demands absolute obedience without regard to a child's individual freedom.

authoritative   a parenting style that emphasizes a balance between a respect for authority and individual freedom.

autoimmune disease   failure of the immune system to recognize certain tissues normally present in the body resulting in an attack against those tissues by the immune system; autoimmune disease includes rheumatic heart disease and rheumatoid arthritis.

autoimmunity   an immune response to self-antigens, which the body normally tolerates.

autonomic ganglia   groups of autonomic nerve cells located outside the central nervous system.

autonomic nervous system   the part of the nervous system that controls involuntary actions.

B lymphocytes   the type of white blood cells that, in response to the presence of an antigen, produce antibodies that attack the antigen, develop a memory for the antigen, and confer long-term immunity to the antigen.

bacteria   (singular bacterium) single-cell organisms with a cell membrane and cytoplasm but no organized nucleus. They bind to the cells of a host organism to obtain food and support.

bag-valve mask (BVM)   ventilation device consisting of a self-inflating bag with two one-way valves and a transparent plastic face mask.

barotrauma   injury caused by pressure within an enclosed space.

basement membrane   a thin sheet of fibers that underlies the epithelia, the membranes that line or cover internal and external body surfaces.

bases   substances that acquire protons during chemical reactions.

basophils   granular white blood cells that, similarly to mast cells, release histamine and other chemicals that control constriction and dilation of blood vessels during inflammation.

benign   not cancerous; not able to spread to other tissues. *See also* malignant.

bilevel positive airway pressure (BiPAP)   air or oxygen delivered under pressure that is higher during inhalation and lower during exhalation.

bioassay   test to ascertain a medication's availability in a biologic model.

bioavailability   amount of a medication that is still active after it reaches its target tissue.

bioequivalence   relative therapeutic effectiveness of chemically equivalent medications.

biologic half-life   time the body takes to clear one-half of a medication.

biotransformation   special name given to the metabolism of medications.

blood-brain barrier   tight junctions of the capillary endothelial cells in the central nervous system vasculature through which only non-protein-bound, highly lipid-soluble medications can pass.

blood tube   glass container with color-coded, self-sealing rubber top.

blood tubing   administration tubing that contains a filter to prevent clots or other debris from entering the patient.

bolus   concentrated mass of medication.

bonding   the formation of a close personal relationship (as between mother and child), especially through frequent or constant association.

bronchi   tubes from the trachea into the lungs.

buccal   between the cheek and gums.

buffer   a substance that tends to preserve or restore a normal acid-base balance by increasing or decreasing the concentration of hydrogen ions.

burette chamber calibrated chamber of Berutrol IV administration tubing that enables precise measurement and delivery of fluids and medicated solutions.

cannula hollow needle used to puncture a vein.

cannulation *see* intravenous (IV) access.

CaO₂ *see* arterial oxygen concentration.

capnography a recording or display of the measurement of exhaled carbon dioxide concentrations over time.

carbon dioxide waste product of the body's metabolism.

carcinogenesis a process of developing a cancer.

carcinoma-in-situ an early form of cancer in which tumor cells have not yet invaded surrounding tissues.

cardiac contractile force the strength of a contraction of the heart.

cardiac output the amount of blood pumped by the heart in 1 minute (computed as stroke volume × heart rate).

cardiogenic shock shock caused by insufficient cardiac output; the inability of the heart to pump enough blood to perfuse all parts of the body.

carrier-mediated diffusion or facilitated diffusion process in which carrier proteins transport large molecules across the cell membrane.

carrier proteins proteins involved in carrying solutes (ions or molecules) across a biologic membrane.

cartilage a type of connective tissue that provides structure and support to other tissues.

cascade a series of actions triggered by a first action and culminating in a final action—typical of the actions caused by plasma proteins involved in the complement, coagulation, and kinin systems.

catabolism the destructive phase of metabolism in which cells break down complex substances into simpler substances with release of energy.

catecholamines epinephrine and norepinephrine, hormones that strongly affect the nervous and cardiovascular systems, metabolic rate, temperature, and smooth muscle.

catheter inserted through the needle/intracatheter Teflon catheter inserted through a large metal stylet.

cation an ion with a positive charge—so called because it will be attracted to a cathode, or negative pole.

cell the basic structural unit of all plants and animals. A membrane enclosing a thick fluid and a nucleus. Cells are specialized to carry out all of the body's basic functions.

cell-mediated immunity the short-term immunity to an antigen provided by T lymphocytes, which directly attack the antigen but do not produce antibodies or memory for the antigen.

cell membrane *also* plasma membrane; the outer covering of a cell.

cellular adaptation physiologic or structural changes to a cell in response to change or stress or a pathological condition.

cellular respiration metabolic processes with a cell that convert nutrients to energy in the form of adenosine triphosphate (ATP) and that subsequently release waste products from the cell.

cellulose a polysaccharide polymer with glucose as its monomer that is the major structural material of plants.

central venous access surgical puncture of the internal jugular, subclavian, or femoral vein.

centrioles cylindrical structures within cells that play an important role in cell division.

chemoreceptors sensory receptors that detect and act on chemical signals—for example, sensing a change in carbon dioxide levels in the blood and responding by causing an increase in respiratory rate to expel the excess carbon dioxide from the body.

chemotactic factors chemicals that attract white cells to the site of inflammation, a process called chemotaxis.

chemotaxis *see* chemotactic factors.

cholinergic pertaining to the neurotransmitter acetylcholine.

chromatin a combination of DNA and other proteins in the nucleus of a cell that condenses to form chromosomes.

chromosomes threadlike structures within the nuclei of cells that carry genetic information.

chronic slow in onset, persisting over a long period of time, as in a chronic disease.

cilia threadlike projections from the surface of cells that move back and forth and can sweep debris such as mucus or dust away from the cell.

circulatory overload an excess in intravascular fluid volume.

cisternae saclike structures within body cells that form part of the structure of rough endoplasmic reticulum (RER) and of the Golgi apparatus and act as carrier vessels that transport proteins from the RER to the Golgi apparatus for further processing.

citric acid cycle a key phase of glucose metabolism, requiring the presence of oxygen, in which pyruvic acid (a product of the breakdown of glucose) is oxidized, resulting in the release of energy in the form of ATP and carbon dioxide as waste. Also called *Krebs cycle* or the *tricarboxylic acid (TCA) cycle*.

clinical presentation the manifestation of a disease; the signs and symptoms of a disease.

clonal diversity the development of receptors, by B lymphocyte precursors in the bone marrow, for every possible type of antigen.

clonal selection the process by which a specific antigen reacts with the appropriate receptors on the surface of immature B lymphocytes, thereby activating them and prompting them to proliferate, differentiate, and produce antibodies to the activating antigen.

clotting system *see* coagulation system.

coagulation system a plasma protein system that results in formation of a protein called fibrin. Fibrin forms a network that walls off an infection and forms a clot that stops bleeding and serves as a foundation for repair and healing of a wound. Also called the *clotting system*.

coenzymes nonprotein substances that bind to enzyme proteins to assist them in biochemical transformations. Also called *cofactors*.

cofactors *see* coenzymes.

collagen proteins that are the main component of connective tissue.

colloid intravenous solutions containing large proteins that cannot pass through capillary membranes.

colloidal solution solution containing large protein molecules that cannot pass through a capillary membrane.

compensated shock　early stage of shock during which the body's compensatory mechanisms are able to maintain normal perfusion.

competitive antagonism　one medication binds to a receptor and causes the expected effect while also blocking another medication from triggering the same receptor.

complement system　a group of plasma proteins (the complement proteins) that are dormant in the blood until activated, as by antigen-antibody complex formation, by products released by bacteria, or by components of other plasma protein systems. When activated, the complement system is involved in most of the events of inflammatory response.

compliance　the stiffness or flexibility of the lung tissue.

complications　abnormalities or conditions that result from another, original disease or problem. Also called *sequelae*.

compound　chemical union of two or more elements.

concentration　weight per volume.

concentration gradient　the gradual change in concentration of a solution over a distance within the solution.

congenital metabolic diseases　diseases affecting the metabolism that are present from birth.

connective tissue　the most abundant body tissue; it provides support, connection, and insulation. Examples: bone, cartilage, fat, blood.

continuous positive airway pressure (CPAP)　air or oxygen delivered under pressure that is maintained at a steady level during both inhalation and exhalation.

contraction　inward movement of wound edges during healing that eventually brings the wound edges together.

conventional reasoning　the stage of moral development during which children desire approval from individuals and society.

Cormack and LeHane grading system　a system for evaluating and scoring airway difficulty based on the portion of the glottic opening and vocal cords that may be seen.

cortisol　a steroid hormone released by the adrenal cortex that regulates the metabolism of fats, carbohydrates, sodium, potassium, and proteins and also has an anti-inflammatory effect.

covalent bond　force holding atoms together that results when atoms share electrons.

cricoid pressure　pressure applied in a posterior direction to the anterior cricoid cartilage; occludes the esophagus.

cricothyroid membrane　membrane between the cricoid and thyroid cartilages of the larynx.

cristae　folds within mitochondria that form shelves within the mitochondria.

crystalloid　intravenous solution that contains electrolytes but lacks the larger proteins associated with a colloid.

cyanosis　bluish discoloration.

cytokines　proteins, produced by white blood cells, that regulate immune responses by binding with and affecting the function of the cells that produced them or of other, nearby cells.

cytoplasm　the thick fluid, or protoplasm, that fills a cell.

cytoskeleton　system of filaments, microtubules, and intermediate filaments that are part of the internal structure of a cell.

cytotoxic　toxic, or poisonous, to cells.

debridement　the cleaning up or removal of debris, dead cells, and scabs from a wound, principally through phagocytosis.

decompensated shock　advanced stages of shock when the body's compensatory mechanisms are no longer able to maintain normal perfusion; also called *progressive shock*.

degranulation　the emptying of granules from the interior of a mast cell into the extracellular environment.

dehydration　excessive loss of body fluid.

delayed hypersensitivity reaction　a hypersensitivity reaction that takes place after the elapse of some time following reexposure to an antigen. Delayed hypersensitivity reactions are usually less severe than immediate reactions.

demand-valve device　a ventilation device that is manually operated by a push button or lever.

denaturation　loss of a protein's three-dimensional shape caused by factors such as heat, chemicals, or pH; the change in the appearance and structure of an egg white when it is cooked is an example of denaturation.

deoxyribonucleic acid (DNA)　double-stranded, helical polymer chain within the nucleus of a cell that carries the genetic information that encodes proteins and enables the cell to reproduce and perform its functions.

desired dose　specific quantity of medication needed.

diagnosis　the process of identifying and assigning a name to a disease in an individual patient or a group of patients with similar signs and symptoms.

diapedesis　movement of white cells out of blood vessels through gaps in the vessel walls that are created when inflammatory processes cause the vessel walls to constrict.

difficult child　an infant who can be characterized by irregularity of bodily functions, intense reactions, and withdrawal from new situations.

diffusion　see simple diffusion. *See also* facilitated diffusion; osmosis.

disaccharides　complex sugars, such as sucrose, lactose, and maltose.

disease　an abnormal structural or functional change within the body.

disinfectant　cleansing agent that is toxic to living tissue.

dissociate　separate; break down. For example, sodium bicarbonate, when placed in water, dissociates into a sodium cation and a bicarbonate anion.

dissociation reaction　any reaction in which a compound or a molecule breaks apart into separate components.

diuretic　an agent that increases urine secretion and elimination of body water; medication used to reduce circulating blood volume by increasing the amount of urine.

DNA　see deoxyribonucleic acid (DNA).

dosage on hand　the amount of medication available in a solution.

dose packaging　medication packages that contain a single dose for a single patient.

down-regulation　binding of a medication or hormone to a target cell receptor that causes the number of receptors to decrease.

drip chamber　clear plastic chamber that allows visualization of the drip rate.

drip rate　pace at which the fluid moves from the bag into the patient.

drop former   device that regulates the size of drops.

drops   (Latin *guttae*, drops *[gutta*, drop*]);* quantity of a solution that falls in one spherical mass.

drug-response relationship   correlation of different amounts of a medication to clinical response.

drugs   foreign substances placed into the human body. *See also* medications.

duration of action   length of time the amount of medication remains above its minimum effective concentration.

dynamic steady state   homeostasis; the tendency of the body to maintain a net constant composition although the components of the body's internal environment are always changing.

dysplasia   a change in cell size, shape, or appearance caused by an external stressor.

dysplastic   having an abnormal appearance, as with a cell seen under a microscope.

dyspnea   an abnormality of breathing rate, pattern, or effort.

ear-to-sternal-notch position   position in which a supine patient's head is elevated to the point where the ear and the sternal notch are horizontally aligned. In the non-obese patient, this position may be called the sniffing position. In the obese patient, this position may be called the ramped position.

easy child   an infant who can be characterized by regularity of bodily functions, low or moderate intensity of reactions, and acceptance of new situations.

ectoderm   the outermost of three germ layers, primitive cell types that develop in the embryo and that will differentiate into the various tissues and organs of the body. *See also* endoderm; germ layers; mesoderm.

edema   excess fluid in the interstitial space.

efficacy   a medication's ability to cause the expected response.

electrolyte   a substance that, in water, separates into electrically charged particles.

electron   negatively charged particle that orbits the nucleus of an atom.

electron shells   levels of orbitals within which electrons rotate around the nucleus of an atom. *See also* orbital.

electron transport chain   carriers embedded on the cristae in the inner membrane of the mitochondria of cells that transfer electrons from one molecule to another, releasing energy in the process.

element   a substance that cannot be separated into simpler substances. An element is defined by its atomic number, the number of protons in its nucleus.

embolus   foreign particle in the blood.

endocrine secretions   secreted substances that are released into the bloodstream or surrounding tissues without the aid of ducts.

endocytosis   process by which substances can enter a cell when a section of the cell's plasma membrane encircles the substance, then pinches off into a vesicle that is released into the cell. *See also* exocytosis.

endoderm   the innermost of three germ layers, primitive cell types that develop in the embryo and that will differentiate into the various tissues and organs of the body. *See also* ectoderm; germ layers; mesoderm.

endoplasmic reticulum   organelle within a cell that is a network of tubules, vesicles, and sacs that interconnect with the plasma membrane, the nuclear envelope, and many of the other organelles of the cell.

endotoxins   molecules in the walls of certain Gram-negative bacteria that are released when the bacterium dies or is destroyed, causing toxic (poisonous) effects on the host body.

endotracheal tube (ETT)   a flexible plastic tube that is inserted into the trachea, usually under laryngoscopy, for the purpose of ventilating the lungs.

endotracheal tube introducer   a device designed to facilitate the introduction of an endotracheal tube; commonly called a gum-elastic bougie. It is a stylet that can be pushed into the glottis and is flexible enough so that the operator can feel the entry. When entry is achieved, the endotracheal tube can then be passed over the introducer and into the glottis.

enema   a liquid bolus of medication that is injected into the rectum.

enteral route   delivery of a medication through the gastrointestinal tract.

enzymes   substances that speed up chemical reactions without themselves being consumed in the process.

enzyme-substrate complex   an enzyme and the substance (substrate) it is bound to and working on.

eosinophils   granular white blood cells that attack parasites and also help to control and limit the inflammatory response.

epithelial tissue   the protective tissue that lines internal and external body tissues. Examples: skin, mucous membranes, the lining of the intestinal tract.

epithelialization   growth of epithelial cells under a scab, separating it from the wound and providing a protective covering for the healing wound.

epithelium   *see* epithelial tissue.

erythrocytes   red blood cells, which contain hemoglobin, which transports oxygen to the cells.

etiology   the study of disease causes; the occurrences, reasons, and variables of a disease.

eukaryotic cells   cells that contain a nucleus and organelles. The cells of most multicellular organisms, including humans, are eukaryotes. *See also* prokaryotic cells.

eustachian tube   a tube that connects the ear with the nasal cavity.

exocrine secretions   secreted substances that are deposited on the surface of the skin or other epithelial surface through ducts.

exocytosis   process by which substances can exit after being encircled by a membrane vesicle. *See also* endocytosis.

exotoxins   toxic (poisonous) substances secreted by bacterial cells during their growth.

expectorant   medication intended to increase the productivity of cough.

extension tubing   IV tubing used to extend a macrodrip or microdrip setup.

extracellular fluid (ECF)   the fluid outside the body cells. Extracellular fluid is comprised of intravascular fluid and interstitial fluid.

extraglottic airway (EGA) device airway device that does not enter the glottis.

extrapyramidal symptoms (EPS) common side effects of antipsychotic medications, including muscle tremors and parkinsonism-like effects.

extravasation leakage of fluid or medication from the blood vessel that is commonly found with infiltration.

extravascular outside the vein.

extubation removing a tube from a body opening.

exudate substances that penetrate vessel walls to move into the surrounding tissues.

facilitated diffusion process in which carrier proteins transport large molecules across the cell membrane.

fermentation the breakdown of glucose without oxygen.

fibrinolytic medication that acts directly on thrombi to break them down; also called *thrombolytic*.

fibroblasts the most abundant cells in connective tissue; cells that secrete collagen proteins that maintain a structural framework for many tissues and play an important role in wound healing.

Fick principle principle stating that the overall movement and utilization of oxygen in the body is dependent on five conditions: adequate concentration of inspired oxygen; appropriate movement of oxygen across the alveolar/capillary membrane into the arterial bloodstream; adequate number of red blood cells to carry the oxygen; proper tissue perfusion; and efficient off-loading of oxygen at the tissue level.

filtration movement of water out of the plasma across the capillary membrane into the interstitial space; movement of molecules across a membrane from an area of higher pressure to an area of lower pressure.

FiO$_2$ concentration of oxygen in inspired air.

first-pass effect the liver's partial or complete inactivation of a medication before it reaches the systemic circulation.

flagella threadlike structures whose undulating movement provides motion to certain bacteria, protozoa, and spermatozoa.

flail chest defect in the chest wall that allows a segment to move freely, causing paradoxical chest wall motion.

free drug availability proportion of a medication available in the body to cause either desired or undesired effects.

free radicals atoms or molecules with an unpaired electron in the outer shell. Most free radicals are highly reactive and cause cell damage, especially oxidative damage.

free water water that is free of solute.

French unit of measurement approximately equal to one-third millimeter.

fructose a five-carbon monosaccharide sugar found in many plants and vegetables as well as honey.

gag reflex mechanism that stimulates retching, or striving to vomit, when the soft palate is touched.

galactose a six-carbon monosaccharide sugar found primarily in dairy products.

gauge the size of a needle's diameter.

general adaptation syndrome (GAS) a sequence of stress response stages: stage I, alarm; stage II, resistance or adaptation; stage III, exhaustion.

germ layers the three primitive cell types (endoderm, ectoderm, mesoderm) that develop in the embryo and that will differentiate into the various tissues and organs of the body. *See also* ectoderm; endoderm; mesoderm.

glottis liplike opening between the vocal cords.

glucagon substance that increases blood glucose level.

glucose a six-carbon monosaccharide sugar that is the principal energy source for the human body.

glycogen a glucose polymer that is primarily stored in the liver and skeletal muscle that can be converted by the body into glucose. *See also* glycogenolysis.

glycogenolysis a process controlled by the hormones glucagon and epinephrine in which stores of glycogen are broken down into glucose to meet a bodily need for glucose. *See also* glycogen.

glycolysis a series of reactions by which a molecule of glucose is converted into two molecules of pyruvic acid, a process that begins the conversion of glucose into energy and that also produces free hydrogen ions that determine the body's pH.

Golgi apparatus organelle within a cell that processes proteins for the cell membrane and other organelles.

granulation filling of a wound by the inward growth of healthy tissues from the wound edges.

granulocytes white cells with multiple nuclei that have the appearance of a bag of granules; also called *polymorphonuclear cells*. Types of granulocytes are neutrophils, eosinophils, and basophils.

granuloma a tumor or growth that forms when foreign bodies that cannot be destroyed by macrophages are surrounded and walled off.

half-life a unit of rate of decay of radioactive isotopes; the time it takes for the decaying parent isotope to decrease by half.

haptens molecules that do not trigger an immune response on their own but can become immunogenic when combined with larger molecules.

hematocrit the percentage of the blood occupied by erythrocytes.

hemoconcentration elevated numbers of red and white blood cells.

hemoglobin an iron-based pigment present in red blood cells that binds with oxygen and transports it to the cells.

hemoglobin-oxygen saturation (SaO$_2$) the amount of oxygen bound to one gram of hemoglobin.

hemolysis the destruction of red blood cells.

hemostasis the stoppage of bleeding.

hemothorax accumulation in the pleural cavity of blood or fluid containing blood.

heparin lock peripheral IV cannula with a distal medication port used for intermittent fluid or medication infusions. Flushes of heparin solution, which inhibit blood coagulation, are used to maintain patency of the device.

hepatic alteration change in a medication's chemical composition that occurs in the liver.

Hgb the amount of hemoglobin present in arterial blood.

high-pressure regulator regulator used to transfer oxygen at high pressures from tank to tank.

histamine   a substance released during the degranulation of mast cells and also released by basophils that, through constriction and dilation of blood vessels, increases blood flow to the injury site and also increases the permeability of vessel walls.

histology   the study of tissues.

histopathology   the study of diseased or abnormal tissues.

HIV (human immunodeficiency virus)   a virus that breaks down the immune defenses, making the body vulnerable to a variety of infections and disorders.

HLA antigens   antigens the body recognizes as self or nonself; present on all body cells except the red blood cells.

hollow-needle catheter   stylet that does not have a Teflon tube but is itself inserted into the vein and secured there.

homeostasis   the natural tendency of the body to maintain a steady and normal internal environment.

Huber needle   needle that has an opening on the side of the shaft instead of the tip.

humoral immunity   the long-term immunity to an antigen provided by antibodies produced by B lymphocytes.

hydrogen bond   a weak bond formed by the attraction between a slightly positively charged hydrogen atom and a slightly negatively charged oxygen atom, as between H_2O water molecules.

hydrolysis   the breakage of a chemical bond by adding water, or by incorporating a hydroxyl (OH^-) group into one fragment and a hydrogen ion (H^+) into the other.

hydrophilic   attracted to water.

hydrophobic   repellent to water.

hydrostatic pressure   blood pressure or force against vessel walls created by the heartbeat. Hydrostatic pressure tends to force water out of the capillaries into the interstitial space.

hypercapnia   an elevated level of plasma CO_2.

hypercarbia   excessive level of carbon dioxide in the blood.

hyperoxia   excessive level of oxygen in certain tissues or in the body as a whole.

hyperplasia   an increase in the number of cells resulting from an increased workload.

hypersensitivity   an exaggerated and harmful immune response; an umbrella term for allergy, autoimmunity, and isoimmunity.

hypertonic   state in which a solution has a higher solute concentration on one side of a semipermeable membrane than on the other side; having a greater concentration of solute molecules; one solution may be hypertonic to another.

hypertrophy   an increase in cell size resulting from an increased workload.

hyperventilation   rapid or deep breathing in excess of the body's needs.

hyperventilation syndrome   excessive CO_2 elimination resulting in respiratory alkalosis, caused by hyperventilation.

hypnosis   instigation of sleep.

hypocapnia   a reduced level of plasma CO_2.

hypodermic needle   hollow metal tube used with the syringe to administer medications.

hypoperfusion   inadequate perfusion of the body tissues, resulting in an inadequate supply of oxygen and nutrients to the body tissues. Also called *shock*.

hypotonic   state in which a solution has a lower solute concentration on one side of a semipermeable membrane than on the other side; having a lesser concentration of solute molecules; one solution may be hypotonic to another.

hypoventilation   reduced rate or depth of breathing that does not meet the body's needs.

hypovolemic shock   shock caused by a loss of intravascular fluid volume.

hypoxemia   decreased partial pressure of oxygen in the blood.

hypoxia   a general oxygen deficiency or oxygen deficiency to a particular tissue or organ.

hypoxic drive   mechanism that increases respiratory stimulation when PaO_2 falls and inhibits respiratory stimulation when PaO_2 climbs.

iatrogenic disease   a disease that results from a medical treatment given for another disease or condition.

idiopathic   of unknown cause, in reference to a disease.

immediate hypersensitivity reaction   a swiftly occurring secondary hypersensitivity reaction (one that occurs after reexposure to an antigen). Immediate hypersensitivity reactions are usually more severe than delayed reactions. The swiftest and most severe such reaction is anaphylaxis.

immune response   the body's reactions that inactivate or eliminate foreign antigens.

immunity   exemption from legal liability; a long-term condition of protection from infection or disease; the body's ability to respond to the presence of a pathogen.

immunogens   antigens that are able to trigger an immune response.

immunoglobulins   antibodies; proteins, produced in response to foreign antigens, that destroy or control the antigens.

induced therapeutic hypothermia (ITH)   the administration of cold IV fluids to cardiac arrest patients to minimize subsequent secondary injury.

inflammation   the body's response to cellular injury; also called the *inflammatory response*. In contrast to the immune response, inflammation develops swiftly, is nonspecific (attacks all unwanted substances in the same way), and is temporary, leading to healing.

inflammatory response   *see* inflammation.

infusion   liquid medication delivered through a vein.

infusion controller   gravity-flow device that regulates fluid's passage through an electromechanical pump.

infusion pump   device that delivers fluids and medications under positive pressure.

infusion rate   speed at which a medication is delivered intravenously.

inhalation   drawing of medication into the lungs along with air during breathing.

injection   placement of medication in or under the skin with a needle and syringe.

inorganic chemicals   chemicals that do not contain the element carbon. *See also* organic chemicals.

insidious   existing without symptoms or with mild symptoms, as a disease that does not seem as serious as it is or as it may become.

insufflate   to blow into.

insulin substance that decreases blood glucose level.

interstitial fluid the fluid in body tissues that is outside the cells and outside the vascular system.

intracatheter *see* catheter inserted through the needle.

intracellular fluid (ICF) the fluid inside the body cells.

intradermal within the dermal layer of the skin.

intramuscular within the muscle.

intraosseous within the bone.

intravascular fluid the fluid within the circulatory system; blood plasma.

intravenous (IV) access surgical puncture of a vein to deliver medication or withdraw blood. Also called *cannulation*.

intravenous fluid chemically prepared solution tailored to the body's specific needs.

intubation passing a tube into a body opening.

ion a charged particle; an atom or group of atoms whose electrical charge has changed from neutral to positive or negative by losing or gaining one or more electrons. (In an atom's normal, nonionized state, its positively charged protons and negatively charged electrons balance each other so that the atom's charge is neutral.)

ion channels hydrophilic pores through a membrane that open and allow certain types of solutes, usually inorganic ions, to pass through.

ionic bond a bond resulting from the attraction between an atom or molecule with a negative charge and an atom or molecule with a positive charge.

ionize to become electrically charged or polar.

irreversible antagonism a competitive antagonist permanently binds with a receptor site.

irreversible shock shock that has progressed so far that no medical intervention can reverse the condition and death is inevitable.

ischemia a blockage in the delivery of oxygenated blood to the cells.

isoimmunity an immune response to antigens from another member of the same species—for example, Rh reactions between a mother and infant or transplant rejections; also called *alloimmunity*.

isotonic state in which solutions on opposite sides of a semi-permeable membrane are in equal concentration; equal in concentration of solute molecules; solutions may be isotonic to each other.

isotopes variants of the same element, having the same number of protons but varying in the number of neutrons. *See also* element.

IV catheter *see* over-the-needle catheter.

kinin system a plasma protein system that produces bradykinin, a substance that works with prostaglandins to cause pain. It also has actions similar to those of histamine (vasodilation and bronchospasm, increased permeability of the blood vessels, and chemotaxis) but acts more slowly than histamine, thus being more important during later stages of inflammation.

Krebs cycle *see* citric acid cycle.

lactose the principal sugar in milk; a disaccharide, it is a combination of glucose and galactose.

laryngoscope instrument for lifting the tongue and epiglottis in order to see the vocal cords.

larynx the complex structure that joins the pharynx with the trachea.

laxative medication used to decrease stool's firmness and increase its water content.

leukocytes white blood cells, which play a key role in the immune system and inflammatory (infection-fighting) responses.

leukotrienes also called *slow-reacting substances of anaphylaxis (SRS-A)*; substances synthesized by mast cells during the inflammatory response that cause vasodilation, vascular permeability, and chemotaxis.

life expectancy based on the year of birth, the average number of additional years of life expected for a member of a population.

lipid bilayer plasma membrane consisting of two layers of phospholipids. Each phospholipid molecule has a hydrophilic head (that attracts water) and a hydrophobic tail (that repels water). In the outer layer, the hydrophilic heads face outward, in contact with the extracellular fluid (ECF). In the inner layer, the hydrophilic heads face inward, in contact with the intracellular fluid (ICF). The hydrophobic tails of both layers face each other and hold the layers of the membrane together.

lipids a broad group of chemicals, not soluble in water, that includes triglycerides, phospholipids, and steroids.

Lipp maneuver a procedure for manually preshaping an Esophageal Tracheal Combitube (ETC).

local limited to one area of the body.

logarithm a base number that is raised to a certain *power*. A common example is $2^3 = 8$, in which 2 is raised to the third power, meaning that 2 (the first power) is multiplied by itself (to the second power, which equals 4), then multiplied by itself again (to the third power, which equals 8)—which may be expressed as $2 \times 2 \times 2 = 8$. In 2^3, 2 is the *base number* and 3 is the *exponent*.

Luer sampling needle long, exposed needle that screws into the vacutainer and is inserted directly into the vein.

lumen the channel through a tube.

lymphocyte a type of leukocyte, or white blood cell, that attacks foreign substances as part of the body's immune response.

lymphokine a cytokine released by a lymphocyte.

lysosome organelle within a cell that degrades and removes products of ingestion and worn out parts of the cell and converts complex nutritional molecules into simple nutritional molecules; sometimes called the cell's "garbage disposal system."

macrodrip tubing administration tubing that delivers a relatively large amount of fluid.

macrophages large white blood cells (matured monocytes) that will ingest and destroy, or partially destroy, invading organisms.

Magill forceps scissor-style clamps with circular tips.

major histocompatibility complex (MHC) a group of genes on chromosome 6 that provide the genetic code for HLA antigens.

malignant cancerous; able to spread to other tissues. *See also* benign.

Mallampati classification system   a system for evaluating and scoring airway difficulty by assessing the tonsillar pillars and uvula.

maltose   a breakdown product of starch; a disaccharide, it is a combination of two glucose molecules.

margination   adherence of white cells to vessel walls in the early stages of inflammation.

mass number   the total number of neutrons and protons in an atom.

mast cells   large cells, resembling bags of granules, that reside near blood vessels. When stimulated by injury, chemicals, or allergic responses, they activate the inflammatory response by degranulation (emptying their granules into the extracellular environment) and synthesis (construction of leukotrienes and prostaglandins).

maturation   continuing processes of wound reconstruction that may occur over a period of years after initial healing, as scar tissue is remodeled and strengthened.

maximum life span   the theoretical, species-specific, longest duration of life, excluding premature or "unnatural" death.

measured volume administration set   IV setup that delivers specific volumes of fluid.

medically clean   careful handling to prevent contamination.

medicated solution   parenteral medication packaged in an IV bag and administered as an IV infusion.

medication injection port   self-sealing membrane into which a hypodermic needle is inserted for medication administration.

medications   agents used in the diagnosis, treatment, or prevention of disease.

memory cells   cells produced by mature B lymphocytes that "remember" the activating antigen and will trigger a stronger and swifter immune response if reexposure to the antigen occurs.

mesoderm   the middle of three germ layers, primitive cell types that develop in the embryo and that will differentiate into the various tissues and organs of the body. *See also* ectoderm; endoderm; germ layers.

metabolic acid-base disorders   metabolic acidosis and metabolic alkalosis; disorders that result from changes in the production of acid or changes in bicarbonate levels within the body.

metabolic acidosis   acidity caused by an increase in acid, often because of increased production of acids during metabolism or from causes such as vomiting, diarrhea, diabetes, or medication.

metabolic alkalosis   alkalinity caused by an increase in plasma bicarbonate resulting from causes including diuresis, vomiting, or ingestion of too much sodium bicarbonate.

metabolism   the total changes that take place during physiologic processes; the body's breaking down of chemicals into different chemicals.

metallic elements   elements that tend to lose electrons. *See also* nonmetallic elements.

metaplasia   replacement of one type of cell by another type of cell that is not normal for that tissue.

metastasis   movement of cancer cells to other areas of the body from the original site.

metered dose inhaler   handheld device that produces a medicated spray for inhalation.

microdrip tubing   administration tubing that delivers a relatively small amount of fluid.

milliequivalent   a unit of measure applied to electrolytes, used as a unit of measure for amounts of very small magnitude.

minimum effective concentration   minimum level of medication needed to cause a given effect.

minute volume (V_{min})   the amount of air (gas) inhaled and exhaled in one minute.

mitochondria   organelles within the cells that are the principal site of conversion of food to energy.

mitosis   cell division with division of the nucleus; each daughter cell contains the same number of chromosomes as the mother cell. Mitosis is the process by which the body grows.

Mix-o-Vial   *see* nonconstituted medication vial.

modeling   a procedure whereby a subject observes a model perform some behavior and then attempts to imitate that behavior. Many believe it is the fundamental learning process involved in socialization.

molarity   moles of solute per liter of solution. A mole is the measure of mass or weight used in chemistry, sometimes defined as "molecular weight."

mole   *see* molarity.

molecule   a substance made up of atoms held together by one or more covalent bonds.

monoclonal antibody   an antibody that is very pure and specific to a single antigen.

monocytes   white cells with a single nucleus; the largest normal blood cells. During inflammation, monocytes mature and grow to several times their original size, becoming macrophages.

monokine   a cytokine released by a macrophage.

monomer   an atom or a small molecule that may bind chemically to other monomers to form a polymer. *See also* polymer.

monosaccharides   simple sugars, such as glucose, fructose, and galactose.

Moro reflex   occurs when a newborn is startled; arms are thrown wide, fingers spread, and a grabbing motion follows; also called *startle reflex.*

mucolytic   medication intended to make mucus more watery.

mucous membrane   lining in body cavities that handle air transport; usually contains small, mucous-secreting cells.

mucus   slippery secretion that lubricates and protects airway surfaces.

multiple organ dysfunction syndrome (MODS)   progressive impairment of two or more organ systems resulting from an uncontrolled inflammatory response to a severe illness or injury.

muscle tissue   tissue that is capable of contraction when stimulated. There are three types of muscle tissue: cardiac (myocardium, or heart muscle), smooth (within intestines, surrounding blood vessels), and skeletal, or striated (allows skeletal movement). Skeletal muscle is mostly under voluntary, or conscious, control; smooth muscle is under involuntary, or unconscious, control; cardiac muscle is capable of spontaneous, or self-excited, contraction.

nare   nostril.

nasal cannula   catheter placed at the nares.

nasal medication   medication administered through the mucous membranes of the nose.

nasolacrimal ducts   tubular vessels that drain tears and debris from the eyes into the nasal cavity.

nasopharyngeal airway (NPA)   uncuffed tube that follows the natural curvature of the nasopharynx, passing through the nose and extending from the nostril to the posterior pharynx.

nasotracheal route   through the nose and into the trachea.

natriuretic peptides (NPs)   peptide hormones synthesized by the heart, brain, and other organs with effects that include excretion of large amounts of sodium in the urine and dilation of the blood vessels.

natural immunity   inborn protection against infection or disease that is part of the person's or species' genetic makeup.

nebulizer   inhalation aid that disperses liquid into aerosol spray or mist.

necrosis   cell death; the sloughing off of dead tissue; a pathological cell change. Four types of necrotic cell change are coagulative, liquefactive, caseous, and fatty. Gangrenous necrosis refers to tissue death over a wide area.

needle adapter   rigid plastic device specifically constructed to fit into the hub of an intravenous cannula.

needle cricothyrotomy   surgical airway technique that inserts a 14-gauge needle into the trachea at the cricothyroid membrane.

negative feedback loop   body mechanisms that work to reverse, or compensate for, a pathophysiologic process (or to reverse any physiologic process, whether pathological or nonpathological).

neoplasia   abnormal or uncontrolled cell growth. *See also* neoplasm.

neoplasm   a tumor that results from neoplasia. *See also* neoplasia.

nerve tissue   tissue that transmits electrical impulses throughout the body.

net filtration   the total loss of water from blood plasma across the capillary membrane into the interstitial space. Normally, hydrostatic pressure forcing water out of the capillary is balanced by oncotic force pulling water into the capillary for a net filtration of zero.

neuroeffector junction   specialized synapse between a nerve cell and the organ or tissue it innervates.

neurogenic shock   shock resulting from brain or spinal cord injury that causes an interruption of nerve impulses to the arteries with loss of arterial tone, dilation, and relative hypovolemia.

neuroglia   glial cells that support, insulate, and protect neurons.

neuroleptanesthesia   anesthesia that combines decreased sensation of pain with amnesia while the patient remains conscious.

neuroleptic   antipsychotic (literally, affecting the nerves).

neuron   nerve cell; cell that transmits electrical impulses.

neurotransmitter   chemical messenger that conducts a nervous impulse across a synapse.

neutron   electrically neutral particle within the nucleus of an atom.

neutrophil   a type of white blood cell; a phagocyte that has the ability to ingest other cells and substances.

noble gases   helium, neon, argon, krypton, xenon, and radon; the only elements that have a full valence shell and thus are very stable.

noncompetitive antagonism   the binding of an antagonist causes a deformity of the binding site that prevents an agonist from fitting and binding.

nonconstituted medication vial/Mix-o-Vial   vial with two containers, one holding a powdered medication and the other holding a liquid mixing solution.

nonmetallic elements   elements that tend to gain electrons. *See also* metallic elements.

normoxia   normal level of oxygen in certain tissues or in the body as a whole.

nuclear envelope   double membrane that encloses the nucleus of a cell.

nuclear pores   openings in the nuclear envelope. *See also* nuclear envelope.

nucleolus   a specialized region of DNA within the nucleus of a cell that is active in the production of ribosomal RNA.

nucleoplasm   the materials on the inside of the nucleus of a cell.

nucleotides   the fundamental building blocks of the nucleic acids, DNA and RNA; nucleotides consist of five-carbon sugar molecules bound to a nitrogen base and a phosphate group.

nucleus   the organelle within a cell that contains the DNA and RNA, or genetic material, proteins, and other components; in the cells of higher organisms, the nucleus is surrounded by a membrane.

ocular medication   medication administered through the mucous membranes of the eye.

oncotic force   a form of osmotic pressure exerted by the large protein particles, or colloids, present in blood plasma. In the capillaries, the plasma colloids tend to pull water from the interstitial space across the capillary membrane into the capillary. Oncotic force is also called *colloid osmotic pressure.*

onset of action   the time from administration until a medication reaches its minimum effective concentration.

open cricothyrotomy   surgical airway technique that places an endotracheal or tracheostomy tube directly into the trachea through a surgical incision at the cricothyroid membrane.

orbital   a specific region within which an electron rotates around the nucleus of an atom. Each orbital has a specific shape and can hold two or more electrons. *See also* electron shells.

organ   a group of tissues functioning together. Examples: heart, liver, brain, ovary, eye.

organ system   a group of organs that work together. Examples: the cardiovascular system, formed of the heart, blood vessels, and blood; the gastrointestinal system, comprising the mouth, salivary glands, esophagus, stomach, intestines, liver, pancreas, gallbladder, rectum, and anus.

organelles structures that perform specific functions within a cell.

organic chemicals chemicals that contain the element carbon. *See also* inorganic chemicals.

organism the sum of all the cells, tissues, organs, and organ systems of a living being. Examples: the human organism, a bacterial organism.

oropharyngeal airway (OPA) semicircular device that follows the curvature of the palate.

osmolality the concentration of solute per kilogram of water. *See also* osmolarity.

osmolarity the concentration of solute per liter of water (often used synonymously with *osmolality*).

osmosis movement of solvent in a solution from an area of lower solute concentration to an area of higher solute concentration.

osmotic diuresis greatly increased urination and dehydration due to high levels of glucose that cannot be reabsorbed into the blood from the kidney tubules, causing a loss of water into the urine.

osmotic gradient the difference in concentration between solutions on opposite sides of a semipermeable membrane.

osmotic pressure the pressure exerted by the concentration of solutes on one side of a membrane that, if hypertonic, tends to "pull" water (cause osmosis) from the other side of the membrane.

osteocytes cells that reside in the lacunae, or cavities, within mature bone and are responsible for the turnover of mineral content of the surrounding bone.

overhydration the presence or retention of an abnormally high amount of body fluid.

over-the-needle catheter/IV catheter semiflexible catheter enclosing a sharp metal stylet.

oxidation the loss of hydrogen atoms or the acceptance of an oxygen atom. This increases the positive charge (or lessens the negative charge) of the molecule; the loss of electrons from one atom to another. *See also* reduction.

oxidize combine with oxygen.

oxygen gas necessary for energy production.

oxygen saturation percentage (SpO$_2$) the saturation of arterial blood with oxygen as measured by pulse oximetry expressed as a percentage.

Pa arterial partial pressure.

PA alveolar partial pressure.

PaCO$_2$ partial pressure of carbon dioxide in the blood.

palmar grasp a reflex in the newborn, which is elicited by placing a finger firmly in the infant's palm.

paradoxical breathing asymmetrical chest wall movement that lessens respiratory efficiency.

parasympatholytic medication or other substance that blocks or inhibits the actions of the parasympathetic nervous system (also called *anticholinergic*).

parasympathomimetic medication or other substance that causes effects like those of the parasympathetic nervous system (also called *cholinergic*).

parenchyma principal or essential parts of an organ.

parenteral route delivery of a medication outside the gastrointestinal tract, typically using needles to inject medications into the circulatory system or tissues.

partial agonist *See* agonist-antagonist.

partial pressure the pressure exerted by each component of a gas mixture.

passive transport movement of a substance without the use of energy.

pathogen a microorganism capable of producing infection or disease.

pathogenesis the sequence of events in the development of a disease.

pathologist a physician who specializes in pathology.

pathology the study of disease and its causes.

pathophysiology the study of the functional changes that occur within living cells and tissues that are associated with or that result from disease or injury.

peptide a protein chain containing less than 10 amino acids. *See also* polypeptide.

peptide bond the force that holds amino acids together; the primary linkage of all protein structures.

perfusion the supplying of oxygen and nutrients to the body tissues as a result of the constant passage of blood through the capillaries.

peripheral vascular resistance the resistance of the vessels to the flow of blood: increased when the vessels constrict, decreased when the vessels relax.

peripheral venous access surgical puncture of a vein in the arm, leg, or neck.

peripherally inserted central catheter (PICC) line threaded into the central circulation via a peripheral site.

permissive a parenting style that takes a tolerant, accepting view of a child's behavior.

peroxisome organelle within a cell within which hydrogen peroxide is degraded.

phagocytes cells that have the ability to ingest other cells and substances, such as bacteria and cell debris. All granulocytes and monocytes are phagocytes.

phagocytosis the process whereby a cell engulfs large particles or bacteria.

pharmacodynamics how a medication interacts with the body to cause its effects.

pharmacokinetics how a medication is absorbed, distributed, metabolized (biotransformed), and excreted; how medications are transported into and out of the body.

pharmacology the study of medications and their interactions with the body.

pharynx a muscular tube that extends vertically from the back of the soft palate to the superior aspect of the esophagus.

phospholipids class of lipids that form the membrane that surrounds cells.

pH scale *pH* is the abbreviation for potential of hydrogen, a measure of relative acidity or alkalinity. The pH scale is inverse to the concentration of acidic hydrogen ions; therefore, the lower the pH the greater the acidity, and the higher the pH the greater the alkalinity. The pH scale ranges from 0 to 14. A normal pH range is 7.35 to 7.45.

physiologic stress a chemical or physical disturbance in the cells or tissue fluid produced by a change in the external environment or within the body.

physiology the functions of an organism; the physical and chemical processes of a living thing.

pinocytosis the process whereby a cell engulfs droplets of fluid.

placental barrier biochemical barrier at the maternal/fetal interface that restricts certain molecules.

plasma the liquid part of the blood.

plasma-level profile describes the lengths of onset, duration, and termination of action, as well as the medication's minimum effective concentration and toxic levels.

plasma membrane the membrane that surrounds a cell.

plasma protein systems complex sequences of actions triggered by proteins present in the blood. For example, immunoglobulins (antibodies) are plasma proteins. Three plasma protein systems involved in inflammation are the complement system, the coagulation system, and the kinin system.

platelets fragments of cytoplasm that circulate in the blood and work with components of the coagulation system to promote blood clotting. Platelets also release serotonin, a vasoconstrictive substance.

pleura membranous connective tissue covering the lungs.

pneumothorax accumulation of air or gas in the pleural cavity.

POGO scoring system a system for evaluating and scoring airway difficulty by the percentage of the glottis that can be visualized.

pOH scale the number of hydroxide ions present in a solution. The pOH is the opposite of pH. *See also* pH scale.

polar bond an unequal covalent bond; a bond in which the sharing of electrons is unequal. *See also* covalent bond.

polar molecule a molecule formed with a polar bond, in which different parts of the same molecule have a different and unequal charge. *See also* polar bond.

polymer a large organic molecule formed by combining many smaller molecules (monomers). An example is the polymer starch, which is largely made up of smaller glucose molecules. *See also* monomer.

polypeptide a protein chain containing more than 10 amino acids. *See also* peptide.

polysaccharides a type of carbohydrate that includes starches, cellulose, and glycogen.

postconventional reasoning the stage of moral development during which individuals make moral decisions according to an enlightened conscience.

postganglionic nerves nerve fibers that extend from the autonomic ganglia to the target tissues.

preconventional reasoning the stage of moral development during which children respond mainly to cultural control to avoid punishment and attain satisfaction.

predisposing factors factors that may lead to or increase the chance of contracting a disease.

prefilled/preloaded syringe syringe packaged in a tamper-proof container with the medication already in the barrel.

preganglionic nerves nerve fibers that extend from the central nervous system to the autonomic ganglia.

preload the amount of blood delivered to the heart during diastole (when the heart fills with blood between contractions); in cardiac physiology, defined as the tension of cardiac muscle fiber at the end of diastole.

primary immune response the initial development of antibodies in response to the first exposure to an antigen in which the immune system becomes "primed" to produce a faster, stronger response to any future exposures.

primary intention simple healing of a minor wound without granulation or pus formation.

prodrug (parent drug) medication that is not active when administered, but whose biotransformation converts it into active metabolites.

prognosis the expected outcome of a disease or injury.

prokaryotic cells cells that do not contain a nucleus and do not contain organelles. Most prokaryotes are surrounded by a rigid cell wall. The cells of most single-cell organisms, such as bacteria, are prokaryotes. *See also* eukaryotic cells.

prostaglandins substances synthesized by mast cells during the inflammatory response that cause vasodilation, vascular permeability, and chemotaxis and also cause pain.

proteins nitrogen-based complex compounds that are the basic building blocks of cells and are essential for the growth and repair of living tissues.

proton positively charged particle within the nucleus of an atom.

prototype medication that best demonstrates the class's common properties and illustrates its particular characteristics.

psychoneuroimmunological regulation the interactions of psychological, neurologic/endocrine, and immunologic factors that contribute to alteration of the immune system as an outcome of a stress response that is not quickly resolved.

psychotherapeutic medication medication used to treat mental dysfunction.

pulmonary embolism blood clot that travels to the pulmonary circulation and hinders oxygenation of the blood.

pulse oximetry a measurement of hemoglobin oxygen saturation in the peripheral tissues.

pulsus paradoxus drop in blood pressure of greater than 10 torr during inspiration.

pus a liquid mixture of dead cells, bits of dead tissue, and tissue fluid that may accumulate in inflamed tissues.

pyrogen foreign protein capable of producing fever.

radioactive decay the breakdown of the nucleus of an unstable atom, resulting in the emission of radiation. *See also* radioactive isotopes.

radioactive isotopes atoms with unstable nuclei that break down and emit radiation, in a process called radioactive decay.

ramped position the ear-to-sternal-notch position in an obese patient. *See also* ear-to-sternal-notch position.

rapid sequence intubation giving medications to sedate (induce) and temporarily paralyze a patient and then performing orotracheal intubation.

receptor specialized protein that combines with a medication resulting in a biochemical effect.

reduction the gain of atoms by one atom from another. *See also* oxidation.

regeneration regrowth through cell proliferation.

repair healing of a wound with scar formation.

resolution the complete healing of a wound and return of tissues to their normal structure and function; the ending of inflammation with no scar formation.

respiration   the exchange of gases between a living organism and its environment.

respiratory acid-base disorders   respiratory acidosis and respiratory alkalosis; disorders that result from an inequality between carbon dioxide generation in the peripheral tissues and carbon dioxide elimination by the respiratory system.

respiratory acidosis   acidity caused by abnormal retention of carbon dioxide resulting from impaired ventilation.

respiratory alkalosis   alkalinity caused by excessive elimination of carbon dioxide resulting from increased respirations.

respiratory rate   number of times a person breathes in 1 minute.

retroglottic airways   extraglottic airway devices that are placed in the esophagus (behind the vocal cords).

Rh blood group   a group of antigens discovered on the red blood cells of rhesus monkeys that is also present to some extent in humans.

Rh factor   an antigen in the Rh blood group that is also known as antigen D. About 85 percent of North Americans have the Rh factor (are Rh positive) while about 15 percent do not have the Rh factor (are Rh negative). Rh positive and Rh negative blood are incompatible; that is, a person who is Rh negative can experience a severe immune response if Rh positive blood is introduced, as through a transfusion or during childbirth.

ribonucleic acid (RNA)   a chemical similar to deoxyribonucleic acid (DNA) that serves as a template for protein synthesis.

ribosome   organelle within a cell that synthesizes polypeptides and proteins.

RNA   *see* ribonucleic acid (RNA).

rooting reflex   occurs when an infant's cheek is touched by a hand or cloth; the hungry infant turns his head to the right or left.

rough endoplasmic reticulum (RER)   parts of the endoplasmic reticulum that contain ribosomes during protein synthesis. *See also* endoplasmic reticulum; ribosome.

saline lock   peripheral IV cannula with a distal medication port used for intermittent fluid or medication infusions. Saline is injected into the device to maintain its patency.

SaO₂   *see* hemoglobin-oxygen saturation.

saturated fatty acids   a class of triglycerides that have a single bond between carbon atoms, leaving room for two hydrogen atoms.

scaffolding   a teaching/learning technique in which one builds on what has already been learned.

secondary immune response   the swift, strong response of the immune system to repeated exposures to an antigen.

secondary intention   complex healing of a larger wound involving sealing of the wound through scab formation, granulation or filling of the wound, and constriction of the wound.

second messenger   chemical that participates in complex cascading reactions that eventually cause a medication's desired effect.

secretory immune system   lymphoid tissues beneath the mucosal endothelium that secrete substances such as sweat, tears, saliva, mucus, and breast milk; also called the *external immune system* or the *mucosal immune system*.

secure attachment   a type of bonding that occurs when an infant learns that his caregivers will be responsive and helpful when needed.

sedation   state of decreased anxiety and inhibitions.

selectively permeable   *see* semipermeable.

Sellick maneuver   *see* cricoid pressure.

semipermeable   referring to a membrane that allows unrestricted movement of some substances across the membrane while restricting the movement of other substances. Also called *selectively permeable.*

septicemia   the systemic spread of toxins through the bloodstream. Also called *sepsis.*

septic shock   shock that develops as the result of infection carried by the bloodstream, eventually causing dysfunction of multiple organ systems.

septum   cartilage that separates the right and left nasal cavities.

sequelae   *see* complications.

serotonin   a substance released by platelets that, through constriction and dilation of blood vessels, affects blood flow to an injured or affected site.

serum   solution containing whole antibodies for a specific pathogen.

sharps container   rigid, puncture-resistant container clearly marked as a biohazard.

shock   *see* hypoperfusion.

side effect   unintended response to a medication.

sign   objective finding that can be identified through physical examination.

simple diffusion   the passive movement of molecules through a membrane from an area of greater concentration to an area of lesser concentration. *See also* facilitated diffusion; osmosis.

sinus   air cavity that conducts fluids from the eustachian tubes and tear ducts to and from the nasopharynx.

slow-reacting substances of anaphylaxis (SRS-A)   *see* leukotrienes.

slow-to-warm-up child   an infant who can be characterized by a low intensity of reactions and a somewhat negative mood.

smooth endoplasmic reticulum (SER)   portion of the endoplasmic reticulum without ribosomes; it provides surface area of the action or storage of key enzymes and their products. *See also* endoplasmic reticulum; enzymes.

sniffing position   the ear-to-sternal-notch position in a non-obese patient. *See also* ear-to-sternal-notch position.

sodium-potassium pump   an enzyme (Na^+-K^+-ATPase); a mechanism of active transport in the plasma membrane, powered by adenosine triphosphate (ATP), that moves sodium ions out of a cell and potassium ions into the cell to help maintain cell potential and regular cellular volume.

solute   a substance dissolved in a solvent, forming a solution. *See also* solvent.

solvent   a substance that dissolves other substances, forming a solution. *See also* solute.

spike   sharp-pointed device inserted into the IV solution bag's administration set port.

Standard Precautions   a strict form of infection control that is based on the assumption that all blood and other body fluids are infectious.

starches   polymers of glucose; carbohydrates.

stem cells   undifferentiated cells in the bone marrow from which all blood cells, including thrombocytes, erythrocytes, and various types of leukocytes, develop; stem cells are also called *hemocytoblasts*.

stenosis   narrowing or constriction.

sterile   free of all forms of life.

steroids   an organic compound, a class of lipid. The dietary fat cholesterol and the sex hormones estradiol and testosterone are examples of steroids.

stock solution   standard concentration of routinely used medications.

stoma   opening in the anterior neck that connects the trachea with ambient air.

stress   a hardship or strain; a physical or emotional response to a stimulus.

stressor   a stimulus that causes stress.

stress response   changes within the body initiated by a stressor.

stroke volume   the amount of blood ejected by the heart in one contraction.

stylet   plastic-covered metal wire used to bend the ETT into a J or hockey-stick shape.

subcutaneous   the layer of loose connective tissue between the skin and muscle.

sublingual   beneath the tongue.

substrate   a substance an enzyme acts on.

sucking reflex   occurs when an infant's lips are stroked.

sucrose   common table sugar; a disaccharide, it is a combination of glucose and fructose.

suction   to remove with a vacuum-type device.

sugars   a class of carbohydrate that can be further classified as simple sugars (monosaccharides) or complex sugars (disaccharides). *See also* disaccharides; monosaccharides.

suppository   medication packaged in a soft, pliable form for insertion into the rectum.

supraglottic airways   extraglottic airway devices that are placed above the vocal cords (above the glottis).

surfactant   substance that decreases surface tension.

sympatholytic   medication or other substance that blocks the actions of the sympathetic nervous system (also called *antiadrenergic).*

sympathomimetic   medication or other substance that causes effects like those of the sympathetic nervous system (also called *adrenergic*).

symptom   subjective complaint; what the patient is experiencing and, possibly, can describe.

synapse   space between nerve cells.

syndrome   a constellation of signs and symptoms commonly found in association with a particular disease or condition.

syringe   plastic tube with which liquid medications can be drawn up, stored, and injected.

systemic   throughout the body.

T cell receptor (TCR)   a molecule on the surface of a helper T cell that responds to a specific antigen. There is a specific TCR for every antigen to which the human body may be exposed.

T lymphocytes   the type of white blood cell that does not produce antibodies but, instead, attacks antigens directly.

teratogenic drug   medication that may deform or kill the fetus.

teratogens   external factors that can affect the development of a fetus.

terminal-drop hypothesis   a theory that death is preceded by a five-year period of decreasing cognitive functioning.

termination of action   time from when the medication's level drops below its minimum effective concentration until it is eliminated from the body.

therapeutic index   ratio of a medication's lethal dose for 50 percent of the population to its effective dose for 50 percent of the population.

therapy regulator   pressure regulator used for delivering oxygen to patients.

thrombocytes   platelets, which are important in blood clotting.

thrombophlebitis   inflammation of the vein.

thrombus   blood clot.

tidal volume (T_V)   the average volume of gas inhaled or exhaled in one respiratory cycle.

tissue   a group of cells that perform a similar function.

tonicity   solute concentration or osmotic pressure relative to the blood plasma or body cells.

topical medications   material applied to and absorbed through the skin or mucous membranes.

total body water (TBW)   the total amount of water in the body at a given time.

total lung capacity (TLC)   maximum lung capacity.

trachea   10- to 12-cm-long tube that connects the larynx to the mainstem bronchi.

transdermal   absorbed through the skin.

trauma   a physical injury or wound caused by external force or violence.

tricarboxylic acid (TCA) cycle   *see* citric acid cycle.

triglycerides   lipids consisting of one molecule of glycerol and three fatty acid molecules that are a rich source of energy for the body.

trocar   a sharp, pointed instrument.

trust vs. mistrust   refers to a stage of psychosocial development that lasts from birth to about 1½ years of age.

tumor   a mass of uncontrolled cell growth. A tumor may be benign (noncancerous) or malignant (cancerous).

turgor   normal tension in a cell; the resistance of the skin to deformation. (In a normally hydrated person, the skin, when pinched, will quickly return to its normal formation. In a dehydrated person, the return to normal formation will be slower.)

turnover   the continual synthesis and breakdown of body substances that results in the dynamic steady state.

unit   predetermined amount of medication or fluid.

unsaturated fatty acids   a class of triglycerides that have a double bond between carbon atoms, leaving room for only one hydrogen atom.

upper airway obstruction   an interference with air movement through the upper airway.

up-regulation   when a medication causes the formation of more receptors than normal.

vaccine   solution containing a modified pathogen that does not actually cause disease but still stimulates the development of antibodies specific to it.

vacuole organelle within a cell that provides temporary storage or transport of substances such as food sources.

vacutainer device that holds blood tubes.

valence electrons electrons found in the outermost shell (valence shell) of an atom.

valence shell the outermost electron shell of an atom. *See also* electron shells.

vallecula depression between the epiglottis and the base of the tongue.

venous access device surgically implanted port that permits repeated access to central venous circulation.

venous constricting band flat rubber band used to impede venous return and make veins easier to see.

ventilation the mechanical process that moves air into and out of the lungs.

Venturi mask high-concentration face mask that uses a Venturi system to deliver relatively precise oxygen concentrations.

vial plastic or glass container with a self-sealing rubber top.

virus an organism much smaller than a bacterium, visible only under an electron microscope. Viruses invade and live inside the cells of the organisms they infect.

volume on hand the available amount of solution containing a medication.